Middle Range Theories

APPLICATION TO NURSING RESEARCH

Middle Range Theories

APPLICATION TO NURSING RESEARCH

Sandra J. Peterson, PhD, RN

Professor and Department Chair

Bethel College

St. Paul, Minnesota

Timothy S. Bredow, PhD, RN

Associate Professor

Bethel College

St. Paul, Minnesota

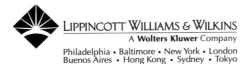

LIPPINCOTT WILLIAMS & WILKINS

A **Wolters Kluwer** Company

Philadelphia • Baltimore • New York • London
Buenos Aires • Hong Kong • Sydney • Tokyo

Senior Acquisitions Editor: Margaret Zuccarini
Associate Managing Editor: Helen Kogut
Editorial Assistant: Carol DeVault
Senior Production Editor: Sandra Cherry Scheinin
Senior Production Manager: Helen Ewan
Managing Editor / Production: Erika Kors

Art Director: Doug Smock
Manufacturing Manager: William Alberti
Compositor: Lippincott Williams & Wilkins
Indexer: Michael Ferreira
Printer: R.R. Donnelley—Crawfordsville

9 8 7 6 5 4 3 2 1

Library of Congress Cataloging-in-Publication Data
Middle range theories : application to nursing research / [edited by] Sandra J. Peterson, Timothy S. Bredow.
    p. ; cm.
Includes bibliographical references and index.
ISBN: 0-7817-4192-0 (alk. paper)
    1. Nursing—Philosophy. 2. Nursing—Research. 3. Nursing. I. Peterson, Sandra J. II Bredow, Timothy S.
[DNLM: 1. Nursing Theory. 2. Nursing Research. WY 86 M6269 2004]
RT84.5M535 2004
610.73′01—dc22
                                                          2003056494

LWW.com

This text is dedicated to nurse scholars, past, present, and future, who provide a vision for the discipline, exercise intellectual rigor in the process of its development, and are committed to the pursuit of excellence in practice.

To my family for their belief that I could do just about anything. It's because of them that I was willing to undertake this project.

Sandra J. Peterson

To four of my former classmates in the Master's of Nursing Program at The University of Iowa. My appreciation is extended to John Folkrod, Mike Catney, Geoff Hodges, and Steve Perrin for helping me understand Dubin and Kaplin and all the nursing theorists we encountered 25 years ago.

Timothy S. Bredow

Contributors

Georgene Gaskill Eakes, EdD, RN
Professor, School of Nursing
East Carolina University
Greenville, North Carolina

Eileen P. Geraci, PhD(Cand.), MA, ANP-C
Associate Professor of Nursing, Department
    of Nursing
Western Connecticut State University
Danbury, Connecticut

Audrey G. Gift, PhD, RN, FAAN
Professor and Associate Dean for Research
    and Doctoral Programs
College of Nursing
Michigan State University
East Lansing, Michigan

Marion Good, PhD, RN
Associate Professor
Frances Payne Bolton School of Nursing
Cleveland, Ohio

Joan E. Haase, PhD, RN
Holmquist Professor in Pediatric Oncology Nursing,
    School of Nursing
Indiana University
Indianapolis, Indiana

Katharine Kolcaba, PhD, RN, C
Associate Professor, College of Nursing
The University of Akron
Akron, Ohio

Diane Kunyk, RN, MN
Project Coordinator, Smoke Free Communities
    Initiative
Capital Health
Edmonton, Alberta, Canada

Marjorie Cook McCullagh, PhD, RN
Assistant Professor, Nursing
North Dakota State University
Fargo, North Dakota

Joanne K. Olson, PhD, RN
Assistant Dean and Professor, Faculty of Nursing
University of Alberta
Edmonton, Alberta, Canada

Mertie L. Potter, ND, ARNP, CS
Associate Professor of Nursing
Saint Anselm College
Manchester, New Hampshire
Nurse Consultant
New Hampshire Hospital
Concord, New Hampshire

Barbara Resnick, PhD, CRNP, FAAN, FAANP
Associate Professor
University of Maryland
Baltimore, Maryland

Marjorie A. Schaffer, PhD, RN
Professor of Nursing
Bethel College
St. Paul, Minnesota

Ellen D. Schultz, PhD, RN
Associate Professor and Department Chair, School
    of Nursing
Metropolitan State University
St. Paul, Minnesota

Perla Werner, PhD
Associate Professor, Department of Gerontology
University of Haifa
Haifa, Israel

Reviewers

Jo Azzarello, PhD, RN
Assistant Professor, College of Nursing
University of Oklahoma
Oklahoma City, Oklahoma

Jeanine Carr, PhD, RN
Associate Professor, College of Nursing
   and Health Sciences
University of Vermont
Burlington, Vermont

Judith A. Cohen, PhD, RN
Associate Professor, College of Nursing
   and Health Science
University of Vermont
Burlington, Vermont

Lucille C. Gambardella, PhD, RN, CS, APN-BC
Chair and Professor, Division of Nursing
Wesley College
Dover, Delaware

Bethany Hall-Long, PhD, RNC, FAAN
Associate Professor, Department of Nursing
University of Delaware
Newark, Delaware

Rebecca L. Hartman, EdD, RN
Professor of Nursing
Indiana University of Pennsylvania
Indiana, Pennsylvania

Catherine Kane, PhD, RN, FAAN
Associate Professor of Nursing and Psychiatric
   Medicine, School of Nursing
University of Virginia
Charlottesville, Virginia

Judith H. Lewis, EdD, RN
Associate Professor and Director
   of Nursing Education
University of Akron College of Nursing
Akron, Ohio

Jean R. Miller, PhD, RN
Professor and Weyker Endowed Chair
   in Thanatology, College of Nursing
University of Rhode Island
Kingston, Rhode Island

Virginia Nehring, PhD, RN
Associate Professor
Wright State University
Dayton, Ohio

Cynthia A. Padula, PhD, RN
Associate Professor, College of Nursing
University of Rhode Island
Kingston, Rhode Island

Linda Ceriale Peterson, EdD, RN
Professor, Sage Graduate School, Department
   of Nursing
The Sage Colleges
Troy, New York

Beth L. Rodgers, PhD, RN, FAAN
Chair and Professor, Foundations
   of Nursing Department
University of Wisconsin – Milwaukee
Milwaukee, Wisconsin

Mary Elizabeth Sadler, PhD, RN
Professor of Nursing and Allied Health, Director
    of Liberal Studies Program
Indiana University of Pennsylvania
Indiana, Pennsylvania

Phyllis Skorga, PhD, RN, CCM
Associate Professor, College of Nursing
    and Health Professions
Arkansas State University
State University, Arkansas

Hélène Sylvain, PhD
Professor
Université du Québec à Rimouski
Rimouski, Québec, Canada

Wendy Woodward, PhD, RN, HNC
Professor, Department of Nursing
Humboldt State University
Arcata, California

Preface

"Middle range theory will create the disciplinary fabric of the new millennium as nurse theorists spin and twist fibers from the past-present into the future" (Liehr & Smith, 1999, The future: Where does nursing theory go from here?, para. 3).

Similar to many initiatives, the creation of this book was motivated by a felt need: the need of students attempting to make connections between their practices, their developing understanding of research, and their use of nursing theory; the need of registered nurses in a degree-completion program trying to develop a research proposal; and the need of graduate students writing a thesis or project. Often these groups find it difficult to relate the research questions or project ideas derived from their practice experiences to the most appropriate nursing theories. Frequently, a middle range theory would best suit the research or projects that are being considered by these students. Unfortunately, until now, there have been limited resources on middle range theories to assist these students with their research.

The needs expressed by students are echoed in the words of nurse scholars represented in the nursing literature. Several authors have identified middle range theory as the preferred direction for knowledge development in the discipline of nursing (Blegen & Tripp-Reimer, 1997; Lenz, 1998; Liehr & Smith, 1999). Suppe (1996) clarified the reciprocal relationship between middle range theory and research, identifying middle range theories as frameworks that guide research, objects to test through research, and scientific end-products that express nursing knowledge. This book hopes to serve the purposes for middle range theory suggested by Suppe.

ORGANIZATION

Part I

Unit I is devoted to an overview of the state of nursing's body of knowledge. Chapter 1 considers the hierarchy of nursing knowledge and particularly the place of middle range theory within that hierarchy (i.e., paradigm, philosophy, conceptual framework, and theories). For each component of the hierarchy, the chapter includes a description of its nature, review of its development, a discussion of its contributions to nursing knowledge, consideration of controversies related to its nature or use, and examples of nurse scholars' work. Chapter 2 emphasizes the analysis and evaluation of middle range theories, including issues to consider in the selection of a middle range nursing theory for research purposes. This chapter also describes a brief evaluative process that is used as a feature throughout the rest of the chapters. Using this evaluation process, readers can compare and contrast their conclusions about the theory as presented in the chapter with those of a nurse scholar who has also used this evaluation process.

Parts II–VI

Parts II–VI are devoted to specific middle range theories. The selected theories are labeled by their developers or by nurse scholars as middle range theories and are the ones most frequently cited in published nursing research. Many of the chapters contain unique nursing theories; some are borrowed from related disciplines, but are, nonetheless, useful to nursing. All theories in the text, however, have the intrinsic capability to be applied to nursing research and address a wide range of phenomena that allow the researcher to consider a variety of nursing research questions.

- Physiological—Pain: Balance of Analgesia and Side Effects; Unpleasant Symptoms
- Cognitive—Self-Efficacy, Reasoned Action
- Emotional—Empathy, Chronic Sorrow
- Social—Social Support, Interpersonal Relations
- Integrative—Modeling and Role-Modeling, Comfort, Heath-Related Quality of Life, Health Promotion, Deliberative Nursing Process, Planned Change, Resilience

SPECIAL FEATURES

Each theory chapter provides the nurse researcher with a variety of tools.

- **Definition of Key Terms:** appears at the beginning of each chapter; provides conceptual definitions to aid the student's understanding of the theory
- **Using Middle Range Theories:** provides examples of how the theory has been used in published research
- **Research Application:** provides a sample application of the theory modeling the research process
- **Analysis Exercise:** appears at the end of each chapter; allows readers to arrive at their own conclusions about the theory and then compare them to a nurse scholar's evaluation
- **Web Resources:** guides the students to valuable Web sites to aid them in their research
- **Instruments:** discussed in the chapters, with specific examples found in Appendix B

Many chapters also contain an extensive bibliography that provides additional references for the development of a review of the literature.

We hope this text provides the readers with the background to appreciate the relationship between nursing theory and research and the specific content to enable them to make use of both in their scholarly work. We also hope the book promotes a sense of excitement about and commitment to the development of nursing's body of knowledge.

REFERENCES

Blegen, M. A. & Tripp-Reimer, T. T. (1997). Implications of nursing taxonomies for middle-range theory development. *Advances in Nursing Science,* 19(3) 37(3). Retrieved December 14, 1999 from *http://web7.infotrac.galegroup.*

Lenz, E. R. (1998). Role of middle range theory for nursing research and practice. Part 1. Nursing research. *Nursing Leadership Forum,* 3(2), 24–33.

Liehr, P. & Smith, M. J. (1999). Middle range theory: Spinning research and practice to create knowledge for the new millennium. *Advances in Nursing Science,* 21(4), 8–91. Retrieved June 11, 2002, from CINAHL/Ovid database.

Suppe, F. (1996, May 10). *Middle range theory: Nursing theory and knowledge development.* Paper presented at the Sixth Rosemary Ellis Scholars Retreat, Cleveland, OH.

Acknowledgments

There are a number of people whose contributions to this text are substantial and without whom it would never have become a reality. Our chapter contributors are amazing scholars and marvelous individuals. Each one produced a chapter that we believe will make a significant contribution to the ongoing development of nursing's body of knowledge, and the process of collaborating with them on this project was uniformly pleasant. They make us even prouder of our profession.

The authors of the critical analysis exercises provided what we believe will be a useful learning tool to those who read this book. The feedback from the nurse scholars who reviewed the chapters was insightful and has improved the book's quality.

Our parent institution, Bethel College in St. Paul, Minnesota, financially supported attendance at the Houghton Institute for Integrative Studies, and provided a timely sabbatical leave. Both activities allowed for the expenditure of the intellectual energy that is so necessary for this type of a project.

The staff at Lippincott Williams & Wilkins was invaluable. Margaret Zuccarini, Senior Acquisitions Editor, recognized the possibilities for a text such as ours. She guided us through proposal development and was a source of much needed encouragement as we began the publication process. Helen Kogut, Associate Managing Editor, provided the structure, the technical expertise, and an ambitious production schedule that enabled us to complete the project in what seemed to us "record time."

And finally we are profoundly grateful for the forbearance of our family and friends (especially husband, Ray Peterson, and wife, Kate Bredow). Our spouses picked up the pieces and filled in the gaps. We are thankful for all of you.

Contents

PART III   Middle Range Theories: Cognitive   95

PART IV   Middle Range Theories: Emotional   149

PART V   # Middle Range Theories: Social   177

PART VI   # Middle Range Theories: Integrative

Overview of Theory

Introduction to the Nature of Nursing Knowledge

SANDRA J. PETERSON

DEFINITION OF KEY TERMS

Concept	Symbolic representation of a phenomenon or set of phenomena
Conceptual model	"Set of abstract and general concepts and the propositions" (Fawcett, 1987, pp. 13–14) that represents a phenomenon of interest
Deduction	Reasoning from the general or universal to the particular or specific
Discipline	A field or branch of knowledge that involves research
Domain	Related components or items that reflect the unified subject matter of a discipline
Empiricism	A philosophical theory of knowledge acquisition through experience, observation, and experiment
Ethics	A branch of philosophy concerned with moral principles
Epistemology	A branch of philosophy concerned with the sources of knowledge of truth and the methods used to acquire it
Induction	Reasoning from the individual or particular to the general or universal
Logic	A branch of philosophy concerned with sound reasoning and validity of thought
Logical positivism	Philosophical perspective that espouses logic, objectivity, falseness/truth, observable and operationally defined concepts, and prediction
Metaparadigm	Global concepts specific to a discipline that are philosophically neutral and stable

DEFINITION OF KEY TERMS

Metaphysics	A branch of philosophy concerned with the study of ultimate cause and underlying nature of that which exists
Metatheory	A philosophical theory about theories, concerned with "logical and methodological foundations of a discipline" (Beckstrand, 1986, p. 503). Examines "how theory affects and is affected by research and practice within nursing, and philosophy and politics outside nursing" (McKenna, 1997, p. 92).
Ontology	Examination of the nature of being or reality
Paradigm	A worldview, a common philosophical orientation, that serves to define the nature of a discipline
Phenomenon	A designation of an aspect of reality
Philosophy	(a) A set of beliefs or values; (b) Science concerned with the study of reality and the nature of being. Comprised of but not limited to aesthetics, epistemology, ethics, logic, and metaphysics.
Science	A systematized body of knowledge that has as its main purpose the discovery of "truths about the world" (Jacox, 1974, p. 4), confirmed through empirical investigation
Theory	"Set of interrelated concepts, based on assumption, woven together through a set of propositional statements" (Fitzpatrick, 1997, p. 37) used to provide a perspective on reality

INTRODUCTION

Two claims can be made about the state of nursing knowledge—it exists in varying degrees of abstraction, and it is characterized by a lack of consistency in the use of its language. Fawcett (1997, 2000) recommends what she refers to as a structural hierarchy of contemporary nursing knowledge to establish the relationships between the various components that comprise nursing's body of knowledge. The components are arranged from most abstract to most concrete in the following order: metaparadigm, philosophy, conceptual model, and theories. The types of theories available to nurses also exist on a continuum from most abstract to most concrete, with grand theories identified as most abstract; practice theories as most concrete; and middle range theories in the logical middle.

There are few components in the hierarchy that appear consistently in the literature with a single label. The terms *conceptual models*, *conceptual frameworks*, and *theories* are sometimes used interchangeably. The terms *grand theory*, *macro theory*, and *general theory* all refer the same level of theory development.

This chapter will address each component of the conceptual hierarchy, with special emphasis on middle range theories. The nature of the component, its development, its contributions to nursing's body of knowledge, and the debates engaged in by nurses in relation to the component will be considered.

PARADIGMS AND METAPARADIGM

The terms *paradigm* and *metaparadigm* are frequently found in the nursing literature. Paradigms provide the basic parameters and framework for organizing a discipline's knowledge. They are the most abstract and least specific means of expressing that knowledge. Paradigms generally are considered to be discipline-specific, philosophical, and mutable. The metaparadigm of a discipline is distinguished from a paradigm in that the metaparadigm is global, philosophically neutral, and fairly stable.

Paradigms

Kuhn introduced the term paradigm and stimulated interest in its use as a method of defining and analyzing the nature of a discipline. He also acknowledged the existence of multiple and conflicting definitions of the term (Kuhn, 1977, p. 294). Kuhn (1996) included the following as the components of paradigms or, as he later referred to them, disciplinary matrices: (a) *symbolic generalizations*; the laws accepted by a scientific community and the language used to express them; (b) *shared commitments to beliefs in particular models*; shared beliefs about and commitment to the prevailing theories of the discipline and the motivation and methods used to create and test them; (c) *values*; shared values that serve to identify what is significant or meaningful to the scientific community; and (d) *exemplars*; the specific problems to be solved and the methods used to solve them. These components of paradigms serve as characteristics of a maturing discipline. Before a paradigm is identified, the facts generated by the discipline and the methods used to generate them are disorganized.

DEVELOPMENT

Paradigms emerge when they are recognized as a dominant way of thinking about the discipline by its scientific community. Kuhn (1996) refers to the emergence of a new paradigm as a revolution in which the new paradigm replaces an older one. "...scientific revolutions are inaugurated by a growing sense, again often restricted to a narrow subdivision of the scientific community, that an existing paradigm has ceased to function adequately in the exploration of an aspect of nature to which that paradigm itself had previously led the way" (Kuhn, 1996, p. 92). Shapere (1980) criticized the notion of revolution, noting that scientific advances can be cumulative in that later sciences build on that which was earlier. This is a more evolutionary perspective on paradigm development. Integration has also been proposed as a form of paradigm development. This form of paradigm development describes a pattern in progress that is created "through accommodation, refinement, and collaboration between thoughts, ideas, and individuals (Meleis, 1997, p. 80). Meleis believes paradigm development in nursing is characterized by this approach.

There are several classifications of paradigms. Parse (1987) identifies two distinct belief systems or paradigms in nursing: totality and simultaneity. The totality paradigm refers to the person as a biopsychosocial and spiritual being who interacts with the environment. In the simultaneity paradigm, the person is considered a unitary being in continual and mutual interrelationships with the environment. Stevens-Barnum (1998) focuses her classification on the nursing act and includes intervention, conservation, substitution, sustenance/support, and enhancement in her paradigm. With intervention, the nurse manipulates the environment to bring about a nurse-determined change for the patient. The nurse in conservation attempts to maintain those elements in the patient's situation considered beneficial. In substitution, the nurse provides for the patient what the patient desires and cannot do for him or herself. The nurse who enables the patient to endure or cope with an altered state of health is functioning within the sustenance/support paradigm of nursing actions. The nurse in enhancement acts to improve the quality of the patient's existence, aiding him/her to experience growth through an illness experience. Other identified paradigm classifications include systems, biobehavioral, holistic, and phenomenological paradigms (King & Fawcett, 1997, p. 32). From these lists of multiple paradigm classifications, it is obvious that competing paradigms exist.

USES

One function of a paradigm is to identify the boundary or limits of the subject matter of concern to a discipline (Kim, 1989). A paradigm also provides a summary of the intellectual and social purposes of the discipline. It provides the "perspective with which essential phenomena of concern are conceptualized" (Kim, 1997, p. 32). A paradigm is considered to represent a worldview, "a coherent and common philosophical orientation" (Sarter, 1988, p. 52).

Therefore paradigms can provide the frames of reference for the construction of nursing theory and the use of nursing and non-nursing theories in nursing research. "Paradigm development is necessary for the enhancement of a discipline, and each one gives rise to several theories (Parse, 1987, p. 2). Paradigms also are important to nursing researchers. Researchers need to be assured that what is being studied will contribute to the body of nursing knowledge. By providing definitions of the discipline's boundaries, paradigms provide researchers with a nursing context for their research. Thus, nursing's paradigms function as a means for nurse theorists and researchers to determine the congruence of their work with the discipline of nursing.

CONTROVERSY

The current debate on the state of the paradigms of nursing focuses on whether unity or multiplicity is preferred. "The paradigm debates have done more to create divisiveness with theoretical nursing than to clearly define our unique mission and facilitate effective communication among nurses" (Thorne et al., 1998, A Unifying Definition, para. 1). There is recognition of inconsistencies within nursing, especially between its professional values and methods of inquiry (Newman, 1996). These inconsistencies are being perpetuated through nursing's educational programs and research practices. For instance, graduate students are prepared in both quantitative and qualitative research methods, perspectives on scientific inquiry that represent quite different paradigms. There is a need for consensus at the macro level about the basic components of the discipline (Northrup, 1992). Thorne and her coauthors propose a generic definition of nursing that integrates a variety of philosophical perspectives. This definition could serve as the basis for a consensus about the core of the discipline of nursing.

> *Nursing is the study of human health and illness processes. Nursing practice is facilitating, supporting, and assisting individuals, families, communities, and/or societies to enhance, maintain and recover health and to reduce and ameliorate the effects of illness. Nursing's relational practice and science are directed toward the explicit outcome of health related quality of life within the immediate and larger environmental contexts (Thorne et al., 1998, A Unifying Definition, para. 2).*

By contrast, Barrett (1992) claims uniformity of perspective is neither possible nor desirable (p. 156) and gives as evidence the variety of viewpoints on the nature of the components of the metaparadigm and of methods of inquiry expressed in the nursing literature. Engebretson (1997) suggests a multiparadigm approach that integrates several paradigms from both the patient and nurse's perspectives (Contemporary Controversies, para. 5). Her work is derived from the Heterdox Explanatory Paradigms Model for health practice. This model is comprised of horizontal and vertical axes, with both axes representing the philosophical dualism between the material and the nonmaterial (Development of the Metaparadigm Model, para. 2–3). On the horizontal axis, arranged on a continuum from logical positivism to metaphysics, are four aspects of healing: mechanical, purification, balance, and supranormal. Represented on the vertical axis are body–mind dualistic types of healing activities: physical manipulation, ingested substances, using energy, psychological activities, and spiritual activities. Engebretson also suggests environment, especially social relationships, as an inclusion in this multiparadigm. She concludes that this multiparadigmatic model provides a means to link holistic theories to biomedical-based nursing practice; promotes flexibility in approaches to working with clients; and is consistent with dialectic methodology, appropriate for theory development and research in nursing.

Metaparadigm

Metaparadigm is defined as the global concepts specific to a discipline and the global propositions that define and relate the concepts (Fawcett, 2000, p. 4). A metaparadigm transcends all specific philosophical or paradigmatic orientations; it must not represent any particular perspective (Fawcett, 1997, 2000). It comprises several domains, often referred to as a typology. These domains are a classification system to identify the constructs or phenomena that are the focus of nursing. A typology of four domains is most common: man/person, health, society/environment, and nursing (Fawcett, 1978; Yura & Torres, 1975). The metaparadigm described by Fawcett is also comprised of four nonrelational and four relational propositions. The nonrelational propositions provide the definitions of the four domains and the relational propositions describe the linkages between the domains. See Table 1-1 for an overview of these propositions.

DEVELOPMENT

A metaparadigm is not so much constructed as it is identified. This identification process occurs through the analysis of the recurring themes of nursing's theories (Sarter, 1988). This analysis is philo-

Table 1-1.   FAWCETT'S RELATIONAL AND NONRELATIONAL PROPOSITIONS OF METAPARADIGM

Nonrelational	1. Person refers to individuals, families, communities, and other groups who are involved in nursing.
	2. Environment refers to the person's social network and physical surroundings and to the setting in which nursing is taking place. It also includes all local, regional, national, cultural, social, political, and economic conditions that might have an impact on a person's health.
	3. Health refers to a person's state of well-being at the time of engagement with nursing. It exists on a continuum from high-level wellness to terminal illness.
	4. Nursing refers to the definition of the discipline, the actions taken by nurses on behalf and/or with the person, and the goals or outcomes of those actions.
Relational	1. Nursing is concerned with the principles and laws that govern life processes, well-being, and optimal functioning of human beings, sick or well.
	2. Nursing is concerned with the patterning of human behavior in the interaction with the environment in normal life events and critical situations.
	3. Nursing is concerned with the nursing actions or processes by which positive changes in health status are effected.
	4. Nursing is concerned with the wholeness or health of human beings, recognizing that they are in continuous interaction with their environment.

Source: Fawcett, J. (2000). *Analysis and evaluation of contemporary nursing knowledge: Nursing models and theories* (3rd ed.). Philadelphia: F. A. Davis, pp. 5–6. Reprinted with permission from F. A. Davis Company, Philadelphia, PA.

sophical in nature and allows for recognition of the "common and coherent philosophical orientation" (p. 52) of the discipline of nursing.

USES

Metaparadigm, or in Kim's (1983) words, a typology, are "boundary-maintaining devices" (p. 19) and as such help delineate nursing's frame of reference. The primary purpose then is to provide a means of focusing on that which is inherently nursing and marginalizing that which is not. This enables nurse practitioners, theorists, and researchers to concentrate their energies on the business of nursing. In addition, the metaparadigm is used for the purpose of analysis, a framework for comparing the perspectives of various nursing theorists (Fawcett, 2000; Fitzpatrick & Whall, 1983; Kim, 1983). For instance, Fitzpatrick and Whall noted that Levine defined health as wholeness, whereas Johnson found health to be a moving state of equilibrium.

CONTROVERSY

By definition, a discipline possesses only one metaparadigm. The controversy involves what that metaparadigm should be. Fawcett (2000) critiqued nine other paradigms using the criteria of distinctiveness, inclusiveness, neutrality, and internationality. The paradigms suggested by Newman; Conway; Kim; Meleis; King; Newman, Sime, and Corcoran-Perry; Malloch, Martinez, Nelson, Predeger, Speakman, Stienbinder, and Tracy; Parse; and Leininger/Watson all failed to meet one or more of the stated criteria. Fawcett's most common criticism was failure of the paradigms to meet the criterion of inclusion. For example, Kim (1983) did not address health; King (1984) eliminated environment and nursing; and Newman and associates (1996) failed to include environment. Obviously, nursing is still in search of a commonly shared metaparadigm and requires further philosophical analysis to arrive at this metaparadigm.

PHILOSOPHY

For a discipline, philosophies represent its beliefs and values, and its mindset or worldview. In that way, philosophies and paradigms (not metaparadigm) are similar. "Nursing philosophy is a statement of foundational and universal assumptions, beliefs, and principles about the nature of knowledge and truth (epistemology) and about the nature of the entities represented in the metaparadigm (i.e., nursing practice and human healing processes [ontology])" (Reed, 1995, Nursing Philosophy: Metaparadigms for Knowledge Development, para. 1). Like other disciplines, nursing has and is reflecting the modern, postmodern, and some would include neomodern thinking, or worldview of its time.

Development

Philosophies emerge as a reflection on the issues of interest to philosophers, primarily logic, ethics, aesthetics, metaphysics, and epistemology. In the 20th century, these reflections or philosophies have been often characterized as either modern or postmodern perspectives. Although modernism and postmodernism do not represent singular philosophies but, rather, a collection of philosophies (Burbules, n.d, para. 2), each possesses commonly occurring themes that can serve as points of contrast. The most basic comparison between the schools of thinking is in their perspectives on metanarratives, defined as efforts to offer "general and encompassing accounts of truth, value, and reality" (Burbules, n.d, para. 5). In modernism, the metanarratives are a primary concern. In postmodernism, metanarratives are dismissed. This dismissal is not necessarily rejection or denial but instead doubt and uncertainty about what metanarratives have to offer. These schools of thought also differ in their view of the nature of problems. In modern thinking, problems are to be solved. In postmodern thinking, they are to be deconstructed, requiring a disassembling of the metanarratives that are entangled in values and beliefs that fail to reveal reality or liberate the oppressed (Reed, 1995, Historical Background: Modernism and Postmodernism, para. 3). Reed (1995) also identified distinctions in epistemology: modernism, concerned with the truth of findings, and postmodernism, concerned with the usefulness of findings. She also suggest a neomodernism perspective for nursing, in which the metanarratives of health and the processes of healing are embraced but also integrated with the postmodern assumptions that knowledge is value-laden and that context is critical.

Within these schools of thought, a variety of philosophies or philosophical schemes have been used to describe the nature of nursing. Adam (1992) identified the following: (a) Socratic—know self; (b) realism—be self; (c) humanism—give self; (d) rationalism—understand self; (e) naturalism—describe self; (f) pragmatism—prove self; (g) idealism—imagine self; and (h) existentialism—choose self (p. 56).

Another schema, proposed by Lerner (1986), which considered the nature of human development, is useful in categorizing nursing philosophies. Three worldviews of most interest are:

1. Mechanistic, in which the machine is the metaphor for the human being. The whole is equal to the sum of the parts, and the goal is a return to equilibrium.
2. Organistic, in which a biologic organism composed of complex interrelated parts is the basic metaphor. The organism is active in a passive environment. Change is probable, goal-directed, and developmental.
3. Developmental–contextual, in which historical events are the metaphor. The individual is immersed in a dynamic context. Change in the person and the environment is ongoing, irreversible, innovative, and developmental. Chaos and conflict are an energy source for change. (Reed, 1995)

Several nursing authors have proposed philosophical or paradigmatic schemes. Hall proposes change and persistence; Parse suggests totality and simultaneity; Newman identifies particulate–deterministic, interactive–integrative, and unitary–transformative; and Fawcett recommends reactive, reciprocal interaction, and simultaneous action. Each provides a refinement of Lerner's classifications that is more specific to the discipline of nursing. A summary of these perspectives is found in Table 1-2.

Uses

Well into the 19th century, the classical Greek thought persisted that philosophy represented humanity's total knowledge (Silva, 1997). The scientific revolution, ushered in by a knowledge explosion related to new thinking about survival of species, cause of disease, nature of matter and energy, and the workings of the human mind, came with new ways of knowing and forms of inquiry. This revolution also resulted in new ways of thinking about philosophy and science. Philosophy is concerned with the nature of being, the meaning and purpose of life, and the theory and limits of knowledge; whereas science is more concerned with causality (Silva, 1997). Philosophy is considered discursive, noninvestigative, and dependent on common experience, contrasting with science, which is considered investigative and dependent on special experience (Simmons, 1992, pp. 16–17). By these definitions, both philosophy and science have contributions to make to nursing's knowledge base, but neither can address all the issues of concern to nursing.

The fields of philosophy suggest a set of questions with relevance to nursing. For instance, ethical nursing questions would be concerned with what is good to do and to seek to attain nursing's goals (Kikuchi, 1992). Epistemological questions would focus on the structure, scope, and reliability of nursing's knowledge, and ontological questions would relate to the meaning of nurses' and clients' realities (Silva, Sorrell, & Sorrell, 1995). But these important questions are ones that cannot be answered through nursing research; they are best addressed through philosophical inquiry.

The contribution the branches of philosophy make to nursing research is more directly related to its methods than to the questions generated. Research requires logic in the use of the research process, with a logical progression from problem identification and hypotheses, to methods, and finally to data analyses and conclusions (Silva, 1997). Epistemology leads nurse researchers to consider the nature of not only evidence obtained through research, but also truth and belief. Metaphysics addresses causality, an important issue for nurse researchers. Ethics are of concern to nurse researchers as they con-

Table 1-2. EXAMPLES OF NURSING'S PHILOSOPHICAL SCHEMES

AUTHOR	CATEGORIZATION OF PERSPECTIVES
Hall (1981)	• *Growth*. Change is natural, proper, and good. It implies progress. Goal of care is on development and adaptive change. • *Persistence*. Change is rare, unnatural, inevitable, and undesirable. Goal of care is to maintain balance and stability.
Parse (1987)	• *Totality*. Man is a total, summative organism, comprised of bio-psycho-social-spiritual features. The environment is a source of external and internal stimuli to which Man must adapt in order to maintain balance and achieve goals. • *Simultaneity*. Man is a unitary being in continuous and reciprocal interrelationships with the environment. Health is an unfolding phenomenon.
Newman, Sime, & Corcoran-Perry (1996)	• *Particulate-deterministic*. Phenomena are specific, reducible, measurable entities. Relationships between and within entities are causal and linear. Change, as a result of prior conditions, can be predicted and controlled. • *Interactive-integrative*. Phenomena include experiences and subjective data. Multiple interrelationships that are contextual and reciprocal exist between phenomena. Change is a function of multiple prior conditions and probalistic relationships. • *Unitary-transformative*. A phenomenon is a unitary, self-organizing field and is identified through pattern recognition and interaction with the larger whole. Change is unidirectional and unpredictable.
Fawcett (1995)	• *Reaction*. Person is viewed as composed of discrete biological, psychological, sociological, and spiritual aspects, who responds in a reactive manner to environmental stimuli. Change occurs when survival is challenged. • *Reciprocal interaction*. Person is holistic, interactive being. Interactions with the environment are reciprocal. Change occurs as a result of multiple factors at varying rates throughout life and can only be estimated, not predicted. • *Simultaneous action*. Person is viewed as a holistic, self-organized field. Person–environment interactions are mutual and rhythmical processes. Change is unpredictable and evolutionary.

Note. These philosophical schemes are also referred to as paradigms.

sider the ethical implications of research problems, research methods, and dissemination of the research findings.

Philosophy, theory, and research are inextricably linked. "...All nursing theory or research derives from or leads to philosophy" (Phillips, 1992, p. 49). Philosophy makes a significant contribution to the development of nursing theories. The conceptual clarification specified by the philosopher of science helps the theorist generate better theories, and the speculation engaged in by the philosopher of science can also suggest the theories of the future (Smart, 1968, p. 17). Analysis of a theory reveals the underlying assumptions and worldview (philosophy). By considering these philosophical statements, nurses can determine the fit between the values and beliefs expressed through the theory and their own. This enables researchers and practitioners to select theories that are philosophically congruent with their own perspectives on nursing. Therefore, philosophy plays a critical role in the formulation of questions important to nursing, the consideration of research methods, and the development of theories and their analysis and use in practice.

Controversy

Similar to the debate over paradigms, the controversy about nursing philosophy centers on the relative value of unity or diversity in nursing thought. Roach (1992) argues that philosophical inquiry in nursing is the pursuit of universal, transcendent principles and suggests metaphysics as the basis for nursing's unity. Others refer to this search for a coherent philosophical foundation in nursing as a pursuit of unity in diversity of thought (Newman, 2002; Phillips, 1992). The diversity of perspectives represented in the variety of existing nursing models requires philosophical inquiry as a means of determining underlying philosophical themes and patterns. This search for the unitary nature of phenomena of concern to nursing will lead to the recognition of core beliefs:

- A holistic view of persons (Phillips, 1992; Roach, 1992)
- A commitment to caring as an expression of the human mode of being (Newman, Sime, & Corcoran-Perry, 1996; Roach, 1992)
- A perspective on education that acknowledges the unity of mind-body-spirit and recognition of the universe of knowledge that is necessary to achieve and makes a contribution to human understanding (Roach, 1992)
- A view of humans in relationship, with awareness of ethical–moral bonds (Roach, 1992).

Though diversity may result in confusion and lack of clarity in nursing's theory-development and research agenda, others believe that a philosophy that represents the worldview of all nurse scientists would be diluted to the point of becoming meaningless and useless (Landreneau, 2002). Diversity of philosophies may be viewed as a more accurate representation of reality, a perspective consistent with postmodern thinking, and may have the potential of stimulating greater creativity and variety in the development of nursing models and theories.

CONCEPTUAL MODELS

The prevailing view is that conceptual models are frameworks of related concepts that delineate phenomena of interest. Adam (1992) claims that they are the cornerstone of nursing's development (p. 61). Conceptual models are considered less abstract and more explicit and specific than philosophies but more abstract and less explicit and specific than theories (Adam, 1992; Alligood & Tomey, 2002; Caper, 1986, 2002; Fawcett, 2000). The term *conceptual model* has been used interchangeably, accompanied by some controversy, with conceptual framework, theoretical framework, conceptual system (King, 1997), philosophy (Adam, 1992), disciplinary matrix, paradigm (Alligood & Tomey, 2002; Fawcett, 1992), theory (Dickhoff & James, 1968; Fitzpatrick & Whall, 1983; Meleis, 1997), and macrotheory (Adam, 1992).

Beginning in the 1960s, conceptual models emerged as nursing attempted to distinguish itself from other disciplines, especially medicine (Kikuchi, 1992; Schlotfeldt, 1992). Since the 1960s, nursing models have been developed, proposed, analyzed, critiqued, and refined. Table 1-3 provides examples of the work of nurse scientists that has been labeled as conceptual models.

Table 1-3. CONCEPTUAL MODELS

MODEL	SELECTED SOURCES
Johnson's Behavioral System Model	Johnson, D. E. (1959). The nature and science of nursing. *Nursing Outlook, 7,* 291–294. Johnson, D. E. (1980). The behavioral system model for nursing. In J. P. Reihl & C. Roy (Eds.), *Conceptual models for nursing practice* (2nd ed., pp. 207–216). New York: Appleton-Century-Crofts. Johnson, D. E. (1990). The behavioral system model for nursing. In Parker, M. E. (Ed.), *Nursing theories in practice* (pp. 23–32). New York: National League for Nursing.
King's General Systems Framework	King, I. M. (1968). A conceptual frame of reference for nursing. *Nursing Research, 17,* 27–31. King, I. M. (1971). *Toward a theory of nursing: General concepts of human behavior.* New York: Wiley. King, I. M. (1981). *A theory for nursing: Systems, concepts, process.* New York: Wiley.
Levine's Conservation Model	Levine, M. E. (1969). The pursuit of wholeness. *American Journal of Nursing, 69,* 93–98. Levine, M. E. (1991). The conservation model: A model for health. In K. M. Schaefer & J. B. Pond (Eds.), *The conservation model: A framework for nursing practice* (pp. 1–11). Philadelphia: F. A. Davis. Levine, M. E. (1996). The conservation principles: A retrospective. *Nursing Science Quarterly, 9*(1), 38–41.
Neuman's Systems Model	Neuman, B. (1982). *The Neuman systems model: Application to nursing education and practice.* Norwalk, CT: Appleton-Century-Crofts. Neuman, B. (1995). *The Neuman systems model* (3rd ed.). Norwalk, CT: Appleton & Lange. Neuman, B. (1996). The Neuman system model in research and practice. *Nursing Science Quarterly, 9*(1), 67–70.
Rogers' Science of Human Beings	Rogers, M. E. (1980). Nursing: A science of unitary man. In J. P. Reihl & C. Roy (Eds.), *Conceptual models for nursing practice* (2nd ed., pp. 207–216). New York: Appleton-Century-Crofts. Rogers, M. E (1990). Nursing: A science for unitary, irreducible human beings: Update 1990. In E. A. M. Barrett (Ed.), *Visions of Rogers' science-based nursing* (pp. 5–11). New York: National League for Nursing. Rogers, M. E (1994). The science of unitary human beings: Current perspectives. *Nursing Science Quarterly, 7,* 33–35.
Roper-Logan-Tierney Model for Nursing	Roper, N., Logan, W., & Tierney, A. (1996). *The elements of nursing: A model for nursing based on a model of living* (4th ed.). Edinburgh: Churchill Livingstone. Roper, N., Logan, W., & Tierney, A. (1983). A nursing model. *Nursing Mirror, 156*(22), 17–19. Roper, N., Logan, W., & Tierney, A. (1997). The Roper-Logan-Tierney model. In P. Hinton-Walker & B. Neuman (Eds.), *Blueprint for use of nursing models.* New York: National League for Nursing.

(Continued)

Table 1-3.   CONCEPTUAL MODELS *(Continued)*

Roy's Adaptation Model	Roy, C. (1971). Adaptation: A conceptual framework for nursing. *Nursing Outlook, 18*(3), 42–45. Roy, C. (1976). *Introduction to nursing: An adaptation model.* Englewood Cliffs, NJ: Prentice-Hall. Roy, C. & Andrews, H. A. (1999). *The Roy adaptation model: The definitive statement.* Norwalk, CT: Appleton & Lange.

In addition to the conceptual model, another type of model found in the nursing literature is the symbolic model. This type of model uses verbal, quantitative, or schematic modes of representing the nature of the phenomena being described (Caper, 1986). The steps in the nursing process could be considered a verbal model. In research studies using path analysis, quantitative models are used to represent the strength of relationships between variables. Schematic models, also called replicas, schemas, or structures, are the most common form of symbolic model (Parse, 1997). Every organizational chart is a schematic model. As such, they can be employed as a means of communicating the relationships between the components of a theory. Many theorists develop a symbolic model to summarize the content of their theories. In addition to descriptive purposes, "the analytical function [of this type] of model prevents use of vague ideas and requires precise analysis of concepts and related data" (King, 1997, p. 23). Several examples of symbolic models are provided in this text as representations of middle range theories, but the focus in this chapter is on conceptual models of nursing.

Development

Conceptual models are typically developed through the three stages of conceptualization or formulation, model formalization, and validation (Young, Taylor, & Renpenning, p. 11). The process can be empirical or intuitive, deductive or inductive. *Empirically*, nurse scholars make observations from practice; *intuitively*, they develop insights; *deductively*, they combine ideas from a variety of areas of inquiry, particularly other theories (e.g., general systems) and scientific bases; and *inductively*, they generalize from specific situations or observations. Conceptual nursing models reflect assumptions, beliefs, and values and, according to Adam (1992), are comprised of six units, with commonly occurring philosophical perspectives. The following list summarizes the units and philosophical perspectives with examples from Johnson's Behavioral System Model.

1. *Goal of nursing*, generally idealistic, pragmatic, and humanistic; for instance, "fostering effective and efficient behavioral functioning" (Johnson, 1990, p. 24).
2. *Conceptualizations of the client*, usually existential and humanistic, and almost certainly holistic, as evidenced by Johnson's eight behavioral subsystems (Grubbs, 1974).
3. *Social role of nurse*, often humanistic and idealistic; for example, nursing is viewed as a service that makes a unique contribution to the health and well-being of individuals—specifically, nurses act to "provide a distinctive service to society" (Grubbs, 1974, p. 160) and "to seek the highest possible level of behavioral functioning [for the patient]" (Grubbs, 1974, p. 161).

4. *Source of difficulty*, primarily pragmatic, because it identifies the scope of nursing's responsibility; for instance, behavioral disequilibrium and unpredictability, indicating a malfunction in the behavioral system (Grubbs, 1974).

5. *Intervention*, typically humanistic, idealistic, and pragmatic; for example, restrict (e.g., set limits on dysfunctional behavior), defend (e.g., use isolation techniques), inhibit (e.g., teach new skills), and facilitate (e.g., provide adequate nutrition) (Grubbs, 1974).

6. *Desired consequences*, also typically humanistic, idealistic, and pragmatic, as evidenced by Johnson's goal of system balance and stability (Grubbs, 1974; Johnson, 1990).

Though Johnson's Behavioral System's Model was used as one example of how these components are addressed in a conceptual model, all the conceptual models found in Table 1-3 consider these six components, each from its unique perspective.

Uses

The development of conceptual models is essential to the professional identity of nursing. The conceptual models delineate the goals and scope of nursing and provide frameworks for considering the outcomes of nursing. In general, they can direct a professional discipline's theory development, practice, education, and research.

Conceptual models can give birth to nursing theories. Fawcett (2000, p. 19) claims that "grand theories are derived directly from conceptual models." Because, by definition, conceptual models are considered more abstract and less specific than theories, several can develop from a single conceptual model. For instance, several grand theories were derived from Roger's conceptual model, the Science of Unitary Human Beings. The Theory of Power as Knowing Participation in Change (Barrett, 1986) is one example of a theory with its origins in Roger's conceptual model. The alternate view is that conceptual models are "not necessary, and, perhaps, not even important for theoretical growth (Rodman, 1980, p. 436). For instance, Leininger's Theory of Cultural Care Diversity and Universality was derived from anthropological concepts, research (the first being a study of the Gadsup people in Papua, New Guinea), and her beliefs about nursing. Peplau's Theory of Interpersonal Relations was based on an integration of theories from the field of psychology and the recorded interactions between student nurses and patients.

In practice, the models have basically provided a framework for implementation of the nursing process (Archibald, 2000, Nursing Models, para. 2). Assessment based on a conceptual model tends to be more comprehensive, focused, and specific (Hardy, 1986). Because of their level of abstraction, models tend to be less effective in prescribing specific nursing interventions. Instead, the conceptual models suggest general areas of nursing action. The unique focus of each conceptual model also implies criteria for determining when problems have been solved, thus aiding the process of evaluation.

Many schools of nursing used conceptual models as a framework for their curricula. The use of nursing's conceptual models ensured that the focus of the students' education was on nursing, not medicine. It provided students with a perspective for considering nursing issues and a language for expressing such. Beginning in the 1960s and through the 1990s, schools of nursing have identified the use of specific conceptual models in their curricula, e.g., Johnson's Behavioral System Model (Harris, 1986), King's General Systems Framework (Brown & Lee, 1980), Neuman's Systems Model (Kilchenstein & Yakulis, 1984), and Roy's Adaptation Model (Brower & Baker, 1976).

Conceptual models can also guide research. "Research is nursing research only if it examines phenomena of special interest to nursing, that is, phenomena that are indicated by one or the other of the conceptual models for nursing" (Adam, 1992, p. 59). Since conceptual models for nursing represent foci of scientific inquiry, they can identify questions for research. For instance, conceptual models generated the following questions: (a) In Johnson's Behavioral System Model, what are the effects of the stage of cancer on the eight behavioral subsystems? (Derdiarian, 1988); (b) In King's General Systems Framework, what factors interfere with goal attainment? (Kameoda & Sugimori, 1993; and (c), In Neuman's System Model, what effect did experience with the model have on the quality of nursing diagnoses? (Mackenzie & Spence Laschinger, 1995). It is important to note that avenues of questioning suggested by conceptual models are not the same as those of empirical testing, which less abstract theories undergo.

Controversy

There are some controversies about the use and usefulness of conceptual models. Although conceptual models cannot be tested or validated because of their level of abstractness (Adam, 1992; Downs, 1982), they can and should be evaluated. Evaluation of conceptual models has revealed some general limitations. They have been criticized for:

- Their level of abstraction, limiting their usefulness
- Rigidity and inflexibility, which inhibits change
- The subjectivity of perspective, which may not be shared by professional colleagues or clients
- The use of a unique language or jargon, requiring specialized education or resulting in confusing communication
- Potential to be used in inappropriate situations and for incorrect purposes (Adam, 1992; Hardy, 1986; Littlejohn, 2002; Tierney, 1998; Young, Taylor, & Renfenning, 2001).

Controversy about the use of conceptual models in relation to theory development is complicated by lack of consistency in labeling the work of nurse scientists. Fawcett's (2000) position is that conceptual models are more abstract and global and less specific than theories. Kramer (1997) identifies conceptual models as a type of theory but claims not all theories are conceptual models. Meleis (1997) concludes that most of the differences between the two are semantic and noted that the nurse scientists themselves referred to their work using a variety of terms. For instance, Rogers called her conceptualization of nursing a science (Science of Unitary Human Beings); Erickson referred to her work as both a theory and a paradigm (Modeling and Role-Modeling: A Theory and Paradigm); and Watson identified her thinking as both philosophy and theory (Watson's Philosophy and Theory of Human Caring). In this book, conceptual models and theories have been treated as distinct entities. Although there is some confusion about the term and some limitations regarding their use, conceptual models have proved valuable for the advancement of nursing research and the development of theories.

THEORY: GENERAL ISSUES

Similar to conceptual models, theories are comprised of concepts and propositions. In a theory, the concepts are defined more specifically and the propositions are more narrowly focused. Though theory and paradigm are sometime used interchangeably, theories differ from both paradigms and philosophies in that they represent what is rather than what should be (Babbie, 1995, pp. 37, 47). A theoretical body of knowledge is considered an essential characteristic of all professions (Johnson, 1974). Therefore, theories serve to further specify the uniqueness or distinctiveness of a profession. "Theories have in fact distinguished nursing from other caring professions by fixing professional boundaries" (Rutty, 1998, Theory, para. 2). The definition of theory by Kerlinger is classic and comprehensive. "Kerlinger (1973) defines theory as follows: A theory is a set of interrelated constructs (concepts, definitions, and propositions) that present a systematic view of phenomena by specifying relations among variables, with the purpose of explaining and predicting phenomena" (King, 1978, p. 11).

In addition to considering the development, uses, and controversies surrounding nursing theories, it is important to address the classifications of theories. Theories can be classified in a number of ways, such as by their purposes, sources, and levels. The three major levels of nursing are grand, middle range, and practice, with middle range theory of special interest as it grows in importance in nursing research and practice.

Development

The development of a theory involves both content and process. Theories are comprised of concepts, and their relationships and are constructed through a variety of processes. The history of theory development in nursing helps provide a context for understanding the ongoing work of nurse scientists in the advancement of nursing's body of knowledge.

COMPONENTS

A variety of terms are used to describe concepts and propositions, the two basic elements of a theory. The terms concept, construct, descriptor, and unit are often used interchangeably, with concept being the most common. Definitions of the concepts can be considered an aspect of the basic element, concept, or as a separate and additional component of a theory. Statements of relationships or propositions refer to the same notion. Also, some scientists include axioms and postulates as other components of a theory, because, though they are relational statements, they are assertions assumed to be true that lay the groundwork for the propositions (Babbie, 1995, p. 48).

Concepts. Concepts are considered the basic building blocks of theory. Kim (1983, p. 8) defines concepts as "a symbolic statement describing a phenomenon or a class of phenomena." In other words, a concept is a mental image of a phenomenon, an idea or construct of an object or action (Walker & Avant, 1995, p. 24). Although there are several more complicated classifications of concepts (or units), basically they can be classified on a continuum of abstractness, which some label primitive, abstract, and concrete (Meleis, 1997) and others global, middle range, and empirical (Moody, 1990). They can also be categorized as property or process concepts (Kim, 1983).

Primitive concepts are those that have a culturally shared meaning (Walker & Avant, 1995, p. 24) or are those that are introduced as new in the theory (Meleis, 1997, p. 252). For instance, in culturally derived concepts, a color is usually primitive because it cannot be defined except by giving examples of another color different from the original color. Grass, leaves, and apples would be examples of green, and sky, bark, and grapefruit would be examples of not green. As an original concept in a new theory, role supplementation in the theory of "Role Insufficiency and Role Supplementation" would be an example of a theory-specific primitive concept (Meleis, 1997, p. 252). Concrete concepts are those that exist in a spatial–temporal reality. They can be defined in terms of primitive concepts. Grass, leaves, apples, sky, bark, and grapefruit would all be examples of concrete concepts. In nursing, touch used by the nurse would be considered a concrete concept. Abstract concepts can be defined by primitive or concrete concepts but are not limited by time or space. "They refer to general cases" (Kim, 1983, p. 8). Communication could be identified as an abstract concept that would be of interest to nursing. Theories can be comprised of both concrete and abstract concepts.

For theories using abstract concepts, operational definitions of those concepts are an important inclusion because the definitions enable the theory to be more easily tested empirically through research. An operational definition "assigns[s] explicit meaning to that [abstract] concept" (Duldt & Giffin, 1985, p. 95). Operational definitions can be (a) experimental, providing specific details necessary to manipulate the concept; (b) measurable, describing the means by which the concept can be measured; (c) administrative, including particular information on how to obtain data about the concept; and (d) evaluative, establishing the criteria for operationalizing the concept and the means of determining the degree to which the criteria are met.

The classification of concepts as property or process is significant because it promotes understanding of the concept as defined by the theorist. Property concepts are those that deal with the state of things, and process concepts are those that relate to the way things happen. Stage of grief would be a property concept, whereas, grieving as the means by which an individual deals with loss would be a process concept. A concept can be considered both a property and process concept, such as communication. In general, theories contain both types of concepts. "The classification system of concepts into property and process types is useful in an analytic sense" (Kim, 1983, p. 10). It provides a clearer sense of the nature of the concepts included in the theory and thus a better understanding of the theory itself.

Propositions. Propositions, defined as statements of the relationships between two or more concepts, provide a theory "with the powers of description, explanation or prediction" (Meleis, 1997, p. 252). Propositional statements can be considered either relational or nonrelational. Relational statements can be either correlational or causal. Nonrelational statements include descriptions of the properties and dimensions of the concept in the definition of the term, proposition (Meleis, 1997).

In propositional statements that are correlational, the assertion is that two or more concepts exist together or are associated. The associations can be positive, negative, or neutral. Orem's Self-care Deficit Nursing Theory provides examples of positive and neutral correlational statements. The nurse affects the movement from the "'present state of affairs' to 'a desirable future state of affairs' by using the 'nursing means' the nurse selects" (Orem, 2001, p. 151) is an example of a positive statement. "Engagement in self-care or dependent-care is affected by persons' valuation of self care measures with respect to life, development, heath, and well-being" (Orem, 2001, p. 146) is an example of a more neutral or directionless statement.

Causal propositional statements establish cause-and-effect relationships. Examples of causal statements are found in Parse's Man-Living-Health Theory of Nursing. "In a nurse–family process, by synchronizing rhythms, the members uncover the opportunities and limitations created by the decisions made in choosing irreplaceable ways of being together. The choices of new ways of being together mobilizes transcendence." (Parse, 1987, p. 170). Causal statements are more difficult to establish than correlational statements and therefore more rare.

"Nonrelational statements serve as adjuncts to relational statements" (Walker & Avant, 1995, p. 25). They provide assertions of the existence of concepts or definitions of concepts of a theory and thus help explain the nature of the theory. An example of an existence proposition would be Parse's statement that the practice methodology of her theory is comprised of three dimensions: illuminating meaning, synchronizing rhythms, and mobilizing transcendence (Parse, 1987, p. 167). Parse also provides definitional propositions, for example, "health is Man's unfolding. It is Man's lived experiences, a non linear entity that cannot be qualified by terms as good, bad, more, or less" (Parse, 1987, p. 160).

The nature of the elements of the theory relates to the purposes for which the theory can be used. Theories with only nonrelational prepositional statements serve to describe, whereas theories with relational prepositional statements have the potential to explain (correlational statements) and predict (causal statements).

PROCESS

Theory development can be accomplished by inductive or deductive processes or by a combination of both. The content of a theory comes from other theories, practice, or research, or a combination of two or more of these sources. Using other theories as a source of generating a theory involves a deductive process, whereas using practice experience or research findings for developing a theory requires an inductive process.

Walker and Avant (1995) describe strategies of theory development that include both inductive and deductive processes. Analysis, synthesis and derivation are applied to concepts, statements, and theories. Analysis is solely an inductive process, whereas synthesis and derivation can involve both inductive and deductive processes (Walker & Avant, 1995, p. 32). Table 1-4 presents a matrix of the purposes of the nine strategies that Walker and Avant (1995) describe in detail in their book, *Strategies for Theory Construction in Nursing*.

Table 1-4. MATRIX OF APPROACHES TO THEORY CONSTRUCTION

	CONCEPT	STATEMENT	THEORY
Analysis	Distinguish between defining and irrelevant attributes of the concept by breaking a concept into simpler elements and considering similarities and differences	Determine how useful, informative, and logically correct the statements are through an orderly examination	Determine the strengths and weaknesses of theory by applying an analytical framework
Synthesis	Generate new ideas by examining data for new insights	Develop statements about relationships through observations of phenomena	Construct a theory from empirical evidence
Derivation	Generate new ways of thinking about phenomena by developing a new vocabulary based on the relationships between phenomena	Formulate statements about a poorly understood phenomenon by clarifying relationships between phenomena	Explain and predict phenomena which are poorly understood or for which no methods of study are known, or for which no theory exists

Source: Walker, L. O. & Avant, K. C. (1995). *Strategies for theory construction in nursing* (3rd ed.). Norwalk, CT: Appleton & Lange.

This process of theory construction is modeled in the work of Lenz, Suppe, Gift, Pugh, and Milligan (1995), as they collaborated on the development of the middle range theory of unpleasant symptoms. For instance the researchers used existing literature for *concept analysis*, examining attributes, characteristics, and dimensions of the concept of dyspnea. The literature review also served as a basis of *concept derivation*, resulting in the identification of pain as an analog of dyspnea. And through *synthesis* of the literature and the researchers' own experiences, they conceptualized dyspnea as having five components: sensation, perception, distress, response, and reporting.

Walker and Avant (1995) identify other theories as a source of additional theory development. Theories from other disciplines are one source of nursing theory content. Peplau made use of psycholanalytic theory and Johnson made use of systems theory, informed by their clinical practices, psychiatric and pediatric nursing, respectively. Nursing theories and conceptual models often give rise to middle range theory. For instance, from Orem's Self-care Deficit Theory came the Theory of Dependent-care Deficit, Theory of Self-care, and Theory of Nursing Systems (Alligood & Tomey, 2002, p. 50).

"Some theories are driven by clinical practice situations and are inductively developed" (Meleis, 1997, p. 230). This grounded theory approach uses observations and analysis of similarities and differences of observed phenomena to develop concepts and establish their relationships. The works of Peplau, Orlando, Travelbee, and Wiedenbach have been associated with this approach.

Research is often cited as the most common and acceptable source for theory development, most often leading to the development of a middle range theory. According to this approach, "theories evolve from replicated and confirmed research findings" (Meleis, 1997, p. 231). This is considered an empirical quantitative approach and involves (a) identifying a phenomenon, listing all its characteristics; (b) measuring these characteristics in a variety of settings; (c) analyzing the results to determine if patterns exist; and (d) formalizing these patterns as theoretical statements (Reynolds, 1971, p. 140). Johnson and Rice's (1974) theory of sensory and distress components of pain was developed using this approach. Qualitative research is often referred to as theory generating. Grounded theory and phenomenology are qualitative approaches to theory development often used by nurse scientists. Fagerhaugh's (1974) theory of pain expression and control is an example of theory developed through qualitative research. McKenna (1997) noted similarities between the quantitative and qualitative approaches: both use inductive methods, and both generally result in the development of middle range theories.

HISTORY

Nursing theory development can trace its roots to the work of Florence Nightingale (Alligood & Tomey, 2002; Dunphy, 2001; Fitzpatrick & Whall, 1983; Meleis, 1997), with her concern for the relationship between health and environment and the nurse's role in that relationship. Hildegard Peplau is credited with being the first contemporary nurse theorist (McKenna, 1997). Other theorists of the 1950s (Henderson [in Henderson and Harmer], 1955; Orem, 1959; Johnson, 1959; Hall, 1959) (McKenna, 1997, p. 95) were influenced by Peplau's conceptualization of interpersonal relationships in nursing. Others were influenced by their involvement at Columbia University's Teachers' College and the practical-oriented philosophy of John Dewey, who served on its staff. From Teachers' College in the 1950s, Abdellah, King, Wiedenbach, and Rogers emerged as nurse theorists (Meleis, 1997). Not all of the work of these nurse scientists would be considered theory by today's definition. The theoretical work that did take place in the 1950s focused on what nurses did, not why they did it, and the conceptual frameworks developed at this time were more often used as a basis for the development of curricula than as a guide for practice. The 1950s also saw the introduction of the journal, *Nursing Research*, which provided a forum for the development of nursing theories and their testing.

In addition to continuing development of individual nursing theories, the 1960s brought a more national and coordinated approach to theory development. Federal financial support became available in 1962 to nurses pursuing doctoral education; the American Nurses Association stated in 1965 that theory development was a significant goal for the profession; and in 1967, Case Western Reserve University sponsored a national nursing symposium, a third of which was devoted to nursing theory. The theorists associated with this decade include "Abdellah et al. (1960), Orlando (1961), Wiedenbach (1964), Levine (1966), Travelbee (1966) and King (1968)" (McKenna, 1997, pp. 95–96). Theorists, particularly Wiedenbach and Orlando, began to consider not only what nurses did but what effect it had on patients. Debate, stimulated by the metatheorists, focused on the issue of the types of theories that nursing should develop rather than the content of theories.

Although nursing theorists continued to develop and publish their work, such as Roy (1970), Rogers (1970), Neuman (1972), Riehl (1974), Adam (1975), Patterson and Zderad (1976), Leininger (1978), Watson (1979) and Newman (1979) (McKenna, 1997, p. 97), the questions posed by metatheorists dominated the decade of the 1970s (Meleis, 1997). Efforts were made to determine what is meant by theory; to identify the structural components of theories; and to clarify the methods of analysis and critique of theory. The previously developed theories were criticized for a failure to include explicated propositions and for their lack of empirical testing (McKenna, 1997, p. 97). The development and use of nursing theories were advanced by (a) the adoption by the National League for Nursing of an accreditation criterion requiring a theory-base to nursing curricula; (b) the formation of two groups (Nursing Theories Conference Group and Nursing Theory Think Tank), that considered application of theory to practice; and (c) the publication of *Advances in Nursing Science*, a journal dedicated to the development of nursing science.

Alligood and Tomey (2001) refer to the 1980s as the Theory Era, even though few new nursing theories emerged. "Only three new nursing theories were published in the 1980s: the work of Parse (1981), Fitzpatrick (1982) and Erickson, Tomlin and Swain (1983) (McKenna, 1997, p. 97). Fawcett's (1984, 1989) explication of a metaparadigm for nursing allowed for the comparative content analysis of theories, and her delineation of the levels of abstraction of nursing knowledge helped nurse scientists and practitioners make the distinctions between grand, middle range, and practice theories. Her work also clarified how nursing grand theory can be derived from nursing conceptual models and how middle range theory can be derived from grand theory. The importance of nursing theory to the profession was well established and the shift by the end of this decade was away from theory development toward theory use (Alligood & Tomey, 2002, p. 9). There was both an increased interest in the relationship between theory and practice and an increased emphasis on the relationship between theory and research.

The decade of the 1990s was hallmarked by the development of the middle range and practice theories. These theories are less abstract and therefore more directly applicable to practice and more easily tested empirically by research. Interest in nursing theory was evidenced by the publication of *Nursing Science Quarterly*, edited by Parse, focusing on theory development and testing and by the increasing number of European-based nursing theory conferences.

Uses

Nurse scientists have worked on the development of nursing theory as part of the process of establishing nursing as a profession with a unique body of knowledge. Nursing theories provide nurses with the language of nursing, a means of communicating the nature of the discipline within and outside the profession. In addition, as a component of nursing knowledge considered less abstract than conceptual frameworks, nursing theories generate more specific research questions and provide greater guidance to nursing practice.

Nursing theories provide nursing-specific identifications, definitions, and interrelationships of concepts. This allows the profession to distinguish itself from the medical and behavioral sciences. For example, in nursing, we speak of unitary human beings, self-care, and the centrality of caring. Through analysis of theories, nursing's metaparadigm emerges, providing us with a common and basic frame of reference for communicating about nursing.

The relationship between nursing theory and research is symbiotic. Research provides for both theory generating and theory testing. Qualitative research seeks to identify and define phenomena of interest to nursing, thus serving as a theory-generating tool. By contrast, quantitative research is a means by which the propositions of theories can be substantiated, thus functioning as a theory-testing tool. Theories then serve as a framework for relating the data generated by research, resulting in a more coherent whole nursing body of knowledge than a collection of isolated facts.

In addition, the greater clarification of concepts and their relationships that nursing theories provide allows researchers to formulate more specific and nursing-relevant research questions. The evidence that is generated through the study of these questions, because of the level of specificity and relevance, in turn is more directly applicable to nursing practice. Parse (1999) challenges nurses "to conduct research to ensure that the practice of nursing serves people in a unique way" (Recommendations, para. 1). It is through nursing theories that the profession identifies its unique service to people. The testing of nursing theories also leads to theory-guided evidence-based practice. "Evidence itself refers to evidence about theories. Similarly, theory determines what counts as evidence" (Fawcett, Watson, Neuman, Walker, & Fitzpatrick, 2001). Thus, theory as it guides research has the potential to provide the evidence that makes nursing practice more efficient and more effective.

Controversy

There are two recurring themes in criticisms of nursing theories: the issue of consistency in labeling and the appropriateness of the sources of the theories used by nurses. The lack of definitional clarity between what is labeled a conceptual model and what is considered a theory is further complicated by confusion over identification of the level of the theory, that is, grand, middle range, or practice. Nurse scientists have not consistently classified the level of the developed theory in the work they publish. This issue is further addressed in the discussion of the middle range level of theory development. In addition, there is some disagreement over the appropriate source of theories to be used by nurses, borrowed or unique. The debate focuses on to what degree nurses can use theories from other disciplines and still advance nursing's unique body of knowledge. The discussion of this issue is integrated into the section on classification of theories by source.

Classifications

Theories differ in their purposes, sources, and, most importantly, levels of abstraction and scope. These differences lead to classifications. The basic purposes of theory are description, explanation, prediction, and/or control. The sources of theory in nursing include those developed by nurse scientists (unique) and those that are used in nursing but come from other disciplines (borrowed). The terms "theory *of* nursing" and "theory *in* nursing" are often used to distinguish between these two sources.

There are multiple terms used to classify the various levels or scope of nursing theories. The broad-scope theories are referred to as "macro," "holistic," "molar," "general," "situation," and, most commonly, "grand." Narrow-scope theories are called "middle range," "circumscribed," or "situation/factor." Theories narrowest in scope are labeled "micro," "molecular," "atomistic," "narrow-range," "phenomena," "prescriptive," "factor," "situation-specific," or "practice" (Babbie, 1995; George, 1995; Parker, 2001; Rinehart, 1978). The most common labels for the levels of nursing theory are grand, middle range, and micro or practice. The level is determined primarily by the theory's degree of abstraction. Examination of the level of abstraction of the "purpose, concept, and definitional components of the theory" (Kramer, 1997, p. 65) allows for the identification of the level of the theory.

PURPOSES

Though theories are designed to describe, explain, predict, and/or control, some nurse scientists claim that only theories that enable nurses to control outcomes are legitimate for a practice discipline (Dickhoff & James, 1968). Descriptive theories are limited to naming and classifying characteristics of the phenomenon of interest, which identify what is happening. Peplau's Theory of Interpersonal Relationships has been labeled a descriptive theory.

Explanatory theories expand the knowledge base by delineating the relationships between characteristics of the phenomenon, clarifying why it is happening. Watson's Theory of Human Caring is considered an explanatory theory. But predictive theories provide the conditions that can result in a preferred outcome, determining how it can intentionally happen. Orlando's Theory of the Deliberative Nursing Process is an example of a predictive theory. Theories whose purpose is to control, often referred to as prescriptive theories, guide action to create an intended result. The three ingredients for this type of theory are content of goal, primary prescription for activity to achieve goal, and list of additional recommendation of activity (Dickhoff & James, 1968, p. 201).

The existence of descriptive and explanatory theories is a necessary precursor to the development of predictive and prescriptive theories. "Predictive theory presupposes the prior existence of more elementary types of theories" (Dickhoff & James, 1968, p. 200). The relationship between the purposes of a theory has been conceptualized in some instances as a hierarchy:

1. Factor-isolating theories (descriptive)
2. Factor-relating theories (descriptive/explanatory)
3. Situation-relating theories (explanatory/predictive)
4. Situation-producing theories (prescriptive) (Dickhoff & James, 1968, pp. 200–201).

SOURCES

The source of theory refers to the discipline from which it developed. The possibilities include theories unique to nursing, theories borrowed from other disciplines, and theories from other disciplines adapted for nursing. The distinctions between these three sources is difficult to make since "the man-made, more-or less arbitrary divisions between the sciences are neither firm nor constant" (Johnson, 1986, p. 117).

Given that the differences between the sources of theory may be less than perfectly precise, unique theory can be defined "as that knowledge derived from the observation of phenomena and the asking of questions unlike those which characterized other disciplines" (Johnson, 1986, p. 118). Many argue that nursing's identity as a profession and, ultimately, its ability to improve nursing practice are dependent on the existence of nursing theories unique to the discipline. Wald and Leonard (1964), the most frequently cited proponents of this position, claimed that to become an independent discipline, nursing was required to develop its own theories rather than borrow theories or apply principles from other disciplines. They expressed concern about nursing's reliance on these borrowed theories.

Wald and Leonard's concerns seem validated by Jacobson's (1987) findings. When nurses with advanced degrees were asked to identify "conceptual models of nursing," responses included Selye's stress model, Piaget's theory of cognitive development, general system's theory, problem solving, and Maslow's hierarchy of needs. All of these examples would be considered borrowed rather than knowledge unique to nursing.

More recent examination of the literature reveals continued reliance on theories from fields other than nursing. Fawcett and Bourbonniere (2001) found that of 90 research studies published in two clinical journals, *Geriatric Nursing* and *Nurse Practitioner* and two research journals, *Nursing Research* and *Research in Nursing and Health*, only nine used nursing conceptual models or theories (p. 314). The borrowed theories or models used in these studies came from psychology, sociology, medicine, dentistry, physiology, biology, education, decision sciences, economics, ethics, epidemiology, management sciences, marketing, and communications.

Borrowed theory is defined "as that knowledge which is developed in the main by other disciplines and is drawn upon by nursing" (Johnson, 1986, p. 118). In past decades, the practice of borrowing theories seemed to be the result of a belief in the superiority of theories "imported" from other disciplines (Meleis, 1997). This perspective was reinforced by nurses whose advanced degrees were in fields other than nursing. Theories from sociology, psychology, education, ecology, physiology, and others were and still are borrowed. The argument for borrowed theories seems to be that theorists and practitioners should not place boundaries on any knowledge that might be useful to nursing because "knowledge does not innately 'belong' to any field of science" (Johnson, 1986, p. 117). Borrowing theories from other disciplines is sometimes referred to as theory adoption and involves the unchanged use of a theory developed from a field other than nursing. The use of unmodified theories from physiology, for instance, acid-base balance, is an example of a completely borrowed theory. Though the need for adopted borrowed theories does exist, there is concern about their prevalence. The preferred approach for the use of borrowed theories seems to be to adapt them to a distinctively nursing perspective.

Adaptation refers to altering the content or structure of a theory that was initially developed for application to a discipline other than nursing. Borrowing and altering theory is seen as necessary "to acquire a means of explanation and prediction about some phenomena that is currently poorly understood, or for which there is no present means to study it, or for which there is no theory at all" (Walker & Avant, 1995, p. 172). Walker and Avant provide a process called theory derivation, which allows nurses to modify the concepts and structures of a theory from another discipline to create a new theory more relevant to nursing. The steps of the process are not considered strictly linear; they are repeated as necessary until the theory being developed is sufficiently complete. Box 1-1 summarizes the steps in theory derivation.

The debate about the value of borrowed theories continues. Fawcett and Bourbonniere (2001) identify premises necessary for a healthy future for the nursing profession. They claim that "the discipline of nursing can survive only if we celebrate our own heritage and utilize nursing knowledge" (p. 311). This premise and the future it suggests is challenged by the ongoing dependence of nurses on perspectives of nursing that are grounded in the knowledge of other disciplines. The solution they suggest is to end nursing's "romance" with borrowed theories. Few would argue that nursing needs to at-

> ### BOX 1-1.   Steps in the Process of Theory Derivation
>
> 1. Become acquainted with the literature that addresses the phenomenon. Evaluate theory in nursing for its adequacy.
> 2. Read extensively in related fields. Look for unusual relationships between the knowledge in those fields and the phenomenon of interest to nursing.
> 3. Choose a parent theory as a source of the derivation. Focus on the theory, or parts of the theory, that best explains or predicts the phenomenon.
> 4. Select the relevant concepts and/or structures. Eliminate those aspects of the theory that are not useful.
> 5. Develop, refine, or redefine the concepts, statements and structures from the parent theory to develop a theory more meaningful for nursing. This requires reflection and creativity
>
> Source: Walker, L. O., & Avant, K. C. (1995). *Strategies for theory construction in nursing* (3rd ed.). (pp. 172–173). Norwalk, CT: Appleton & Lange.

tend to the ongoing development of its unique body of knowledge; perhaps not for the sole purpose of divorcing itself from other disciplines, but for creating a body of knowledge that could be shared across disciplines. Thus nursing theory could be borrowed.

GRAND THEORY

Grand theories, as the most abstract of the three identified levels, attempt "to create a view of the whole of nursing" (Liehr & Smith, 1999, Juxtaposition with Grand Nursing theory, para. 1). They address the nature, mission, and goals of nursing care (Meleis, 1997) in a general fashion and are created through the observations and/or insights of the theorist. The development of grand theories served to differentiate the discipline of nursing from the medical model, stimulated the expansion of nursing knowledge (McKenna, 1997), and provided a general "structure for the organization of nursing knowledge" (Orem, 2001, p. 139). Orem also claimed that the unstructured nature of grand or general theories allows for a wide range of knowledge available to practitioners and scholars within a nursing-specific frame of reference. McKenna (1997) outlined the benefits of grand theories to include (a) a guide for practice as an alternative to practicing solely by tradition or intuition; (b) a framework for education by suggesting a focus and a structure for curricula; and (c) an aid to the professionalization of nursing by providing a basis of practice.

More than 50 grand theories have been identified (McKenna, 1997, p. 93), although that number may vary based on the label assigned to the work. Because of their level of abstraction, there has been some difficulty in distinguishing between grand theories, philosophies, and conceptual models. Examples of nursing theories that have been designated as grand include Leininger's Theory of Culture Care Diversity and Universality, Newman's Theory of Health as Expanding Consciousness, Parse's Theory of Human Becoming (Fawcett & Bourbonniere, 2001; Fawcett, 1997; Parker, 2001), and King's Theory of Goal Attainment (Alligood & Tomey, 2002; Fawcett, 1997). Parker (2001) also identifies Orem's Self-care Deficit, Roger's Science of Human Beings, and Roy's Adaptation Model as theories, whereas Fawcett (1997) and Alligood and Tomey (2002) label these nursing scientists' work as conceptual models. Orem (2001) refers to her work as a general theory. Table 1-5 provides sources of information about specific grand theories.

Table 1-5.   EXAMPLES OF GRAND THEORIES WITH SOURCES OF INFORMATION

THEORY	PRIMARY SOURCES OF INFORMATION
King's Theory of Goal Attainment	King, I. M. (1981). *A theory of goal attainment: Systems, concepts, process.* New York: Wiley. King, I. M. (1990). Health the goal for nursing. *Nursing Science Quarterly, 3,* 123. King, I. M. (1992). King's theory of goal attainment. *Nursing Science Quarterly, 5,* 19. King, I. M. (1994). Quality of life and goal attainment. *Nursing Science Quarterly, 7,* 29. King, I. M. (1996). The theory of goal attainment in research and practice. *Nursing Science Quarterly, 9,* 61. King, I. M. (1997). King's theory of goal attainment in practice. *Nursing Science Quarterly, 10,* 180–185.
Leininger's Theory of Culture Care and Universality	Leininger, M. M. (1970). *Nursing and anthropology: Two worlds blend.* New York: Wiley. Leininger, M. M. (1978). *Transcultural Nursing: Concepts, theories, and practices.* New York: Wiley. Leininger, M. M. (1985). Transcultural care diversity and universality: A theory of nursing. *Nursing and Health Care, 6,* 208–212. Leininger, M. M. (1988). Leininger's theory of nursing: Cultural care diversity and universality. *Nursing Science Quarterly, 1,* 152–160. Leininger, M. M. (1991). *Cultural care diversity and universality: A theory of nursing.* New York: National League for Nursing. Leininger, M. M. (1995). *Transcultural nursing: Concepts, theories, research, and practice.* Columbus, OH: McGraw Hill College Custom Series.
Newman's Theory of Health as Expanding Consciousness	Newman, M. A. (1986). *Health as expanding consciousness.* St. Louis: Mosby. Newman, M. A. (1990). Newman's theory of health as praxis. *Nursing Science Quarterly, 3,* 37–41. Newman, M. A. (1994). *Health as expanding consciousness* (2nd ed.). Boston: Jones & Bartlett. Newman, M. A. (1997). Evolution of a theory of health as expanding consciousness. *Nursing Science Quarterly, 10,* 22–25.
Orem's Self-care Deficit Theory	Orem, D. E. (1971). *Nursing: Concepts of practice* (2nd ed.). New York: McGraw Hill. Orem, D. E. (1983). *The self-care deficit theory of nursing.* New York: Wiley. Orem, D. E. (1987). *Orem's general theory of nursing.* Philadelphia: W. B. Saunders. Orem, D. E., & Taylor, S. G. (1986). *Orem's general theory of nursing.* New York: National League for Nursing. Orem, D. E. (2001). *Nursing: Concepts of practice* (6th ed.). New York: McGraw Hill.

Table 1-5. EXAMPLES OF GRAND THEORIES WITH SOURCES OF INFORMATION

THEORY	PRIMARY SOURCES OF INFORMATION
Parse's Theory of Human Becoming	Parse, R. R. (1981). *Man-living-health: A theory of nursing.* New York: Wiley.
	Parse, R. R. (1987). *Nursing science: Major paradigms, theories, and critiques.* Philadelphia: W. B. Saunders.
	Parse, R. R. (1992). Human becoming: Parse's theory of nursing. *Nursing Science Quarterly, 5,* 35–42.
	Parse, R. R. (1994). Quality of life: Sciencing and living the art of human becoming. *Nursing Science Quarterly, 7,* 16–21.
	Parse, R. R. (1996). Reality: A seamless symphony of becoming. *Nursing Science Quarterly, 9,* 181–183.
	Parse, R. R. (1997). The human becoming theory: The was, is, and will be. *Nursing Science Quarterly, 10,* 32–38.
	Parse, R. R. (1998). *The human becoming school of thought.* Thousand Oaks, CA: Sage.

The level of abstraction makes it difficult to test grand theories empirically. In fact, Donnelly (2001), citing the work of Lundh, Soder, and Waerness, 1988, claimed that because the theories were abstract and normative "rather than facilitating research development [they] actually made research development in nursing 'more difficult'" (p. 337). This conclusion is supported in part by the findings of Moody et al. (1988) that in nursing practice research published from 1977 to 1986, fewer than 13% of the 720 studies identified were linked to one of the grand theories.

Grand theories seem better able to serve as a basis for the development of the more specific theories of the middle and practice range, which can undergo empirical testing. For instance, the middle range theory, "A Theory of Sentient Evolution" was derived from Roger's Science of Unitary Human Beings (Parker, 1989). In addition, grand theories have fulfilled the important functions of distinguishing nursing from other helping professions and providing legitimization to its science. But because of their success in fulfilling these functions, grand theories have become less necessary and the focus of theory development has changed to the middle range theories (Suppe, 1996a).

MIDDLE RANGE THEORY

Compared to grand theories, middle range theories are less abstract. Merton (1968), whose work served to promote the development of middle range theories, described them as lying between "the minor but necessary working hypotheses that evolve in abundance during day to day research and the all-inclusive systematic efforts to develop a unified theory...." (p. 39). Consistent with Merton's conceptualization, nurse authors have described middle range theories in comparison to grand theories as:

- Narrower in scope (Fawcett, 2000; Liehr & Smith, 1999; McKenna, 1997; Meleis, 1997; Parker, 2001; Walker & Avant, 1995)

- Concerned with less abstract, more specific phenomena (Fawcett, 2000; Meleis, 1997)
- Comprised of fewer concepts and propositions (Fawcett, 2000; McKenna, 1997; Walker & Avant, 1995)
- Representative of a limited or partial view of nursing reality (Jacox, 1974; Liehr & Smith, 1999; Young, Taylor, & Renpening, 2001)
- More appropriate for empirical testing (Liehr & Smith, 1999; McKenna, 1997; Meleis, 1997; Parker, 2001; Walker & Avant, 1995)
- More applicable directly to practice for explanation and implementation (McKenna, 1997; Walker & Avant, 1995; Young, Taylor, & Renpening, 2001)

These attributes make middle range theories attractive to nurses who wish to engage in theory-based research and practice.

The appeal of these theories to nurse researchers and practitioners is demonstrated by their proliferation in the past 15 years. Lenz (1996) identified a number of the middle range theories developed in the 1980s and 1990s. Table 1-6 provides a partial listing of theories used by nurses in research and/or practice that have been considered to be middle range. The table also includes one reference for each theory.

Although not included in the table, Peplau's Theory of Interpersonal Relationships, Orlando's Theory of Deliberative Nursing Process, and Watson's Theory of Human Caring (Fawcett, 2000; Fawcett & Bourbonniere, 2001; Jones, 2001) have been labeled middle range theories. Also not included in the

Table 1-6. EXAMPLES OF MIDDLE RANGE THEORIES

TYPE	THEORY	REFERENCE
Physiologic	Acute pain	Good, M. A. (1998). A middle range theory of acute pain management: Use in research. *Nursing Outlook, 46,* 120–124.
	Chronotherapeutic intervention for postsurgical pain	Auvil-Novak, S. E. (1997). A mid-range theory of chronotherapeutic intervention of postsurgical pain. *Nursing Research, 46,* 66–71.
	Dyspnea	Gift, A. G. (1992). Dyspnea. *Northern Clinics of North America, 25,* 955–965.
	Perimenopausal process	Quinn, A. A. (1991). A theoretical model of the perimenopausal process. *Journal of Nurse-Midwifery, 36*(1), 25–29.
	Unpleasant symptoms	Lenz, E. R., Pugh, L. C., Milligan, R. A., Gift, A. G., & Suppe, F. (1997). The middle range theory of unpleasant symptoms: An update. *Advances in Nursing Science, 19,* 14–27.
Cognitive	Health belief*	Champion, V. L. (1985). Use of the health belief model in determining frequency of breast self-examination. *Research in Nursing Health, 8,* 373–379.
	Social learning theory*	Bandura, A. (1986). *Social foundations of thought and action: A social cognitive theory.* Englewood Cliffs, NJ: Prentice-Hall.

Table 1-6.   EXAMPLES OF MIDDLE RANGE THEORIES

TYPE	THEORY	REFERENCE
Emotional	Chronic sorrow	Eakes, G. G., Burke, M. L., & Hainsworth, M. A. (1998). Middle-range theory of chronic sorrow. *Image, 30,* 179–184.
	Empathy	Olson, J., & Hanchett, E. (1997). Nurse expressed empathy, patient outcomes, and development of a middle range theory. *Image, 29,* 71–76.
	Fulfillment	Kylma, J., & Vehvilainen-Julkunen, K. (1995). Hope in nursing research: A meta-analysis of the ontotological and epistemological foundations of research on hope. *Journal of Advanced Nursing, 25*(2), 364–371.
	Grief	Chapman, K. J., & Pepler, C. (1998). Coping, hope and anticipatory grief in family members with palliative home care. *Cancer Nursing, 21*(4), 226–234.
	Hope	Morse, J. M., & Doberneck, B. (1995). Delineating the concept of hope. *Image, 27*(4), 277–285.
	Personal risking	Hitchcock, J. M., & Wilson, H. S. (1992). Personal risking: Lesbian self-disclosure of sexual orientation to professional health care providers. *Nursing Research, 41,* 178–183.
	Postpartum depression	Beck, C. T. (1993). The lived experience of postpartum depression: A substantive theory of postpartum depression. *Nursing Research, 42,* 42–48.
	Resilience	Polk, L. V. (1997). Toward a middle range theory of resilience. *Advances in Nursing Science, 19,* 1–13.
	Uncertainty	Mishel, M. H. (1991). Reconceptualization of the uncertainty in illness theory. *Image, 2,* 256–261.
	Uncertainty of illness	Deane, K. A., & Degner, L. F. (1998). Information needs, uncertainty, and anxiety in women who had a breast biopsy with benign outcome. *Cancer Nursing, 21*(2), 117–126.
Social	Bureaucratic caring	Ray, M. (1989). The theory of bureaucratic caring for nursing practice in the organizational culture. *Nursing Administrative Quarterly, 13*(2), 31–42.
	Caring through relation and dialogue	Sanford, R. C. (2000). Caring through relation and dialogue: A nursing perspective for patient education. *Advances in Nursing Science, 22*(3), 1–15.
	Coercion in the development of behavior*	Patterson, G. R. (1982). Coercive family process. Eugene, OR: Castoglia.
	Entry into nursing home as a status passage	Chenitz, W. C. (1983, March/April). Entry into a nursing home as status passage: A theory to guide nursing practice. *Geriatric Nursing,* 92–97.

(continued)

Table 1-6.   EXAMPLES OF MIDDLE RANGE THEORIES *(Continued)*

TYPE	THEORY	REFERENCE
	Home Care	Smith, C. E., Pace, K., Kochinda, C., Kleinbeck, S., Koehler, J., & Popkess-Vawter, S. (2002). Caregiver effectiveness model evolution to a midrange theory of home care: A process for critique and replication. *Advances in Nursing Science, 25*(1), 50–64.
	Informed caring	Swanson, K. M. (1993). Nursing as informed caring for the well-being of others. *Image, 25*(4), 352–357.
	Maternal role attainment	Mercer, R. T. (1986). *First time motherhood: Experiences from teens to forties.* New York: Springer.
	Negotiating partnerships	Powell-Cope, G. M. (1994). Family caregivers of people with AIDS: Negotiating partnerships with professional health care providers. *Nursing Research, 43,* 324–330.
	Quality of family caregiving	Phillips, L. R., & Rempusheski, V. F. (1986). Caring for the frail elderly at home: Toward a theoretical explanation of the dynamics of poor quality family caregiving. *Advances in Nursing Science, 8*(4), 62–84.
	Self-transcendence	Reed, P. (1991). Toward a nursing theory of self-transcendence: Deductive reformulation using developmental theories. *Advances in Nursing Science, 12,* 64–74.
Integrative	Experiencing transitions	Meleis, A. I., Sawyer, L. M., Im, E., Messias, D. K., & Schumacher, K. (2000). Experiencing transitions: An emerging middle range theory. *Advances in Nursing Science, 23*(1), 12–28.
	Health promotion	Pender, N. J. (1987). *Health promotion in nursing practice.* Norwalk, CT: Saunders.
	Illness constellation	Morse, J. M., & Johnson, H. K. (1991). In *The Illness Experience: Dimensions of Suffering.* Newbury Park, CA: Sage.
	Interaction model of client behavior	Cox, C. L. (1982). An interaction model of client behavior: A theoretical prescription for nursing. *Advances in Nursing Science, 5*(1), 41–56.

* Theories used in nursing research that are not nursing developed theories.

table are the middle range theories derived directly and specifically from nursing's major conceptual models and grand theories. Middle range theories have been developed from Johnson's Behavioral System Model, Levine's Conservation Principles, Roger's Science of Unitary Beings, and Roy's Adaptation Model (Alligood & Tomey, 2002). Table 1-7 provides examples of these middle range theories.

Table 1-7. Middle Range Theories Derived from Conceptual Models

CONCEPTUAL MODEL	MIDDLE RANGE THEORY
Johnson's Behavioral System Model	Theory of a Restorative Subsystem Theory of Sustenal Imperatives
Levine's Conservation Principles	Theory of Redundancy Theory of Therapeutic Intention
Rogers' Science of Unitary Human Beings	Theory of Perception of Dissonant Pattern
Roy's Adaptation Model	Theory of the Physiologic Mode Theory of the Self-concept Mode Theory of the Interdependence Mode Theory of the Role Function Mode

Source: Alligood, M. R., & Tomey, A. M. (2002). *Nursing theory: Utilization & application.* (pp. 46–54). St. Louis: Mosby. With permission from Elsevier Science.

Development of Middle Range Theory

Liehr and Smith (1999) outlined the relationships between the intellectual processes and the sources of content related to the development of middle range theories, which included:

- Inductive theory, building theory through research
- Deductive theory, building from grand nursing theories
- Combining existing nursing and non-nursing theories
- Synthesizing theories from published research findings
- Developing theories from clinical practice guidelines (Approaches for Generating Middle Range Theory, para. 1).

Qualitative research, particularly phenomenological and grounded theory studies, has served as a source of middle range theory development. Ten qualitative studies conducted through the Nursing Consortium for Research on Chronic Sorrow provided a foundation for the development of the middle range theory of chronic sorrow (Eakes, Burke, & Hainsworth, 1998). The research findings of these and of other studies underwent concept analysis as part of the process of developing this theory.

Several conceptual models and grand theories have served as the foundation for the development of middle range theories. For instance, the middle range theory of homecare effectiveness was based on Roy's Adaptation Model (Smith et al., 2002). The work of the theorists resulted in increased specificity of the conceptualization of Roy's interdependence mode.

Theories from nursing have been combined with those from other disciplines to create middle range theories. Mercer used Rubin's work on maternal role attainment (i.e., attachment and role identity during pregnancy and early infancy) and integrated role and developmental theories from the field of psychology to arrive at her Theory of Maternal Role Attainment (Meighan, 2002). She also conducted a number of research studies on the subject, the findings of which were reflected in the theory.

Published research findings have been cited as the most common source for constructing middle range theories of nursing (Lenz, 1998). The development of Online Social Support Theory is an example of this approach (LaCoursiere, 2001). Synthesized research findings from various patient populations (e.g., patients diagnosed with cancer or cardiovascular illness) that reflected the perspectives of those involved with the use of online social support (i.e., patient, caregiver, and nurse) served as a foundation for LaCoursiere's theory.

Clinical practice and clinical practice guidelines are sources of middle range theory development. Peplau is credited with introducing the use of clinical data in the development of her theory, the Theory of Interpersonal Relations. She based her understanding of the stages of the nurse–patient relationship on the observations of interactions between student nurses and psychiatric patients. The guidelines established by the Agency for Health Care Policy and Research for the management of acute pain were used by Good and Moore in the development of the theory of a balance between analgesia and side effects in the management of pain.

It is important to note that most of the nurses involved in the development of middle range theories used more than one approach. As part of arriving at the creation of the middle range theory, often findings from previous research studies were reviewed and analyzed, conceptual models and theories were considered, and additional research was conducted that targeted the phenomenon of most interest.

Uses of Middle Range Theory

Middle range theory has been found to be useful in both research and practice. "Theory can serve a heuristic function to stimulate and provide the rationale for studies, as well as help guide the selection of research questions and variables" (Lenz, 1998, p. 26). Middle range theories also can assist practice by facilitating understanding of client's behavior, suggesting interventions, and providing possible explanations for the degree of effectiveness of the interventions.

Reviews of published studies reveal a fairly extensive use of middle range theory in nursing research, most often middle range theories from other disciplines (Lenz, 1998). This is particularly evident when comparing how frequently middle range theories and grand theories of nursing are cited in the nursing research literature. Of 173 studies included in *Nursing Research* from January 1994 through June 1997, only 79 (45.7 %) identified any theory. Of the 79 studies that identified a theory, 25 were nursing theories and 54 were middle range theories borrowed from other disciplines, most frequently from psychology. Nursing's middle range theories accounted for most of the nursing theories used in the studies, 22 of the 25 (Lenz, 1998, p. 27).

Though middle range theory has great potential for guiding nursing practice, the nursing literature suggests that the potential has not been fully realized. Many authors note a gap between theory and practice. And when applications of theory to practice are included in the literature, it is more likely to be a grand rather than a middle range theory (Lenz, 1998). An informal survey of ten clinical nurse specialists and five staff nurses, conducted by Lenz, revealed few who were able to identify theories they were using in their practice. She attributes this to several factors: (a) the busyness of practicing nurses that does not allow time for consideration of the theoretical bases for their actions; (b) educational programs that do not help students learn the connections between theory and practice; (c) clinical environments that do not value theory-based practice; and (d) the lack of availability and usability of information on middle range theories. Nurse theorists need to address the last factor by producing literature describing their theories in understandable terms, identifying the theories' implications for practice, and placing that information in practice-oriented journals.

Controversy Surrounding Middle Range Theory

The identification of middle range theories is not unambiguous. For instance, Chenitz, primary author of Entry into a Nursing Home as Status Passage, labeled it practice theory, whereas others considered it middle range theory (Liehr & Smith, 1999, Analysis of the Middle Range Theory Foundation, para.2). "The question about what constitutes theory at the middle range is not a black and white issue for which a precise and clear definition can be offered. Middle range theory holds to a given level of abstraction. It is not too broad nor too narrow, but somewhere in the middle" (Leihr & Smith, 1999, Analysis of the Middle Range Theory Foundation, para. 3). To reduce confusion, nurse theorists are encouraged to clearly identify their work as middle range and provide a name that represents its conceptual components (Liehr & Smith, 1999; Sanford, 2000).

The imprecision of what constitutes a middle range theory is only one of several criticisms of middle range theory. In addition to lack of definitional clarity, middle range theory has been criticized for distinguishing itself from grand theories by its ability to be tested, using a logical positivistic idea of testability. Suppe (1996b) suggests an alternative approach to considering the testability of middle range theory. He rejects the widely accepted notion of theories as a set of propositions and proposes the idea that theories are "*state-transitions systems* modeling the behaviors of real world systems within the theory's *scope*" (Suppe, 1996b, p. 10). By this conceptualization of theories, operational concepts become descriptors; the values of these concepts become state specifications; and the propositions become specifications of state-transition relations (Suppe, 1996b, p. 11). The purpose of testing using this understanding of the nature of theories is delineating the scope of the middle range theory rather than subjecting a hypothesis to statistical analysis or qualitative data to coding. The basic research question is for what systems does the theory work and for what systems does it not, a question of scope. This type of research question is well suited to the testing of middle range theories.

Since Merton (1968) first promoted the notion of middle range theories, they have been criticized as being intellectually unambitious. Critics argue that their scope and suggested methods of inquiry are too limited. Merton countered that middle range theory was addressing just the questions that the discipline of sociology was asking, and that middle range theories can undergo the same systematic empirical testing that both more and less abstract theories can (pp. 63–64).

Another criticism of middle range theories is that their increasing numbers can lead to fragmentation of nursing's knowledge base into unrelated and distinct theories. This claim could be as legitimately made about either grand or micro theories. Merton acknowledged that risk and proposed consolidating theories to create groups of like theories at the middle range (Whall, 1996). Nurse scientists have addressed this issue. The identification of a metaparadigm is an attempt to create some conceptual cohesion for nursing's knowledge base. In addition, there has been an intentional effort to relate middle range theories to nursing's conceptual models, grand theories, and taxonomies. For instance, the middle range theory of Therapeutic Intention is clearly linked to Levine's Conservation Principles. Nurse scientists have proposed anchoring middle range theories to nursing's taxonomies of: (a) *diagnoses*, North American Nursing Diagnosis Association (NANDA); (b) *interventions*, Nursing Interventions Classification (NIC); and (c) *outcomes*, Nursing Outcomes Classification (NOC) (Blegan & Tripp-Reimer, 1997) and have identified a structure to accomplish that linkage (Tripp-Reimer, Woodworth, McCloskey, & Bulechek, 1996). Others consider these taxonomies as types of middle range theories rather than frameworks for categorizing the theories because they consist of concepts, definitions of concepts, propositional statements, and assumptions (Whall, 1996). As taxonomies, these middle range theories could not be considered unrelated and fragmented aspects of nursing's knowledge base. Nurse scientists continue to recommend persistence in efforts to "create an association between the proposed theory and a disciplinary perspective in nursing" (Liehr & Smith, 1999).

Nurse researchers have been denounced for making use of middle range theories from disciplines other than nursing. This was certainly true of nursing research published from the mid 1970s to the mid 1980s. During this period, more than half of the studies made use of theories or models from disciplines other than nursing (Moody et al., 1988). The increasing number of nursing middle range theories is reversing that trend. Liehr and Smith (1999) found 22 middle range nursing theories published in the decade from 1988 to 1999 through a CINAHL search. These theories met a number of criteria, including identification by the author that the theory was of the middle range. The criticism that nurse researchers use middle range theories from disciplines other than nursing is also being addressed by a call to continue to develop theories in the midlevel of scope and abstractness. "Situating middle range theory at the forefront for practice and research is critical to epistemologic and ontologic growth in nursing" (Sanford, 2000, Recommendation 5, para. 1).

PRACTICE THEORY/MICRO THEORY/SITUATION-SPECIFIC THEORY

The literature includes a confusing variety of terms to refer to the level of theory that is considered less abstract, more specific, and narrower in scope than middle range theory. *Practice theory* seems to be the most commonly used term (Jones, 2001; McKenna, 1997; Walker & Avant, 1995). Suppe (1996b), Kramer (1997), and Parker (2001) referred to both practice and micro theory, and Suppe discussed some of the distinctions between the two terms. The term *micro theory* was also used by Kim (1983), Duldt and Giffin (1985), Chinn and Kramer (1999), and by George (1995) and Young, Taylor, and Renpenning (2001), who both cited Chinn and Kramer. The most recently introduced term is *situation-specific theory* (Im & Meleis, 1999; Meleis & Im, 2001).

Practice theory can trace its origins to the work of metatheorists Dickhoff and James (1968). Their position is that because nursing is a profession, its theory must have an action orientation that can shape reality to create a desired goal. "The major contention here is that theory exists finally for the sake of practice" (p. 199).

Several authors have provided a list of the components of a practice theory. As stated earlier, Dickhoff and James referred to this goal-oriented theory as "situation-producing" and identified its essential elements as: "1) goal-content specified as aim for activity; 2) prescriptions for activity to realize the goal-content; and 3) a survey list to serve as a supplement to present prescription and preparation for future prescription for activity toward the goal-content" (p. 201). Jones (2001, p. 376) interprets these elements to include the use of nursing diagnosis and outcomes classification systems as components of practice theory. Walker and Avant (1995) and Kramer (1997) referred to these three components in their definitions of practice theory and both suggested additional considerations. Walker and Avant claim that without a basis in situation-relating (predictive) theories, it would require a liberal definition of theory to identify practice or situation-producing theory as theory. They suggest that it would be more legitimate to refer to practice theory as nursing practices (pp. 12–13). Kramer identifies a similar issue, the importance of connecting practice theory to the more encompassing knowledge structures of nursing as identified by metatheory. To the traditional understanding of practice theory she adds theory about nursing practice (e.g., administrative and educational theories). This is not a commonly occurring use.

Like other levels of theory, practice theories as situation producing are derived from middle range theories, practice experiences, and empirical testing. Middle range theories are the source of the prescriptions that are directed at the specified goal (McKenna, 1997; Parker, 2001; Walker & Avant, 1995) and if not specifically derived from these middle range theories, at the very least, practice theories should identify how the concepts from both levels of theory are interrelated. Practice theory also develops from the clinical experiences of nurses that have been subjected to the process of reflection. Reflection on practice leads to insights that can serve as a foundation for developing theory. It provides a real world basis for the creation of practice theory. Research is also an important source of practice theories. Walker and Avant (1995) note the contributions of the Conduct and Utilization of Research in Nursing project in the formulation of practice theories. This project, initiated in 1975, identified a need for change in practice and summarized the relevant research to arrive at research-based principles for nursing interventions. There were ten practice theories or protocols that were considered during the project. Examples of the protocols that were developed include (a) lactose-free diet, (b) sensation information: distress, (c) intravenous cannula-change regiment, and (d) prevention of decubiti by means of small shifts of body weight (Haller, Reynolds, & Horsley, 1979, p. 47).

Micro theory, a term identified as interchangeable with practice theory (Parker, 2001), is included in the writings of Kim (1983), Suppe (1996b), and Chinn and Kramer (1995). Kim's definition of micro theory as a set of "theoretical statements, usually hypotheses, that deal with narrowly defined phenomena" (p. 13) suggests a research-based theory. Suppe (1996b) also identifies hypothesis testing as a primary feature of micro theories and claims that this fact provides the primary distinction between micro theory and middle range theory, both of which could be considered practice theories (pp. 12–13). According to Suppe, the term micro theory is found with increasing frequency in the literature to refer to theories that are too limited in scope to be considered middle range. He provided a hypothetical example of a micro theory of pain management for a hospitalized patient with acute postamputation pain, who was treated with PCA morphine, with possible Valium potentiation, focusing on pain intensity and addiction outcomes (Suppe, 1996b, p. 12). Kim (1983) provided examples of what she labeled as micro theories, i.e., maternal attachment, pressure sores, wound healing, and positioning. Other examples of this level of theory development found in the literature include alcoholism recovery in lesbian women (Hall, 1990), quality of care (Nielson, 1992), milieu therapy for short-stay units (LeCuyer, 1992), caring for patients with chronic skin disease (Kirkevold, 1993), therapeutic touch (Green, 1998), exercise as self-care (Ulbrich, 1999), and ecological view of protection (Shearer, 2002).

Im and Meleis (1999) use the term situation-specific to refer to that level of nursing theory that focuses on specific nursing phenomena with direct application to nursing practice. There are a number of features that distinguish situation-specific theories from either grand or middle range theories. They exhibit "(1) a lower level of abstraction, (2) reflection of specific nursing phenomenon, (3) context, (4) readily accessible connection to nursing research and practice, (5) reflection of diversities in nursing phenomena, and (6) limitation of generalization" (Properties of situation-specific theories, para. 1). A somewhat unique quality of situation-specific theories is their emphasis on sociopolitical, cultural, and historical contexts, demonstrated by the theory of menopausal transition of Korean immigrant women described by Im and Meleis.

In addition to the debate on the term to use in referring to this level of theory, the controversies about practice theory center on whether it is a theory, and if so, whether it is needed. Walker (1986) suggests that, based on a definition of practice theory as sets of principles or directives, the terms policy, procedure, or principles of practice might be more appropriate. Her conclusion is based on an understanding of theory as a "systematic description and explanation" (p. 28). Walker's position seems consistent with the increasingly popular phenomena of research utilization and evidence-based practice. Berkstrand's (1986) contention is that practice theory is unnecessary. She claims that "all the theoretical knowledge relevant to practice can be discovered within existing systems of knowledge such as metatheory, philosophy, science, and ethics." Collins and Fielder (1986) respond to Beckstrand's conclusion by emphasizing the unique issues that nursing theories must address. They assert that Beckstrand's position does not consider the nurse's responsibility for caring for the client as a "particular" individual. Nursing still has a need for "a nursing theory that will set out the kinds of nursing practice and the particular set of moral ideals that nursing practice seeks to bring about" (Collins & Fielder, 1986, p. 510). The increasing number of practice theories or their semantic equivalent identified in the literature in the 1990s seems to be supporting, if not a need, at least an interest in this level of theory development.

SUMMARY

The development of nursing knowledge is an ongoing process, though debates continue on the direction that this development should take. For instance, there are differences of opinion on whether diversity or unity of paradigms and philosophies is preferred. The language of nursing science is not firmly established or used consistently; there still is not consensus on the use of some of the terms that refer to the components of the structural hierarchy of nursing knowledge. One term used fairly consistently in the literature is middle range theory, and it is the development of this level of theory verified by research and useful for practice that is the focus of the efforts of many nurse scientists.

WEB RESOURCES

Philosophy
1. *http://www-ksl.stanford.edu/kst/what-is-an-ontology.html* provides expanded definition of ontology and links to several on-line articles.
2. The site *http://www.formalontology.it/index.htm* traces historical development and lists relevant readings.

Theory
There are several Internet sites that provide links to the home pages of individual nursing theorists. These home pages often include biographical information and bibliographies of the theorists' publications, and sometime provide descriptions of the theories, reviews of their published work, and the E-mail addresses of the theorists.

The links to theorists include but are not limited to:

Faye Abdellah
Anne Boykin and
    Savina Schoenhofer
Helen Erickson,
    Evelyn Tomlin, and
    Mary Ann Swain
Joyce Fitzpatrick
Lydia Hall
Virginia Henderson
Dorothy Johnson
Ionnis Kalofissudi
Imogene King
Kathy Kolcaba
Madeleine Leininger
Myra Levine
Alaf Meleis
Ramona Mercer

Betty Neuman
Margaret Newman
Florence Nightingale
Ida Jean Orlando
Josephine Paterson and
    Loretta Zderad
Nola Pender
Hildegard Peplau
Joan Riehl-Sisca
Martha Rogers
Sister Callista Roy
Nancy Roper, Winifred
    Logan, and Alison
    Tierney
Cornelia Ruland
Jean Watson
Ernestine Wiedenbach

WEB RESOURCES

Theory

The following Internet sites provide links to the theorists and to other nursing theory pages:

1. *http://www.sandiego.edu/nursing/theory* organizes its links to the web pages of the nurse scientists by categorizing them as general theories, middle range theories, and models. In addition to links to middle range theories, the site provides a description of this level of theory development. Other features included are discussion forums and lists of resources (books and videos).

2. *http://www.healthsci.clayton.edu/eichelberger/nursing.htm* includes a list of theory books, links to electronic resources and advice for searching on-line for information on nursing theories, in addition to the links to specific theorists.

3. *http://www.enursescribe.com/nurse_theorists.htm* classifies the nurse theorists as models: adaptation, anthropological, energy fields, humanist, self-care and systems. There are also sections devoted to the early nurse theorists, middle range theories, and book reviews.

4. *http://www.valdosta.edu/nursing/history_theory/theory.html* focuses on links to nursing theorists and other nursing theory pages.

These sites can also be located through a web search on "nursing theory."

Another source of information on nursing theorists, though not an Internet site, is the video series, *The Nurse Theorists: Portraits in Excellence.* The individual videos provide biographical information and description of the theory, with an interview of the theorists conducted by Jacqueline Fawcett. The following theorists are included in this series: Johnson, King, Levine, Neuman, Orem, Rogers, Roy, Leininger, Newman, Orlando, Parse, Peplau, Watson, Rubin, Henderson, and Nightingale. This resource is available from Fuld Institute for Technology in Nursing Education (FITNE) at their address, 5 Depot Street, Athens, OH 455701, their telephone numbers, 1-800-691-8480 or 740-592-2511, or on-line at *http://fitne.net.*

REFERENCES

Adam, E. (1992). Contemporary conceptualization of nursing: Philosophy or science? In J. F. Kikuchi & H. Simmons (Eds.), *Philosophic inquiry in nursing* (pp. 55–63). London: Sage.

Alligood, M. R., & Tomey, A. M. (2002). *Nursing theory: Utilization & application* (2nd ed.). St. Louis: Mosby.

Archibald, G. (2000). A postmodern nursing model. *Nursing Standard 14* (34), 40–42.

Babbie, E. (1995). *The practice of social research* (7th ed.). Belmont, CA: Wadsworth.

Barrett, E. (1986). Investigation of the principle of helicy: The relationship of human filed motion and power, In V. Mailinski (Ed.), *Explorations on Martha Rogers' Science of Unitary Human Beings* (pp. 173–184). Norwalk, CT: Appleton-Century-Crofts.

Barrett, E. A. M. (1992). Diversity reigns. *Nursing Science Quarterly, 5*(4), 155–157.

Berkstrand, J. (1986). A critique of several conceptions of practice theory in nursing. In L. H. Nicholl (Ed.), *Perspectives on nursing theory* (pp. 494–504). Boston: Little, Brown and Company.

Blegan, M. A., & Tripp-Reimer, T. (1997). Implications of nursing taxonomies for middle-range theory development. *Advances in Nursing Science, 19*(3), 37(13). Retrieved December 14, 1999 from Health Reference Center–Academic database.

Brower, H. T. F., & Baker, B. J. (1976). Using the adaptation model in a practitioner curriculum. *Nursing Outlook, 24,* 686–689.

Brown, S. T., & Lee, B. T. (1980). Imogene King's conceptual framework: A proposed model for continuing nursing education. *Journal of Advanced Nursing, 5,* 467–473.

Burbules, N. C. (n.d). Postmodern doubt and philosophy of education. Retrieved June 6, 2002, from University of Illinois at Urbana-Champaign Web site: *http://www.ed.uiuc.edu/EPS/PES-Yearbook/95_docs/burbules.html.*

Caper, C. F. (1986). Some basic facts about models, nursing conceptualizations, and nursing theories. *The Journal of Continuing Education in Nursing, 16* (5), 149–154.

Chinn, P. & Kramer, M. (1995). *Theory and nursing: A systematic approach* (4th ed.). St Louis: Mosby Year-Book.

Chinn, P. L. & Kramer, M. K. (1999). *Theory and nursing: Integrated nursing knowledge* (5th ed.). St. Louis: Mosby.

Collins, R. C., & Fielder, J. H. (1986). Beckstrand's concept of practice theory: A critique. In L. H. Nicholl (Ed.), *Perspectives on nursing theory* (pp. 505–511). Boston: Little, Brown and Company.

Derdiarian, A. K. (1988). Sensitivity of the Derdiarian behavioral system model instrument to age, sit, and stage of cancer: A preliminary validation study. *Scholarly Inquiry for Nursing Practice, 2,* 103–121.

Dickhoff, J., & James, P. (1968). A theory of theories: A position paper. *Nursing Research, 17*(3), 197–203.

Donnelly, E. (2001). An assessment of nursing theories as guides to scientific inquiry. In N. L. Chaska (Ed.), *The nursing profession: Tomorrow and beyond.* (pp.331–344). Thousand Oaks, CA: Sage.

Downs, F. S. (1982). A theoretical question. *Nursing Research, 3*, 259.

Duldt, B. W., & Giffin, K. (1985). *Theoretical perspectives for nursing.* Boston: Little, Brown and Company.

Dunphy, L. H. (2001). Florence Nightingale care actualized: A legacy for nursing. In M. E Parker, *Nursing theories and nursing practice* (pp. 31–53). Philadelphia: F. A. Davis.

Eakes, G. G., Burke, M. L., & Hainsworth, M. A. (1998). Middle-range theory of chronic sorrow. *Image, 30* (2), 179–184.

Engebretson, J. (1997). A multiparadigm approach to nursing. *Advances in Nursing Science, 20*(1), 21–33. Retrieved June 3, 2002 from CINAHL/OVID database.

Fagerhaugh, S. Y. (1974). Pain expression and control on a burn care unit. *Nursing Outlook, 22*, 645–650.

Fawcett, J. (1995). *Analysis and evaluation of contemporary nursing knowledge: Nursing models and theories* (3rd ed.). Philadelphia: F. A. Davis.

Fawcett, J. (1997). The structural hierarchy of nursing knowledge: Components and their definitions. In I.M. King & J. Fawcett. (Eds.), *The language of nursing theory and metatheory* (pp.11–17). Indianapolis, IN: Sigma Theta Tau.

Fawcett, J. (2000). *Analysis and evaluation of contemporary nursing knowledge: Nursing models and theories* (4th ed.). Philadelphia: F. A. Davis.

Fawcett, J., & Bourbonniere, M. G. (2001). Utilization of nursing knowledge and the future of the discipline. In N. L. Chaska (Ed.), *The nursing profession: Tomorrow and beyond.* (pp.311–320). Thousand Oaks, CA: Sage.

Fitzpatrick, J., & Whall, A. (1983). *Conceptual models of nursing.* Bowie, MD: Robert J. Brady.

George, J. B. (1995). *Nursing theories: The base for professional nursing practice* (4th ed.). Norwalk, CT: Appleton & Lange.

Green, C. A. (1998). Critically exploring the use of Rogers' nursing theory of unitary beings as a framework to underpin therapeutic touch practice. *European Nurse, 3*(3), 158–169.

Grubbs, J. (1974). An interpretation of the Johnson behavioral system model for nursing practice. In J. P. Riehl & C. Roy, *Conceptual models for nursing practice* (pp. 160–206). New York: Appleton-Century-Crofts.

Hall, B. A. (1981). The change paradigm in nursing: Growth versus persistence. *Advances in Nursing Science, 3*(4), 1–6.

Hall, J. M. (1990). Alcoholism recovery of lesbian women: A theory in development. *Scholarly Inquiry for Nursing Practice, 4*(2), 109–122.

Haller, K. B., Reynolds, M. A., & Horsley, J. A. (1979). Developing research-based innovation protocols: Process, criteria, and issues. *Research in Nursing and Health, 2,* 45–51.

Hardy, L. K. (1986). Janforum: Identifying the place of theoretical frameworks in an evolving discipline. *Journal of Advanced Nursing 11*, 103–107.

Harris, R. B. (1986). Introduction of a conceptual model into a fundamental baccalaureate course. *Journal of Nursing Education, 25*, 66–69.

Im, E. O., & Meleis, A. (1999). Situation-specific theories: Philosophical roots, properties, and approach. *Advances in Nursing Science, 22*(2), 11–24. Retrieved June 3, 2002 from CINAHL/OVID database.

Jacobson, S. F. (1987). Studying and using conceptual models of nursing. *Image: Journal of Nursing Scholarship, 19*(2), 78–82.

Jacox, A. (1974). Theory construction in nursing: An overview. *Nursing Research, 23*(1), 4–13.

Johnson, D. E. (1974). Development of theory: A requisite for nursing as a primary health profession. *Nursing Research 23*, (5), 372–377.

Johnson, D. E. (1986). Theory in nursing: Borrowed and unique. In L. H. Nicholl (Ed.), *Perspectives on nursing theory* (pp. 117–121). Boston: Little, Brown and Company.

Johnson, D. E. (1990). The behavioral system model for nursing. In M. E. Parker (Ed.), *Nursing theories in practice* (pp. 23–32). New York: National League for Nursing.

Johnson, J. E., & Rice, V. H. (1986). Sensory and distress components of pain. *Nursing Research, 23*, 203–209.

Jones, D. A. (2001). Linking nursing language and knowledge development. In N. L. Chaska (Ed.), *The nursing profession: Tomorrow and beyond.* (pp.373–386). Thousand Oaks, CA: Sage.

Kameoda, T., & Sugimori, M. (1993, June). Application of King's goal attainment theory in Japanese clinical setting. Paper presented at the meeting of Sigma Theta Tau International's Sixth International Nursing Research Congress, Madrid, Spain.

Kikuchi, J. F. (1992). Nursing questions that science cannot answer. In J. F. Kikuchi & H. Simmons (Eds.), *Philosophic inquiry in nursing* (pp. 26–37). Newbury Park, CA: Sage.

Kilchenstein, L., & Yakulis, I. (1984). The birth of a curriculum: Utilization of the Neuman health care system model in an integrated baccalaureate program. *Journal of Nursing Education, 23*, 126–127.

Kim, H. S. (1983). *The nature of theoretical thinking in nursing.* Norwalk, CT: Appleton-Century-Crofts.

Kim, H. S. (1989). Theoretical thinking in nursing: Problems and Perspectives. *Recent Advances in Nursing, 24,* 106–122.

Kim, H. S. (1997). Terminology in structuring and developing nursing knowledge. In I. M. King & J. Fawcett (Eds.), *The Language of nursing theory and metatheory* (pp.27–35). Indianapolis, IN: Sigma Theta Tau.

King, I. M. (1978). The "why" of theory development. In National League for Nursing, *Theory development: What, why, how?* (pp. 11–16). New York: National League for Nursing.

King, I. M. (1984). Philosophy of nursing education: A national survey. *Western Journal of Nursing Research, 6,* 387–406.

King, I. M. (1997). Knowledge development for nursing: A process. In I. M. King & J. Fawcett (Eds.). *The language of nursing theory and metatheory* (pp. 19–25). Indianapolis, IN: Sigma Theta Tau.

King, I. M., & Fawcett, J. (Eds.). (1997). *The language of nursing theory and metatheory.* Indianapolis, IN: Sigma Theta Tau.

Kirkevold, M. (1993). Toward a practice theory of caring for patients with chronic skin disease. *Scholarly Inquiry for Nursing Practice, 7*(1), 37–57.

Kramer, M. K. (1997). Terminology in theory: Definitions and comments. In I. M. King & J. Fawcett (Eds.), *The language of nursing theory and metatheory* (pp.61–71). Indianapolis, IN: Sigma Theta Tau.

Kuhn, T. S. (1977). *The essential tension.* Chicago: Chicago University Press.

Kuhn, T. S. (1996). *The structure of scientific revolutions* (3rd ed.). Chicago: Chicago University Press.

LaCoursiere, S. P. (2001). A theory of online social support. *Advances in Nursing Science, 24*(1), 60–77.

Landreneau, K. J. (2002). Response to: 'The nature of philosophy of science, theory and knowledge relating to nursing and professionalism." *Journal of Advanced Nursing, 38* (3). 283–285. Retrieved November 6, 2002 from CINAHL/OVID database.

LeCuyer, E. A. (1992). Milieu therapy for short stay units: A transformed practice theory. *Archives of Psychiatric Nursing, 6*(2), 108–116.

Lenz, E. R. (1996). Role of middle range theory for research and practice. Paper presented at the Proceedings of the Sixth Rosemary Ellis Scholars' Retreat, Frances Payne Bolton School of Nursing, Case Western Reserve University, Cleveland, OH.

Lenz, E. R. (1998). Role of middle range theory for nursing research and practice. Part 1. Nursing research. *Nursing Leadership Forum, 3*(1), 24–33.

Lenz, E. R., Suppe, F., Gift, A. G., Pugh, L. C., & Milligan, R. A. (1995). Collaborative development of middle-range theories: Toward a theory of unpleasant symptoms. *Advances in Nursing Science, 17*(3), 1–13.

Lerner, R. M. (1986). *Concepts and theories of human development* (2nd ed.). New York: Random House.

Liehr, P., & Smith, M. J. (1999). Middle range theory: Spinning research and practice to create knowledge for the new millennium. *Advances in Nursing Science, 21*(4), 81–91. Retrieved June 11, 2002 from CINAHL/OVID database.

Littlejohn, C. (2002). Are nursing models to blame for low morale? *Nursing Standard, 16*(17), 39–41.

Mackenzie, S., & Spence Laschinger, H. (1995). Correlates of nursing diagnoses in public health nursing. *Journal of Advanced Nursing, 21*(4), 772–777.

McKenna, H. (1997). *Nursing theories and models.* London: Routledge.

Meighan, M. (2002). Mercer's maternal role attainment theory in nursing practice. In M. R. Alligood & A. M. Tomey (Eds.), *Nursing theory: Utilization & application.* (2nd ed.). (pp.367–383). St. Louis: Mosby.

Meleis, A. I. (1997). *Theoretical nursing: Development and progress* (3rd ed.). Philadelphia: Lippincott-Raven.

Meleis, A. I., & Im, E. (2001). From fragmentation to integration in the discipline of nursing: Situation-specific theories. In N. L. Chaska (Ed.), *The nursing profession: Tomorrow and beyond* (pp.881–891). Thousand Oaks, CA: Sage.

Merton, R. K. (1968). *On social theory and social structure.* New York: Free Press.

Moody, L. E. (1990). *Advancing nursing science through research* (Vol. 1). Newbury Park, CA: Sage.

Moody, L. E., Wilson, N. E., Smyth, K., Schwartz, R., Tittle, M., & Van Cott, M. L. (1988). Analysis of a decade of nursing practice research: 1977–1986. *Nursing Research, 37*(6), 374–379.

Newman, M. (1996). Prevailing paradigms in nursing. In J. W. Kenney (Ed.), *Philosophical and theoretical perspectives for advanced nursing practice* (pp.302–307). Boston: Jones and Bartlett.

Newman, M. (2002). The pattern that connects. *Advances in Nursing Science, 24*(3), 1–7.

Newman, M. A., Sime, A. M. & Corcoran-Perry, S. A. (1996). The focus of the discipline of nursing. In J. W. Kenney (Ed.), *Philosophical and theoretical perspectives for advanced nursing practice.* (pp.297–301). Boston: Jones and Bartlett.

Nielson, P. A. (1992). Quality of care: Discovering a modified practice theory. *Journal of Nursing Care Quality, 6*(2), 63–76.

Northrup, D. T. (1992). A unified perspective within nursing. *Nursing Science Quarterly, 5*(4). 154–155.

Orem, D. E. (2001). *Nursing: Concepts of practice* (6th ed.). St. Louis: Mosby.

Parker, K. P. (1989). The theory of sentience evolution: A practice-level theory of sleeping, waking, and beyond waking patterns based on the science of unitary human beings. *Rogerian Nursing Science News, 2*(1), 4–6.

Parker, M. E. (2001). *Nursing theories and nursing practice.* Philadelphia: F. A. Davis.

Parse, R. R. (1987). *Nursing science: Major paradigms, theories, and critiques.* Philadelphia: W. B. Saunders.

Parse, R. R. (1997). The language of nursing knowledge: Saying what we mean. In King, I. M. & Fawcett, J. (Eds.) *The language of nursing theory and metatheory* (pp.73–77). Indianapolis, IN: Sigma Theta Tau.

Parse, R. R. (1999). Nursing science: the transformation of practice. *Journal of Advanced Nursing, 30*(6), 1383–1387. Retrieved November 6, 2002, from OVID/CINAHL database.

Phillips, J. R. (1992). The aim of philosophical inquiry in nursing: Unity or diversity of thought. In J. F. Kikuchi & H. Simmons (Eds.), *Philosophic inquiry in nursing* (pp. 45–50). Newbury Park, CA: Sage.

Reed, P. G. (1995). A treatise on nursing knowledge development for the 21st century: Beyond postmodernism. *Advances in Nursing Science 17* (3), 70–84. Retrieved June 3, 2002, from CINAHL/OVID database.

Reynolds, P. D. (1971). *A primer for theory construction.* Indianapolis, IN: Bobbs-Merrill.

Rinehart, J. M. (1978). The "how" of theory development in nursing. In National League for Nursing, *Theory development: What, why, how?* (pp. 67–74). New York: National League for Nursing.

Roach, M. S. (1992). The aim of philosophical inquiry in nursing: Unity or diversity of thought. In J. F. Kikuchi & H. Simmons (Eds.), *Philosophic inquiry in nursing* (pp. 38–44). Newbury Park, CA: Sage.

Rodman, H. (1980). Are conceptual frameworks necessary for theory building? The case of family sociology. *The Sociology Quarterly, 21*, 429–441.

Rutty, J. E. (1998). The nature of philosophy of science, theory and knowledge relating to nursing and professionalism. *Journal of Advanced Nursing, 28*(2), 243–250. Retrieved July 16, 2002, from OVID/CINAHL database.

Sanford, R. C. (2000). Caring through relation and dialogue: A nursing perspective for patient education. *Advances in Nursing Science, 22*(3), 1–15. Retrieved April 15, 2002, from CINAHL/OVID database.

Sarter, B. (1988). Philosophical sources of nursing theory. *Nursing Science Quarterly, 1*(2), 52–59.

Schlotfeldt, R. M. (1992). Answering nursing's philosophical questions: Whose responsibility is it? In J. F. Kikuchi and H. Simmons (Eds.), *Philosophic inquiry in nursing* (pp. 97–104). Newbury Park, CA: Sage.

Shapere, D. (1980). The structure of scientific revolutions. In G. Gutting (Ed.), *Paradigms & revolutions* (pp. 27–38). Notre Dame, IN: University of Notre Dame Press.

Shearer, J. E. (2002). The concept of protection: A dimen-sional analysis and critique of a theory of protection. *Advances in Nursing Science, 25*(1), 65–78.

Silva, M. C. (1997). Philosophy, science, theory, interrelationships and implications for nursing research. *Image: Journal of Nursing Scholarship, 29* (3), 210–213. Retrieved June 7, 2002, from CINAHL/OVID database.

Silva M. C., Sorrell, J. M., & Sorrell, C. D. (1995). From Carper's ways of knowing to ways of being: An ontological philosophical shift. *Advances in Nursing Science, 18* (1), 1–13.

Simmons, H. (1992). Philosophic and scientific inquiry: The interface. In J. F. Kikuchi & H. Simmons (Eds.), *Philosophic inquiry in nursing* (pp. 9–25). Newbury Park, CA: Sage.

Smart, J. J. C. (1968). *Between science and philosophy.* New York: Random House.

Smith, C. E., Pace, K., Kochinda, C., Kleinbeck, S., Koehler, J., & Popkess-Vawter, S. (2002). Caregiver effectiveness model evolution to a midrange theory of home care: A process for critique and replication. *Advances in Nursing Science, 25*(1), 50–64.

Stevens-Barnum, B. J. (1998). *Nursing theory: Analysis, application, evaluation* (5th ed.). Philadelphia: Lippincott Williams & Wilkins.

Suppe, F. (1996a, May). Middle-range theory: Nursing theory and knowledge development. Paper presented at the Proceedings of the Sixth Rosemary Ellis Scholars' Retreat, Frances Payne Bolton School of Nursing, Case Western Reserve University, Cleveland, OH.

Suppe, F. (1996b, July). *Middle-range theories: Historical and contemporary perspectives.* (Available from Institute for Advanced Study, Indiana University, Poplars 335, Bloomington, IN 47405).

Thorne, S., Canam, C., Dahinten, S., Hall, W., Henderson, A., & Kirkham, S. R. (1998). Nursing's metaparadigm concepts: Disimpacting the debates. *Journal of Advanced Nursing, 27*(6), 1257–1268. Retrieved June 3, 2002, from OVID/CINAHL database.

Tierney, A. J. (1998). Nursing models: Extant or extinct? *Journal of Advanced Nursing, 28*(1), 77–85. Retrieved June 3, 2002, from CINAHL/OVID database.

Tripp-Reimer, T., Woodworth, G., McCloskey, J. C., & Bulechek (1996). The dimensional structure of nursing interventions. *Nursing Research, 45*(1), 10–17.

Ulbrich, S. L. (1999). Nursing practice theory of exercise as self-care. *Image, 31*(1), 65–70. Retrieved August 1, 2002, from CINAHL/OVID database.

Wald, F. S., & Leonard, R. C. (1964). Towards development of nursing practice theory. *Nursing Research, 13,* 309–313.

Walker, L. O. (1986). In L. H. Nicholl (Ed.). *Perspectives on nursing theory* (pp. 26–38). Boston: Little, Brown and Company.

Walker, L. O., & Avant, K. C. (1995). *Strategies for theory construction in nursing* (3rd ed.). Norwalk, CT: Appleton & Lange.

Whall, A. L. (1996, May). Overview of middle-range theory. Paper presented at the Proceedings of the Sixth Rosemary Ellis Scholars' Retreat, Frances Payne Bolton School of Nursing, Case Western Reserve University, Cleveland, OH.

Young, A., Taylor, S. G., & Renpenning, K. (2001). *Connec-*

tions: Nursing research, theory, and practice. St. Louis: Mosby.

Yura, H., & Torres, G. (1975). Today's conceptual frameworks within baccalaureate nursing programs. In National League for Nursing, *Faculty-curriculum development part III: Conceptual frameworks—its meaning and functioning* (pp. 17–30). New York: National League for Nursing.

Analysis, Evaluation, and Selection of a Middle Range Nursing Theory

TIMOTHY S. BREDOW

DEFINITION OF KEY TERMS

Adequacy Determines how completely the theory addresses the topics it claims to address. Establishes if there are holes or gaps that need to be filled in by other work or further refinement of the theory. Addresses if the theory accounts for the subject matter under consideration.

Clarity Addresses if the theory clearly states the main components to be considered. Determines if it is easily understood by the reader.

Complexity Reviews how many concepts are involved as key components in the theory. Decides how complicated is the description of the theory, and if it can it be understood without lengthy descriptions and explanations: considers the number of variables being addressed, exists on a continuum from parsimony–limited number of variables to complex–extensive number of variables.

Consistency Addresses whether the theory maintains the definitions of the key concepts throughout the explanation of the theory. Determines if it has congruent use of terms, interpretations, principles, and methods throughout.

Discrimination Addresses whether the hypothesis generated by the theory led to research results that could not be

DEFINITION OF KEY TERMS

	arrived at using some other nursing theory. Determines how unique the theory is to the area of nursing that it addresses. Decides if it has precise and clear boundaries, definitive parameters of the subject matter.
External criticism	Considers the fit between the theory and criteria external to the theory, such as the social environment and the prevailing views on the nursing metaparadigm. Criticism here is dependent on individual preference. It depends on reasonableness and perceptions of the evaluator.
Internal criticism	Deals with the criteria concerning the inner workings (internal dimensions) of the theory and how the theory's components fit with each other
Logical development	Resolves the questions: "Does the theory logically follow a line of thought of previous work that has been shown to be true or does it launch out into unproven territory with its assumptions and premises"? Do the conclusions proceed in a logical fashion? Are the arguments well supported?
Nursing metaparadigm	Global concepts that identify the phenomena of nursing, including person, environment, health, and nursing (Fawcett, 1995)
Pragmatic	Determines if the theory can be operationalized in real life settings
Reality convergence	Determines if the theory's underlying assumptions ring true. Decides if the theory's assumptions represent the real world, and if it represents the real world of nursing. Does the theory reflect the real world as understood by the reader?
Scope	Determines how broad or narrow is the range of phenomena that this theory covers. Does it stay in a narrow range of scope to keep it a middle range theory? (narrower implies more applicable to practice; wider implies more global and all encompassing)
Significance	Will the result of the research that is conducted because of the hypotheses generated by the theory have any impact on the way nurses carry out nursing

INTRODUCTION

Middle range nursing theories can help nurses and graduate nursing students alike meet and accomplish their goals of carrying out sound nursing research. When nursing theories are analyzed and evaluated in a thorough, systematic fashion, it is easier to determine which middle range nursing theory will provide the proper guidance and direction for the research under consideration. This chapter should help graduate student nurses and research nurses deal with the problem of how to analyze, evaluate, and choose a middle range nursing theory for their assignments, and apply it to their research interests.

Theory analysis is the systematic examination of what was personally written over time by the theory author(s) about the theory. When performing a middle range theory analysis, the component parts are identified and the relationship of these components to each other and to the whole theory are examined. This analysis can provide the nurse researcher a thorough understanding about the theory. Theory evaluation is the identification of the theory's same components and judging them against a set of predetermined criteria. The criteria used for judging theories are not standardized within the field of nursing, but, rather, have evolved over time, and are different depending on who is presenting the evaluation. Nonetheless, a thorough evaluation of a middle range theory will help the nurse researcher determine the robustness of the theory and the goodness of fit for application to a particular research project.

Over the years, nursing theorists have emerged with different theoretical positions and theories proposing how various nursing concepts and the nursing metaparadigm are uniquely linked. Most of these theorists have constructed theories of nursing that could be termed grand theories, while later theorists have constructed middle range nursing theories. There are now more than 50 different grand nursing theories for nursing researchers to choose from (McKenna, 1997) and several dozen middle range nursing theories.

HISTORICAL BACKGROUND

Historically, nursing theorists worked hard to explain the nature of nursing, carving out a differentiated scientific field to call their own. At the same time, nursing researchers wanted nursing theory to be constructed to aid the generation of testable research hypothesis and also have the ability to affect the practice of nursing. As nursing theory developed and progressed through different stages of maturity, so did the evaluation process of what constitutes sound nursing theory.

In the past, nurses had Nightingale's environmental model, the medical model, and borrowed theories to use as a basis for nursing research. Through the 1960s, 70s, and 80s, several different grand nursing theories and some middle range theories were developed for nurses to use as a basis for their research. In the 1990s and beyond, many more middle range theories have emerged, allowing nurses to move away from using Nightingale, the medical model, borrowed theories, and grand nursing theories. When compared to grand theories, middle range theories contain fewer concepts, with relationships that are adaptable and concrete enough to be tested. Middle range theories have a particular substantive focus and consider only a limited aspect of reality. For example, Orem's Self-care Deficit grand nursing theory would consider patients who are unable to carry out the activities of daily living and provide nursing care necessary to aid them back to a level of living where they were able to provide self care. The middle range theory of unpleasant symptoms would use this same situation and consider the actual unpleasant symptom that was causing the problem for the patient. It would address the patient's symptom as a consideration for a multidimensional approach to health care symptom management. Kolcaba states "that for these reasons middle range theories are particularly cogent as nursing science addresses the challenges of the 21st century" (2001, p. 86). The use of many different middle range nursing theories for research purposes became a relatively new and exciting possibility for nurses during the 1990s. Now, researchers are expanding the knowledge base of nursing by enhancement of nursing's frameworks and theories (Parse, 2001). Because of this evolutionary process of theory building, nurses need to understand the historical roots for the analysis and evaluation of grand and middle range nursing theory. Additionally, understanding the process of analysis and evaluation provides insight to the evaluator about the strengths and weaknesses of the individual theory itself, as well as its possible use and application to nursing research and practice.

Meleis (1997, p. 245) states that "nurses have always evaluated theories." She provides the reasons why evaluation of theory is an essential component of nursing research:

1. To decide which theory is more appropriate to use as a framework for research
2. To identify effective theories for guiding a research project
3. To compare and contrast different explanations of the same phenomenon
4. To identify epistemological approaches of a discipline through attention to the sociocultural context of the theorist and the theory
5. To assess the ontological beliefs and schools of thought in a discipline
6. To define research priorities (Meleis, 1997).

THEORY ANALYSIS

Theory Analysis by Early Authors

The analysis of nursing theory has evolved over time as nurses have proposed increasingly sophisticated methods for reviewing and analyzing nursing theory. Three "early approaches" to theory analysis by Duffy and Muhlenkamp, Hardy, and Chinn and Jacobs will be discussed followed by a discussion of "recent approaches" by Barnum, Meleis, and Fawcett.

In 1974, Duffy and Muhlenkamp wrote that nursing theory should be examined using four distinct questions. They suggested looking at the origin of the problem, the methods used in the pursuit of knowledge, the subject matter, and the kind of outcomes of testing generated by this theory.

These four questions when used alone to examine a nursing theory provided a fairly good evaluation of the theory; however, additional evaluation questions were proposed when the theory was used for research. Their additional questions for analyzing a nursing theory for nursing research included:

- Does it generate a testable hypothesis, and is it complete in terms of subject matter and perspective?
- Are the biases or values underlying the theory made explicit?
- Are the relationships among the propositions made explicit and is it parsimonious?

With all of these questions in hand, a nurse could do what was thought, at the time, to be a thorough and complete assessment of any particular nursing theory to be used for nursing research.

During the same period of time, Hardy (1974) developed another way to analyze nursing theories. Her analysis method contained some unique criteria when compared to Duffy and Muhlenkamp's and included more criteria related to the process and outcome of theory evaluation. Her evaluation criteria identified the need for the theory to have adequacy, meaning, logic, and pragmatism. She wanted the theory to provide empirical evidence, have the ability to be generalized, contribute to further understanding, and be able to predict outcomes.

These two positions within the same historical time period contain some unique as well as overlapping criteria for the analysis and evaluation of nursing theory.

In the 1980s, Chinn and Jacobs (1983) proposed a combination of the previous two positions and recommended five brief criteria for evaluating nursing theories. They stated that a theory could be evaluated by asking if it had clarity, simplicity, generality, empirical applicability, and consequences. Clarity was further expanded to include semantic clarity, semantic consistency, structural clarity, and structural consistency. Apparently they felt that semantics and clarity were becoming issues in the nursing community, and they were attempting to address these particular issues.

Recent Approaches to Theory Analysis

In addition to consideration of criteria for evaluation of theories, nursing theorists have proposed steps for the analysis process of nursing theories. Barnum, Meleis, and Fawcett all present several steps for the analysis of a nursing theory.

Recognizing the underlying assumptions of a theoretical work is an analyst's first task in understanding the theory (Barnum, 1998; Meleis, 1997). These assumptions may not be stated but may be inferred by the reader on the basis of other statements made about the given nursing theory in other publications and writings. However, recognizing underlying assumptions may not be possible for some middle range theories, because many of these middle range theories are not constructed by any one particular nursing author but are the work of multiple authors. It then becomes difficult to understand all of the different assumptions from the variety of publications written by them. Additionally, not all middle range theories are named after some nursing author or even have a particular author's name attached to the theory. For example, most of the middle range theories contained in this text do not have a theorist name attached to them, yet they have proved useful in the furthering of nursing understanding. Additionally, there are middle range theories such as Quality of Life or Reasoned Action that are borrowed from other disciplines unrelated to nursing but are used by nurses to describe and build the understanding of nursing. Nonetheless, there are some middle range theories that do have information available about the underlying assumptions, and for them, it is important to understand and relate these assumptions to the research problem.

Barnum (1990, p. 22) asserts that analysis of a theory demands that the analyst "dig beneath the surface for a deeper insight into a thesis in all its meaning and implications." This "reading between the lines" work may be difficult for some nurses as they may not be comfortable with criticism at this level. Meleis (1997) would like to see reviews of theorists, their education, experience, professional network, and the socio-cultural context of their theories. Because theory development in nursing did not take place in a vacuum, Meleis (1997) feels that it is important to carefully consider the paradigmatic origins of the theory through careful analysis of the references and citations cited by the author. In addition, she wants the analysis to include a thorough review of the assumptions, concepts, propositions, and hypothesis that the author employed. Additionally, she wants the theory to be examined for beginnings. Analysis of beginnings looks at where the theory started. Did it begin in the mind of the theorist as an attempt to explain what ought to be, or did it arise out of experience and explain what is? Fawcett (1995) suggests that analysis needs to include a thorough review of all the author's original works and presentations. However, for some middle range theories, because they are relatively new to the field of nursing, there may not be enough published work produced by a particular author or group of authors for the analyst to read and grasp this level of understanding about the theory's meaning and implications.

Barnum believes that the analyst should determine who or what performs an activity within the theory, as well as to determine whom or what is the recipient of the activity. A third area that should be evaluated in each theory is in what context the activity is performed and what the end point of the activity is. Two additional concepts that need to be addressed include the procedures that guide the activity and the energy source of the activity. Other concepts Barnum considered essential for theory analysis include nursing acts, the patient, and health (1998). Also included for good theory analysis are the relationship of nursing acts to the patient, the relationship of nursing acts to health, and the relationship of the patient to health. These concepts from Barnum are closely associated with the nursing metaparadigm that includes the concepts of nursing, person, health, and environment.

Barnum presents several devices for theory analysis. These devices use common nursing concepts to define nursing theory elements and their interrelationships. They also include determination of the level of theory development, descriptive or explanatory, and the need to discriminate nursing acts from nonnursing acts. Barnum (1990) adds that every nursing theory is based upon one or more dominant principles. These dominant principles contain an idea that is essential for stating or explaining a theory. It is important to identify and to consider the nature of each key principle. A principle is a fundamental or basic concept with an explanatory function. It explains the basis upon which the theory rests. The theorist's interpretation of reality if it is given should be analyzed by asking, "What is reality like?" Many of these considerations were geared towards the analysis of grand theories and have to be adapted for use when considering middle range theories. For example, if a middle range theory has been formulated over time by several authors, then it will be difficult, if not impossible, to determine the theorist's interpretation of reality.

Meleis includes internal dimensions as a criterion of her method of theory analysis. Internal dimensions include assumptions and concepts upon which the theory is built. She includes several units of analysis as part of this inquiry. Her units of analysis include content, context, and methods, and are similar to the units of analysis contained in Barnum's list. Other items unique to Meleis include the rationale, the system of relations, beginnings, scope, goals, and abstractness. Examining the rationale of a theory's construction provides clarification of how the elements of the theory are united. Meleis (1997) wants the analyst to discover the theory's system of relations. This is accomplished by asking the following question, "Do relations explain elements or do the elements explain relations?" (Meleis, 1997 p. 258) The scope of a theory determines how broad or narrow is the range of phenomena that the theory covers. Middle range theories keep their scope narrow, helping to make the theory more applicable to research and practice. The scope of a theory also deals with the breadth of the explanations it attempts to accomplish. The scope is narrower, more specific, and concrete for middle range theories than it is for grand theories (Fawcett, 1999).

The goals of a theory also need to be examined. Does the theory attempt to describe, explain, predict, or prescribe? Each theory must attempt to accomplish at least one of these goals. Middle range theories can be classified as falling into three distinct categories. These categories are descriptive, explanatory, or predictive (Fawcett, 2000). These three categories are closely aligned with the definition given by Meleis (1997) for a grand theory that includes describing, explaining, and predicting different phenomena.

Abstractness is another point that Meleis says is necessary to examine when analyzing a theory. Analyzing abstractness is an attempt to determine the width of the gaps between the theories, propositions, concepts, and reality. In middle range theories, this gap should be small, or nonexistent, since middle range theories deal with what is and not with what ought to be.

Fawcett (2000) has several recommendations for theory analysis that are similar to Meleis's and Barnum's. She has two additional components to consider. They are theory context and theory content. Theory context is the environment in which the theory's nursing action takes place. It tells about the nature of the nurses' world and may describe the nature of the client environment. Theory context is also concerned with which nursing metaparadigm concepts are addressed by the theory (Fawcett, 2000). In middle range theories, the focus of the theory may be purposefully limited to just one of the nursing metaparadigm concepts, such as in Pain Theory.

Theory content identifies the theory elements that are the subject matter of the theory. The content is stated through the concepts and propositions (Fawcett, 2000). Middle range theories should have their content well defined and their concepts clearly stated in the description of the theory.

A theory's process refers to the activities that either the nurse or the client has to perform to implement the theory. This should be a strength of middle range theories as they give clear direction to some process or activity carried out in application of the theory in research or practice.

THEORY EVALUATION

Barnum's Theory Evaluation Recommendations

Barnum (1990, p. 20) states "a thorough criticism (both analysis and evaluation) of a theory requires that attention be given to both aspects of internal and external criticism." Internal criticism refers to the internal construction of how the components of the theory fit together, while external criticism considers the theory and its relationship to people, nursing, and health. Internal criticism requires the reviewer to answer the following questions:

- Given the theorist's underlying assumptions, does the theory logically follow?
- Is the theory consistent with and logical in light of the underlying assumptions?

For external criticism, the reviewer would ask the following questions:

- Do the theory's underlying assumptions ring true?
- Do the assumptions represent the "real world" out there, especially the real world of nursing?

Barnum's criteria for evaluating theories include both internal and external criticism based on specific criteria. Her criteria for judging theories for internal criticism include clarity, consistency, adequacy, logical development, and level of theory development. Her criteria for judging theories using external criticism include reality convergence, utility, significance, discrimination, scope of theory, and complexity (Barnum, 1998).

Internal criticism is first evaluated by deciding the clarity of the theory. Two questions should be answered to determine clarity:

- Does the theory clearly state the main components to be considered?
- Is it easily understood by the reader?

Next on Barnum's list is consistency. Two more questions help to determine if the theory is consistent:

- Does the description of the theory continue to maintain the definitions of the key concepts throughout the explanation of the theory?
- Does it have congruent use of terms, interpretations, principles, and methods?

The next criterion is adequacy. Three questions help to determine if the theory is adequate. They are:

- How completely does the theory speak to the topics it claims to address?
- Are there holes or gaps that need to be filled in by other work or further refinement of the theory?
- Does it account for the subject matter under consideration?

Her fourth criterion is logical development. The quality of this criterion is determined by asking three questions.

- Does the theory logically follow a line of thought of previous work that has been shown to be true or does it launch out into unproven territory with its assumptions and premises?
- Do the conclusions proceed in a logical fashion?
- Are the arguments well-supported?

The final criterion for evaluating the internal portion of the theory is the level of the theory development.

- Is it in early development, just at the stage of naming its elements or has it been around a long time and is able to explain or even predict outcomes?
- How often have different nurse researchers conducted independent research studies applying the theory to different situations and reported the findings in the literature?

Barnum (1998, p. 178) states that "external criticism evaluates a nursing theory as it relates to the real world of man, of nursing and of health." She recommends that the following criteria should be considered: reality convergence, utility, significance, and capacity for discrimination. In addition two other criteria may be included. They are scope and complexity (Barnum, 1998).

Reality convergence deals with how well the theory builds upon the premises from which it is derived and then relates that to reality. Some nursing theorists build on past work and remain within the framework of traditional thinking. Other nurse theorists deconstruct the past and develop a new framework to build upon. These theorists are termed deconstructionists. Deconstructionists start with a different set of presuppositions than the historical nursing leaders did, and the resulting nursing theories may not represent the same world view of nursing as described in the past. At this point, the person doing the evaluation may choose to disagree as to whether a particular theory achieves reality convergence, based primarily on the differences between the beliefs and values that he holds to be true and those proposed by the theory. This part of theory evaluation may have more applicability to grand theories than middle range theories, but is an important point to consider as new and different middle range theories are developed in the future.

Utility simply requires that the theory be useful to the nurse researcher employing it. It should suggest subject material that could be investigated and lend itself to methods of inquiry. Middle range theories generally lend themselves to a greater ease of usefulness by nurse researchers than grand nursing theories. This is because they tend to be very narrow in scope and focused on specific concepts, like health promotion, pain, and quality of life.

The significance of a nursing theory depends upon the extent to which it addresses the phenomena of nursing and lends itself to further research.

Discrimination is the capacity to differentiate nursing from other health-related disciplines through the use of well-defined boundaries. The boundaries need to be clear and precise so that judgements can be made about any given action performed by a nurse.

Barnum includes the scope of a theory as a necessary criterion for external criticism. Important questions to consider here are: Does it have a narrow range of scope to help identify it as a middle range theory and does that narrow focus make it easier to use in a research setting?

Complexity is the final criterion in Barnum's list. Complexity is at the opposite pole from the criterion of parsimony. The level of complexity is determined by the number of variables. Middle range nursing theories are less complex than grand nursing theories because they deal with fewer variables, resulting in a fewer number of relationships between the concepts.

Meleis's Theory Evaluation Recommendations

Meleis (1997) provides a complex model for theory evaluation. It includes several integral parts: theory description, theory support, theory analysis, and theory critique. She proposes that this complete model represents the necessary elements needed to thoroughly evaluate a theory. Meleis begins the description of her model by listing two criteria that help describe the theory. These two criteria are structural and functional components. Within the criterion of structural components, there are separate units of analysis to consider. The first is assumptions. Assumptions are "givens" in the theory and are based on the theorist's values. They are not subject to testing but lead to the set of propositions that are to be tested. In nursing theories, there are many assumptions made about the concepts included in the nursing metaparadigm and, additionally, to the concepts of human behavior, life, death, and illness. Again, it must be stated that it will not be possible to find the assumptions of all middle range theories.

Another part of Meleis' theory description includes functional components. A functional assessment of a theory carefully considers the anticipated consequences of the theory and its purposes. The units of analysis of the functional components are the theory's focus, i.e., the client, nursing, health, nurse–patient interactions, the environment, nursing problems, and nursing therapeutics (p. 251).

Meleis offers several questions to ask when considering the functional components of a nursing theory (p. 254). They include the following:

1. Who does the theory act upon?
2. What definitions does the theory offer for the elements of the nursing metaparadigm?
3. Does the theory offer a clear idea of what the sources of nursing problems are?
4. Does the theory provide interventions for nurses?
5. Are there guidelines for intervention modalities?
6. Does it provide guidelines for the role of the nurse?
7. Are the consequences of the nurse's actions articulated?

Meleis feels that these criteria are consistent with the ones offered by Barnum.

Another major area of theory evaluation for Meleis is theory support. She includes theory testing in this area. Theory testing consists of four separate tests, including tests of utility, tests of nonnursing propositions, tests of concepts, and tests of propositions.

A final area of evaluation in the model is what Meleis calls theory critique. Theory critique is made up of several criteria. Many of her criteria are similar to ones developed by Barnum but some are unique to Meleis. The duplicated criteria similar to Barnum's are clarity, consistency, simplicity/complexity, and usefulness. Some unique criteria are tautology/teleology, and diagrams.

Tautology considers evaluating the needless repetition of an idea in separate parts of the theory. Overuse of repetition can confuse a reader and make the theory explanation unclear.

Teleology is assessed by considering the extent to which causes and consequences are kept separate in the theory. Meleis (1997) says teleology occurs when the theorist defines concepts by consequences and then introduces totally new concepts, rather than getting to the definitions of the original concepts. As this process continues, there is never a clear definition of the theory's concepts, and the theory remains unclear.

Diagrams are useful to visually see the interrelationship of the concepts to each other before doing research. They can be especially useful for reviewing the strength of statistical correlations between the theories concepts.

Fawcett's Theory Evaluation Recommendations

Fawcett (2000) made the following recommendations to be used for the evaluation of nursing theories. Her criteria include significance, internal consistency, parsimony, testability, empirical adequacy, and pragmatic adequacy. She also recommends that the evaluation of a theory requires judgements to be made about the extent to which a theory satisfies the criteria.

Significance may be determined by asking the following questions: "Are the metaparadigm concepts and propositions addressed by the theory explicit?" In middle range theories, all aspects of the metaparadigm for nursing are not always covered, and that should not detract from its use by nursing researchers. "Are the philosophical claims on which the theory is based explicit?" Here again, some middle range theories will be devoid of philosophical claims. "Is the conceptual model from which the theory was derived explicit?" "Are the authors of antecedent knowledge from nursing and adjunctive disciplines acknowledged and are bibliographical citations given?" (Fawcett, 2000, p. 504).

Fawcett's second criterion of internal consistency requires that all the elements of the theory are congruent. These elements may include conceptual model, and theory concepts and propositions. Additionally, Fawcett suggests that semantic clarity and consistency is required for internal consistency to be maintained. She proposes the following questions be asked when evaluating the internal consistency of a theory: Are the content and the context of the theory congruent? Do the concepts reflect semantic clarity and consistency? Do the theory propositions reflect structural consistency? (Fawcett, 2000).

Parsimony is concerned with whether the theory is stated clearly and concisely. This criterion is met when the statements clarify rather than obscure the topic of interest. This is as important in middle range theory as it is in grand theory. Even though the scope of the theory may be narrow in a middle range theory, it is still important to be clear and concise in the explanations of the concepts.

The goal of theory development in nursing is the empirical testing of interventions that are specified in the form of middle range theories (Fawcett, 2000). The concepts of a middle range theory should be observable and the propositions measurable. Fawcett (2000, p. 506) suggests that the following questions should be asked when evaluating the testability of a middle range theory: Does the research methodology reflect the middle range theory? Are the middle range theory concepts observable through instruments that are appropriate empirical indicators of those concepts? Do the data analysis techniques permit measurement of the middle range theory propositions?

Empirical adequacy is the fifth step that Fawcett says is necessary in the evaluation of nursing theories. This step requires that assertions made by the theory are congruent with empirical evidence found through studies done using the theory as a basis for research. It usually takes more than one research study to establish empirical adequacy. The end result of using empirical adequacy is to establish the level of confidence in the theory from the best studies yielding empirical results. The question to be considered here is "Are the middle range theory's assertions harmonious with the research studies' empirical results?"

The final and sixth step in Fawcett's framework for evaluation of nursing theories is the criterion of pragmatic adequacy. This criterion evaluates the extent of how well the middle range theory is utilized in clinical practice. The criterion also requires that nurses fully understand the full content of the theory. Additionally, the theory should help move resulting nursing action towards favorable client outcomes. Ask the following questions when evaluating a theory for pragmatic adequacy:

- Do nurses need special education and skill training to apply the theory in clinical practice?
- Is it possible to derive clinical protocols from the theory?
- How often has the theory been used as the basis of nursing research?
- Do favorable outcomes result from using the theory as a basis for nursing actions? (Fawcett, 2000).

Kolcaba's Theory Evaluation Recommendations

The most recent contribution to this discussion of theory evaluation comes from Kolcaba. According to Kolcaba (2002), there are several criteria that determine a good middle range theory. Her criteria involve evaluation and do not mention steps for theory analysis. They include questions concerning the theories concepts and propositions, and whether or not they are specific to nursing. She also wants to determine if the theory has components that are readily operationalized and can be applied to many situations.

She asserts that a middle range theory's propositions can range from causal to associative, depending on their application. The assumptions provided fit the middle range theory. The theory should be relevant for the potential users. The middle range theory should be oriented to outcomes that are important for patients and not merely describe what nurses do. Finally, Kolcaba thinks that middle range theory should describe nursing-sensitive phenomena that are readily associated with the deliberate actions of nurses.

It is evident that there are several distinct differences between the analysis and evaluation process for grand theories and middle range theories. At the same time, there are several similarities. Many of the principles applied to the analysis and evaluation of grand theories can be readily applied to middle range theories and, with some minor modification, can be used to determine the adequacy of a middle range theory. With this in mind, the next section will address the selection of a middle range theory for use in nursing research.

SELECTING A THEORY FOR NURSING RESEARCH

Before starting to write a proposal, Fawcett (1999) suggests that each investigator become familiar with the research topic and the conceptual model that will guide the study. She reiterates that this is done by an immersion into the literature and a thorough study of the research topic. Additionally, a comprehensive literature search should be done several months before making a proposal of the study. This much time must be given to allow the proper amount of time for reading and thinking about both the content of the proposed study and the conceptual model to provide the basis for the study. It is during this time that the most appropriate middle range theory can be decided upon for use in the research.

As nurse researchers shift away from using grand nursing theories and begin to consider using middle range theories, the philosophical underpinnings of the theory itself become of decreased importance. The emphasis shifts from the philosophical basis of the nursing theory to how the middle range theory is applied in research and practice. Thus, time previously spent with the philosophy and background of the theorist can now be devoted to making sure of the proper fit between the research questions to be studied and the middle range theory. Each nurse researcher should ask the following questions about the middle range theory proposed for use in his or her research:

- Does the theory seem to fit the research that you wish to do?
- Is it readily operationalized?
- What has been the primary application for this theory in the past?
- Where has the theory in question been applied and used before?
- How well has the theory performed at describing, predicting and/or explaining the phenomena that it relates to?
- Does the theory relate to and address the research hypothesis in its description and explanation?
- Does the hypothesis flow from the research problem?
- Does the theory address the primary and secondary research questions?
- Are the theories assumptions congruent with the assumptions that are made for this research?
- Is it oriented to outcomes that are critical to patients and does not describe what nurses perform?
- Are tools available to test relationships of the theory or do they need to be developed?

The nurse researcher should consider several different middle range theories as possibilities for use. A thorough analysis and evaluation of these theories in question should be done before selecting one.

Subsequently, the nurse researcher should become familiar with all aspects of the theory, using the questions provided in the discussion above. It is essential to have a sound understanding and be in total agreement with the theory selected before beginning the study. This is accomplished by becoming immersed in the literature about the middle range theory in question, and arriving at a thorough and complete understanding of the theory before using it. The nurse researcher should try to understand the middle range theory by identifying all the major concepts. The definitions of these concepts, in turn, should be studied for this particular theory, to make sure the meanings have not been changed slightly over time as they are described in the literature.

Additionally, the major concepts should be examined to determine how they relate to each other. Next, the researcher needs to decide if he/she can accept the premises, rationale, and presuppositions that the nursing theory are based upon before adopting it for use (McKenna, 1997). Finally, it is necessary to determine what means of measurement have been used with previous studies employing this theory. It will be important to know if new measurement tools will need to be obtained or if similar tools can be employed for the study at hand.

It is evident that to decide upon and use a middle range theory effectively in nursing research, the potential nurse researcher must do a thorough analysis and evaluation of the middle range nursing theory. The following analysis exercise will provide the guidance for conducting an evaluation of a middle range theory before selecting it for use in a research study.

MIDDLE RANGE THEORY EVALUATION PROCESS

This evaluation process, to be applied at the end of each subsequent chapter as an intellectual educational exercise, is a synthesis of the works of the authors reviewed above. After careful review of the theory presented in each chapter, taking into consideration the examples given where the middle range theory is applied in practice and the case study provided, the reader should be able carry out this theory evaluation, taking into account the following criteria listed here with their definitions. Answer the questions posed for each criterion. Summarize the findings in a concluding paragraph for both internal and external criticism. Finally, make a judgment as to whether this theory could be adapted for use in research. Start the process by evaluating internal criticism.

Internal Criticism
Adequacy: How completely does the theory address the topics it claims to address? Are there holes or gaps that need to be filled in by other work or further refinement of the theory? Does it account for the subject matter under consideration?
Clarity: Does the theory clearly state the main components to be considered? Is it easily understood by the reader?
Consistency: Does the description of the theory address whether the theory maintains the definitions of the key concepts throughout the explanation of the theory? Does it have congruent use of terms, interpretations, principles, and methods?
Logical development: Does the theory logically follow a line of thought of previous work that has been shown to be true, or does it launch out into unproven territory with its assumptions and premises? Do the conclusions proceed in a logical fashion? Are the arguments well supported?
Level of theory development: Is it consistent with the conceptualization of middle range theory?

External Criticism

Complexity: How many concepts are involved as key components in the theory? How complicated is the description of the theory? Can it be understood without lengthy descriptions and explanations? (considers the number of variables being addressed, exists on a continuum from parsimony–limited number of variables to complex–extensive number of variables).

Discrimination: Is this theory able to produce hypotheses that will lead to research results that could not be arrived at using some other nursing theory? How unique is this theory to the area of nursing that it addresses? Does it have precise and clear boundaries, definitive parameters of the subject matter?

Reality convergence: Do the theories underlying assumptions ring true? Do these assumptions represent the real world? Do they represent the real world of nursing? Does the theory reflect the real world as understood by the reader?

Pragmatic: Can the theory be operationalized in real-life settings?

Scope: How broad or narrow is the range of phenomena that this theory covers? Does it stay in a narrow range of scope to keep it a middle range theory? (narrower implies more applicable to practice; wider implies more global and all encompassing)

Significance: Will the result of the research that is conducted because of the hypothesis generated by the theory have any impact on the way nurses carry out nursing interventions in the real world or does it merely describe what nurses do? Does the theory address issues essential, not irrelevant, to the discipline?

Utility: Is the theory able to be used to generate hypotheses that are researchable by nurses?

After completing the evaluation based on the criteria listed above, compare and contrast responses to the ones done by contributors for each chapter listed in Appendix A at the end of the text.

WEB RESOURCES

The Hardin Library for the Health Sciences Electronic Resources Homepage has full text journals, subject-specific web resources, governmental and statistical resources, medical databases, and more. You can access it at *http://www.lib.uiowa.edu/hardin/md/nurs.html*. Advice for searching nursing theory references can be found at *http://www.wwnurse.com/topsites/topsites.cgi?ID=364*.

REFERENCES

Barnum, B. (1950). *Nursing theory, analysis application, evaluation* (3rd ed.). Glenview, IL: Scott, Foresman, Little Brown.

Barnum, B. (1998). *Nursing theory: Analysis, application and evaluation* (5th ed.). Philadelphia: Lippincott Williams & Wilkins.

Chinn, P. & Jacob, M. (1983). *Theory and nursing: A systematic approach*. St.Louis: Mosby

Duffy, M., & Muhlenkamp, A. (1974). A framework for theory analysis. *Nursing Outlook, 22*(9), 570–574.

Fawcett, J. (1995). *Analysis and evaluation of conceptual models of nursing* (3rd ed.). Philadelphia: F.A. Davis.

Fawcett, J. (1999). *The relationship of theory and research* (3rd ed.). Philadelphia: F.A. Davis.

Fawcett, J. (2000). *Analysis and evaluation of contemporary nursing knowledge: Nursing models and theories.* Philadelphia: F.A. Davis.

Hardy, M. (1974). Theories: Components, development, evaluation. *Nursing Research, 23*(2), pp. 100–107.

Kolcaba, K. (2001). Evolution of the middle range theory of comfort for outcomes research. *Nursing Outlook 49*(2), 86–92.

McKenna, H. (1997). *Nursing theories and models.* London: Routledge.

Meleis, A. (1997). *Theoretical nursing: Development & progress.* (3rd ed.). Philadelphia: Lippincott-Raven.

Parse, R. (2001). Rosemary Rizzo Parse the human becoming school of thought. In M. Parker (Ed.), *Nursing theories and nursing practice.* Philadelphia: F. A. Davis.

BIBLIOGRAPHY

Alligood, M. R., & Marriner-Tomey, A. M. (2002). *Nursing theory: Utilization & application*. (2nd ed.) St. Louis: Mosby.

Barns, B., (1999). *Nursing theories' conceptual and philosophical foundations*. New York: Springer Publishing Company.

Chinn, P., & Kramer, M. (1999). *Theory and nursing: Integrated knowledge development*. (5th ed) St. Louis: Mosby.

Chinn, P., & Kramer, M. (1995). *Theory and nursing: A systematic approach*. (4th ed.). St. Louis: Mosby.

Dubin, R. (1978). *Theory building*. New York: The Free Press.

Fawcett, J. (1993). *Analysis and evaluation of nursing theories*. Philadelphia: F. A. Davis.

Fawcett, J. (1995). *Analysis and evaluation of conceptual models of nursing*. (3rd ed.). Philadelphia: F. A. Davis

Fawcett, J. (1993). *Analysis and evaluation of nursing theories*. Malinski, V., & Barrett, E.. (Eds.). (1994). *Martha E. Rogers: Her life and her work*, Philadelphia: F. A. Davis.

Fawcett, J. (1999). *The relationship of theory and research* (3rd ed.) Philadelphia: F. A. Davis.

Fawcett, J. (2000). *Analysis and evaluation of contemporary nursing knowledge: Nursing models and theories*. Philadelphia: F. A. Davis.

Gift, A. (1997). *Clarifying concepts in nursing research*. New York: Springer Publishing Company.

George, J. (1995). *Nursing theories: The base for professional nursing practice*. (4th ed.). Norwalk, CT: Appleton & Lange.

Greenwood, J. (Ed.). (2000). *Nursing theory in Australia: Development and application*. Sydney: Harper Collins.

Huck, S., & Cormier, W. (1996). *Reading statistics & research*. New York: Harper Collins College Publishers.

Kim, H., Kollak, I., & Parker, M. (Eds). (1990). *Nursing theories in practice*. New York: National League for Nursing, Publ. # 15-2350.

McKenna, H. (1997). *Nursing models and theories*. London: Routledge.

McQuiston, C. & Webb, A. (Eds). (1995). *Foundations of nursing theory*. Thousand Oaks, CA: Sage Publications.

Meleis, A. I. (1997). *Theoretical nursing: Development and progress*. (3rd ed.). Philadelphia: Lippincott-Raven.

Nicoll, L. H. (1992). *Perspectives on nursing theory*. J. B. Lippincott.

Nolan, M., & Grant, G. (1992). Middle range theory building and the nursing theory-practice gap: A respite case study. *Journal of Advanced Nursing, 17,* 217–223.

Parker, M. E. (2000). *Nursing theories and nursing practice*. Philadelphia: F. A. Davis.

Parker, M. (Ed). (1990). *Nursing theories in practice*. New York: National League for Nursing.

Parker, M. (Ed). (1993). *Patterns of nursing theories in practice*. New York: National League for Nursing, Publ. # 15-2548.

Tomey, A. M., & Alligood, M. R.(Eds). (2002). *Nursing theorists and their work* (5th ed.). St. Louis: Mosby.

Walker, L. O., & Avant, K. C. (1997). *Strategies for theory construction in nursing*. New York: Appleton-Century-Crofts.

Wesley, R. L. (1995). *Nursing theories and models* (2nd ed.). Springhouse, PA: Springhouse.

Whall, A. (1996). The structure of nursing knowledge: Analysis and evaluation of practice, middle range and grand theory. In Fitzpatrick, J., and Whall, A. (Eds.). *Conceptual models of nursing: Analysis and application* (3rd ed.) Norwalk, CT: Appleton & Lange.

Winstead-Fry, P. (Ed.) (1986). *Case studies in nursing theory*. New York: National League for Nursing.

Young A., Taylor, S. G., & Renpenning, K. (2001). *Connections: Nursing research, theory and practice*. St. Louis: Mosby.

Middle Range Theories: Physiological

Pain: A Balance Between Analgesia and Side Effects

MARION GOOD

DEFINITION OF KEY TERMS

Analgesia	Pain relief
Balance between analgesia and side effects	Patient satisfaction with relief of pain and relief or absence of side effects
Identification of lack of pain/side-effect relief	Pain intensity greater than mutual goal; side-effect intensity unacceptable to patient/nurse
Intervention, reassessment, and reintervention	Immediate intervention for pain and side effects; reassessment when peak effect is expected, and reintervention if pain and side effects are still unacceptable
Mutual goal-setting	Mutually agreed-upon, safe, realistic goals for relief
Nonpharmacological adjuvant	Complementary nursing therapies for pain relief of relaxation, music, imagery, massage, or cold
Pain	An unpleasant sensory and affective experience associated with tissue damage
Pharmacological adjuvant	Analgesic given as a supplement
Patient teaching	Patient instruction encouraging attitudes, expectations, and action in reporting pain; obtaining medication, preventing pain during activity, and use of complementary therapies
Potent pain medication	Opioid analgesic or local anesthetic given systemically or by epidural for acute pain
Regular assessment of pain and side effects	Report of pain and side effects every 2 hours until under control, and then every 4 hours
Side effects	Unpleasant sensory and affective experiences associated with adverse effects of pain medication

INTRODUCTION

Multiple theories have been developed to explain and manage pain. Pain is the most common reason that people seek health care. Although pain is known to be a part of life, it is compelling in its unpleasantness and is sometimes overwhelming in its effect. Patients who are in pain endure considerable suffering and are at risk for long-term adverse effects that include slower wound healing, downregulation of the immune system, and metastasis of tumor cells (Padgett, Marucha, & Sheridan, 1998; Page, 1996; Page, Ben-Eliyahu, Yirmiya, & Liebeskind, 1993; Zeller, McCain, & Swanson, 1996). There are many different types of pain: acute pain of injury, surgery, labor, and sickle cell crisis; chronic pain of musculoskeletal or gastrointestinal disorders; procedural pain of lumbar puncture, venipuncture, and chest tube removal; cancer pain from the enlarging tumor, its metastases, or its treatment; and pain in infants, the critically ill, and at the end of life. Health care professionals today have a duty and an obligation to identify the source, to treat the cause, and to relieve the pain. Researchers have an obligation to test interventions for relief.

To study pain, researchers have experimentally induced it in animals and humans using noxious stimuli such as heat, cold, constriction, and sharpness. In animal research, surgically exposed pain pathways provide information about the transmission of noxious impulses to the thalamus, sensory cortex, and limbic system. However, in animals, the affective component of pain is difficult to discern. In contrast, when conducting human laboratory studies of induced pain, researchers do not measure pain invasively, but they can easily obtain a report of the affective component of pain. Experimentally induced pain in human beings, however, does not have the holistic physical and emotional impact over time that clinical pain does. Experimental pain does not limit life functions and arouse fears as the pain of illness and surgery do. Clinical studies are needed.

HISTORICAL BACKGROUND

To those who experience pain, there is no mystery as to how it feels. Health professionals who study pain or care for persons in pain may or may not have experienced similar pain themselves. They must believe the patient who tells them what it is like, and know that the quality, intensity, duration, and trajectory of pain will vary depending on the type of pain and the person experiencing it.

Theories of Pain Mechanism

The earliest pain theory was illustrated by Descartes in his 17th-century drawing of a child whose foot was too close to a fire. Pain transmission was drawn as a direct cord ascending from the foot through the back to the brain. Descartes described it as similar to pulling a rope to ring a bell (Melzack & Wall, 1962, 1965). Years later, in 1895, von Frey published evidence that led to the specificity theory of pain. He proposed the existence of nerve fibers specific to pain, which, if stimulated, would invariably allow impulses to travel to the pain centers in the brain and result in the experience of pain. This implied a direct one-to-one relationship between the noxious stimulus and the sensation of pain. However, physiological evidence does not support this model of an invariant relationship, nor do all types of pain fit into it. Referred pain and phantom pain are notable exceptions. The specificity theory was followed by pattern theories proposing that stimulus intensity, temporal–spatial transmission patterns, central summation, and input control were critical to pain. These early theories, however, focused only on sensory pain and did not take into account the complexity of the human organism, particularly the interactive functions of the brain and spinal cord. As a group, early theories lacked anything to unify them (Melzack & Wall, 1965). Beecher (1959) described extensively wounded American soldiers who completely denied pain because they were so elated to be alive and to be going home. These descriptions showed the theoretical insight that pain was more complex than simply the transmission of impulses along nerve pathways. It had a psychological component that could attenuate the transmission of impulses (Melzack & Wall, 1965).

GATE CONTROL THEORY

A major watershed or turning point in pain theory was the paradigm shift initiated by the gate control theory that Melzack and Wall published in 1965. Melzack was a psychologist who was searching for a more comprehensive understanding of pain; one that included the brain. He linked with Wall, a neurophysiologist who had described lamina II in the dorsal horn of the spinal cord, where nociceptive impulses were modified by neural input from other areas of the central nervous system (CNS). Together they created the gate control theory, which unified several sensory pain theories and added the affective, motivational, and central control elements. Touch, attention, and emotion were then theoretically capable of increasing or decreasing pain by descending mechanisms from the brain to the dorsal horn.

ENDOGENOUS ANALGESIC THEORIES

Discoveries of endogenous opiates in the periaqueductal gray area of the brain, opioid receptors in the CNS, and later catecholemines, serotonin, and neuropeptide receptors all produced new theories that some scientists viewed as refuting the gate control theory. Others viewed them as explanatory mechanisms for descending control of noxious impulse transmission. Today, descending control is known to occur through neurons, neurotransmitters, opioid receptors, and also indirectly through the sympathetic nervous system. The gate is no longer localized solely in lamina II of the dorsal horn, but the "gate" has been broadened to refer to repeated modulation, filtering, and abstraction of input in many areas of the CNS via numerous mechanisms (Melzack, 1982). Recently, Melzack traced the evolution of the gate control theory and presented his new neuromatrix theory of pain that encompasses current knowledge about the CNS (Melzack, 1996).

The gate control theory and theories of endogenous analgesic factors, however, are only descriptive and explanatory theories of pain mechanisms. They contain propositions of how pain occurs, and how it is modulated within the body. These theories offer valuable insight into ways that health professionals can interface with pain. The theories are suggestive of therapeutic relationships, but they do not specify effective interventions and are therefore not prescriptive theories. Prescriptive theories are needed for the discipline of nursing because nurses intervene to improve health as an important part of their mission (Dickhoff & James, 1968).

Shift in Focus to Pain Relief

A second watershed in pain theory was a paradigm shift from theories of the mechanisms of pain to theories of relief. These included explanatory and prescriptive theories of opioids and of nonopioids such as local anesthetics and nonsteroidal anti-inflammatory drugs (NSAIDs). Health professionals have known for years that opioids, whether taken orally or injected into blood vessels, muscles, or epidural space, provide potent relief for moderate to severe pain. There is evidence that even ancient peoples used opium for pain during disease and surgery (Keyser, 2002). The explanatory theory (mechanism) for this effect was later found to be attachment of opioids to mu and kappa opioid receptors in the CNS.

NSAIDs, including aspirin, ibuprofen, acetaminophen, and ketorolac, have a different mechanism. Acting at the site of the tissue injury, NSAIDs decrease the release of inflammatory substances that sensitize the nerve fibers to respond to the painful stimuli. NSAIDs do not bind to opioid receptors and do not produce the same side effects as opioids. Therefore, when they are used as adjuvants, they can be opioid sparing, but some could also interfere with blood clotting. Ketorolac is an intravenous NSAID, given IV to provide moderate relief. It is often used to add a second mechanism of relief when using opioids after surgery.

In the discipline of nursing, there are middle range descriptive theories of pain from the perspective of both patients and expert nurses (Mahon, 1994; Morse, Bottorff, & Hutchinson, 1995; Simon, Baumann, & Nolan, 1995). Qualitative themes obtained from patients have characterized chronic pain as dominating and seemingly endless (Mahon, 1994); it results in vulnerable feelings and thoughts of suicide and death (Morse et al., 1995). Expert nurses have also differentiated between acute and chronic pain (Simon et al., 1995).

Broad descriptive theories include pain as one of several major concepts. The theory of unpleasant symptoms generalizes across symptoms of pain, dyspnea, nausea, and fatigue, based on the commonalities of these symptoms (Lenz, Pugh, Milligan, Gift, & Suppe, 1997). The theory of comfort care proposes that nursing action and health-seeking behavior of patients can satisfy the basic human need for relief, ease, or transcendence (Kolcaba, 1994). Other nursing theories are focused on nurse and patient facilitators and barriers to relief (Greipp, 1992), analgesic delivery according to pain diurnal rhythms (Auvil-Novak, 1997), and nurse education for pain management (Dalton & Blau, 1996).

Development of Integrated, Prescriptive Approach

A third paradigm shift was the notion that pain alleviation by nurses requires an integrated prescriptive approach that includes patient teaching, analgesic medication, nonpharmacologic methods, *and* expert nursing care. Do patients need analgesics alone? What can provide additional relief? What patient teaching and what nursing actions produce effective relief? Integrated prescriptive pain theories specify the actions that nurses must take to deliver both pharmacological and nonpharmacological therapies that are effective for relief. There is an integrative pain alleviation theory for adults (Good & Moore, 1996) and one for children (Huth & Moore, 1998). Good and Moore proposed a middle range prescriptive acute pain theory of a balance between analgesia and side effects (Good, 1998; Good & Moore, 1996). The theory prescribes patient participation, analgesic administration plus nonpharmacological adjuvants, and nursing actions to reduce acute pain. The theory for children adds prescriptions for assessment of developmental level, coping strategies, and cultural background (Huth & Moore, 1998). The theory for adults will be described in more detail.

Acute Pain Management Guidelines

The theory of a balance between analgesia and side effects was developed from the acute pain management guidelines published by the Agency for Health Care Policy and Research (Acute Pain Management Guideline Panel, 1992). The guidelines were published to address the long-standing problem of the inadequate treatment of acute pain following surgery and trauma. The guideline panel was cochaired by two pain management researchers, Ada K. Jacox, RN, PhD, FAAN, from nursing, and Daniel B. Carr, MD, from anesthesiology. Other members of the panel were experts in pain management from medicine or nursing specialties, such as surgery, pain management, cancer, neurology, pediatrics, physiology, psychology, pharmacy, physical therapy, ethics, religion, and also a consumer representative who had suffered burn pain.

The panel undertook the task of reviewing and synthesizing the research literature and, whenever research support was lacking, they added their collective expert opinion. They wrote a concise but comprehensive book, *Clinical Practice Guideline Acute Pain Management: Operative or Medical Procedures and Trauma*. For adult care, they supplemented the book with a pamphlet for nurses, "Quick Reference Guide for Clinicians Acute Pain Management in Adults: Operative Procedures" and a pamphlet for patients, "Pain Control after Surgery, A Patient's Guide." For care of children and adolescents, they supplemented the book with a "Quick Reference Guide for Clinicians, Acute Pain Management in Infants, Children, and Adolescents: Operative and Medical Procedures." These were the first of many federal guidelines published by the Agency for Health Care Policy and Research (AHCPR) for a variety of health conditions, which later included guidelines for cancer pain and back pain. The pain guidelines can be obtained on-line at *http://www.ahcpr.gov/clinic/cpgonline.htm*.

The acute pain guidelines give detailed direction for health professionals to use in clinical practice. The goals are to reduce the incidence and severity of pain, to educate patients for communication of pain, to enhance patient satisfaction, and to contribute to fewer postoperative complications. The comprehensive book mentioned above includes sections on the literature, the empirical evidence for relieving pain, the process of pain assessment and reassessment, pharmacological management, and patient education. There are also sections on pain management in children, adolescents, older adults, substance abusers, and burn victims. The AHCPR acute pain guidelines served as a foundation for the development of the pain theory, A Balance Between Analgesia and Side Effects.

DEFINITION OF THEORY CONCEPTS

The major concepts of the theory, A Balance Between Analgesia and Side Effects, are found in Table 3-1, along with theoretical definitions and examples of operational definitions that can be used in research. In addition, Figure 3-1 is a graphic representation of the theory. Acute pain is conceptualized as a multidimensional phenomenon occurring after surgery or trauma that includes sensory and affective dimensions. *Pain* in alert adults is what the person reports. The sensory component of pain following damage to body tissues is the localized physical perception of hurt. It is ordinarily termed "sensation of pain" (Good, 1995; Johnson, 1973; Price, McGrath, Rafii, & Buckingham, 1983). The affective component of pain is the unpleasant emotion associated with the sensation and has been named "distress of pain" (Ceccio, 1984; Flaherty & Fitzpatrick, 1978; Good, 1995; Johnson, 1973), "anxiety" (Good, 1995), or "unpleasantness" (Price, Harkins, & Baker, 1987; Price et al., 1983). The sensory and affective components of pain affect each other (Casey & Melzack, 1967; Jacobsen, 1938; Johnson & Rice, 1974; Rathbone, 1943; Sternbach, 1984), and can be measured in terms of intensity magnitude (Good et al., 2001).

Patient teaching and mutual goal setting are addressed first because of the key relationships between these concepts and some of the other variables. Nurses should conduct patient teaching to encourage effective attitudes and accurate expectations of pain, and to educate patients to report pain, obtain

Table 3-1. CONCEPTS WITH THEORETICAL AND OPERATIONAL DEFINITIONS

CONCEPTS	THEORETICAL DEFINITIONS	OPERATIONAL DEFINITIONS (EXAMPLES)
OUTCOMES		
Balance between analgesia and side effects	Patient satisfaction with relief of pain and relief or absence of side effects	Patient report of safe and satisfying pain relief with few or no side effects
Pain	An unpleasant sensory and affective experience associated with tissue injury following surgery or trauma	Pain intensity on a visual analogue scale
Side effects	Unpleasant sensory and affective experiences associated with pain medication	Opioid Side Effects Scale (Good et al., 2001–2005)
PROPOSITION 1		
Patient teaching	Patient instruction, encouraging attitudes, expectations, and action in reporting pain, obtaining medication, preventing pain during activity and using complementary therapies	Documentation of nurse instruction, or patient use of audio/videotape
Mutual goal-setting	Mutually agreed-upon, safe, realistic, goals for relief	Nurse discussions with patient daily, including documentation.
PROPOSITION 2		
Potent pain medication	Opioid analgesic or local anesthetic given systemically or by epidural for acute pain	Drug, dose, frequency, route, and method of administration
Pharmacological adjuvant	Analgesic given as a supplement	Drug, dose, frequency, route, and method of administration
Nonpharmacological adjuvant	Complementary nursing therapies: relaxation, music, imagery, massage, or cold for pain relief	Technique, dose, frequency, given, and mastery of use
PROPOSITION 3		
Regular assessment of pain and side effects	Report of pain and side effects every 2 hours until under control, and then every 4 hours	Pain rating scale Opioid Side Effects Scale
Identification of inadequate relief of pain and side effects	Pain/side effect intensity greater than mutual goal	Number and intensity of side effects that are unacceptable to patient/nurse
Intervention, reassessment, and reintervention	Immediate intervention for pain and side effects; reassessment when peak effect is expected, and reintervention if pain and side effects are still unacceptable	Nurse documentation

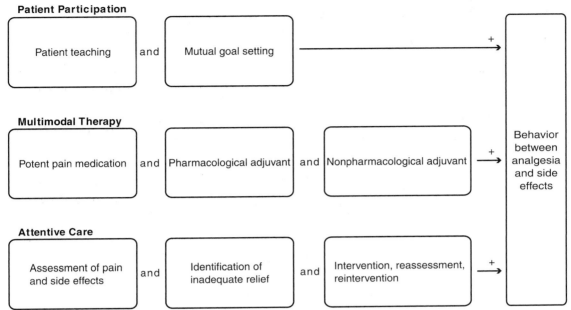

Figure 3-1. The middle range theory of a balance between analgesia and side effects prescribes nursing actions to encourage patient participation in using multimodal therapy with attentive care. Adapted from Good, M. (1998). A middle range theory of acute pain management: Use in research. *Nursing Outlook, 46*(3), 120–124. Good, M., & Moore, S. M. (1996). Clinical practice guidelines as a new source of middle-range theory: Focus on acute pain. *Nursing Outlook, 44*(2), 74–79.

medication and use adjuvants. Nurses should initiate dialogue for mutual goal setting each day to set a realistic relief goal that is acceptable to the patient.

The concept of *potent pain medication* refers to the major method of relief which may be opioids delivered by patient-controlled analgesia, or by subcutaneous intramuscular (IM) or IV injection. However, opioid analgesics have side effects of nausea, vomiting, drowsiness, and respiratory depression. In addition, dependence can occur. Therefore, to avoid these side effects, patients often take less analgesic than is needed for relief (Acute Pain Management Guideline Panel, 1992). Epidural analgesia can be achieved with the use of opioids, local anesthetics, or both; these are injected into the epidural space of the spinal cord. Side effects of epidural analgesia includes numbness of the lower extremities.

Pharmacological adjuvants may be given because their unrelated mechanism of action increases relief, yet "spares" the use and the side effects of strong analgesics. For example, peripheral-acting NSAIDs have been used in combination with centrally acting opioids to achieve greater effects (Acute Pain Management Guideline Panel, 1992). In addition, NSAIDs may be used as rescue doses for unrelieved or breakthrough pain.

Nonpharmacological adjuvants to analgesic medication can include relaxation techniques (Good et al., 1999; Roykulcharoen, 2002), music (Good et al., 1999), hypnosis (Olness, 1989), guided imagery with self-efficacy messages (Tusek, Church, Strong, Grass, & Fazio, 1997; Tusek, Cwynar, & Cosgrove, 1999), or guided imagery with messages for pleasant images (Albert, 2002; Huth, 2001; Locsin, 1988) (Box 3-1). Music can be soft, soothing, sedative instrumental music (Good, Picot, Salem, Chin, Picot, & Lane, 2000), and can be combined with relaxation or guided imagery. Studies are needed to compare sedative music to favorite music of any kind and to music with faster tempos, and also to compare the effects of various musical instruments and various cultural preferences. Nonpharmacological adjuvants can be studied during emergency treatment, following surgery and trauma, during labor, and during painful procedures. As nonpharmacological interventions are found to be effective in acute pain populations, they can also be investigated in chronic pain populations, in which relief over a longer period of time is needed.

Regular pain and side effect assessment is about actions the nurse takes to identify patient symptoms. The theory further specifies the need to treat these symptoms rather than simply record them. *Identification of inadequate pain relief and side effects* requires the nurse to believe the patient's report and know what is inadequate relief, despite the wide variation in patient response to pain and to analgesic medication. Treating the symptoms can be done in hospitals by seeking and using rescue orders, which could include a range of doses (1–2 mg, for example), or an adjuvant or rescue medication when the usual dose is insufficient. The nurse also can encourage the use of nonpharmacological interventions. *Interventions* should be followed by *reassessment* at the expected time of the greatest effect of the intervention, and *reintervention* if pain is still not relieved.

When testing a middle range theory, more specific concepts and testable hypotheses can be deducted from the more general concepts and prepositions (Good, 1998). *A balance between analgesia and side effects* is the general outcome. A researcher may wish to deduct more specific outcome concepts to study. To do this, the researcher would think of more specific components of the concept and state their relationships to the general concept. For example, the concept of side effects is a subset of the *balance between analgesia and side effects* outcome. Analgesia is the opposite of pain. Sensation and distress of pain can be deducted and studied individually if pain is conceptualized as a sensory and affective phenomenon (Good, 1998).

BOX 3-1. Nonpharmacological Adjuvants

RELAXATION

Jaw relaxation (Good, 1995; Good et al., 1999)

Autogenic phrases (Green, Green, & Norris, 1979)

Progressive muscle relaxation (Snyder, Pestka, & Bly, 2002)

Systematic relaxation (Roykulcharoen, 2003)

Slow rhythmic breathing

GUIDED IMAGERY

Self efficacy imagery (Tusek et al., 1997)

Pleasant imagery (Locsin, 1988)

Hypnosis (Olness, 1981)

MUSIC

Sedative music (Good et al., 1999, 2001)

Favorite music

Tempos (fast or slow)

Instruments

DESCRIPTION OF THE THEORY OF PAIN: A BALANCE BETWEEN ANALGESIA AND SIDE EFFECTS

The theory of a balance between analgesia and side effects is the first integrative prescriptive middle range pain management theory. Although the AHCPR acute pain guidelines, discussed earlier, are detailed, the theory provides a broader and more parsimonious overview. Its general principles of acute pain management serve as a framework for research and also as a guide for nursing practice with adults. The theorists expect practitioners to use the overall principles, along with the detailed knowledge contained in the adult acute pain guidelines and any new empirical evidence that has emerged since that time. These principles for practice are called "propositions" when theorizing or testing them through research. This terminology is a matter of function: principles for practice and theoretical propositions to test in research. With the idea that the purpose of theory is research and the purpose of research is theory, but the purpose of both is practice, this theory with its principles/propositions is organized for additional research and for teaching and communicating pain management to nurses. New research findings will add to the theory.

Further, the theory presents a new perspective: that the best pain management practice is an integrated one that combines analgesic medications with nonpharmacological adjuvants, careful nursing care, and patient participation. The goal of the theory is to achieve a balance between analgesia and side effects, which is a more holistic relief outcome than analgesia alone. The goal, then, is to balance pain relief and side effects of opioids by using the principles so that there is greater pain relief with fewer symptoms of side effects.

The assumptions of the theory are presented in Box 3-2. They are fairly narrow so that prescriptions can be specific. The theorists meant the theory to be tested and used clinically in adults having moderate to severe acute pain after surgery or trauma. The theory has limits; it does not address the treatment of pain in children, elders, or those with special kinds of acute pain. However, middle range theories have been or can be developed for these phenomena as well.

Propositions

The theory has three prescriptive propositions that can be summarized. In acute pain, patient participation, multimodal interventions, and attentive care are needed for a balance between analgesia and side effects.

BOX 3-2. Assumptions of the Theory of a Balance Between Analgesia and Side Effects

1. The nurse and physician collaborate to effectively manage acute pain.
2. Systemic opioid analgesics or epidural opioids or anesthetic agents are indicated.
3. Medication for side effects is given as needed.
4. Patients are adults with ability to learn, set goals, and communicate symptoms.
5. Nurses have current knowledge of pain management.

The first proposition is about patient participation. It proposes that patient teaching and goal setting contribute to a balance between analgesia and side effects (see Figure 3-1). This proposition is supported by meta-analyses for patient teaching (Devine, 1992; Devine & Cook, 1986; Shuldham, 1999) and expert opinion for goal setting (Acute Pain Management Guideline Panel, 1992). Patient teaching is a key concept to consider when trying to improve outcomes. Patient teaching should include ways to obtain medication, report pain, and use a nonpharmacological adjuvant.

The second proposition is about multimodal intervention. It proposes that nurses use potent pain medication plus pharmacological and nonpharmacological adjuvants to achieve a balance between analgesia and side effects. The effect on pain has empirical support published by the Acute Pain Management Guideline Panel and Good and colleagues (Good, Stanton-Hicks et al., 1999; Good et al., 2001; Good, Anderson, Stanton-Hicks, Grass, & Makii, 2002; Good, Stiller, et al., 1999).

The third proposition is about attentive care. It proposes that nurses assess, intervene, reassess, and reintervene to achieve a balance between analgesia and side effects. The effect on pain is supported by 20 years of research showing that pain is inadequately treated and by findings that regular assessment alone does not produce relief (Good, Auvil-Novak, & Group, 1994). Intervention, reassessment after a strategic interval, and reintervention by increasing the dose of analgesic and/or adding an adjuvant are needed and should continue until a satisfactory balance is attained (Good & Moore, 1996). Any part of the theory can be examined in research: one concept, new relationships between concepts, part of a proposition, all of a proposition, or the whole theory. In addition, the application to nursing practice or education can be studied.

APPLICATIONS OF THE THEORY

Research Support for the Theory

The theory is currently being tested further in two studies funded by the National Institute of Nursing Research (NINR). This support exemplifies the national interest and support for nursing research on pain management (Good, Anderson, Wotman, & Albert, 2001–2005). In the latest study, a short patient-teaching tape that is specific to pain control is being compared with a relaxation and music tape and a third tape that combines them.

The relaxation and music audio tapes provided an average of up to a mean of 31% more relief than PCA alone in the first NINR study (Good et al., 1999), and the patient-teaching tape was added in the second study to lower pain even more. In the second study, which is also funded by NINR, the patient-teaching tape encourages patients to dismiss fears of opioid dependency, to use their patient-controlled analgesia system (PCA), and to communicate pain with their nurse until relief is obtained. Postoperative abdominal surgery patients are encouraged to use the randomly assigned tape as much as possible the first 2 days. Pain and side effects are being measured four times a day and will be analyzed longitudinally. In addition, there are five cross-sectional pre- and posttests in which pain is being measured before and after 20 minutes of listening to the tape (or lying in bed for controls). In some of these, saliva samples are being obtained to determine the effects of the intervention on stress (salivary cortisol) and immune factors (salivary IgA). In addition, complications and rate of recovery from surgery will be measured and related to minutes of tape use as recorded on a timing device.

This study is expected to demonstrate that relaxation, music, and patient teaching for pain management reduce pain and side effects over time during the first 2 postoperative days. Secondarily, the effects on recovery will be explored. If the theory is supported, patients undergoing surgery will have more options, sufficient pain relief, and will go home in better physical condition.

The results are expected to support the theory in three ways. First, they are expected to support the proposition that patient teaching contributes to lower pain; second, they are expected to support the proposition that pharmacological and nonpharmacological interventions reduce pain; and third, they also reduce side effects more than analgesics alone. The goal is to relieve postoperative pain, using the optimal pharmacological and nonpharmacological blend to achieve a balance between analgesia and side effects.

Using Middle Range Theories 3-1 summarizes earlier findings supporting the theory's propositions.

 3-1 USING MIDDLE RANGE THEORIES

The theory of a balance between analgesia and side effects was first tested in a large randomized clinical trial sponsored by the National Institute of Nursing Research from 1994 to 1998. This study was published first as a cross-sectional study in 1999 and later as a repeated measures study in 2001. The researchers wanted to test the effects of jaw relaxation, soft music, and the combination of relaxation and music on postoperative pain in abdominal surgical patients who were receiving patient-controlled analgesia. Patients were recruited from the preadmission testing departments of five hospitals in northeast Ohio, and were tested at ambulation and rest on postoperative days 1 and 2. Patients marked the visual analogue sensation and distress of pain scales for self-reported pain before and after listening to the tapes during 15 minutes of rest, and at four times during ambulation each day. Patients in the control group did not receive a tape but were asked to rest in bed during the test and to ambulate according to hospital practice during the test at ambulation. All patients were told they could use PCA as much as they desired. In this cross-sectional study, the researchers used multivariate analysis of covariance (MANCOVA), with the pretests as the covariate, and sensation and distress as the multivariate- dependent variable. They found that the three nonpharmacological interventions as a group resulted in significantly less pain (10%–31%) than the control group, and that the three interventions were not different from one another in their effect. Posthoc univariate analysis of covariance (ANCOVA) with sensation or distress as a single dependent variable was then used; it found that compared to controls, the combination of relaxation and music resulted in significantly less sensation and distress of pain at each of 12 data points. Jaw relaxation and music, used separately, reduced pain at most data points, with mixed findings at the after-ambulation point, probably due to increased pain and loss of mental focus on relaxation while getting back into bed.

Longitudinal analysis was done across the same data points, with repeated measures MANCOVA (Good et al., 2001). The interventions were found to be effective across each day (day 1 and 2) and across each activity (ambulation and rest), and the effects were similar at ambulation and rest. Based on these studies, the researchers reported support for the part of the theory that they tested: in addition to strong medication, the three nonpharmacological interventions reduced pain. Side effects and pharmacological adjuvants were not studied nor was the balance itself. The concept of pain was deducted from the concept of the balance between analgesia and side effects.

Good, M., Stanton-Hicks, M., Grass, J. A., Anderson, G. C., Choi, C. C., Schoolmeesters, L., & Salman, A. (1999). Relief of postoperative pain with jaw relaxation, music, and their combination. *Pain, 81*(1–2), 163–172.

Good, M., Stanton-Hicks, M., Grass, J. A., Anderson, G. C., Lai, H. L., Roykulcharoen, V., & Adler, P. A. (2001). Relaxation and music to reduce postsurgical pain. *Journal of Advanced Nursing, 33*(2), 208–215.

Suggestions for Additional Research

This theory is useful for intervention research with experimental designs in clinical populations. Such studies are called randomized controlled trials (RCT). The theory is useful in alert adult populations in which pain is incompletely controlled by medication alone, and side effects may preclude taking increased amounts of analgesic medication. The theory should be used with adults who are able to learn, set goals, and communicate symptoms. The cornerstone is the first proposition of the theory: that patient teaching and goal setting are needed for the *balance between analgesia and side effects.*

The theory is prescriptive, but can be combined with the gate control theory used to explain the mechanism of effect. The gate control mechanism is that therapies such as music, relaxation techniques, and guided imagery relax and distract, allowing the brain to exert descending control of the transmission of noxious impulses (Good et al., 1999). It is possible that the theory could be extended to chronic pain populations, and the interventions could be tested in pain that persists for a longer period of time.

Research Application 3-1 demonstrates the integration of gate control mechanisms in a study of pain after abdominal surgery.

3-1 RESEARCH APPLICATION

A nurse researcher is conducting a study in which the research question is "What is the effect of relaxation and music, patient teaching for pain management, and the combination of both on postoperative pain, side effects of opioids, stress, and secretory immunoglobulin A?" The human subjects committees of the school of nursing, the university, and the hospital have approved the study. Using an RCT, the researcher reviews the surgery schedule each day to identify males and females scheduled for major abdominal surgery who meet the criterion for age (18–75 years) and are expecting to receive general anesthesia and patient-controlled analgesia (PCA).

(continued)

3-1 RESEARCH APPLICATION

(continued)

The researcher arrives at the hospital at 6:00 AM and introduces herself to Mr. Green, who has been admitted to the surgical waiting area for a 7:30 AM colectomy for cancer, but has not yet received any premedication that would compromise his ability to give consent.

After obtaining written informed consent, the nurse conducts a brief interview and teaches Mr. Green to use the Sensation and Distress of Pain Visual Analogue Scales (Good et al., 2001). The researcher uses a computerized minimization program to randomly assign Mr. Green to one of four groups, while balancing the groups on potentially confounding variables such as age, sex, race, type of surgery, chronic pain, smoking, alcohol use, and time of surgery (Zeller, Good, Anderson, & Zeller, 1997). The groups are: (a) relaxation and music; (b) patient teaching for pain management; (c) the combination of the two; and (d) the control group, which receives the usual care. Mr. Green's assignment is the combination of relaxation, music, and patient teaching. He then listens to the 9-minute teaching tape giving him instruction in using the jaw relaxation technique and offering him a choice among six types of sedative instrumental music (Gaston, 1951). He listens to 20 seconds of each type of music: synthesizer, harp, piano, orchestra, jazz, and inspirational. Mr. Green chooses the inspirational music.

After surgery, Mr. Green is taken to his postoperative room, and the nurse researcher goes to the bedside to conduct the first pretest-posttest. She asks him to rate the intensity of his sensation and distress of pain on the dual VAS scales, and then she obtains pulse and respirations. She gives him the tape and recorder, and plays his assigned tape for 20 minutes. The tape reviews his role in pain management, guides him in the use of a relaxation technique, and plays soft inspirational music for 20 minutes. The researcher asks him to rate his pain again for the posttest and records his pulse and respirations. She shows Mr. Green and his wife and daughter how to use the tape recorder and encourages him to use it as much as possible for the rest of the day, evening, and even during the night. The idea is to get pain under control early in the postoperative period and keep it controlled.

For the next two days at 8 AM, 12 noon, 4 PM, and 8 PM, a research nurse or graduate student comes to the bedside to ask about pain and side effects of opioids. In addition, at 10 AM and 2 PM each day, the research nurse conducts 20-minute pre- and posttests. On day 2, she also collects pretest and posttest saliva specimens. The patient's chart is reviewed at each visit for medications and other factors that could confound the outcome. At 8 AM on the 3rd day, the research nurse conducts a structured interview, asking about demographics and information on contextual variables that might confound the outcome. Mr. Green is thanked for participating in the study and for his contribution to nursing knowledge about pain management. A $20 gift certificate is mailed to subjects who complete the study.

The data recorded on the questionnaire is coded and entered into an SPSS statistical program file by graduate student assistants who are learning to become researchers. The principal investigator and the project manager will analyze the data to determine whether or not

(continued)

(continued) **3-1 RESEARCH APPLICATION**

the interventions reduce pain, side effects of opioids, stress, and/or improve immunity. The findings will be written up in a manuscript and sent to a peer-reviewed research journal for publication. The results are expected to support the theory by finding that patient teaching contributes to lower pain, and that patient teaching for using pharmacological and nonpharmacological interventions reduces pain and side effects.

INSTRUMENTS USED IN EMPIRICAL TESTING

There are many pain scales used to measure pain. In an effort to capture and study the experience of pain, researchers have created so many scales that it is difficult to compare scores across studies, making synthesis of the literature difficult. For example, a five-point scale cannot be easily equated to an eight-point scale.

Different scales, however, are needed to measure the experience of each type of pain (e.g., acute, chronic, cancer, labor, and pediatric pain). For example, the pain of advanced cancer patients is qualitatively, quantitatively, and temporally different from the pain of arthritis or labor. Nurses, who are sensitive to these differences, have been instrumental in creating new instruments to measure pain, but now must consider some sort of standardization across studies so that they can be compared. Different scales are also needed for each component of pain (e.g., sensory and affective pain).

Some scales contain both numeric intensity measures and descriptors such as "mild," "moderate," and "severe" to guide responses of subjects. Examples of these combinations are the 0–10 Numeric Pain Intensity Scale and the 0–10 Numeric Pain Distress Scale (Acute Pain Management Guideline Panel, 1992). Visual analogue scales (VAS) have a horizontal line with no numbers and only descriptive anchors at each end (Good, et al., 2001).

The Word–Graphic Rating Scale for adolescents and children is a horizontal line with five verbal descriptors under the line, but no numbers or upright lines (Good et al., 2001; Savedra, Tesler, Holzemer, & Ward, 1989). This scale may produce more evenly distributed scores than numerical scales, but the presence of the words may still serve as a clustering factor, even when patients are told to mark anywhere along the line (Good et al., 2001; Savedra, Tesler, Holzemer, & Ward, 1989). Patients notice the numbers and verbal descriptors and tend to make their mark near them.

Another solution may be to identify the widely used and sensitive VAS as a "gold standard," and administer it, followed by a brief descriptor scale *and* a scale that researchers think is most specific to the health condition. This would provide specificity as well as sensitivity to the type of pain experienced, but could also be used to standardize all three measures of pain in various populations and increase communication and synthesis across studies. This combination would also permit analysis of criterion-related validity of the scales when compared to the gold standard, and concurrent validity when the other scales are compared. Although the McGill Pain Questionnaire contains three measures, including a descriptive scale, VAS and a numerical-description rating scale, it could be used for standardization in this manner. Table 3-2 lists instruments and indicates the type of pain measured by each.

Table 3-2. INSTRUMENTS TO MEASURE PAIN

CATEGORY	ABBREVIATION	NAME OF SCALE AND CITATION
Pain	VAS	Visual Analogue Scale [a]
Sensory pain	-	VAS Sensation of Pain Scale [b]
Sensory pain	-	Numeric Pain Intensity Scale [c]
Sensory pain	-	Descriptive Pain Intensity Scale [d]
Affective pain	-	VAS Distress of Pain Scale [e]
Affective pain	-	Numeric Pain Distress Scale [f]
Affective pain	-	Descriptive Pain Distress Scale [g]
Affective pain	-	VAS Unpleasantness Scale [h]
Affective pain	-	VAS Anxiety of Pain Scale [i]
Affective pain	MPQ	McGill Pain Questionnaire [j]
Total pain	MPQ-PRI	Pain Rating Index (PRI)
Sensory pain	PRI-sensory	Sensory subscale
Affective pain	PRI-affective	Affective subscale
Pain intensity	MPQ-NWC	Number of Words Chosen
Pain intensity	MPQ-PPI	Present Pain Index
Pain intensity	MPQ-VAS	Visual Analogue Scale
Total, sensory, & affective pain	MPQ-SF	McGill Pain Questionnaire–Short Form [k]
Chronic pain	UAB	University of Alabama–Birmingham Pain Behavior Scale [l]
Chronic pain	WHYMPI	West Haven–Yale Multidimensional Pain Inventory [m]
Cancer pain	BPI	Brief Pain Inventory [n]
Cancer pain, relief, mood	MPAC	Memorial Pain Assessment Card [o]
24-hour time-intensity	-	Keele's Pain Chart [p]
Labor pain	-	Behavioral Index for Assessment of Labor Pain [q]
Children's pain	-	Poker Chip Scale [r]
Children's pain	-	Word-Graphic Rating Scale [s]
Children's pain	-	Oucher Scale [t]
Children's pain	-	Wong-Baker Faces Scale [u]
Young children's pain	FLACC	Faces, legs, activity, cry, consolability [v]

- = no abbreviation;

[a, b, e] Good et al., 2001; [b, c, d, e, f, g, r, s] Acute Pain Management Guidelines, 1992; [h] Price et al.,1983; [i] McCormack, et al., 1988[s]; [j, k] Melzack, 1975; [l] Richards et al., 1982; [m] Kerns, Turk, & Rudy, 1985; [n] Daut, Cleeland, & Flanery, 1983; [o] Fishman et al., 1986; [p] Keele, 1948; [q] Bonnel & Boureau, 1985; [t] Beyer, Denyes, & Villarruel, 1992; [u] Wong & Baker, 1988; [v] Merkel, Voepel-Lewis, Shayevitz, & Malviya, 1997.

SUMMARY

Pain is a universal human experience that has been known since the first human experienced illness, trauma, or labor. Although pain has been studied descriptively for more than a century, it has only recently been studied from a prescriptive nursing perspective. The middle range prescriptive pain management theory of a balance between analgesic and side effects reflects the nursing mission to intervene effectively and holistically to relieve pain, suffering, and to prevent their long-term effects. Nurse researchers who wish to study pain with this theory can test it further and provide support and creative extensions of the theory. Practicing nurses can use the evidence-based principles for effective relief of acute pain in their patients.

ANALYSIS EXERCISE

Using the criteria presented in Chapter 2, critique the Theory of a Balance Between Analgesia and Side Effects. Compare your conclusions about the theory with those found in Appendix A. A researcher who has worked with the theory completed the analysis found in the Appendix.

Internal Criticism
1. Clarity
2. Consistency
3. Adequacy

4. Logical development
5. Level of theory development

External Criticism
1. Reality convergence
2. Utility
3. Significance
4. Discrimination
5. Scope of theory
6. Complexity

WEB RESOURCES

1. National Institute of Nursing Research (NINR): *http://www.nih.gov/ninr*
2. National Center for Complementary and Alternative Medicine: *http://www.nccam.nih.gov*
3. Sigma Theta Tau International Nursing Society, Virginia Henderson International Nursing Library; keyword, "pain": *http://www.stti.iupui. edu/library/librarysearch.html*
4. The American Pain Society (APS) is the leading US organization committed to pain management. The mission is to advance pain-related research, education, treatment, and professional practice. It is a multidisciplinary society of basic and clinical scientists, clinicians and others: *http://www.ampainsoc.org*

5. The American Pain Society publishes: Journal of Pain: *http://www.ampainsoc.org/ pub/bulletin/jan01/commu1.htm* APS Bulletin: *http://www.ampainsoc.org/pub/ bulletin* It has recently released the guidelines for managing acute and chronic pain of arthritis: *http://www.ampainsoc.org/pub/arthritis.htm* and sickle cell disease: *http://www. ampainsoc.org/pub/sc.htm*
6. The International Association for the Study of Pain (IASP) is the largest multidisciplinary international organization in the field of pain and is dedicated to furthering research and improving patient care. Currently, IASP has 6744 individual members from 107 countries. *http://www.iasp-pain.org*

WEB RESOURCES

7. PAIN is the official publication of the IASP. It publishes original research on the nature, mechanisms, and treatment of pain of multidisciplinary interest. *http://www.elsevier.nl/inca/publications/store/5/0/6/0/8/3/index.htt*

8. American Association of Pain Management Nurses (ASPMN) is an organization of professional nurses dedicated to promoting and providing optimal care of patients with pain through education, standards, advocacy, and research (7794 Grow Drive, Pensacola, FL 32514, (888) 34-ASPMN, Fax: (850) 484-8762, e-mail: aspmn@puetzamc.com) *http://www.aspmn.org*

9. Pain Management Nursing (PMN) is a peer-reviewed journal, indexed in Index Medicus. It reports the unique nursing focus on pain management. Original and review articles from experts offer insight into clinical practice, advocacy, education, administration, and research. Additional features are practice guidelines and pharmacology updates: *http://www.harcourthealth.com*

10. The European Journal of Pain is a multidisciplinary international journal. It aims to become a global forum on major aspects of pain and pain management: *http://intl.elsevier-health.com/journals/eujp/subscribe.cfm*

11. Alternative therapies: *http://www.holisticonline.com/hol_alt-therapies.htm*

12. Mind–body therapy: *http://www.holisticonline.com/hol_mindcontrol.htm*

13. The Cancer Pain & Symptom Management Nursing Research Group is an innovative, group of researchers focused on the generation and dissemination of knowledge related to the pain and other symptoms in persons with cancer and those at the end-of-life. *http://www.son.washington.edu/departments/bnhs/pain*

14. Clinical Practice Guidelines Online can be accessed through an electronic full-text retrieval system called HSTAT (Health Services Technology Assessment Text) at the National Library of Medicine: *http://www.ahcpr.gov/clinic/cpgonline.htm*

REFERENCES

Acute Pain Management Guideline Panel. (1992). *Acute pain management: Operative or medical procedures and trauma. Clinical practice guideline*. Rockville, MD: Agency for Health Care Policy and Research, Public Health Service, U. S. Department of Health and Human Services. (Vol. AHCPR No. 92-0032).

Albert, R. E. (2002). *Effect of guided imagery and music on pain during laceration repair in the emergency department*. Unpublished dissertation, Case Western Reserve University, Cleveland OH.

Auvil-Novak, S. E. (1997). A middle-range theory of chronotherapeutic intervention for postsurgical pain. *Nursing Research, 46*(2), 66–71.

Beecher, H. K. (1959). *Measurement of subjective responses: Quantitative effects of drugs*. New York: Oxford University Press.

Beyer, J. E., Denyes, M. J., & Villarruel, A. M. (1992). The creation, validation, and continuing development of the Oucher: A measure of pain intensity in children. *Journal of Pediatric Nursing, 7*(5), 335–346.

Bonnel, A. M., & Boureau, F. (1985). Labor pain assessment: Validity of a behavioral index. *Pain, 22*(1), 81.

Casey, K. L., & Melzack, R. (1967). Neural mechanisms of pain: A conceptual model. In E. L. Way (Ed.), *New concepts in pain and its clinical management* (pp. 13–31). Philadelphia: F. A. Davis.

Ceccio, C. M. (1984). Postoperative pain relief through relaxation in elderly patients with fractured hips. *Orthopaedic Nursing, 3*(3), 11–14.

Dalton, J. A., & Blau, W. (1996). Changing the practice of pain management: An examination of the theoretical basis of change. *Pain Forum, 5*(4), 266–272.

Daut, R. L., Cleeland, C. S., & Flanery, R. C. (1983). Development of the Wisconsin brief pain questionnaire to assess pain in cancer and other diseases. *Pain, 17*, 197–210.

Devine, E. C. (1992). Effects of psychoeducational care for adult surgical patients: A meta-analysis of 191 studies. *Patient Education and Counseling, 19*, 129–142.

Devine, E. C., & Cook, T. D. (1986). Clinical and cost saving effects of psychoeducational interventions with surgical patients: A meta analysis. *Research in Nursing and Health, 9*, 89–105.

Dickhoff, J., & James, P. (1968). A theory of theories: A position paper. *Nursing Research, 17*(3), 197–203.

Fishman, B., Pasternak, S., Wallenstein, S. L., Houde, R.W., Holland, J. C., & Foley, K. M. (1987). The Memorial Pain Assessment Card: A valid instrument for the evaluation of cancer pain. *Cancer, 60*(5), 1151–1158.

Flaherty, G. G., & Fitzpatrick, J. J. (1978). Relaxation technique to increase comfort level of postoperative patients: A preliminary study. *Nursing Research, 27*(6), 352–355.

Gaston, E. T. (1951). Dynamic music factors in mood changes. *Music Educators Journal, 37*, 42–44.

Good, M. (1995). A comparison of the effects of jaw relaxation and music on postoperative pain. *Nursing Research, 44*(1), 52–57.

Good, M. (1998). A middle range theory of acute pain management; use in research. *Nursing Outlook, 46*(3), 120–124.

Good, M., Stanton-Hicks, M., Grass, J. A., Lai, H. L., Roykulcharoen, V., & Adler, P. A. (2001). Jaw relaxation, music, and the combination reduce postoperative pain across days and activities. *Journal of Advanced Nursing, 33*(2), 208–215.

Good, M., Anderson, G., Stanton-Hicks, M., Grass, J., & Makii, M. (2002). Relaxation and music reduce pain following gynecological surgery. *Pain Management Nursing, 3*(2), 61–70.

Good, M., Anderson, G. C., Wotman, S., & Albert, J. (2001–2005). Supplementing relaxation and music for postoperative pain. National Institute of Nursing Research. (National Institutes of Health, Bethesda, MD, Grant number R013933).

Good, M., Auvil-Novak, S., & Group, M. (1994). *Pain and its management: One year after the guidelines.* Paper presented at the AHSR & FSHR Annual Conference, June 12–14. Health Services Research, San Diego, CA.

Good, M., & Moore, S. M. (1996). Clinical practice guidelines as a new source of middle-range theory: Focus on acute pain. *Nursing Outlook, 44*(2), 74–79.

Good, M., Picot, B., Salem, S., Chin, C., Picot, S., & Lane, D. (2000). Cultural responses to music for pain relief. *Journal of Holistic Nursing, 18*(3), 245–260.

Good, M., Stanton-Hicks, M., Grass, J. M., Anderson, G. C., Choi, C. C., Schoolmeesters, L., & Salman, A. (1999). Relief of postoperative pain with jaw relaxation, music, and their combination. *Pain, 81*(1–2), 163–172.

Good, M., Stiller, C., Zauszniewski, J., Stanton-Hicks, M., Grass, J., & Anderson, G. C. (2001). Sensation and distress of pain scales: Reliability, validity and sensitivity. *Journal of Nursing Measurement, 9*(3), 219–238.

Green, E. E., Green, A. M., & Norris, P. A. (1979). Preliminary observation on a new-drug method for control of hypertension. *Journal of the South Carolina Medical Association, 75*(11), 575–582.

Greipp, M. E. (1992). Undermedication for pain: An ethical model. *Advances in Nursing Science, 15*(1), 44–53.

Huth, M. M. (2001). *Guided imagery to reduce postoperative pain in children.* Unpublished dissertation, Case Western Reserve University, Cleveland, OH.

Huth, M. M., & Moore, S. M. (1998). Prescriptive theory of acute pain management in infants and children. *Journal of the Society of Pediatric Nursing, 3*(1), 23–32.

Jacobsen, E. (1938). *Progressive relaxation.* Chicago: University of Chicago Press.

Johnson, J. E. (1973). Effects of accurate expectations about sensations on the sensory and distress components of pain. *Journal of Personality and Social Psychology, 27*, 261–275.

Johnson, J. E., & Rice, V. H. (1974). Sensory and distress components of pain: Implications for the study of clinical pain. *Nursing Research, 23*, 203–209.

Keele, K. D. (1948, July 3). The pain chart. *Lancet, 2*, 6–8.

Kerns, R. D., Turk, D. C., & Rudy, T. E. (1985). The West Haven–Yale Multidimensional Pain Inventory (WHYMPI). *Pain, 23*(4), 345.

Keyser, J. (2002, August 11). Archaeologists uncover ancient drug trade. *The Plain Dealer*, 3.

Kolcaba, K. Y. (1994). A theory of holistic comfort for nursing. *Journal of Advanced Nursing, 19*, 1178–1184.

Lenz, E. R., Pugh, L. C., Milligan, R. A., Gift, A., & Suppe, F. (1997). The middle-range theory of unpleasant symptoms: An update. *Advances in Nursing Science, 19*(3), 14–27.

Locsin, R. (1988). Effects of preferred music and guided imagery music on the pain of selected postoperative patients. *ANPHI Papers, 23*(1), 2–4.

Mahon, S. M. (1994). Concept analysis of pain: Implications related to nursing diagnoses. *Nursing Diagnosis, 5*(1), 14–25.

McCormak, H. M., del Horne, D. J., & Sheather, S. (1988). Clinical applications of visual analogue scales: A critical review. *Psychological Medicine, 18*, 1007–1009.

Melzack, R. (1975). The McGill Pain Questionnaire: Major properties and scoring methods. *Pain, 1*, 277–299.

Melzack, R. (1982). Recent concepts of pain. *Journal of Medicine, 13*, 147–160.

Melzack, R. (1996). Gate control theory. *Pain Forum, 5*(2), 128–138.

Melzack, R., & Wall, P. D. (1962). On the nature of cutaneous sensory mechanisms. *Brain, 85*, 331.

Melzack, R., & Wall, P. D. (1965). Pain mechanisms: A new theory. *Science, 150*(3699), 971–979.

Merkel, S. I., Voepel-Lewis, T., Shayevitz, J. R., & Malviya, S. (1997). The FLACC: A behavioral scale for scoring postoperative pain in young children. *Pediatric Nursing, 23*(3), 293–297.

Morse, J. M., Bottorff, J. L., & Hutchinson, S. (1995). The paradox of comfort. *Nursing Research, 44*(1), 14–19.

Olness, K. (1981). Self-hypnosis as adjunct therapy in childhood cancer: Clinical experience with 25 patients. *American Journal of Pediatric Hematology Oncology, 3*, 313–321.

Olness, K. (1989). Hypnotherapy: A cyberphysiologic strategy in pain management. *Pediatric Clinics of North America, 36*(4), 873–884.

Padgett, D. A., Marucha, P. T., & Sheridan, J. F. (1998). Restraint stress slows cutaneous wound healing in mice. *Brain, Behavior, and Immunity, 12*(1), 64–73.

Page, G. G. (1996). The medical necessity of adequate pain management. *Pain Forum, 5*(4), 227–233.

Page, G. G., Ben-Eliyahu, S., Yirmiya, R., & Liebeskind, J. C. (1993). Morphine attenuates surgery-induced enhancement of metastatic colonization in rats. *Pain, 54*(1), 21–28.

Price, D. D., Harkins, S. W., & Baker, C. (1987). Sensory-affective relationships among different types of clinical and experimental pain. *Pain, 28,* 297–307.

Price, D. D., McGrath, P. A., Rafii, A., & Buckingham, B. (1983). The validation of visual analogue scales as ratio scale measures for chronic and experimental pain. *Pain, 17*(1), 45–56.

Rathbone, J. L. (1943). *Relaxation.* Teachers College, Columbia University, New York.

Richards, J. S., Nepomuceno, C., Riles, M., & Suer, Z. (1982). Assessing pain behavior: The UAB pain behavior scale. *Pain, 14*(4), 393.

Roykulcharoen, V. (2003). The effect of a systematic relaxation technique on postoperative pain in Thailand. Unpublished dissertation, Case Western Reserve University, Cleveland, Ohio.

Savedra, M. C., Tesler, M. D., Holzemer, W. L., & Ward, J. A. (1989). *Adolescent pediatric pain tool (APPT): Preliminary user's manual.* San Francisco: University of California.

Shuldham, C. (1999). A review of the impact of pre-operative education on recovery from surgery. *International Journal of Nursing Studies, 36*(2), 171–177.

Simon, J. M., Baumann, M. A., & Nolan, L. (1995). Differential diagnostic validation: Acute and chronic pain. *Nursing Diagnosis, 6*(2), 73–79.

Snyder, M., Pestka, E., & Bly, C. (2002). Progressive muscle relaxation. In M. Snyder & R. Lindquist (Eds.), *Complementary/Alternative therapies in nursing* (4th ed., pp. 310–319). New York: Springer.

Sternbach, R. A. (1984). Acute vs. chronic pain. In R. Melzack & P. D. Wall (Eds.), *Textbook of pain* (pp. 173–177). New York: Churchill Livingstone.

Tusek, D. L., Church, J. M., Strong, S. A., Grass, J. A., & Fazio, V. W. (1997). Guided imagery: A significant advance in the care of patients undergoing elective colorectal surgery. *Diseases of the Colon and Rectum, 40*(2), 172–178.

Tusek, D. L., Cwynar, R., & Cosgrove, D. M. (1999). Effect of guided imagery on length of stay, pain and anxiety in cardiac surgery patients. *Journal of Cardiovascular Management, 10*(2), 22–28.

Wong, D. L., & Baker, C. M. (1988). Pain in children: Comparison of assessment scales. *Pediatric Nursing, 14*(1), 9–17.

Zeller, J. M., McCain, N. L., & Swanson, B. (1996). Psychoneuroimmunology: An emerging framework for nursing research. *Journal of Advanced Nursing, 23,* 657–664.

Zeller, R., Good, M., Anderson, G. C., & Zeller, D. (1997). Strengthening experimental design by balancing confounding variables across eight treatment groups. *Nursing Research, 46*(6), 345–349.

This chapter was supported in part by the National Institute of Nursing Research, NIH, Grant Number R01 NR3933 (1994–2005), to M. Good, PhD, Principal Investigator, and by the General Clinical Research Center, Case Western Reserve University.

Unpleasant Symptoms

AUDREY GIFT

DEFINITION OF KEY TERMS

Performance	Performance is the outcome or effect of the symptom experience. It includes functional and cognitive activities. Functional performance includes activities of daily living (ADLs), social interaction, and role performance. Quality of life is a part of performance.
Physiological factors	Physiological factors are the normal or abnormal functioning of bodily systems. They may include indicators of disease severity, comorbidities, nutritional balance, or hydration.
Psychological factors	Psychological factors include the mental state or mood, affective reaction to illness, and the degree of uncertainty and knowledge about the symptoms and their possible meaning.
Situational factors	Situational factors include aspects of the social and physical environment that surround the person and may influence the experience and reporting of symptoms. They also include environmental factors, such as heat, humidity, noise, light, and air quality. They may include socioeconomical factors, marital status, social support, and lifestyle behaviors, such as exercise and diet.
Unpleasant symptoms	Symptoms are the perceived indicators of change in normal functioning as experienced by patients. They are the subjective indicators of threats to health.

INTRODUCTION

The Theory of Unpleasant Symptoms (TOUS) is a relatively new middle range nursing theory—the original concept paper appeared in 1995 and was revised in 1997. It was developed and intended for application and use by nurses. The theory uniquely allows for the presence of multiple symptoms and implies that management of one symptom will contribute to the management of other symptoms.

HISTORICAL BACKGROUND

The TOUS originated when Drs. Linda Pugh and Audrey Gift were writing a chapter for the *Nursing Clinics of North America*. The chapter was to be titled "Dyspnea and Fatigue," Gift writing the dyspnea section and Pugh the fatigue section. They began meeting to develop a common outline for the two sections of the chapter. Working on the chapter outline, they realized that they were similar in their thinking about the two symptoms. Each had hypothesized antecedent or influencing factors that would impact their symptom. Each had hypothesized their symptom to occur in the context of environmental or situational factors that would influence the reporting of the symptom. Additionally, each had hypothesized the symptom as influencing performance. Also, they were both familiar enough with the pain literature to know that similar models had been proposed for pain.

In addition to noting similar models for the symptoms, they realized that similar interventions, such as the use of progressive muscle relaxation, had been proposed and tested for both the symptom of dyspnea and fatigue. These management techniques were similar to those proposed for the management of pain. Thus, they imagined that if a nurse had one model that helped her or him to understand all symptoms and how to manage them, it would advance nursing practice. They decided to call that model the Theory of Unpleasant Symptoms.

After completing the "Dyspnea and Fatigue" chapter, Drs. Gift and Pugh began to work on developing the TOUS. However, they were not able to successfully describe their model in a manner acceptable for publication. After having the manuscript rejected by two journals, they decided they needed collaborators more experienced at writing about theory. They contacted Dr. Elizabeth Lenz, who was an expert on theory development and had done research related to pain in the cardiac patient, and asked her to collaborate on the development of the TOUS. Because the focus of the manuscript was changed to further develop the model, requiring extensive revision of the manuscript, it was agreed that Dr. Lenz would be first author. Since Dr. Pugh had developed many of her ideas about fatigue in her collaboration with Dr. Milligan, she was invited to collaborate on the development of the TOUS. Dr. Lenz took the lead to call the collaborators together to further develop the model. She also contacted Dr. Suppe, a philosopher with much experience related to nursing science. The authors began meeting regularly to develop the model, assign writing tasks, and discuss each other's work. The collaboration became a source of idea development for the authors, and the meetings continued after the manuscript was accepted for publication (Lenz, Suppe, Gift, Pugh, & Milligan, 1995).

It was in the later meetings that work began on the revision of the model. The desire was to make the model less linear and reflect the dynamic clinical situation the authors had observed. The collaborators reviewed the symptom literature once again and began to redesign the model. The work accelerated when there was a call for theory revision manuscripts, and the collaborators decided to publish their update. The second article was published 2 years after the first article (Lenz, Pugh, Milligan, Gift, & Suppe, 1997). Thus, the TOUS originated from clinical observations, a review of the symptom research literature, and a sharing among investigators. Refining the theory and communicating those ideas to the nursing community required the collaboration of those with an in-depth understanding of a clinical population who regularly experienced symptoms, those who knew the research literature related to at least one symptom, as well as those with expertise in theory development and skill in writing theoretical articles.

DEFINITION OF THEORY CONCEPTS

While some use symptoms simply as a means to identify and characterize the underlying disease, most symptom models established in the nursing literature conceptualize theories more holistically and include physiological, psychological, cognitive, and/or social aspects. Symptoms are seen as belonging to the lived experience of the illness rather than being a precise map of the underlying disease (Benner & Wrebel, 1989). Symptom theories within the nursing literature focus on the symptom experience or are designed to provide a framework for symptom management.

Nociceptive Model of Dyspnea

An example of a symptom theory that is focused on the symptom experience is the nociceptive model of dyspnea (Steele & Shaver, 1992). This theory is characterized as an ecological model of dyspnea because it provides a psychosocial framework for guiding nursing science, allowing for the interactive effects of multiple individual and environmental influences. It includes multiple feedback loops, with internal and external variables, and biobehavioral outcomes that reflect multiple dependencies. Environmental factors that affect symptoms include living conditions, economic status, air quality, work and family demands, as well as perceived social support. Individual factors include disease severity, duration of disease, trajectory of disease process, vulnerability, and resilience, as well as the nature of the symptom experience. Biobehavioral outcomes include individual adaptations, life management strategies, and tolerance for the symptom.

Symptom Interpretation Model

Another model of the symptom experience is the Symptom Interpretation Model (SIM), which focuses on cognition from an intrapersonal perspective (Teel, Meek, McNamara, & Watson, 1997). It includes conceptual identification, use of knowledge structures, and reasoning. An individual's knowledge of a symptom and the meaning attached are critical to understanding outcomes relative to the symptom.

Three major constructs of the model are input, interpretation, and outcome. Input includes the recognition of a disturbance in the human system. It must be of sufficient magnitude and impact to stimulate an awareness of something being different. The repetition of the stimulus affects the threshold at which the stimulus is brought to awareness to initiate interpretation and cognitive appraisal. Awareness is shaped by personal history, current context, and individual factors.

Interpretation, the second construct in the SIM model, is the naming of the sensation and attaching meaning to the symptom by activating stored information and reasoning about the symptom. Three elements of appraisal are critical to symptom recognition and discrimination. They consist of conceptual identification, knowledge structures, and reasoning. Conceptual identification is a judgment about the similarity between a disturbance and established knowledge structures. Knowledge structures include definitions, exemplars, prototypes, and mental models that are needed for symptom interpretation. Reasoning is the third component of interpretation. It involves a comparative process in which similarity is determined between an input and knowledge structure. Comparisons are made to worst symptom experiences (exemplars) and typical symptom patterns (prototype), leading to the interpretation of symptoms.

Outcome, the third major construct in the SIM model, involves having the individual make decisions about the sensation and doing something or nothing about it. Consequences of these outcome actions and behaviors are fed back into the interpretation of the symptom, modifying knowledge, and affecting future symptom interpretations. Over time, the individual recognizes patterns that inform future responses. The outcome component of the SIM is whether or not an individual is going to take action and what action is taken. The meaning attached to the sensation influences the outcome. The SIM explains the process the patient goes through in interpreting symptoms and deciding management strategies. It also points to potential patient education topics, such as focusing on the meaning of symptoms in specific situations.

Model of Chronic Dyspnea

While the SIM focuses on the cognitive processes that influence symptom interpretation, it does not model the symptom experience over time. The only known model to examine changes in perception and behavior that occur when a symptom is experienced continuously over time is the Model of Chronic Dyspnea (McCarley, 1999). In this model, dyspnea is seen from a longitudinal perspective, as waxing and waning over time, occasionally increasing greatly, only to eventually return to baseline, but with the baseline (usual dyspnea) slowly increasing over time. The model has three components: physiologic antecedents, dyspnea, and the consequences of dyspnea. The physiologic antecedents are conceptualized as being of lesser importance in chronic dyspnea than in acute dyspnea. The main focus of this model is the ever-present dyspnea, which is depicted as having a gradually increasing baseline interspersed with episodes of acute dyspnea. Acute episodes are precipitated by physical, environmental, or psychoemotional factors. The consequences of chronic dyspnea include reduced activities, fatigue, depression, and social isolation. Reduced activity results in physical deconditioning, leading to dyspnea at a lower level of activity. There is also the constant threat of a bout of acute dyspnea. This threat contributes further to the decrease in physical activities and the downward spiral of physical deconditioning.

Model for Symptom Management

The most comprehensive symptom model that focuses on symptom management is the Model for Symptom Management proposed by the faculty at the University of California at San Francisco, School of Nursing (UCSF-SON Symptom Management Faculty Group, 1994). This model views the patient's symptom experience, the symptom management strategies, and the symptom outcomes as interrelated. The patient's symptom experience is seen as an interaction of symptom perception, symptom evaluation, and the response to symptoms. Symptoms are managed by the patient, family, health care provider and/or the health care system. The outcomes of symptom management include functional status, emotional status, self-care ability, financial status, quality of life, mortality, morbidity and comorbidity, and health service use. The advantage of this model is that it identifies ways in which the health care provider can intervene to assist the patient in the management of symptoms. It suggests a multidimensional approach to symptom management.

The Theory of Unpleasant Symptoms

Most models of symptoms focus on one symptom, such as pain. The focus is also on the intensity of the symptom, not the quality, distress, or duration. The TOUS is unique in its portrayal of multiple symptoms occurring together and relating to each other in a multiplicative manner. Symptoms occurring together are depicted as catalyzing each other. Thus, this theory uniquely allows for the presence of multiple symptoms and implies that management of one symptom will contribute to the management of other symptoms.

DESCRIPTION OF THE THEORY
OF UNPLEASANT SYMPTOMS

The TOUS focuses on the symptom experience, with multiple symptoms occurring together, rather than one symptom in isolation. The symptoms are seen as multiplicative, rather than additive. Symptoms have antecedent factors such as physiological factors, psychological factors, and environmental factors. These antecedents are interactive and reciprocal.

Symptoms can be considered alone or in combination. Symptoms have the dimensions of intensity (severity), timing (frequency, duration, and relationship to events), distress (the person's reaction to the sensation), and quality (descriptors used to characterize the symptom, location of the symptom, or response to intervention). The quality dimension may be especially difficult, depending on the culture and language of the patient, and the number of symptoms experienced at the same time.

The antecedent factors are categorized as physiological, psychological, or situational. Physiological antecedents are commonly what characterize the severity of the disease, such as comorbidities, abnormal blood studies, or other pathological findings. Stages of disease may also be a physiological antecedent factor. Psychological factors affecting the symptom experience may include the person's

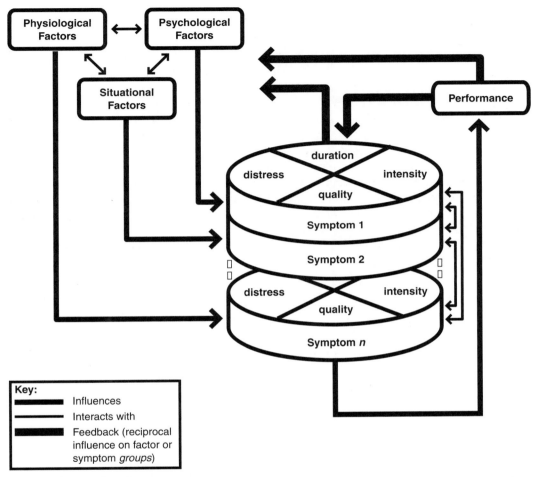

■ Figure 4.1 Theory of unpleasant symptoms.

mood, level of depression, affective reaction to disease, degree of uncertainty regarding the symptoms, and meaning ascribed to the symptoms. Situational factors refer to the social and physical environment that may affect patients' symptom experience and their reporting of that experience, including social support, marital status, and resources.

In the TOUS, symptoms affect performance. Performance includes functional (physical activity, ADLs, social, and role performance) and cognitive performance (ability to concentrate, problem solve and/or think). Cognitive functioning is also seen as a consequence of symptoms. Those who experience more symptoms are likely to have impaired cognitive functioning.

4-1 USING MIDDLE RANGE THEORIES

The TOUS can be used to examine an individual symptom and determine the antecedents and consequences of the symptom.

Fatigue is a common symptom in patients with renal failure and on hemodialysis. However, there is little research available regarding this symptom, and little to guide the nurse in caring for hemodialysis patients. In a descriptive correlation study of 39 hemodialysis patients using self-report and blood tests, these researchers explored the antecedents and consequences of the symptom of fatigue. They found fatigue to be associated with sleep problems, poor physical health, and depression, but not associated with biochemical or situational factors. They proposed a modification of the TOUS similar to the 1997 update of the model, in which the physiological and psychological factors are seen as interacting to cause fatigue, and fatigue, in turn, affecting performance.

McCann, K., & Boore, J. (2000). Fatigue in persons with renal failure who require maintenance haemodialysis. *Journal of Advanced Nursing, 32*(5), 1132–1142.

In the updated version of the theory (Lenz et al., 1997), symptoms are seen as occurring together and interacting with each other, as are antecedent factors. See Figure 4-1 for a model of TOUS. An interaction and reciprocal relationship between the antecedent factors and symptoms is also hypothesized. While symptoms are seen as influencing performance, performance is, likewise, seen as affecting symptoms. See Using Middle Range Theories 4-1 and 4-2 for examples of the theory's use.

4-2 USING MIDDLE RANGE THEORIES

The TOUS has been used to design an experimental intervention aimed at reducing fatigue. The intervention involved two home visits by a professional community health nurse and a telephone call from a lactation consultant. The structure of the visits to the new mothers was based on the influencing factors as outlined in the TOUS. It included an assessment of the physiological, psychological, and situational factors that could influence fatigue during the postpartum period. Mothers were then taught strategies to reduce their fatigue. Those who received the intervention were significantly less fatigued than those who did not receive the intervention.

Pugh, L. C., & Milligan, R. A. (1998) Nursing intervention to increase the duration of breastfeeding. *Applied Nursing Research, 11*(4), 190–194.

Assessment of Symptoms

The distress associated with a symptom relates to both the symptom itself and the individual's interpretation. This may result in over- or under-reporting of a symptom. Appropriate symptom assessment depends on the symptom involved, the underlying disease or other cause of the symptom, the stage of the illness, and the patient's prognosis. The medical history is an important part of the assessment, including physical and emotional conditions or symptoms, medications, and previous and current family/living situation, including caregiver needs. Symptoms should be characterized by assessing their rate of onset (sudden or gradual), the factors precipitating or alleviating them, the frequency, intensity, duration, quality, and the distress felt by the patient as a result of the symptom (Meek et al., 1999).

A careful physical examination focusing on possible underlying causes of the symptoms should be performed. Signs supporting progression of the underlying condition should be sought. Is the patient anxious or agitated? Is he or she anemic or cyanotic? Particular attention needs to be paid to signs associated with clinical syndromes. Physical exams, laboratory tests, and interventional procedures need to be undertaken, noting the stage of the illness and treatment being prescribed (Zeppetella, 1998).

Diagnostic tests helpful in determining the etiology of the symptom are advised. Since many symptoms are contextual and related to movement or exercise, it is important to assess these parameters as well.

INSTRUMENTS USED IN EMPIRICAL TESTING

Symptom measures can either focus on one symptom or include multiple symptoms that are commonly seen in a specific disease entity. Some symptom measures focus only on physical symptoms, while others include both physical and emotional symptoms. Symptom measures may focus only on presence or absence, intensity or frequency, rather than all the dimensions described in the TOUS.

Single Symptom Assessment

Several individual symptoms have been studied over time by a variety of nurses and other health care providers. As a result of this interest, investigators have developed tools for assessing and measuring these particular individual symptoms. Some of these single symptom assessment scales will be discussed next.

VISUAL ANALOGUE SCALE

Single symptom measures can be focused only on the intensity of the symptom or on multiple symptom dimensions. A valid symptom measure that focuses on intensity is a visual analogue scale (VAS). This scale was first introduced for the measurement of feelings (Aitken, 1969). It has been validated as a measure of pain, dyspnea, fatigue, and other symptoms. It consists of a 100-mm line (placed either horizontally or vertically) with anchors indicating the low and high end of the scale. The patient is asked to mark the intensity of the symptom on the continuum. Scoring the measure involves measuring the distance (in millimeters) from the lowest end of the line to the patient's mark.

The VAS validated as a measure of dyspnea (VADS) consists of a 100-mm vertical VAS with anchors of "shortness of breath as bad as can be" at the top and "no shortness of breath" at the bottom. Concurrent validity of this scale has been established with COPD patients, using both a horizontal VAS and a measure of airway obstruction (Gift, Plaut, & Jacox, 1986). Construct validity was established, using the contrasted-groups approach between those expected to have dyspnea and those not expected to have dyspnea. Differences between the two groups were significant for both COPD and asthmatic patients (Gift, 1989). Drawbacks of the VADS are (1) the scale is limited in discerning the different dimensions of dyspnea (Mancini & Body, 1999) and (2) the comparison of ratings between individuals may be problematic because the anchors may be discerned as qualitatively different for each individual (Mahler & Jones, 1997).

NUMERIC RATING SCALE

The Numeric Rating Scale (NRS) has patients rate the intensity of their pain or shortness of breath by choosing a number on a scale from zero, the lowest intensity of the symptom to 10, the highest intensity of the symptom. The NRS can be administered either in the written or verbal form and is extremely easy to administer and score. This scale has been used clinically as a measure of pain or dyspnea and is a valid measure of these symptoms (Gift & Narsavage, 1998).

MULTIDIMENSIONAL FATIGUE INVENTORY

The Multidimensional Fatigue Inventory (Smets, Garssen, Bonke, & de Haas, 1995; Smets, Garssen, Schuster-Uitterhoeve, & de Haas, 1993) is an example of a scale that focuses on only one symptom but does so in a comprehensive manner, to explore general fatigue, physical fatigue, reduced activity, reduced motivation, and mental fatigue.

MCGILL PAIN QUESTIONNAIRE (MPQ)

The MPQ was developed by Melzack (1975) at McGill University, with a focus on pain description. The MPQ permits measurement of the sensory, affective, and evaluative dimensions of pain and provides information on the relative intensity of each, as well as several measures of the patient's evaluation of the overall intensity of the pain (Melzack, 1983). The words used to describe pain are classified in three quality categories: (1) sensory (including temporal, spatial, pressure, thermal, and other properties); (2) affective (including tension, fear, and autonomic properties of the pain experience); and (3) evaluative (words describing overall intensity).

These are followed by four miscellaneous items. In addition, patients are asked to rate their present pain intensity (PPI) based on a 0-to-5 scale. Repeated administrations of the questionnaire to cancer patients have established the reliability of the MPQ. The consistency index (average of the individuals' repeated scores) was high, ranging from 66% to 80%. Factor analytical techniques have been used to demonstrate that the affective and evaluative categories are distinctly different from each other.

MAGNITUDE ESTIMATION

Another approach to symptom measurement is the use of magnitude estimation, which determines the change in the symptom that is needed to have the patient report a change in intensity. The magnitude estimation technique was originally used by Borg (1982) as a measure of perceived exertion. The different intervals between the descriptors were designed to reflect the nonlinearity between a perceived load and a physical load. It has been used in the rating of pain and dyspnea. Magnitude estimates of breathlessness made using a modified Borg scale were highly reproducible after 1 week of the study and at the end of the 40-week study period (Wilson & Jones, 1991). Measurements of dyspnea made with the Borg scale appeared to have greater stability than VAS measurements and to correlate better with expiratory volume (V_E). The use of descriptors on the modified Borg scale, or any graphic rating scale, can detract from the reliability of the measure.

Multiple Symptom Assessment

In addition to single symptom inventories, several tools have been developed to assess multiple symptoms with just one assessment. Several of these multiple-symptom inventory tools will be discussed next.

MEMORIAL SYMPTOM ASSESSMENT SCALE

The Memorial Symptom Assessment Scale is one of the most comprehensive symptom scales. It includes 24 symptoms, both physical and psychological, and asks the subject to indicate the presence or absence of each of the symptoms. In addition, for all symptoms indicated as occurring, the subject is asked the frequency, intensity, and distress the symptom causes them. Additionally, eight longer-lasting symptoms that commonly occur in the cancer patient are listed, and the subject is requested to indicate how severe the symptom was and how much he or she was distressed by the symptom. This scale was developed and tested on 246 patients with a variety of cancers. A factor analysis found three factors that were labeled as psychological, high-prevalence physical, and low-prevalence physical. High correlations with the clinical status and quality-of-life measures further supported the validity of the scale. Reliability was established using Cronbach's alpha (Portenoy et al., 1994). The scale has recently been demonstrated to be of value in the assessment of symptoms in other patient populations as well.

SYMPTOM DISTRESS SCALE

The Symptom Distress Scale (SDS) is another example of a measure that includes multiple symptoms. In this scale, patients are asked to rate each symptom on a five-point response format, ranging from 1 (normal or no distress) to 5 (extensive distress). Evidence for validity and alpha reliability (.82 for the total scale) has been reported (McCorkle & Young, 1978). This is one of the most frequently used measures, often with advanced disease and palliative care.

Activity Symptom Assessment

This category of measures refers to instruments requiring some activity or report of activity to indicate the intensity of the symptom. Such measures are often referred to as functional scales because they require the patient's report of activities. The symptom of dyspnea is often measured with such a scale. The scales' emphasis on physical activity make them inappropriate for use in those who are in critical care or at the end stage of disease. They are often used in a rehabilitation setting.

BRITISH MEDICAL RESEARCH COUNCIL SCALE

One activity measure is the British Medical Research Council Scale, a listing of five levels of activities that provoke dyspnea. The patient reads the descriptive phrases for each level and selects the number with the activity level that provokes dyspnea for them. The five-point scale was originally developed by Fletcher in 1952 and later modified. It focuses on the patient's report of dyspnea either while walking distances on a level or climbing stairs. The patient selects from among the five grades of activity and levels of assistance needed to indicate what results in dyspnea. There is, however, a lack of clear limits between grades, and it may subsequently be difficult to establish an improvement in dyspnea following a therapeutic intervention. The modified Medical Research Council Scale (MRCS) method is a five-point scale based on degrees of various physical activities that precipitate breathlessness (Table 4-1).

TABLE 4-1. MODIFIED MEDICAL RESEARCH COUNCIL DYSPNEA SCALE

GRADE	DESCRIPTION
0	Not troubled with breathlessness except with strenuous exercise
1	Troubled by shortness of breath when hurrying on the level or walking up a slight hill
2	Walks slower than people of the same age on the level because of breathlessness or has to stop for breath when walking at own pace or on the level
3	Stops for breath after walking about 100 yards or after a few minutes on the level
4	Too breathless to leave the house or breathless when dressing or undressing.

Source: Task Group on Surveillance for Respiratory Hazards in the Occupational Setting. ATS News (1982); 8, 12–16.

(UCSD) SHORTNESS OF BREATH QUESTIONNAIRE

University of California at San Francisco Dyspnea (UCSD) Shortness of Breath Questionnaire is a 24-item, self-administered questionnaire measuring dyspnea during the past week. Patients are asked three questions about their overall limitations due to dyspnea and to rate how short of breath they get while performing 21 activities. The rating uses a six-point Likert scale—0=not at all to 5=maximally or unable to do because of breathlessness. Patients are asked to rate activities they have never performed by estimating the amount of dyspnea they would experience if they performed the activity (Archibald & Guidotti, 1987). Test–retest reliability was examined (Eakin, Sass-Dambron, Ries, & Kaplan, 1995). Internal consistency was demonstrated using a Cronbach's alpha and found to be .92 (Eakin et al., 1995). Concurrent validity was demonstrated using FEV_1, the Quality of Well-being Scale, the CES-D, and the 6MWD (Eakin, Prewitt, Ries, & Kaplan, 1994).

Selection of Instruments

The use of a particular symptom-measurement instrument in a research study is dependent upon the needs of the researcher for assessment to adequately answer the research question study. Review Research Application 4-1 provides an example of how the TOUS may be used, and how symptoms can be assessed using a single-symptom assessment measure.

SUMMARY

Having symptoms as the focus of nursing care, rather than simply being an indication of the underlying "cause" of another problem, is new to the nursing literature. The use of middle range theories to

4-1 RESEARCH APPLICATION

A nurse researcher is interested in reducing pain postoperatively in hip-replacement patients. The researcher decides to use the TOUS to structure the preoperative teaching class. The class has components related to all aspects of the model, such as physiological factors that can be controlled to reduce pain postoperatively, psychological factors, and social or environmental factors that will help patients manage their pain postoperatively. Patients are taught to characterize their pain according to the intensity, frequency, distress, and quality of the sensation, and to record the sensation, so they can note the changes that occur after medication and over time as they recover. They are taught to note other symptoms that may accompany the pain. In addition, patients are told what to expect related to their performance after surgery, and how to gradually increase what they do as the pain is relieved. The effectiveness of this preoperative teaching is assessed by having patients rate their pain using a visual analogue pain scale (VAS) during the postoperative period and comparing it to pain ratings in those not exposed to the teaching.

guide the management of symptoms is even newer. They serve the useful purpose of guiding the practitioner to focus on more than the sensation and its intensity but, rather, to have a more comprehensive approach, including the context in which the symptom occurs. The situational aspects that contribute to the symptom experience need further study. We know that there are environmental, social, and cultural factors that play a part in the interpretation of symptoms, but more detail is needed to guide the clinician in planning nursing care. Although the symptom models advocate the assessment of multiple symptoms rather than only one, such as pain, few clinical settings implement that assessment in their routine patient care.

The effects of symptoms on patient performance are just beginning to be identified. Symptoms affect all aspects of performance, not just the physical aspects. Because proper management of symptoms can be expected to affect patients physically, psychologically, and socially, it is important for nurses to develop their science in this area.

ANALYSIS EXERCISE

Using the criteria presented in Chapter 2, critique the TOUS. Compare your conclusions about the theory with those found in Appendix A. An experienced nurse has completed the analysis found in Appendix A.

Internal Criticism
1. Clarity
2. Consistency
3. Adequacy

4. Logical development
5. Level of theory development

External Criticism
1. Reality convergence
2. Utility
3. Significance
4. Discrimination
5. Scope of theory
6. Complexity

WEB RESOURCES

1. American Academy of Pain Management: *http://www.aapainmanage.org/*
2. American Pain Society: *http://www.ampainsoc.org/*
3. American Thoracic Society Consensus Statement on Dyspnea: *http://www.olivija.com/dyspnea/*
4. NIH Research Workshop: Symptoms in Terminal Illness: *http://www.nih.gov/ninr/wnew/ symptoms_in_terminal_illness.html*
5. Research Center for Symptom Management at UCSF/SON: *http://nurseweb.ucsf.edu/www/rcsm.htm*

6. Theory of Unpleasant Symptoms journal article: e-library to search Advances in Nursing Science. Vol 19, page 14, 3/1/1997 and download one article free. *http:// ask.elibrary.com/login.asp?c=&host=ask% 2 Eelibrary%2Ecom&script=%2Fgetdoc%2 Easp&query=pubname%3DAdvances%5Fin%5 FNursing%5FScience%26puburl%3Dhttp%7EC% 7E%7ES%7E%7ES%7Ewww%2Easpenpub%2 Ecom%7ES%7Eans%2Ehtm%26querydocid%3 D29089530%40urn%3Abigchalk%3AUS%3 BLib%26dtype%3D0%7E0%26dinst%3D0%26 refid%3Dalleffort&title=&pubname=Advances%5Fin%5FNursing%5FScience&author=&date=*

REFERENCES

Aitken, R.C.B. (1969). Measurement of feelings using visual analogue scales. *Proceedings of Research Social Medicine, 62,* 989–993.

Archibald, C. J., & Guidotti, T. L. (1987). Degree of objectivity measured impairment and perceived shortness of breath with activities of daily living in patients with chronic obstructive pulmonary disease. *Canadian Journal of Rehabilitation 1*(1), 45–54.

Benner P. E. & Wrebel J. (1989) *The primacy of caring: Stress and coping in health and illness* (pp. 199–200). Menlo Park, CA: Addison-Wesley Publishing Co.

Borg, G. (1982). Psychophysical bases of perceived exertion. *Medicine and Science in Sports and Exercise,* 14, 377–381.

Eakin, E., Prewitt, L. M., Ries, A., & Kaplan, R. (1994). Validation of the UCSD Shortness of Breath questionnaire. *Journal of Cardiopulmonary Rehabilitation,* 14, 322–323.

Eakin, E., Sassi-Dambron, D. E., Ries, A., & Kaplan, R. (1995). Reliability and validity of dyspnea measures in patients with obstructive lung disease. *International Journal of Behavioral Medicine, 2*(2), 118–134.

Gift, A.G., & Narsavage, G. (1998).Validity of the numeric rating scale as a measure of dyspnea. *American Journal of Critical Care, 7*(3), 200–204.

Gift, A. G., Plaut, S. M., & Jacox, A. K. (1986). Psychologic and physiologic factors related to dyspnea in subjects with chronic obstructive pulmonary disease. *Heart & Lung,* 15, 595–602.

Hutchinson, S. A., & Wilson, H. S. (1998). The Theory of Unpleasant Symptoms and Alzheimer's disease. *Scholarly Inquiry for Nursing Practice: An International Journal, 12*(2), 143–158.

Lenz, E., Pugh, L. C., Milligan, R. A., Gift, A., & Suppe, F. (1997). The middle range theory of unpleasant symptoms: An update. *Advances in Nursing Science, 19*(3), 14–27.

Lenz, E., Suppe, F., Gift, A. G., Pugh, L. C., & Milligan, R. A. (1995). Collaborative development of middle-range nursing theories: Toward a theory of unpleasant symptoms. *Advances in Nursing Science, 17*(3), 1–13.

Mahler, D. A., & Jones, P. W. (1997). Measurement of dyspnea and quality of life in advanced lung disease. *Clinical Chest Medicine, 18*(3), 457–469.

Mancini, I., & Body, J. J. (1999). Assessment of dyspnea in advanced cancer patients. *Supportive Care in Cancer, 7*(4), 229–232.

McCann, K., & Boore, J. (2000). Fatigue in persons with renal failure who require maintenance haemodialysis. *Journal of Advanced Nursing, 32*(5), 1132–1142.

McCarley, C. (1999). A model of chronic dyspnea. *Image: Journal of Nursing Scholarship, 31*(3), 231–236.

McCorkle R. & Young, K. (1978). Development of a symptom distress scale. *Cancer Nursing, 1,* 373–378.

Meek, P. M., Schwartzstein, R. M., Adams, M. M., Altose, M. D., Breslin, E. H., Carrieri-Kohlman, V., Gift, A., Hanley, M. V., Harver, A., Jones, P. W., Killian, K., Knebel, A., Lareau, S. C., Mahler, D. A., Meek, O'Donnell, D., Schwartzstein, R. M., Steele, B., Stuhlbarg, M., & Titler, M. (1999). Dyspnea: Mechanisms, assessment, and management: A consensus statement. *American Journal of Respiratory and Critical Care Medicine, 159,* 321–340.

Melzack, R. (1975). The McGill Pain Questionnaire: Major properties and scoring methods. *Pain, 1,* 277–299.

Melzack, R. (1983). The McGill Pain Questionnaire. In Melzack, R (Ed.). *Pain measurement and assessment.* New York: Raven Press, 41–47.

Portenoy, R. K., Thaler, H. T., Kornblith, A. B., Lepore, J. M., Friedlander-Klar, H., Kiyasu, E., Sobel, K., Coyle, N., Kemeny, N., Norton, L., & Scher, H. (1994). The Memorial Symptoms Assessment Scale: An instrument for the evaluation of symptom prevalence, characteristics and distress. *European Journal of Cancer, 30A*(9), 1326–1336.

Pugh, L. C., & Milligan, R. A. (1998). Nursing intervention to increase the duration of breastfeeding. *Applied Nursing Research, 11*(4), 190–194.

Smets, E., Garssen, B., Bonke, B., & de Haas, J. (1995). The Multidimensional Fatigue Inventory (MFI): Psychometric qualities of an instrument to assess fatigue. *Journal of Psychosomatic Research, 39*(5), 315–325.

Smets, E., Garssen, B., Schuster-Uitterhoeve, A., & de Haas, J. (1993). Fatigue in cancer patients. *British Journal of Cancer, 68,* 220–224.

Steele, B., & Shaver, J. (1992). The dyspnea experience: Nociceptive properties and a model for research and practice. *Advances in Nursing Science, 15*(1), 64–76.

Task Group on Surveillance for Respiratory Hazards in the Occupational Setting. ATS News (1982); 8: 12–16.

Teel, C. S., Meek, P., McNamara, A. M., & Watson, L. (1997). Perspectives unifying symptom interpretation. *Image: Journal of Nursing Scholarship, 29*(2), 175–181.

University of California at San Francisco, School of Nursing, Symptom Management Faculty Group. (1994). A model for symptom management. *Image: Journal of Nursing Scholarship, 26*(4), 272–276.

Wilson, R. C., & Jones, P. W. (1991). Differentiation between intensity of breathlessness and the distress it evokes in normal subjects during exercise. *Clinical Science,* 80, 65–70.

Zeppetella, G. (1998). The palliation of dyspnea in terminal disease. *The American Journal of Hospice and Palliative Care, 15*(6), 322–330.

BIBLIOGRAPHY

Aaronson, L. et al. (1999). Defining and measuring fatigue. *Image, 31*(1), 45–50.

Acheson, A., & MacCormack, D. (1997). Dyspnea and the cancer patient—an overview. *Canadian Oncology Nursing Journal, 7*(4), 209–213.

Algase, D. L., Newton, S. E., & Higgins, P. A. (2001). Nursing theory across curricula: A status report from Midwest nursing schools. *Journal of Professional Nursing, 17*(5), 248–255.

Blegen, M. A., & Tripp-Reimer, T. (1997). Implications of nursing taxonomies for middle-range theory development. *Advanced Nursing Science, 19*(3), 37–49.

Bredin, M., Corner, J., Krishnasamy, M., Plant, H., Bailey, C., & A'Hern, R. (1999). Multicentre randomized controlled trial of nursing intervention for breathlessness in patients with lung cancer. *British Medical Journal, 318*, 901–904.

Brown, M., Carrieri, V., Janson-Bjerklie, S., & Dodd, M. (1986). Lung cancer and dyspnea: The patient's perception. *Oncology Nursing Forum, 13*(5), 19–24.

Carrieri-Kohlman, V., Gormley, J. M., Douglas, M. K., Paul, S. M., & Stulbarg, M. S. (1996). Differentiation between dyspnea and its affective components. *Western Journal of Nursing Research, 18*, 626–642.

Cella, D., Passik, S., Jacobsen, P., & Breitbart, W. (1998). Progress toward guidelines for the management of fatigue. *Oncology, 12*(11A), 369–377.

Cimprich, B. (1992). Attentional fatigue following breast cancer surgery. *Research in Nursing & Health, 15*, 199–207.

Cody, W. K. (1999). Middle-range theories: Do they foster the development of nursing science? *Nursing Science Quarterly, 12*(1), 9–14.

Cooley, M. E. (2000). Symptoms in adults with lung cancer: A systematic research review. *Journal of Pain and Symptom Management, 19*(2), 137–153.

Deets, C. (1998). Nursing—A maturing discipline? *Journal of Professional Nursing, 14*(2), 65.

Dodd, M., Janson, S., Facione, N., Faucett, J., Froelicher, E. S., Humphreys, J., Lee, K., Miaskowski, C., Puntillo, K., Rankin, S., & Taylor, D. (2001). Advancing the science of symptom management. *Journal of Advanced Nursing, 33*(5), 668–676.

Dodd, M., Miaskowski, C., & Paul, S. (2001). Symptom clusters and their effect on the functional status of patients with cancer. *Oncology Nursing Forum. 28*(3) 465–470.

Donnelly, S., & Walsh, D. (1995). The symptoms of advanced cancer. *Seminars in Oncology, 22*(2, Suppl. 3), 67–72.

Drevdahl, D. (1999). Sailing beyond: Nursing theory and the person. *Advanced Nursing Science, 21*(4), 1–13.

Ducharme, F., Ricard, N., Duquette, A., Levesque, L., & Lachance, L. (1998). Empirical testing of a longitudinal model derived from the Roy adaptation model. *Nursing Science Quarterly, 11*(4), 149–159.

Dudley-Brown, S. L. (1997). The evaluation of nursing theory: A method for our madness. *International Journal of Nursing Studies, 34*(1), 76–83.

Gift, A. G. (1989). Validation of a vertical visual analogue scale as a measure of clinical dyspnea. *Rehabilitation Nursing, 14*, 323–325.

Gift, A. G. (1991). Psychologic and physiologic aspects of acute dyspnea in asthmatics. *Nursing Research, 40*, 96–199.

Gift, A. G., Jablonski, A., Stommel, M., & Given, C. W. (in press). Symptom clusters in patients with lung cancer. *Oncology Nursing Forum.*

Gift, A. G., Moore, T., & Soeken, K. (1992). Relaxation to reduce dyspnea and anxiety in COPD patients. *Nursing Research, 41*, 242–246.

Given, C. W., Stommel, M., Given, B., Osuch, J., Kurtz, M. E., & Kurtz, J. C. (1993). The influence of cancer patients' symptoms and functional status on patients' depression and family caregivers' reaction and depression. *Health Psychology, 12*, 277–285.

Good, M. (1998). A middle-range theory of acute pain management: Use in research. *Nursing Outlook, 46*(3), 120–124.

Hann, D., Jacobson, P., Azzarillo, M., & Martin, S. (1998). Measurement of fatigue in cancer patients: Development and validation of the fatigue symptom inventory. *Quality of Life Research, 7*, 301–311.

Higgins, P. A. (1998). Patient perception of fatigue while undergoing long-term mechanical ventilation: Incidence and associated factors. *Heart & Lung, 27*(3), 177–183.

Higgins, P. A., & Moore, S. M. (2000). Levels of theoretical thinking in nursing. *Nursing Outlook, 48*, 179–183.

Hopp, J. P., & Duffy, S. A. (2000). Racial variations in end-of-life care. *Journal of the American Geriatrics Society, 48*, 658–663.

Hupcey, J. A., Morse, J. M., Lenz, E., & Tason, M. C. (1996). Wilsonian methods of concept analysis: A critique. *Scholarly Inquiry for Nursing Practice, 10*, 185–210.

Kurtz, M. E., Given, B. A., Kurtz, J. C., & Given, C. W. (1994). The interaction of age, symptoms and survival status on physical and mental health of patients with cancer and their families. *Cancer, 74*, 2071–2078.

LaMontagne, L. L., Pressler, J. L., & Salisbury, M. H. (1996). Scholarly mission: Fostering scholarship in research, theory and practice. *N & HC—Perspectives on Community, 17*(6), 298–302.

Lee, K., Hicks, G., & Nino-Murcia, G. (1991). Validity and reliability of a scale to assess fatigue. *Psychiatry Research, 36*, 291–298.

Liehr, P., & Smith, M. J. (1999). Middle range theory: Spinning research and practice to create knowledge for the new millennium. *Advance Nursing Science, 21*(4), 81–91.

Mahler, D. A., Harver, A., Lentine, T., Scott, J. A., Beck, K., & Schwartzstein, R. M. (1996). Descriptors of breathlessness in cardiorespiratory diseases. *American Journal of Respiratory and Critical Care Medicine, 154*, 1357–1363.

Mahler, D. A., Harver, A., Rosiello, R., & Daubenspeck, J. A. (1989). Measurement of respiratory sensation in interstitial lung disease: Evaluation of clinical dyspnea ratings and magnitude scaling. *Chest, 96*(4), 767–771.

Mahler, D. A., Matthay, R. A., Snyder, P. E., Wells, C. K., & Loke, J. (1985). Sustained release theophylline reduces dyspnea in non-reversible obstructive airway disease. *American Review of Respiratory Disease, 131*, 22–25.

Mahler, D. A., & Wells, C. K. (1988). Evaluation of clinical methods for rating dyspnea. *Chest, 93*(3), 580–586.

Mahler, D., Weinberg, D., Wells, C., & Feinstein, A. (1984). The measurement of dyspnea: Contents, interobserver agreement and physiologic correlates of two new clinical indexes. *Chest, 85*(6), 751–758.

McCorkle, R. (1983). Symptom distress, current concerns and mood disturbances after diagnosis of life-threatening disease. *Social Science Medicine, 17*, 431–438.

Meek, P. M., Lareau, S. C., & Anderson, D. (2001). Memory for symptoms in COPD patients: How accurate are their reports? *European Respiratory Journal,18*, 1–8.

Morse, J. M. (1995). Exploring the theoretical basis of nursing using advanced techniques of concept analysis. *Advances in Nursing Science, 17*, 31–46.

Morse, J. M., Hupcey, J., Mitcham, C., & Lenz, E. (1996). Concept analysis in nursing research: A critical appraisal. *Scholarly Inquiry for Nursing Practice, 10*, 257–281.

Morse, J. M., Hutchinson, S. A., & Penrod, J. (1998). From theory to practice: The development of assessment guides from qualitatively derived theory. *Qualitative Health Research, 8*(3), 329–340.

Morse, J. M., Mitcham, C., Hupcey, J. E., & Tason, M. C. (1996). Criteria for concept evaluation. *Journal of Advanced Nursing, 24*, 385–390.

Nield, M. (2000). Dyspnea self-management in African Americans with chronic lung disease. *Heart & Lung, 29*, 50–55.

Noseda, A. J., Schmerber, J., Priogogine, T., & Yernault, J. C. (1992). Perceived effect on shortness of breath of an acute inhalation of saline or terbutaline: Variability and sensitivity of a visual analogue scale in patients with asthma or COPD. *European Respiratory Journal, 5*, 1043–1053.

Parshall, M. B., Welsh, J. D., Brockopp, D. Y., Heiser, R. M., Schooler, M. P., & Cassidy, K. B. (2001). Dyspnea duration, distress, and intensity in emergency department visits for heart failure. *Heart & Lung, 30*(1), 47–56.

Perreault, M., & Saillant, F. (1996). Nursing sciences and social sciences: Dialog and mutual enrichment. *Sciences Sociales et Sante, 14*(3), 7–16.

Piper, B., Dibble, S., Dodd, M., Weiss, M., Slaughter, R., & Paul, S. (1998). The Revised Piper Fatigue Scale: Psychometric evaluation in women with breast cancer. *Oncology Nursing Forum, 25*(4), 677–684.

Portenoy, R. K., Thaler, H. T., Kornblith, A. B., Lepore, J., Ffiedlander-Klar, H., Kiyasu, E., et al. (1994). The Memorial Symptom Assessment Scale: An instrument for the evaluation of symptom prevalence, characteristics and distress. *European Journal of Cancer, 30A*, 1326–1336.

Pugh, L. (1993). Childbirth and the measurement of fatigue. *Journal of Nursing Measurement, 1*, 57–66.

Redeker, N. S., Lev, E. L., & Ruggiero, J. (2000). Insomnia, fatigue, anxiety, depression and quality of life of cancer patients undergoing chemotherapy. *Scholarly Inquiry for Nursing Practice, 14*(4), 275–290.

Ruland, C. M., & Moore, S. M. (1998). Theory construction based on standards of care: A proposed theory of the peaceful end of life. *Nursing Outlook, 46*(4), 169–175.

Sarna, L., & Brecht, M. (1997). Dimensions of symptom distress in women with advanced lung cancer: A factor analysis. *Heart & Lung, 26*(1), 23–30.

Schneider, R. (1998). Reliability and validity of the Mutidimensional Fatigue Inventory (MFI-20) and the Rhoten Fatigue Scale among rural cancer outpatients. *Cancer Nursing, 21*, 370–373.

Schwartz, A. (1998). The Schwartz Cancer Fatigue Scale: Testing reliability and validity. *Oncology Nursing Forum, 25*(4), 711–717.

Shih, F. J., & Chu, S. H. (1999). Comparisons of American-Chinese and Taiwanese patients' perceptions of dyspnea and helpful nursing actions during the intensive care unit transition from cardiac surgery. *Heart & Lung, 28*(1), 41–54.

Simon, P., Schwartzstein, R. M., Weiss, J. W., Fencl, V., Teghtsoonian, M., & Weinberger, S. E. (1990). Distinguishable types of dyspnea in patients with shortness of breath. *American Review of Respiratory Disease, 142*, 1009–1014.

Smith, M. C. (1999). Caring and the science of unitary human beings. *Advanced Nursing Science, 21*(4), 14–28.

Vainio, A., Aurinen, A., & Members of the Symptom Prevalence Group. (1996). Prevalence of symptoms among patients with advanced cancer: An international collaborative study. *Journal of Pain and Symptom Management,* *12*(1), 3–10.

Van der Molen, B. (1995). Dyspnoea: A study of measurement instruments for the assessment of dyspnoea and their application for patients with advanced cancer. *Journal of Advanced Nursing, 22*(5), 948–956.

Weaver, T. E., & Narsavage, G. L. (1992). Physiological and psychological variables related to functional status in COPD. *Nursing Research, 41,* 286–291.

Wolfe, J., Grier, H. E., Klar, N., Levin, S. B., Ellenbogen, J. M., Salem-Schatz, S., Emanuel, E. J., & Weeks, J. C. (2000). Symptoms and suffering at the end of life in children with cancer. *The New England Journal of Medicine, 342*(5), 326–333.

Zhou, Q., O'Brien, B., & Soeken, K. (2001). Rhodes Index of Nausea and Vomiting—Form 2 in pregnant women. *Nursing Research, 50*(4), 251–257.

Middle Range Theories: Cognitive

Self-Efficacy

BARBARA RESNICK

DEFINITION OF KEY TERMS

Mastery experience	The most influential source of self-efficacy information is the interpreted result of one's prior performance, or mastery experience. Individuals engage in tasks and activities, interpret the results of their actions, use the interpretations to develop beliefs about their capability to engage in subsequent tasks or activities, and act in concert with the beliefs created.
Outcome expectations	The belief that if a specific behavior is completed, there will be a certain outcome. Bandura postulates that because the outcomes an individual expects are the result of the judgments of what he or she can accomplish, outcome expectations are unlikely to contribute to predictions of behavior.
Self-efficacy	Peoples' judgments of their capabilities to organize and execute courses of action required to attain designated types of performances. Self-efficacy beliefs provide the foundation for human motivation, well-being, and personal accomplishment.
Social persuasions	Individuals also create and develop self-efficacy beliefs as a result of the social persuasions they receive from others. These persuasions can involve exposure to verbal judgments of others.
Somatic and emotional states	Somatic and emotional states, such as anxiety, stress, arousal, and mood, also provide information about efficacy beliefs. People can gauge their degree of confidence by the emotional state they experience as they contemplate an action.

DEFINITION OF KEY TERMS

Vicarious experience   In addition to interpreting the results of their actions, people form their self-efficacy beliefs through the vicarious experience of observing others perform tasks. This source of information is weaker than mastery experience in helping to create self-efficacy beliefs, but when people are uncertain about their own abilities or when they have limited prior experience, they are more likely influenced by observation reactions.

INTRODUCTION

The links between health and lifestyle behavior (i.e., smoking, physical activity, weight, and diet) are now well supported. The challenge is, however, how to best help individuals change behavior to promote health and well-being. Understanding the determinants of health behaviors and the mechanisms linking health and behavioral processes is an essential step in designing interventions to support health-promoting behaviors and to eliminate those that can impair health.

Theories are judged by their explanatory and predictive power. The value of psychological theory must also be judged by the ability of the theory to change people's lives for the better. Self-efficacy theory provides a body of knowledge for social applications to varied health-related activities. The broad scope and variety of applications attests to the explanatory and operative generality of this theory.

Individuals can exercise influence over what they do. Most human behavior, however, is determined by many interacting factors. Individuals are contributors to, rather than determiners of, what happens to them. The power to make things happen should be distinguished from the mechanics of how things are made to happen. Based on their understanding of what is within the power of humans to do and beliefs about their own capabilities, people try to generate courses of action to suit given purposes. Because control is central in human lives, many theories have been proposed. Peoples' levels of motivation, affective states, and actions are based more on what they believe than on what is objectively true. Therefore, it is the person's belief in his or her causative capabilities that is the major focus of behavior.

The theory of self-efficacy is based on the belief that what people think, believe, and feel affects how they behave. The natural and extrinsic effects of their actions, in turn, partly determine their thought patterns and affective reactions and behavior. Freedom of choice is central to the theory. Freedom is considered as the exercise of self-influence. This is achieved through reflective thought, use of the knowledge and skills at one's command, and other tools of self-influence.

Many prior theories developed to understand behavior were focused on an inborn drive for control (i.e., self-determination or mastery). Theories stating that striving for personal control is an expression of an innate drive tend to ignore how human efficacy is developed and the impact this has on behavior. The fact that all individuals try to influence some of the things that affect them does not necessarily mean that this is solely driven by an innate motivator. Understanding of whether the individual controls behavior by an inborn drive or is pulled by an anticipated benefit is central to behavior change. Most human behavior, however, is determined by many interacting factors. The theory of self-efficacy, derived from social cognitive theory, has proven to be a useful guide in understanding behavior and facilitating behavior change.

HISTORICAL BACKGROUND

The theory of self-efficacy was derived from social cognitive theory. Social cognitive theory favors a conception of interaction based on triadic reciprocity. In this model of reciprocal determinism, behavior, cognitive and other personal factors, and environmental influences all operate interactively as determinants of each other. In this triadic reciprocal determinism, there is mutual action between causal factors. Reciprocity does not, however, mean symmetry in the strength of bidirectional influences. Nor is there a specific pattern of influences. There are times when environmental factors may be the driving force in behavior, and other times when the individual's behavior and its intrinsic feedback are the central factors in determining behavior. Generally, however, when situational constraints are weak, personal factors serve as the predominant influence in the regulatory system.

The initial work in the development of the theory of self-efficacy tested the assumption that psychological procedures could result in behavior change by altering an individual's level and strength of self-efficacy expectations. Studies of the treatment of snake phobias demonstrated that certain interventions, such as performance of a behavior and observing others perform a behavior, strengthen self-efficacy expectations to perform that behavior. In the early studies, Bandura manipulated variables and observed outcomes. The interventions resulted in increased self-efficacy expectations, and positive behavioral changes occurred.

The theory of self-efficacy was initially developed in the late 1970s, and its early use in nursing focused on recovery from cardiovascular events in the 1980s (Gortner, 1988). With the increased focus on middle range theories versus models of nursing care, the theory of self-efficacy was increasingly recognized by nurse researchers as a useful way to guide research and to develop interventions for clinical use.

Cognitions do not arise in a vacuum, and Bandura (1977, 1986, 1995) suggested that individuals' conceptions about themselves are developed and verified through four different processes: (1) direct experience of the effects produced by their actions; (2) vicarious experience; (3) judgments voiced by others; and (4) derivation of further knowledge of what they already know by using rules of inference. External influences play a role in the development of cognitions as well as in their activation.

Initial Theory Development and Research

Early research using the theory of self-efficacy tested the assumption that psychological procedures could result in behavioral change by altering an individual's level and strength of self-efficacy. In the initial study (Bandura, Adams, & Beyer, 1977), 33 subjects with snake phobias were randomly assigned to different treatment conditions: (1) enactive attainment, which included actually touching the snakes; (2) role modeling, or seeing others touch the snakes; and (3) the control group. Results suggested that self-efficacy was predictive of subsequent behavior, and enactive attainment resulted in stronger and more generalized (to another snake) self-efficacy expectations.

Expansion of the early research included three additional studies (Bandura, Reese, & Adams, 1982): (1) 10 subjects with snake phobias; (2) 14 subjects with spider phobias; and (3) 12 subjects with spider phobias. Similar to the initial self-efficacy study, enactive attainment and role modeling were effective interventions for strengthening self-efficacy expectations and impacting behavior. The study of 12 subjects with spider phobias also considered the physiological arousal component of self-efficacy. Pulse and blood pressure were measured as indicators of fear arousal when interacting with spiders. After interventions to strengthen self-efficacy expectations (enactive attainment and role modeling), heart rate decreased and blood pressure stabilized.

This early self-efficacy research was in an ideal controlled setting in that the individuals with snake phobias were unlikely to seek out opportunities to interact with snakes when away from the laboratory setting. Therefore, there was controlled input of efficacy information. While this ideal situation is not possible in the clinical setting, the theory of self-efficacy has been used to study and predict health behavior change and management in a variety of settings.

At the core of this theory is the assumption that people can exercise influence over what they do. Based on reflective thought, generative use of the knowledge and skills to perform a specific behavior, as well as other tools of self-influence, a person will decide how to behave (Bandura, 1995). It has also been suggested that to determine one's self-efficacy, the individual must have the opportunity for self-evaluation, or the comparison of individual output to some sort of evaluative criterion (White, Kjelgaard, & Harkins, 1995). It is this comparison process that provides the individual with a sense of how likely it is that he or she can achieve a given level of performance.

DEFINITION OF THEORY CONCEPTS

Human Agency

The role of intentionality in self-efficacy theory is essential and is described as personal agency. Personal or human agency refers to acts done intentionally. Actions intended to serve a certain purpose can cause quite different things to happen. Effects are not the characteristics of the individual's actions; they are the consequences of those actions. The power to originate actions for given purposes is the key feature of personal agency.

Human agency operates largely on the basis of control beliefs. That is, in daily life individuals formulate solutions for tasks at hand. They act on their thoughts and later analyze how well their thoughts served them in managing events. An individual reflects on his or her experiences in executing courses of action as well as on the consequences of those actions. In social cognitive theory, human agency operates within an interdependent causal structure involving triadic reciprocal causation (Figure 5-1). In this model of causality, internal personal factors in the form of cognitive affective and biological events, behavior, and environmental influences all operate as interacting determinants that influence each other bidirectionally. The relative influence of each of these factors will vary for different activities and under different circumstances.

Self-Efficacy and Outcome Expectations

Bandura (1977, 1986) suggests that outcome expectations are based largely on the individual's self-efficacy expectations. The types of outcomes people anticipate generally depend on their judgments of how well they will be able to perform the behavior. That is, individuals who consider themselves to be

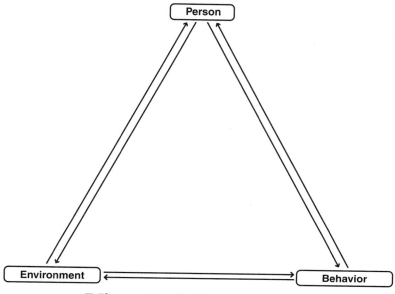

■ **Figure 5.1.** Triadic reciprocal causation.

highly efficacious will expect favorable outcomes. Expected outcomes are highly dependent on self-efficacy judgments; therefore, Bandura postulated that, on their own, expected outcomes may not add much to the prediction of behavior.

Bandura differentiated between two components of self-efficacy theory: judgments of personal efficacy or self-efficacy, and outcome expectancy. Self-efficacy is a comprehensive summary or judgment of perceived capability for performing a specific task. Self-efficacy is a dynamic construct, because the efficacy judgment changes over time as new information and experiences are acquired. Self-efficacy beliefs also involve a mobilization component. That is, self-efficacy reflects a process that involves the construction and orchestration of adaptive performance to fit changing circumstances. Individuals who have the same skills may perform differently based on their use, combination, and sequencing of the skills. Outcome and self-efficacy expectations were differentiated because an individual can believe that a certain behavior will result in a specific outcome; however, they may not believe that they are capable of performing the behavior required for the outcome to occur. For example, Mrs. White may believe that rehabilitation will result in her being able to go home independently, yet she may not believe she is capable of walking across the room. Therefore Mrs. White may not participate in the rehabilitation program or be willing to practice ambulation.

Bandura (1986) does state that there are instances when outcome expectations can be dissociated from self-efficacy expectations. This occurs either when no action will result in a specific outcome, or the outcome is loosely linked to the level or quality of the performance. For example, if Mrs. White knows that *even* if she regains functional independence by participating in rehabilitation, she will still be discharged to a skilled nursing facility rather than back home, her behavior is likely to be influenced by her outcome expectations (discharge to the skilled nursing facility). In this situation, no matter what Mrs. White's performance is, the outcome is the same. Thus, outcome expectancy may influence her behavior independent of her self-efficacy beliefs.

Expected outcomes also are partially separable from self-efficacy judgments when extrinsic outcomes are fixed. For example, when a nurse provides care to six patients during an 8-hour shift, the nurse receives a certain salary. When the same nurse cares for 10 patients during that shift, the same salary is received. This could negatively impact performance. It is also possible for an individual to believe he or she is capable of performing a specific behavior, but not believe that the outcome of performing that behavior is worthwhile. For example, older adults in rehabilitation may believe that they are capable of performing the exercises and activities involved in the rehabilitation process, but they may not believe that performing the exercises will result in improved functional ability. Some older adults believe that resting rather than exercising will lead to recovery. In this situation, outcome expectations may have a direct impact on performance.

Some researchers found that perceived self-efficacy expectations predicted behavior much better than outcome expectations (Barling & Abel, 1983; Godding & Glasgow, 1985; Jenkins, 1985). Conversely, other researchers demonstrated the important impact of outcome expectations regarding predicting behavior (Condiotte & Lichtenstein, 1981; Grembowski et al., 1993; Jette et al., 1998; Resnick, Palmer, Jenkins, & Spellbring, 2000; Resnick & Spellbring, 2000; Stanley & Maddux, 1986; Strecher, DeVellis, Becker, & Rosenstock, 1986).

Stanley and Maddux (1986) included both outcome expectations (referred to as response efficacy) and outcome value, or a more general consideration of the outcome, in an investigation of participation in health-promoting behaviors. The results suggest that self-efficacy and outcome expectations both significantly predicted behavior ($R^2 = .17$ and .26 respectively). However, outcome value did not add significantly to the model. In both quantitative and qualitative research (Resnick, 1994, 1996, 1998a, 2000a, 2001; Resnick & Spellbring, 2000) has repeatedly demonstrated that, with regard to older adults, outcome expectations explain behavior beyond the influence of self-efficacy expectations. It is likely, as concluded by Strecher et al. (1986), that outcome expectations and self-efficacy are both important determinants of health behavior. Which one is more important in any given situation may depend on the features of the situation, such as the cost of performing the activity or the perceived certainty of its benefit or outcome.

Sources of Self-Efficacy Information

Bandura suggested that knowledge of one's self-efficacy is based on four informational sources: (1) enactive attainment, which is the actual performance of a behavior; (2) vicarious experience or visualizing other similar people perform a behavior; (3) verbal persuasion or exhortation; and (4) physiological state or physiological feedback during a behavior, such as pain or fatigue. The cognitive appraisal of these factors results in a perception of confidence in the individual's ability to perform a certain behavior. The performance of this behavior reinforces self-efficacy expectations (Bandura, 1995).

ENACTIVE ATTAINMENT

Enactive attainment has been described as the most influential source of efficacy information (Bandura, 1986; Bandura & Adams, 1977). There has been repeated empirical verification that actually performing an activity strengthens self-efficacy beliefs. Specifically, the impact of enactive attainment has been demonstrated with regard to:

1. Snake phobias (Bandura, 1977; Bandura, Adams, Hardy, & Howells, 1980; Bandura et al., 1982)
2. Smoking cessation (Colletti, Supnick, & Payne, 1985; Condiotte & Lichtenstein, 1981; McIntyre, Lichtenstein, & Mermelstein, 1983)
3. Exercise behaviors and performance of functional activities (Ewart, Taylor, Reese, & DeBusk, 1983; Kaplan, Atkins, & Reinsch, 1984; McAuley, Courneya, & Lettunich, 1991; Resnick, 1998a, 1998b; Robertson & Keller, 1992)
4. Weight loss (Chambliss & Murray, 1979).

Enactive attainment generally results in strengthening self-efficacy expectations better than the other informational sources. However, performance alone does not establish self-efficacy beliefs. Other factors, such as preconceptions of ability, the perceived difficulty of the task, the amount of effort expended, the external aid received, the situational circumstance, and past successes and failures all affect the individual's cognitive appraisal of self-efficacy (Bandura, 1995; Gist & Mitchell, 1992). An older adult who strongly believes he is able to independently bathe and dress because he has been doing so for 90 years will not likely alter self-efficacy expectations if he wakes up with severe arthritic changes one morning and is consequently unable to put on a shirt. However, repeated failures to perform the activity will impact self-efficacy expectations. The relative stability of strong self-efficacy expectations is important. Otherwise, an occasional failure or setback could severely impact self-efficacy expectations and impact behavior.

VICARIOUS EXPERIENCE

Self-efficacy expectations are also influenced by vicarious experiences or seeing other similar people successfully perform the same activity (Bandura et al., 1980; Kazdin, 1979). There are some conditions, however, which impact the influence of vicarious experience. If the individual has not been exposed to the behavior of interest or has had little experience with it, vicarious experience is likely to have a greater impact (Takata & Takata, 1976). Additionally, when clear guidelines for performance are not explicated, personal efficacy will be more likely to be impacted by the performance of others.

VERBAL PERSUASION

Verbal persuasion involves verbally telling an individual that he or she has the capabilities to master the given behavior. Empirical support for the influence of verbal persuasion, in addition to the early research of individuals with phobias (Bandura & Adams, 1977), has been demonstrated with regard to adoption of health-promoting behavior (Meyerowitz & Chaiken, 1987), recovery from postmyocardial infarction (Ewart et al., 1983), in performing functional activities (Resnick, 1998b), and in exercising (Resnick, 2002). Persuasive health influences lead people with a high sense of efficacy to intensify efforts at self-directed change with regard to reducing risky health behavior (Meyerowitz & Chaiken, 1987). For example, in patients with postmyocardial infarction, verbal persuasion by a physician and a nurse resulted in increasing self-efficacy beliefs regarding sexual activity, lifting, and general exertion. The counseling, or verbal persuasion had the greatest impact on the activities that were not actually performed while in the hospital (Ewart et al., 1983).

PHYSIOLOGICAL FEEDBACK

Individuals rely in part on information from their physiological state to judge their abilities. Physiological indicators are especially important in relation to coping with stressors, physical accomplishments, and health functioning. Individuals evaluate their physiological state, or arousal, and if aversive, they may avoid performing a particular behavior. For example, if an older adult has a fear of falling or getting hurt when walking, this high arousal state can debilitate performance and make the individual feel incapable of performing the activity. Likewise, if the rehabilitation activities result in fatigue, pain, or shortness of breath, these symptoms may be interpreted as physical inefficacy, and the older adult may not feel capable of performing the activity.

Interventions can be used to alter the interpretation of physiological feedback and help individuals cope with the sensations, including: (1) visualizing mastery, which eliminates the emotional reactions to a given situation and can strengthen self-efficacy expectations, resulting in improvement in performance (Bandura & Adams, 1977); (2) enhancing physical status (Bandura, 1995); and (3) altering the interpretation of bodily states (Meichenbaum, 1974).

DESCRIPTION OF THE THEORY OF SELF-EFFICACY

The theory of self-efficacy states that perceived self-efficacy, defined as an individual's judgment of his or her capabilities to organize and execute courses of action, is a determinant of performance (Figure 5-2). The theory of self-efficacy must be considered within the context of reciprocal determinism as described above. The four sources of information that can potentially influence self-efficacy and outcome expectations interact with characteristics of the individual and the environment. Ideally, self-efficacy and outcome expectations are strengthened by these experiences and thereby influence behavior. At the core of this theory is the assumption that people can exercise influence over what they do. A person will decide how to behave based on reflective thought, generative use of knowledge and skills to perform a specific behavior, as well as other tools of self-influence. Moreover, to determine one's self-efficacy, the individual must have the opportunity for self-evaluation or the comparison of individual output to some sort of evaluative criterion (White, Kjelgaard, & Harkins, 1995). This comparison process provides the individual with a sense of how likely it is that he or she can achieve a given level of performance.

Using the experiences or informational sources indicated above, it has been suggested that three processes are involved in the ultimate formation of self-efficacy expectations: (1) analysis of task requirements; (2) attributional analysis of experience; and (3) assessment of personal and situational resources/constraints (Gist & Mitchell, 1992). The analysis of task requirements involves consideration of what it takes to perform an activity at various levels. The attributional analysis of experience involves the individual's judgments or attributions about why a particular performance level occurred. For example, an individual might believe that she was able to jog when tired because she had strong muscles. The individual also considers the specific resources/constraints for performing the task at various levels. This assessment includes consideration of personal factors such as skill level, anxiety, or desire, as well as situational factors, such as competing demands or distractions that impinge on future performance. All three of these assessment processes are impacted by the individual's familiarity with the behavior and by the nature of the task itself.

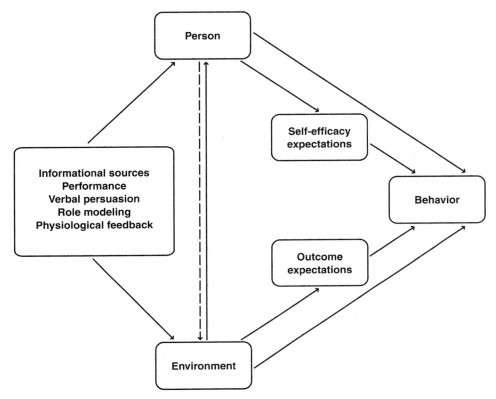

■ **Figure 5-2.** Model of theory of self-efficacy.

APPLICATIONS OF THE THEORY

Research

During the past 10 years, there have been approximately 400 articles in nursing journals that focus on the measurement and use of self-efficacy expectations and/or outcome expectations to predict behavior. While the focus of the studies range from management of chronic illnesses to education of nurses and parental training, the majority have been related to chronic health problems and participation in health-promoting activities such as exercise, smoking cessation, and weight loss (Table 5-1). The majority of these descriptive studies explore the relationship between self-efficacy expectations and behavior. A smaller number, however, have tested interventions developed to strengthen efficacy expectations related to the behavior of interest. What is most important regarding the use of the theory of self-efficacy in nursing research is that the researcher maintains the behavioral specificity of self-efficacy expectations and behavior. That is, measures should be developed to fit specifically with the be-

Table 5-1.   USE OF SELF-EFFICACY IN NURSING RESEARCH

AREA OF FOCUS	REFERENCE
Nurse Care Practices	Dilorio & Price, 2001; Ben-Ami et al., 2001; Rabinowitz et al., 1996; O'Brien & Page, 1994
Managing chronic illness Asthma and COPD	Siela, 1998; Sterling, 1999; Scherer et al., 1998; Scherer & Schmieder, 1996, 1997; Zimmerman et al., 1996; Van Der Palen et al., 2001
Diabetes	Bernal et al., 2000; Bijl et al., 1999; Johnson, 1996; Lo, 1998; Leonard et al., 1998; Remley & Cook-Newell, 1999
Depression	Kurlowicz, 1998; Perraud, 2000
Urinary incontinence	Broome, 1999
Cognitive impairment	McDougall, 2000; Mowat & Laschinger, 1994
Cancer	Boehm et al., 1995; Lev, 1997; Lev, Paul & Owen, 1999; Davis et al., 1994; Hammond et al., 1999; Keefe et al., 1997; Lorig & Holman, 1998
Arthritis	Rejeski et al., 1998; Borsody et al., 1999; Jeng & Braun, 1997
Cardiac	Perkins & Jenkins, 1998
Osteoporosis	Ali, 1998; Horan et al., 1998
Pain	Patel, 1998; Lin & Ward, 1996
Epilepsy	DiIorio et al., 1994
HIV	Sharts-Hopko, Regan-Kubinski, Lincoln & Heverly, 1996
Wound healing	Johnson, 1995
Nursing Education Math	Andrew, 1998; Hodge, 1999
Undergraduate, graduate and continuing education	Harvey & McMurray, 1994; Murdock & Neafsey, 1995; Nugent et al., 1999; Parsons, 1999
Mentoring	Hayes, 1998
Student	Goldenberg et al., 1997
Transcultural Care	Jeffreys & Smodlaka, 1999; Smith, 1998
Health Promotion Practices	Adderley-Kelly & Green, 1997; DiIorio et al., 2000; Fletcher & Banasik, 2001; Hale & Trumbetta, 1996; Kowalski, 1997; Moseley, 1999; Lindberg, 2000; Plotnikoff et al., 2000; Resnick, 1998a, 1998b; Resnick & Jenkins, 2000; Van Der Plight & Richard, 1994

Table 5-1. USE OF SELF-EFFICACY IN NURSING RESEARCH

AREA OF FOCUS	REFERENCE
Pre- and Postoperative Care	Moon & Backer, 2000; Oetker-Black, 1996; Parent & Fortin, 2000; Pellino et al., 1998
Drug Abuse	Washington, 1999; 2001
Maternal Child	Dilks & Beal, 1997; Drummond & Rickwood, 1997; Dennis & Faux, 1999; Gross et al., 1994; Hanson, 1998; Sinclair & O'Boyle, 1999

havior that is being considered, and efficacy and outcome expectations should be related to a specific behavioral outcome (i.e., exercise, smoking cessation).

SELF-EFFICACY STUDIES RELATED TO MANAGING ACUTE AND CHRONIC ILLNESS

Self-efficacy studies related to chronic illness both described and tested theory-based interventions. Many of the studies focused on self-efficacy in cardiac patients. Descriptive studies considered the relationship between self-efficacy and the rehabilitation activities of cardiac patients (Allen, Becker, & Swank, 1990; Jeng & Braun, 1994; Jenkins, 1985; Perkins, 1991; Schuster & Waldron, 1991). Jenkins (1985), basing his work on prior research on self-efficacy in cardiac patients (Ewart et al., 1983; Taylor, Bandura, Ewart, Miller & DeBusk, 1985), found self-efficacy expectations related to only two rehabilitation behaviors (walking and resting) when measured at four different periods during postmyocardial infarction recovery. For male patients following cardiac surgery, self-efficacy related to performance of activities of daily living at discharge was the best predictor of 6-month functional status (Allen et al., 1990). Perkins (1991), in a similar study of males postcardiac surgery, found self-efficacy measured prior to discharge correlated with participation in all cardiac-recovery behaviors except work. Schuster and Waldron (1991) included consideration of gender differences in their study of the impact of self-efficacy expectations on attendance in a cardiac rehabilitation program. On admission to the program, men had stronger self-efficacy expectations. Among participants who had not had bypass surgeries, men with high self-efficacy and women with low self-efficacy had fewer days of program attendance. In participants who had undergone bypass surgery, there was no relationship between attendance and self-efficacy for either sex. Jeng and Braun (1994) also considered the impact of self-efficacy expectations on participation in cardiac rehabilitation programs.

Several studies have been conducted to determine the effect of interventions on self-efficacy expectations (Gillis et al., 1993; Gulanick, 1991). Forty patients who had cardiac surgery or who experienced a myocardial infarction were randomly assigned to: (a) a treatment group receiving stress testing, teaching, and exercise training; (b) a treatment group receiving stress testing and exercise training but not teaching; or (c) a control group. There were statistically significant differences regarding self-efficacy between the groups before the treatment. Following the interventions, the treatment groups had higher self-efficacy expectations than the control group, but these differences were not statistically different. Nurse researchers have also used self-efficacy expectations to increase physical activity in patients with heart failure (Borsody, Courtney, Taylor & Jairath, 1999), and in those who have had percutaneous transluminal coronary angioplasty.

The example in Using Middle Range Theories 5-1 describes the influence of an intervention on self-efficacy expectations and behavioral outcomes.

Several studies have considered self-efficacy expectations in adults with diabetes. In a descriptive study of 142 inpatients with diabetes, Hurley and Shea (1992) reported that self-efficacy expectations regarding general management of diabetes, insulin, and diet management were predictive of follow-up diabetic self-care behaviors 4 weeks after discharge. An intervention study considering self-efficacy expectations regarding diabetic self-care (diet and exercise activities) was done in a group of 102 older adults who volunteered to participate in a diabetes self-care program (Glasgow et al., 1992). Although the intervention resulted in an improvement in self-management skills of older diabetic adults, there was no increase in self-efficacy expectations following the intervention.

Continued research in the area of diabetes management has focused on self-management and self-care issues (Bernal, Woolley, Schensul, & Dickinson, 2000; Bijl, Poelgeest-Eeltink, & Shortridge-Baggett, 1999; Lo, 1998). Specifically, the relationship between self-efficacy expectations and meal planning for adolescents was explored (Remley & Cook-Newell, 1999), as was maternal self-efficacy related to diabetes management in children (Leonard, Skay, & Rheinberger, 1998).

Building off the early work by Kaplan et al., (1984), nurse researchers have continued to focus on managing chronic obstructive pulmonary disease (COPD). In particular, research has focused on exploring the relationship between self-efficacy expectations and managing the associated shortness of breath in COPD and asthma (Scherer & Schmieder, 1996; Siela, 1998). Interventions such as educational programs and rehabilitation for COPD have been implemented and tested to determine if the in-

---

 5-1 USING MIDDLE RANGE THEORIES

Based on the self-efficacy interventions developed by Gortner, Rankin and Wolfe (1988), a large experimental study of the recovery of 156 patients following cardiac surgery was conducted. During their acute hospital stay, participants were randomized to receive one of the following interventions: (a) routine information about recovery after cardiac surgery or (b) routine information plus a slide/tape program on family coping and conflict resolution, with a brief counseling session and a weekly follow-up telephone call to monitor recovery. Efficacy expectations and the behaviors of walking, climbing, lifting, as well as general activity level, were monitored via telephone at 4, 8, 12, and 24 weeks. Based on repeated measures analyses, main effects of treatment were significant for increasing self-efficacy expectations for walking (p=.013), and actual walking performance (p=.01). Posthoc analyses demonstrated significantly higher levels of lifting (p=.001) and general activity (p=.003) between 4 and 8 weeks. Significant main effects of time were noted across all aspects of self-efficacy expectations, although there was little increase after the 8th week. Overall, this study provided some support for the impact of specific interventions to strengthen self-efficacy expectation, as well as the influence of self-efficacy on behavioral outcomes following cardiac surgery.

Gortner, S. & Jenkins, L. (1990). Self-efficacy and activity level following cardiac surgery. *Journal of Advanced Nursing*, 15, 1132–1138.

terventions result in increased self-efficacy expectations and decreased symptomatology (Scherer & Schmieder, 1996; Scherer & Shimmel, 1997; Van der Palen, Klein, & Seydel, 1997; Zimmerman, Brown, & Bowman, 1996). As with diabetes, consideration has also been given to the impact of parental self-efficacy expectations regarding the management of childhood asthma (Sterling, 1999).

Self-efficacy theory has been used repeatedly in nursing literature to explore the relationship between self-efficacy expectations and management of chronic musculoskeletal problems, including osteoarthritis (Lorig & Holman, 1998), rheumatoid arthritis (Smarr et al., 1997), hip fracture (Ruiz, 1992), chronic low back pain (Lin & Ward, 1996), and fibromyalgia (Buckelew et al., 1996). Interventions studies have focused on strengthening self-efficacy expectations related to the management of pain (Keefe et al., 1997), joint protection (Hammond, Lincoln, & Sutcliffe, 1999), medication management and performance of daily activities (Taal, Rasker, & Wiegman, 1996).

Resnick (1994, 1996, 1998a, 1999, 2000a), using combined quantitative and qualitative approaches, demonstrated that self-efficacy expectations and outcome expectations influence older adults' participation in functional activities and exercise. Based on these findings, interventions were developed to strengthen self-efficacy and outcome expectations related to these activities (Resnick, 1998a, 1998b, 2002; Resnick, Magaziner, Orwig, & Zimmerman, 2002).

The relationship between mood and cognition and self-efficacy expectations has also been studied in older adults. Self-efficacy expectations related to coping with depression (Perraud, 2000), as well as the exploration of the self-efficacy for caregivers regarding coping with individuals with cognitive impairment (Mowat & Laschinger, 1994), has been explored. Interventions to strengthen self-efficacy expectations related to cognition and thereby improve cognitive ability have also been tested (McDougall, 2000).

Nurse researchers in oncology identified relationships between self-efficacy expectations and health-promotion and disease-prevention behaviors and adaptation to cancer. Strong self-efficacy expectations, for example, predict intention to quit smoking, increased participation in screening programs, and adjustment to cancer diagnosis (Boehm et al., 1995; Lev, 1997; Lev, Paul, & Owen, 1999). Increased self-efficacy is associated with increased adherence to treatment, increased self-care behaviors, and decreased physical and psychological symptoms.

Less frequently studied is the impact of self-efficacy expectations on ulcer healing, particularly leg ulcerations (Johnson, 1995), and urinary incontinence (Broome, 1999). Self-efficacy beliefs are unlikely to change wound healing. Rather, the focus of self-efficacy should be on the behavior(s) needed to promote healing of a wound, for example, or the management of a disease. Beliefs about the ability to perform the required behavior (self-efficacy) and beliefs in the benefit of doing this behavior (response efficacy) are likely to make the individual more willing to perform the behavior. For example, if the patient believes that she is capable of wearing a compression dressing (putting it on, for example) and believes that it will improve wound healing, it is more likely that she will actually wear the dressing.

SELF-EFFICACY STUDIES RELATED TO HEALTH PROMOTION/MATERNAL/CHILDCARE

Self-efficacy theory has directed research in nursing regarding a variety of health promotion activities. These studies focus on: (1) exercise in middle-aged adults (Fletcher & Banasik, 2001), older adults (Resnick, 2000a, 2001; Resnick et al., 2000), and individuals with diabetes (Plotnikoff, Brez, & Holz, 2000); (2) smoking cessation (Lev, et al., 1999); (3) cancer prevention, specifically related to breast cancer (Adderly, Kelly, & Green, 1997); (4) safe sexual activity in adults (Dilorio, Dudley, Soet, Watkins & Maibach, 2000) and adolescents (Van der Pligt & Richard, 1994); (5) education related to pre- and postop care for cardiac surgeries (Parent & Fortin, 2000), and orthopedic surgeries (Moon & Backer, 2000; Pellino et al., 1998); and (6) changing behavior related to drug dependence (Washington, 1999, 2001). Self-efficacy theory has likewise driven research in the area of maternal child nursing specifically related to childbirth activities (Dilks & Beal, 1997; Drummond & Rickwood, 1997; Sinclair & O'Boyle, 1999), breast feeding (Dennis & Faux, 1999), maternal expectations for care of toddlers (Gross, Conrad, Fogg, & Wotke, 1994) and care of children with asthma (Hanson, 1998).

While the majority of these studies were descriptive, some tested the impact of self-efficacy–based interventions specifically to see if the interventions influenced self-efficacy and outcome expectations and ultimately changed behavior. Resnick (2002), for example, developed and tested the WALC intervention (Table 5-2) to determine if this intervention strengthened self-efficacy and outcome expectations for walking in a group of older adults. The results indicated that those exposed to the intervention had stronger self-efficacy expectations and increased walking/exercise during a 6-month period (Resnick, 2002).

Nursing Education

In addition to a clinical focus, self-efficacy–based research has guided the exploration of educational techniques for nursing. Studies of undergraduates have focused on self-efficacy expectations related to math and science (Andrew, 1998; Hodge, 1999) and clinical skills (Dilorio & Price, 2001; Ford-Gilboe, 1997; Goldenberg, Iwasiw, & MacMaster, 1997; Mandorin & Iwasiw, 1999). The impact of

Table 5-2. WALC INTERVENTION

PNEUMONIC	INTERVENTION
W: Walk	Participants were visited weekly by the nurse practitioner and encouraged to walk at least 3 times per week for 20 minutes.
A: Address uncomfortable sensations associated with exercise	At each weekly visit attempts were made to decrease any unpleasant sensations associated with exercise, such as pain, fatigue, or shortness of breath.
L: Learn about exercise	At each weekly visit the nurse practitioner reviewed a simple investigator-developed booklet about exercise for older adults, which reviewed the benefits of exercise and how to overcome the barriers to exercise.
	The nurse practitioner worked with the participants to develop short- and long-term goals related to exercise, and these were reviewed weekly and updated as appropriate.
C: Cueing for exercise	During the first visit of the month, the nurse practitioner provided the participants with a calendar that depicted exactly what exercise to do each day.

self-efficacy expectations for the new advanced practice nurse has also been explored (Beraducci & Lengacher, 1998), as has teacher and mentor self-efficacy expectations (Hayes, 1998; Nugent, Bradshaw, & Kito, 1999).

Nursing Practice

Translation of research findings into practice is not often done in a timely fashion. This is particularly true of research findings that focus on behavior change. There is, however, evidence to demonstrate that the theory of self-efficacy can help direct care in a variety of areas relevant to nursing. In particular, the theory of self-efficacy has been particularly helpful for motivating individuals to participate in health-promoting activities, such as regular exercise, smoking cessation, weight loss, and regular cancer screenings. Resnick (1999, 2001, 2002) has developed and implemented a variety of clinical programs based on the theory of self-efficacy to encourage exercise activity in older adults. The Seven Step Approach to Developing and Implementing an Exercise Program for community-dwelling older adults incorporates the theory of self-efficacy. The seven steps include (1) Education, (2) Exercise prescreening, (3) Setting Goals, (4) Exposure to Exercise, (5) Role Models, (6) Verbal Encouragement, and (7) Verbal Reinforcement/Rewards, all of which focus on strengthening self-efficacy and outcome expectations (Resnick, 2000).

The theory of self-efficacy also guides the recommended steps for developing and implementing restorative-care nursing programs (Fleishell & Resnick, 2000). Based on the theory of self-efficacy, a two-tiered approach was developed as a practical way to implement a successful restorative care nursing program (Resnick, Allen, & Ruane, 2002). The two-tiered approach focuses first on teaching nursing assistants how to perform restorative-care activities and how to motivate older adults to engage in these activities. The second tier focuses on the residents and the implementation of techniques to motivate these individuals to perform the necessary restorative-care tasks.

Similarly, self-efficacy theory was used to guide the development of cardiac rehabilitation programs (Jeng & Braun, 1994). For patients to achieve the greatest benefit from cardiac rehabilitation programs, nurses must help them to modify unhealthy behaviors. The theory of self-efficacy provides a systematic direction that allows the nurse to interpret, modify, and predict the patient's behaviors.

Changes in lifestyle are also commonly needed for individuals who must learn to live with chronic illness. The ease with which such changes occur depends on the individual's self-efficacy and outcome expectations. Self-efficacy theory has also been used to help patients manage chronic disease, such as COPD and cancer. A self-management program for COPD, for example, was developed and incorporates a 6-week, nurse-directed, self-management program geared toward strengthening self-efficacy expectations related to managing dyspnea (Scherer & Shimmel, 1996).

INSTRUMENTS USED IN EMPIRICAL TESTING

Self-efficacy is situation specific and dynamic, in that it focuses on beliefs about personal abilities in a specific setting or on a particular behavior, such as dieting or exercise. Additionally, self-efficacy varies in magnitude or difficulty, strength, or degree of confidence, and generality, which is the ability to generalize about one's self-efficacy from one situation to another. Instruments to measure self-efficacy are developed to include these three parameters (Bandura, 1986; Dilorio, Faherty, & Manteuffel, 1992;

O'Leary, 1985). Because self-efficacy is highly context or situation dependent, measurement tools must be developed with respect to a specific task or activity. No single standardized measure of self-efficacy will be appropriate for all studies, and researchers often need to develop new or significantly revised measures in each investigation.

Generally, operationalization of self-efficacy expectation has been based on Bandura's (1977) early work with snake phobias. This approach included a paper-and-pencil measure, with a series of activities in a specific behavioral domain listed from least to most difficult. The respondents first indicated whether or not they could perform the activity, and then evaluated the degree of confidence they had in performing the activity. Respondents were given a 100-point scale, divided into 10-unit intervals, ranging from 0, which is completely uncertain, to 10, which is completely certain, to identify the extent of confidence they had in performing the activity. Additionally, generality was measured by evaluating the individual's ability to generalize self-efficacy to other similar behaviors (initially, ability to tolerate snakes was translated to ability to tolerate spiders).

Item/Scale Characteristics

The majority of the self-efficacy scales developed have continued to use the format described by Bandura. Most commonly, researchers attempted to measure the strength of self-efficacy using the confidence continuum. There have been some alternative-response formats used that differ from the 0 to 10 (corresponding to 0% through 100%) confidence continuum. These include a rating scale that consists of choices from 1 to 5 or 1 to 4, and, in some cases, a yes/no format. Bandura, and others working in close association with him, continue to encourage the 0-to-10 format, although this is not based on empirical evidence of its greater accuracy.

Another important issue in the measurement of self-efficacy relates to administration of the measure. The majority of self-efficacy scales have been paper-and-pencil tests (Vispoel, 1990). This type of administration was suggested to give the participant optimum privacy and to encourage honesty. Some researchers have developed the scales to be given either as self-administered measures or as an interview (Jenkins, 1985). However, little research has explored whether or not there is a significant difference in using one or the other approach.

Because self-efficacy is dynamic in nature, measurement of self-efficacy is designed to be administered at different points. Additionally, it is important when measuring self-efficacy to be certain to (1) rate self-efficacy expectations before any behavior is measured, or any other scale given that could influence the individual's self-efficacy expectation; (2) include a measure of the behavior of interest that corresponds to the items in the self-efficacy scale; and (3) only measure self-efficacy in respondents who can realistically perform the activity; otherwise, it is a measure of wishful thinking, rather than a belief in one's ability to realistically perform a behavior (Bandura, 1977, 1986).

Development of Self-Efficacy Measures: Selected Examples

At least 90 different self-efficacy measures have been identified in the literature, covering a wide range of content (Vispoel, 1990). The majority of scales have been associated with school-related and health-related content; however, self-efficacy related to careers, military competency, computer use, and general self-efficacy have also been developed. There are, for example, self-efficacy scales for adults with arthritis (Lomi & Nordholm, 1992; Lorig, Chastain, Ung, Shoor, & Holman, 1989), epilepsy (Dilorio, Faherty, & Manteuffel, 1992), those recovering from cardiac events (Hickey, Owen, & Froman, 1992; Jenkins, 1985), orthopedic events (Ruiz, 1992); those that consider overall physical function (Ryckman, Robbins, Thornton, & Cantrell, 1982; Schuster & Waldron, 1991), asthma management (Wigal, Stout, Brandon, Winder, McConnaughy, Creer, & Kotses, 1993), and COPD (Wigal, Creer, & Kotses, 1991); and outcome expectation scales focusing on functional ability (Resnick, 1998b), exercise (Resnick & Jenkins, 2000); and adherence to osteoporosis medication (Resnick, Wehren, & Orwig, 2003). Because self-efficacy and outcome expectations are behavior specific, it is essential to use an appropriate measure that truly reflects the behavior of interest. Examples of measures developed and used in nursing research are listed in Table 5-3. In-depth examples for how these measures can be developed and tested are provided to serve as a template for how this can be done.

THE SELF-EFFICACY FOR FUNCTIONAL ABILITY (SEFA) SCALE

The SEFA scale (Resnick, 1999) is a nine-item measure that asks participants to rate their confidence in their ability to perform functional activities (with or without an assistive device). Specifically, these activities include bathing, dressing, transferring, toileting, ambulating, and climbing stairs. Traditionally, self-efficacy measures are ordered hierarchically, from the easiest to the most difficult. There is, however, individual variation regarding which functional task is the most difficult to perform. Therefore, random ordering of the items in the SEFA was done

The SEFA scale was administered using an interview format. Participants were instructed to listen to the statement and then use numbers from 0 to 10 (with 0 being no confidence and 10 being very confident) to rate present beliefs in their ability to perform functional activities. The scale was scored by getting a mean score (i.e., summing scores for each activity and dividing by the number of activities). Evidence of reliability and validity of the SEFA based on three studies (Resnick, 1998a; 1998b) is described in Table 5-4.

THE SELF-EFFICACY FOR EXERCISE (SEE) SCALE

The SEE scale (Resnick & Jenkins, 2000) is a revision of McAuley's (unpublished) self-efficacy-barriers-to-exercise measure. The self-efficacy-barriers-to-exercise measure is a 13-item instrument that focuses on self-efficacy expectations related to the ability to continue exercising in the face of barriers to exercising. This measure was initially developed for sedentary adults in the community who participated in an outpatient exercise program (including biking, rowing, and walking). The revision of McAuley's self-efficacy-barriers-to-exercise measure was based on a combined quantitative and qualitative study exploring factors that influenced adherence to a regular walking program for older adults (Resnick & Spellbring, 2000). The participants in this exploratory study identified several items on the self-efficacy-barriers to exercise measure that were not relevant to them: (a) the impact of a vacation on exercise activity; (b) getting to the exercise location; (c) feeling self-conscious about ones' appearance while exercising; and (d) lack of encouragement from the leader. These questions were therefore removed from the initial measure. There were two questions that participants felt were repetitive (both related to the individuals' interest in the activity), and these questions were combined into a single item (item 5) on the revised measure. Qualitative interviews indicated that past experiences with ex-

Table 5-3. SELF-EFFICACY MEASURES IN NURSING RESEARCH

AUTHOR	MEASURE
Ali, 1998	Hormone Replacement Theory Self-Efficacy Scale
Bijl, Poelgeest-Eeltink, Shortridge-Baggett, 1999	Self-Efficacy in New Nurse Educators
Broome, 1999	Self-Efficacy for Pelvic Muscle Exercise
Corbett, 1999	Diabetes Self-Efficacy
DeGeest, Abraham, Gemoets & Evers, 1994	Long-Term Medication Behavior Scale
Dennis & Faux, 1999	Breast Feeding Self-Efficacy
Dilorio & Price, 2001	Neuroscience Self-Efficacy
Fletcher & Banasik, 2001	Exercise Self-Efficacy
Froman & Owen, 1999	Physical and Mental Self-Efficacy
Hale & Trumbetta, 1996	Women's Self-Efficacy and Sexually Transmitted Disease
Hanson, 1998	Parental Self-Efficacy and Asthma Self-Efficacy
Hayes, 1998	Mentoring NP Student Self-Efficacy
Horan et al., 1998	Osteoporosis Self-Efficacy Scale
Jeffreys & Smodlaka, 1999	Transcultural Self-Efficacy Scale
Lev & Owen, 1999	Self-Care and Self-Agency Self-Efficacy
Lin & Ward, 1996	Self-Efficacy and Outcome Expectation in Coping with Chronic Low Back Pain
Madorin & Iwasiw, 1999	Self-Efficacy of Baccalaureate Nurses
Moseley, 1999	Food Pyramid Self-Efficacy
Oetker-Black, 1996	Preop Self-Efficacy
Perraud, 2000	Depression Coping Self-Efficacy Scale
Remley & Cook-Newell, 1999	Meal Planning Self-Efficacy
Resnick & Jenkins, 2000	Self-Efficacy for Exercise
Resnick, 1999	Self-Efficacy for Functional Activities
Sinclair & O'Boyle, 1999	Childbirth Self-Efficacy

ercise, identification of goals, personality, sensations associated with exercise, such as pain and mood, all influenced exercise activity. Therefore, appropriate items relevant to these issues (items 1, 3, and 9) were added to the SEE measure. Initial reliability and validity testing was done using a sample of 187 older adults living in a continuing-care retirement community, and supported evidence of reliability and validity of this measure (Resnick & Jenkins, 2000).

TABLE 5-4. DESCRIPTIVE STATISTICS OF PILOT SAMPLE

VARIABLE	STUDY I Frequency (%) (N = 51 participants in rehabilitation program)	STUDY II Frequency (%) (N = 77 participants in rehabilitation program)	STUDY III Frequency (%) (N = 44 residents in long-term care facility)
Gender			
Males	11 (22%)	22 (29%)	7 (16%)
Females	40 (78%)	55 (71%)	37 (84%)
Marital Status			
Married	20 (39%)	-	8 (12%)
Widowed	30 (59%)	-	50 (73%)
Never Married	1 (2%)	-	11 (15%)
Race			
White	44 (86%)	63 (82%)	44 (100%)
Black	7 (14%)	14 (18%)	
Age	77 ± 8	78 ± 7.2	88 ± 6.4
SEFA (admission)	5.9 ± 1	5.6 ± 2	5.6 ± 2.9
SEFA (discharge)	8.3 ± .8	8.8 ± 1.5	
Functional	50 ± 6.8	44 ± 8.5	59 ± 18.5
Performance	65 ± 5.8	63 ± 7.8	

THE SELF-EFFICACY FOR OSTEOPOROSIS MEDICATION ADHERENCE (SEOMA) SCALE

Prior research exploring the development of long-term medication behavior self-efficacy expectations resulted in the identification of three major categories that influence adherence (De Geest, Abraham, Germoets, & Evers, 1994). These categories include (1) personal attributes, such as emotions, perceived health status, and confidence in the physician; (2) environmental factors, such as routine, distraction, cost, and social support; and (3) task-related and behavioral factors, such as medication aids, schedules, knowledge about the medication, drug delivery system, and side effects. To build on these findings, focus groups were held to identify the issues around adherence (i.e., particularly the barriers and challenges to adherence) to osteoporosis medication for older adults. Box 5-1 lists the most common challenges identified by the older adults that influence adherence. Based on these findings, the self-efficacy measures for osteoporosis medication adherence were developed.

The SEOMA scale (Resnick, Wehren, & Orwig, 2003) is a 14-item measure that addresses the many challenges associated with taking medication for osteoporosis. Examples of these challenges include adherence in light of side effects, such as constipation or stomach upset, or reluctance due to the high cost of the treatment. To complete the SEOMA, the participant was instructed to listen to a statement and then use numbers from 0 to 10, with 0 being not confident, and 10 being very confident, to rate present self-efficacy expectations related to adhering to his or her osteoporosis medication. Initial reliability and validity testing provided support for the reliability and validity of this measure (Resnick et al., 2003).

BOX 5-1. Factors That Influence Adherence to Osteoporosis Medication	
Stomach upset	Lack of knowledge as to need for the
Fear of stomach upset/ulceration	medication
Inconvenience of AM schedule	Constipation
Cost	Belief that it isn't necessary because of low
Uncertainty about the effects	risk of disease

OUTCOME EXPECTATIONS FOR EXERCISE (OEE) SCALE

The OEE is a nine-item scale that was developed based on several previously tested measures that focused on the outcome expectations and benefits associated with exercise in adults (Sechrist, Walker, & Pender, 1987; Steinhardt & Dishman, 1989), as well as qualitative and quantitative studies that identified the specific benefits of exercise to older adults (Conn, 1998; Melillo et al., 1996; Resnick & Spellbring, 2000; Schneider, 1997; Sharon, Hennessy, Brandon, & Boyette, 1997). In these studies, older adults reported that exercise made them feel better and walk better, improved their blood pressure control, and decreased pain, while at the same time accomplishing something, enjoying the activity, and experiencing an overall sense of well-being. While many of the same concepts were included in earlier versions of measures that focused on the benefits of exercise, the items for the OEE were written using the older adults' *own words* to describe the benefits they derived from exercise. Five of the items reflected physical benefits and four focused on mental health benefits. Item 9 was included in the measure because there has been a strong emphasis in the lay literature suggesting that exercise increases bone strength and prevents osteoporosis.

To complete the OEE scale, the participant is asked to listen to a statement about exercise and to (1) strongly agree, (2) agree, (3) neither agree nor disagree, (4) disagree, or (5) strongly disagree with the stated outcomes or benefits of exercising. The following nine statements are included: (1) Makes me feel better physically (physical health); (2) Makes my mood better in general (mental health); (3) Helps me feel less tired (physical health); (4) Makes my muscles stronger (physical health); (5) Is an activity I enjoy doing (mental health); (6) Gives me a sense of personal accomplishment (mental health); (7) Makes me more alert mentally (mental health); (8) Improves my endurance in performing my daily activities (physical health); and (9) Helps to strengthen my bones (physical health). Mean scores were obtained as they were done in the self-efficacy measure. There was sufficient evidence of the reliability and validity of both of these measures (Resnick et al., 2003).

The Research Application 5-1 provides an example of the use of the OEE Scale to determine the effectiveness of an intervention on self-efficacy and increased exercise in older adults.

SUMMARY

Empirical testing using the theory of self-efficacy has provided significant support for the importance of self-efficacy and outcome expectations regarding behavior and changing behavior. There is also some support for the effectiveness of specific interventions that have been tested to strengthen both self-efficacy and outcome expectations and thereby improve or change behavior. It is important to note, how-

5-1 RESEARCH APPLICATION

A researcher wants to examine the effect of several approaches that could be used to promote physical exercise in attendees at senior centers. The hypothesis to be tested in this study is: There are increased self-efficacy outcome expectations and self-initiated physical exercise in elderly women from senior centers who participate in an exercise class with telephone follow-up when compared to those who attend a didactic class with telephone follow-up, or exercise class without telephone follow-up.

Thirty subjects each from three senior centers in a metropolitan area are to be recruited and randomly assigned to one of three groups: (a) exercise class with telephone follow-up; (b) didactic class with telephone follow-up; and (c) exercise class without telephone follow-up. Each senior center will offer all three interventions. To be included in the study, participants must be female, between ages 70 to 85 years old, and without physical limitations as determined by a physician.

Before being randomly assigned to a treatment group, each subject keeps an exercise diary for 1 week and completes Outcome Expectations for Exercise (OEE) scale. Those who are assigned to the exercise class with telephone follow-up attend four weekly 30-minute classes in which exercises are demonstrated and they participate. In addition, a staff member from the senior center will call each participant every other week to inquire about how her personal exercise program is progressing. The phone calls are to continue for a period of 2 months. Participants assigned to the didactic class with telephone follow-up attend four weekly 30-minute class sessions in which the benefits of exercise in the elderly are emphasized. They also receive a pamphlet with instructions on specific exercises. Their telephone follow-up is identical to that of the group participating in a physical exercise class. The third group of participants also attend four weekly 30-minute classes in which exercises are demonstrated, and they participate but receive no telephone follow-up.

During the period of the study, all participants keep an exercise activity diary, recording daily the frequency and duration of exercise. The OEE will be readministered at 4, 6, 8, and 12 weeks after initiation of the interventions. The exercise diaries are to be collected at the same time and the total amount of exercise in minutes per week tabulated. ANOVA with follow-up t-tests, using Tukey's Wholly Significant Difference test will be used to test the hypothesis.

ever, that these studies also serve as a reminder that self-efficacy and outcome expectations may not be the *only* predictors of behavior. Other variables, such as tension/anxiety, barriers to behavior, and other psychosocial constructs likewise influence behavior. Bandura (1986) recognized that expectations alone will not result in behavior change if there are no incentives to perform, inadequate resources, or external constraints. Certainly, an individual may believe he or she can participate in a rehabilitation program but may not have the resources (i.e., transportation or money) to do so.

Self-efficacy theory is situation-specific. It is difficult, therefore, to generalize an individual's self-efficacy expectations from one type of behavior to another. If an individual has high self-efficacy regarding diet management, this may or may not translate to persistence in an exercise program. Consequently, it is essential to use appropriate self-efficacy measures, or develop an appropriate measure that is relevant to the behavior of interest. This requires the preliminary work of understanding behavior, particularly the challenges associated with performance and the consequences (both positive and negative) of performance of the behavior.

Self-efficacy and outcome expectations measures should be developed to comprehensively include a series of activities/challenges listed in order of increasing difficulty. It is important to carefully construct these scales and establish evidence of reliability and validity. Because self-efficacy and outcome expectations can be influenced by the many sources of efficacy expectations (e.g., performing a behavior), in most situations, it is not appropriate to estimate reliability using test–retest reliability. Although useful in research as either predictors or outcomes of behavior, these scales can be used as the foundation for assessing an individual's self-care abilities in a particular area. Interventions can then be developed that are relevant for that individual.

As with most research findings, use of the theory of self-efficacy, assessments of individual self-efficacy and outcome expectations, and implementation of interventions to strengthen self-efficacy or outcome expectations in real-world settings is slow. Measurement tools can be used clinically to evaluate the individual's efficacy expectations, and the health care provider can then implement appropriate interventions to strengthen expectations. For example, if completion of the OEOMA indicated that the individual did not believe that taking osteoporosis medication strengthens bones, appropriate interventions would focus on educational sessions that reviewed the impact of osteoporosis medication on bone and bone density.

There are several areas of self-efficacy–based research that have not yet been comprehensively addressed. Consistently, there has been a lack of consideration of outcome expectations, and most researchers ignore this component of the theory. Regarding exercise in older adults, however, outcome expectations have been better predictors of exercise behavior than self-efficacy expectations (Jette et al., 1998; Resnick et al., 2000). Increased focus is needed on outcome expectations because this can have a significant influence on the types of interventions developed to strengthen efficacy expectations and alter behavior.

Consideration also needs to be given to the influence of self-efficacy and outcome expectations to not only initiate behavior, but more importantly, to maintain adherence to that behavior. Most of the current work in this area considers the immediate influence of self-efficacy and outcome expectations, or the impact of these expectations over a relatively short time frame.

ANALYSIS EXERCISE

Using the criteria presented in Chapter 2, critique the Theory of Self-Efficacy. Compare your conclusions about the theory with those found in Appendix A. A researcher who has worked with the theory completed the analysis found in the Appendix.

Internal Criticism
1. Clarity
2. Consistency
3. Adequacy
4. Logical Development
5. Level of Theory Development

External Criticism
1. Reality Convergence
2. Utility
3. Significance
4. Discrimination
5. Scope of Theory
6. Complexity

WEB RESOURCES

1. Interventions Enhancing Self-Efficacy
   *http://www.positivepractices.com/
   InterventionsEnhancingSel.html*
2. Information on Self-Efficacy in a Community
   of Scholars
   *http://www.emory.edu/EDUCATION/mfp/
   efficacy.html*
   Comprehensive review of the theory of self-efficacy provided by Dr. Bandura, plus complete book chapters from previously published books on the theory by Dr. Bandura. In addition, there are PowerPoint slides available (English and Spanish) that review the theory, define components within the theory, and address the use of the theory in specific areas (i.e., education).
3. Self-Efficacy Measures
   *http://www.vangaurd.edu/faculty/ddege/man/
   amoeba.web/index*
   Comprehensive list of many different types of self-efficacy measures, such as self-efficacy for computer use and in the area of education. Covering the life span, these tools include a multitude of health behaviors.

REFERENCES

Adderly-Kelly, T., Rabin, S., & Azulai, S. (1997). Breast cancer education, self-efficacy, and screening in older African American women. *Journal of the National Black Nurses Association, 9*(1), 45–57.

Ali, N. (1998). Hormone replacement therapy self-efficacy scale. *Journal of Advanced Nursing, 28*(5), 1115–1119.

Allen, J. K., Becker, D. M., & Swank, R. T. (1990). Factors related to functional status after coronary artery bypass surgery. *Heart Lung, 19*(4), 337–343.

Andrew, S. (1998). Self-efficacy as a predictor of academic performance in science. *Journal of Advanced Nursing, 27*(3), 596–603.

Bandura, A. (1977). Self-efficacy: Toward a unifying theory of behavioral change. *Psychological Review, 84,* 191–215.

Bandura, A. (1986). *Social Foundations of Thought and Action.* Englewood, NJ: Prentice Hall.

Bandura, A. (1995). *Self-Efficacy in Changing Societies.* New York: Cambridge University Press.

Bandura, A. (1997). *Self-Efficacy: The Exercise of Control.* New York: W.H. Freeman.

Bandura, A., & Adams, N. (1977). Analysis of self-efficacy theory of behavioral change. *Cognitive Therapy and Research, 1*(4), 287–308.

Bandura, A., Adams, N., & Beyer, J. (1977). Cognitive processes mediating behavioral change. *Journal of Personality and Social Psychology, 35*(3), 125–149.

Bandura, A., Adams, N., Hardy, A., & Howells, G. (1980). Tests of the generality of self-efficacy theory. *Cognitive Therapy and Research, 4,* 39–66.

Bandura, A., Reese, L., & Adams, N. (1982). Microanalysis of action and fear arousal as a function of differential levels of perceived self-efficacy. *Journal of Personality and Social Psychology, 43,* 5–21.

Barling, J., & Abel, M. (1983). Self-efficacy beliefs and tennis performance. *Cognitive Therapy and Research, 7,* 371–376.

Ben-Ami, S., Shaham, J., Rabin, S., Melzer, A., & Ribak, J. (2001). The influence of nurses' knowledge, attitudes and health beliefs on their safe behavior with cytotoxic drugs in Israel. *Cancer Nursing, 24*(3), 192–200.

Berarducci, A., & Lengacher, C. (1998). Self-efficacy: An essential component of advanced practice nursing. *Nursing Connections, 11*(1), 55–67.

Bernal, H., Woolley, S., Schensul, J., & Dickinson, J. (2000). Correlates of self-efficacy in diabetes self-care among Hispanic adults with diabetes. *Diabetes Educator, 26,* 673–680.

Bijl, J., Poelgeest-Eeltink, A., & Shortridge-Baggett, L. (1999). The psychometric properties of the diabetes management self-efficacy scale for patients with type 2 diabetes mellitus. *Journal of Advanced Nursing, 30*(2), 352–359.

Boehm, S., Coleman-Burns, P., Schlenk, E., Funnell, M. M., Parzuchowski, J., & Powel, I. J. (1995). Prostate cancer in African American men: Increasing knowledge and self-efficacy. *Journal of Community Health Nursing, 12*(3), 161–169.

Borsody, J., Courtney, M., Taylor, K., & Jairath, N. (1999). Using self-efficacy to increase physical activity in patients with heart failure. *Home Healthcare Nurse, 17*(2), 113–118.

Broome, B. (1999). Development and testing of a scale to measure self-efficacy for pelvic muscle exercises in women with urinary incontinence. *Urology Nursing, 19*(4), 258–268.

Buckelew, S. P., Huyset, B., Hewett, J. E., Parker, J. C., Johnson, J. C., Conway, R., & Kay, D. R. (1996). Self-efficacy predicting outcome among fibromyalgia subjects. *Arthritis Care Research, 9*(2), 82–88.

Chambliss, C., & Murray, E. (1979). Efficacy attribution,

locus of control, and weight loss. *Cognitive Therapy and Research, 3,* 349–353.

Colletti, G., Supnick, J., & Payne, A. (1985). The smoking self-efficacy questionnaire (SSEQ): Preliminary scale development and validation. *Behavioral Assessment, 6*(3), 234–238.

Condiotte, M., & Lichtenstein, E. (1981). Self-efficacy and relapse in smoking cessation programs. *Journal of Consulting Clinical Psychology, 49,* 648–658.

Conn, V. (1998). Older adults and exercise. *Nursing Research, 47,* 180–189.

Corbett, C. (1999). Research-based practice implications for patients with diabetes. Part II: Diabetes self-efficacy. *Home Healthcare Nurse, 17*(9), 587–596.

Davis, P., Busch, A. J., Lowe, J. C., Taniguchi, J., & Djkowich, B. (1994). Evaluation of a rheumatoid arthritis patient education program: Impact on knowledge and self-efficacy. *Patient Education and Counseling, 24*(1), 55–61.

De Geest, S., Abraham, I., Gemoets, H., & Evers, G. (1994). Development of the long term medication behavior self-efficacy scale: Qualitative study for item development. *Journal of Advanced Nursing, 19,* 233–238.

Dennis, C., & Faux, S. (1999). Development and psychometric testing of the Breastfeeding Self-Efficacy Scale. *Research in Nursing and Health, 22*(5), 399–409.

Dilks, F., & Beal, J. (1997). Role of self-efficacy in birth choice. *Journal of Perinatal and Neonatal Nursing, 11*(1), 1–9.

Dilorio, C., Dudley, W., Soet, J., Watkins, J., & Maibach, E. (2000). A social cognitive based model for condom use among college students. *Nursing Research, 49*(4), 208–214.

Dilirio, L., Faherty, B., & Manteuffel, B. (1992). Instrument to measure self-efficacy in individuals with epilepsy. *Journal of Neuroscience Nursing, 24*(1), 9–13.

Dilorio, C. & Price, M. (2001). Description and use of the neuroscience nursing self-efficacy scale. *Journal of Neuroscience Nursing, 33*(3), 130–135.

Drummond, J., & Rickwood, D. (1997). Childbirth confidence: Validating the childbirth self-efficacy inventory (CBSEI) in an Australian sample. *Journal of Advanced Nursing, 26*(3), 613–622.

Ewart, C., Taylor, G., Reese, L., & DeBusk, R. (1983). Effects of early post-myocardial infarction exercise testing on self-perception and subsequent physical activity. *American Journal of Cardiology, 51,* 1076–1080.

Fleishell, A., & Resnick, B. (2000). *Staying Alive: Minimizing Loss and Maximizing Potential. Manual for Restorative Care Nursing Programs.* Published by Joanne Wilson's Gerontological Nursing Ventures, Laurel, MD.

Fletcher, J., & Banasik, J. (2001). Exercise self-efficacy. *Clinical Excellence for Nurse Practitioners, 5*(3), 134–143.

Ford-Gilboe, M. (1997). Family strengths, motivation, and resources as predictors of health promotion behavior in single-parent and two-parent families. *Research in Nursing and Health, 20*(3), 205–217.

Gillis, C., Gortner, S., Hauck, W., Shinn, J., Sparacino, P., & Tompkins, C. (1993). A randomized clinical trial of nursing care for recovery from cardiac surgery. *Heart & Lung, 22*(2), 125–133.

Gist, M., & Mitchell, T. (1992). Self-efficacy: A theoretical analysis of its determinants and malleability. *Academy of Management Review, 17*(2), 183–211.

Glasgow, R., Toobert, D., Hampson, S., Brown, J., Lewinston, P., & Donnelly, J. (1992). Improving self-care among older patients with Type II diabetes: The sixty something study. *Patient Education and Counseling, 19,* 61–70.

Godding, P., & Glasgow, R. (1985). Self-efficacy and outcome expectations as predictors of control in health status. *Cognitive Therapy and Research, 9,* 27–35.

Goldenberg, D., Iwasiw, C., & MacMaster, E. (1997). Self-efficacy of senior baccalaureate nursing students and preceptors. *Nurse Educator Today, 17*(4), 303–310.

Gortner, S., & Jenkins, L. (1990). Self-efficacy and activity level following cardiac surgery. *Journal of Advanced Nursing, 15,* 1132–1138.

Gortner, S., Rankin, S., & Wolfe, M. (1988). Elders' recovery from cardiac surgery. *Progress in Cardiovascular Nursing, 3*(2), 54–61.

Grembowski, D., Patrick, D., Diehr, P., Durham, M., Beresford, S., Kay, E., & Hecht, J. (1993). Self-efficacy and health behavior among older adults. *Journal of Health and Social Behavior, 34,* 89–104.

Gross, D., Conrad, B., Fogg, L., & Wotke, W. (1994). A longitudinal model of maternal self-efficacy, depression, and difficult temperament during toddlerhood. *Research in Nursing and Health, 17*(3), 207–215.

Gulanick, M. (1991). Is phase 2 cardiac rehabilitation necessary for early recovery of patients with cardiac disease? A randomized, controlled study. *Heart & Lung, 20*(1), 9–15.

Hale, P., & Trumbetta, S. (1996). Women's self-efficacy and sexually transmitted disease preventive behaviors. *Research in Nursing and Health, 19*(2), 101–110.

Hammond, A., Lincoln, N., & Sutcliffe, L. (1999). A crossover trial evaluating an educational-behavioral joint protection programme for people with rheumatoid arthritis. *Patient Education and Counseling, 37*(1), 19–32.

Hanson, J. (1998). Parental self-efficacy and asthma self-management skills. *Journal of Society of Pediatric Nurses, 3*(4), 146–154.

Harvey, V., & McMurray, N. (1994). Self-efficacy: A means of identifying problems in nursing education and career progress. *International Journal of Nursing Studies, 31*(5), 471–485.

Hayes, E. (1998). Mentoring and nurse practitioner student self-efficacy. *Western Journal of Nursing Research, 20*(5), 521–535.

Hickey, M., Owen, S., & Froman, R. (1992). Instrument development: Cardiac diet and exercise self-efficacy. *Nursing Research, 41*(6), 347–351.

Hodge, M. (1999). Do anxiety, math self-efficacy and gender affect nursing students' drug dosage calculations? *Nurse Educator, 24*(4), 36, 41.

Horan, M., Kimm, K., Gendler, P., Froman, R., & Patel, M. (1998). Development and evaluation of an osteoporosis self-efficacy scale. *Research in Nursing and Health, 21*(5), 395–403.

Hurley, D., & Shea, C. (1992). Self-efficacy: Strategy for enhancing diabetes self-care. *Diabetes Educator, 18*(2), 146–150.

Jeffreys, M., & Smodlaka, I. (1999). Construct validation of the transcultural self-efficacy tool. *Journal of Nurse Educator, 38*(5), 222–227.

Jeng, C., & Braun, L. T. (1997). Bandura's self-efficacy theory: A guide for cardiac rehabilitation nursing practice. *Journal of Holistic Nursing, 12*(4), 425–436.

Jenkins, L. (1985). Self-efficacy in recovery from myocardial infarction. Unpublished Doctoral Dissertation. University of Maryland, Baltimore, MD.

Jette, A., Rooks, D., Lachman, M., Lin, T., Levensen, C., Heislein, D., Giorgetti, N. M., & Harris, B. A. (1998). Effectiveness of home-based, resistance training with disabled older persons. *Gerontologist, 38*, 412–422.

Johnson, J. A. (1996). Self-efficacy theory as a framework for community pharmacy-based diabetes education programs. *Diabetes Educator, 22*(3), 237–241.

Johnson, M. (1995). Healing determinants in older people with leg ulcers. *Research in Nursing and Health, 18*(5), 393–403.

Kaplan, R., Atkins, C., & Reinsch, S. (1984). Specific efficacy experiences mediate exercise compliance in patients with COPD. *Health Psychology, 3*(3), 223–242.

Kazdin, A. (1978). Behavioral modification and role modeling. *Child Behavior Therapy, 1*(1), 13–36.

Keefe, F. J., Lefebvre, J. C., Maixner, W., Salley, A. N., & Caldwell, D. S. (1997). Self-efficacy for arthritis pain: Relationship to perception of thermal laboratory pain stimuli. *Arthritis Care Research, 10*(3), 177–184.

Kowalski, S. (1997). Self-esteem and self-efficacy as predictors of success in smoking cessation. *Journal of Holistic Nursing, 15*(2), 128–142.

Kurlowicz, L. H. (1998). Perceived self-efficacy, functional ability, and depressive symptoms in older patients. *Nursing Research, 47*(4), 219–226.

Leonard, B., Skay, C., & Rheinberger, M. (1998). Self-management development in children and adolescents with diabetes: The role of maternal self-efficacy and conflict. *Journal of Pediatric Nursing, 13*(4), 224–233.

Lev, E.L. (1997). Bandura's theory of self-efficacy: Applications to oncology. *Image: Scholarly Inquiry for Nursing Practice, 11*(1), 21–37.

Lev, E., Paul, D., & Owen, S. (1999). Age, self-efficacy and change in patients' adjustment to cancer. *Cancer Practitioner, 7*(4), 170–176.

Lin, C., & Ward, S. (1996). Perceived self-efficacy and outcome expectancies in coping with chronic low back pain. *Research Nursing and Health, 19*(4), 299–310.

Lindberg, C. (2000). Knowledge, self-efficacy, coping and condom use among urban women. *Journal of the Association of Nurses AIDS Care, 11*(5), 80–90.

Lo, R. (1998). A holistic approach in facilitation adherence in people with diabetes. *Australian Journal of Holistic Nursing, 5*(1), 10–18.

Lomi, C., & Nordholm, L. (1992). Validation of a Swedish version of the arthritis self-efficacy scale. *Rheumatology, 21*(5), 231–237.

Lorig, K., Chastain, R., Ung, E., Shoor, S., & Holman, H. (1989). Development and evaluation of a scale to measure perceived self-efficacy in people with arthritis. *Arthritis and Rheumatism, 32*(1), 37–44.

Lorig, K., & Holman, H. (1998). Arthritis self-efficacy scales measure self-efficacy. *Arthritis Care Research, 11*(3), 155–157.

Macnee, C. L., & Talsma, A. (1995). Predictors of progress in smoking cessation. *Public Health Nursing, 12*(4), 242–248.

Madorin, S., & Iwasiw, C. (1999). The effects of computer-assisted instruction on the self-efficacy of baccalaureate nursing students. *Journal of Nurse Educators, 38*(6), 282–285.

McAuley, E., Courneya, K., & Lettunich, J. (1991). Effects of acute and long-term exercise on self-efficacy responses in sedentary, middle-aged males and females. *The Gerontologist, 31*(4), 534–542.

McDougall, G. (2000). Memory improvement in assisted living elders. *Issues in Mental Health Nursing, 21*(2), 217–233.

McIntyre, K., Lichtenstein, E., & Mermelstein, R. (1983). Self-efficacy and relapse in smoking cessation: A replication and extension. *Journal of Consulting and Clinical Psychology, 51*, 632–633.

Melillo, K., Futrell, M., Williamson, E., Chamberlain, C., Bourque, A., MacDonnell, M., & Phaneuf, J. (1996). Perceptions of physical fitness and exercise activity among older adults. *Journal of Advanced Nursing, 23*, 542–547.

Meichenbaum, D. (1974). Self-instructional strategy training: A cognitive prosthesis for the aged. *Human Development, 17*, 273–280.

Meyerowitz, C., & Chaiken, H. (1987). The impact of self-efficacy on risky health behaviors. *Behavioral Research and Therapy, 25*(5), 267–273.

Moon, L., & Backer, J. (2000). Relationships among self-efficacy, outcome expectancy, and postoperative behaviors in total joint replacement patients. *Orthopedic Nursing, 19*(2), 77–85.

Moseley, J. (1999). Reliability and validity of the Food Pyramid Self Efficacy Scale: Use in coronary artery bypass patients. *Progress of Cardiovascular Nursing, 14*(4), 130–135.

Mowat, J., & Laschinger, H. K. (1994). Self-efficacy in caregivers of cognitively impaired elderly people: A concept analysis. *Journal of Advanced Nursing, 19*(6), 1105–1113.

Murdock, J. E., & Neafsey, P. J. (1995). Self-efficacy measurements: An approach for predicting practice outcomes in continuing education? *Journal of Continuing Education in Nursing, 26*(4), 158–165.

Nugent, K., Bradshaw, M., & Kito, N. (1999). Teacher self-efficacy in new nurse educators. *Journal of Professional Nursing, 15*(4), 229–237.

O'Brien, S., & Page, S. (1994). Self-efficacy perfectionism and stress in Canadian nurses. *Canadian Journal of Nursing Research, 26*(3), 49–61.

Oetker-Black, S. (1996). Generalizability of the Preoperative Self-Efficacy Scale. *Applied Nursing Research, 9*(1), 40–44.

O'Leary, A. (1985). Self-efficacy and health. *Behavioral Research and Therapy, 23*(4), 437–450.

Parent, N., & Fortin, F. (2000). A randomized, controlled trial of vicarious experience through peer support for male first time cardiac surgery patients: Impact on anxiety, self-efficacy expectation, and self-reported activity. *Heart and Lung, 29*(6), 389–400.

Parsons, L.C. (1999). Building RN confidence for delegation decision-making skills in practice. *Journal of Nurses Staff Development, 15*(6), 263–269.

Pellino, T., Tluczek, A., Collins, M., Trimborn, S., Norwick, H., Engelke, Z., & Broad, J. (1998). Increasing self-efficacy through empowerment: Preoperative education for orthopaedic patients. *Orthopedic Nursing, 17*(4), 48-51, 54–59.

Perkins, S. (1991). Self-efficacy and mood status in recovery from percutaneous transluminal coronary angioplasty. Unpublished doctoral dissertation. University of Kansas, Kansas City.

Perkins, S., & Jenkins, L. (1998). Self-efficacy expectation, behavior performance and mood status in early recovery from percutaneous transluminal coronary angioplasty. *Heart and Lung, 27*(1), 37–46.

Perraud, S. (2000). Development of the Depression Coping Self-efficacy Scale (DCSES). *Archives of Psychiatric Nursing, 14*(6), 276–284.

Plotnikoff, R., Brez, S., & Hotz, S. (2000). Exercise behavior in a community sample with diabetes: Understanding the determinants of exercise behavioral change. *Diabetes Educator, 26*(3), 450–459.

Rabinowitz, S., Kushnir, T., & Ribak, J. (1996). Preventing burnout: Increasing professional self-efficacy in primary care nurses in a Balint Group. *AAOHN Journal, 44*(1), 28–32.

Rejeski, W. J., Ettinger, W. H., Martin, K., & Morgan, T. (1998). Treating disability in knee osteoarthritis with exercise therapy: A central role for self-efficacy and pain. *Arthritis Care Research, 11*(2), 94–101.

Remley, D., & Cook-Newell, M. (1999). Meal planning self-efficacy index for adolescents with diabetes. *Diabetes Educator, 25*(6), 883–886.

Resnick, B. (1994). The wheel that moves. *Rehabilitation Nursing, 19,* 140.

Resnick, B. (1996). Motivation in geriatric rehabilitation. *Image: The Journal of Nursing Scholarship, 28,* 41–47.

Resnick, B. (1998a). Efficacy beliefs in geriatric rehabilitation. *Journal of Gerontological Nursing, 24,* 34–45.

Resnick, B. (1998b). Functional performance of older adults in a long term care setting. *Clinical Nursing Research, 7,* 230–246.

Resnick, B. (1999). Reliability and validity testing of the self-efficacy for functional activities scale. *Journal of Nursing Measurement, 7*(1), 5–20.

Resnick, B. (2000a). Functional performance and exercise of older adults in long-term care settings. *Journal of Gerontological Nursing, 26*(3), 7–16.

Resnick, B. (2000b). A Seven Step Approach to Starting an Exercise Program for Older Adults. *Patient Education and Counseling, 39,* 243–252.

Resnick, B. (2001). Testing a model of exercise behavior in older adults. *Research in Nursing and Health, 24,* 83–92.

Resnick, B. (2002). Testing the impact of the WALC intervention on exercise adherence in older adults. *Journal of Gerontological Nursing, 28*(6), 32–40.

Resnick, B., Allen, P., & Ruane, K. (2002). Testing the effectiveness of a restorative care program. *Long-term Care Interface, 1*(3), 11–14.

Resnick, B., & Fleishell, A. (1999). Restoring quality of life. *Advance for Nurses, 1,* 10–12.

Resnick, B., & Jenkins, L. (2000). Reliability and validity testing of the self-efficacy for exercise scale. *Nursing Research, 49,* 154–159.

Resnick, B., & Jenkins, L. (2000). Testing the reliability and validity of the self-efficacy for exercise scale. *Nursing Research, 49*(3), 154–159.

Resnick, B., Palmer, M. H., Jenkins, L., & Spellbring, A. M. (2000). Path analysis of efficacy expectations and exercise behavior in older adults. *Journal of Advanced Nursing, 31*(6), 1309–1315.

Resnick, B., & Spellbring, A. M. (2000). Understanding what motivates older adults to exercise. *Journal of Gerontologic Nursing, 26*(3), 34–42.

Resnick, B., Wehren, L., & Orwig, D. (2003). Testing the reliability and validity of the SEOMA and OEOMA. *Journal of Orthopaedic Nursing, 3*(4), 11–15.

Robertson, D., & Keller, C. (1992). Relationship among health beliefs, self-efficacy and exercise adherence in patients with CAD. *Heart and Lung, 21*, 56–63.

Ruiz, B. (1992). Hip fracture recovery in older women: The role of self-efficacy and mood. Unpublished doctoral dissertation, University of California, San Francisco.

Ryckman, R., Robbins, M., Thornton, B., & Cantrell, P. (1982). Development and validation of a physical self-efficacy scale. *Journal of Personality and Social Psychology, 42*(5), 891–900.

Scherer, Y., & Schmieder, L. (1996). The role of self-efficacy in assisting patients with chronic obstructive pulmonary disease to manage breathing difficulty. *Clinical Nursing Research, 5*(3), 243–255.

Scherer, Y., & Shimmel, L. (1996). The effect of a pulmonary rehabilitation program on self-efficacy, perceptions of dyspnea, and physical endurance. *Heart and Lung, 26*(1), 15–22.

Scherer, Y., Schmieder, L., & Shimmel, S. (1998). The effects of education alone and in combination with pulmonary rehabilitation on self-efficacy in patients with COPD. *Rehabilitation Nursing, 23*(2), 71–77.

Schneider, J. (1997). Self-regulation and exercise behavior in older women. *Journal of Gerontology, 52*, P235–P241.

Schuster, P., & Waldron, J. (1991). Gender differences in cardiac rehabilitation patients. *Rehabilitation Nursing, 16*(5), 248–253.

Sechrist, K., Walker, S., & Pender, N. (1987). Development and psychometric evaluation of the exercise benefits/barriers scale. *Research in Nursing & Health, 10*, 357–365.

Sharon, B., Hennessy, C., Brandon, L., & Boyette, L. (1997). Older adults' experiences of a strength training program. *Journal of Nutrition, Health & Aging, 1*, 103–108.

Sharts-Hopko, N., Regan-Kubinski, M., Lincoln, P., & Heverly, M. (1996). Problem-focused coping in HIV-infected mothers in relation to self-efficacy, uncertainty, social support, and psychological disease. *Image: Journal of Nursing Scholarship, 28*(2), 107–111.

Siela, D. (1998). Self-efficacy in managing dyspnea in COPD. *Perspectives of Respiratory Nursing, 9*(1), 9,12.

Sinclair, M., & O'Boyle, C. (1999). The Childbirth Self-efficacy Inventory: A replication study. *Journal of Advanced Nursing, 30*(6), 1416–1423.

Smith, L. (1998). Cultural competence for nurses: Canonical correlation of two culture scales. *Journal of Cultural Diversity, 5*(4), 120–126.

Stanley, M., & Maddux, J. (1986). Cognitive process in health enhancement: Investigation of a combined protection motivation and self-efficacy model. *Basic and Applied Social Psychology, 7*(2), 101–113.

Steinhardt, M., & Dishman, R. (1989). Reliability and validity of expected outcomes and barriers for habitual physical activity. *Journal of Occupational Medicine, 31*, 536–546.

Sterling, Y. (1999). Parental self-efficacy and asthma self-management. *Journal of Child and Family Nursing, 2*(4), 280–281.

Strecher, V., DeVellis, B., Becker, M., & Rosenstock, I. (1986). The role of self-efficacy in achieving health behavior change. *Health Education Quarterly, 13*(1), 73–91.

Taal, E., Rasker, J., & Wiegman, O. (1996). Patient education and self-management in the rheumatic diseases: A self-efficacy approach. *Arthritis Care Research, 9*(3), 229–238.

Takata, C., & Takata, T. (1976). The influence of models on the evaluation of ability: 2 functions of social comparison processes. *Japanese Journal of Psychology, 47*(2), 74–82.

Taylor, C., Bandura, A., Ewart, C., Miller, N., & DeBusk, R. (1985). Exercise testing to enhance wives' confidence in their husband's cardiac capability soon after clinically uncomplicated acute MIs. *American Journal of Cardiology, 55*, 635–638.

Van der Palen, J., Klein, J., Zielhuis, G., Van Herwaarden, C., & Seydel, E. (2001). Behavioural effect of self-treatment guidelines in a self-management program for adults with asthma. *Patient Education Counseling, 43*(2), 161–169.

Van der Pligt, J., & Richard, R. (1994). Changing adolescents' sexual behavior: Perceived risk, self-efficacy and anticipated regret. *Patient Education and Counseling, 23*(3), 187–196.

Vispoel, W. (1990). Measuring self-efficacy: The state of the art. Paper presented at the Annual Meeting of the American Educational Research Association. (Boston, MA, April 16-20, 1990).

Washington, O. (1999). Effects of cognitive and experiential group therapy on self-efficacy and perceptions of employability of chemically dependent women. *Issues in Mental Health Nursing, 20*(3), 181–198.

Washington, O. (2001). Using brief therapeutic interventions to create change in self-efficacy and personal control of chemically dependent women. *Archives of Psychiatric Nursing, 15*(1), 32–40.

White, P., Kjelgaard, M., & Harkins, S. (1995). Testing the contribution of self-evaluation to goal-setting effects. *Journal of Personality and Social Psychology, 69*(1), 69–79.

Wilgal, J. K., Creer, T. L., & Kostes, H. (1991). The COPD self-efficacy scale. *Chest, 99*(5), 1193–1196.

Wigal, J., Stout, C., Brandon, M., Winder, J., McConnaughy, K., Creer, T., & Kotses, H. (1993). The knowledge, attitude and self-efficacy asthma questionnaire. *Chest, 104*(4), 1144–1148.

Zimmerman, B., Brown, S., & Bowman, J. (1996). A self-management program for chronic obstructive pulmonary disease: Relationship to dyspnea and self-efficacy. *Rehabilitation Nursing, 21*(5), 253–257.

Reasoned Action and Planned Behavior

PERLA WERNER

DEFINITION OF KEY TERMS

Perceived power	The subjective perception of the power of a specific factor to facilitate or inhibit the performance of the behavior
Subjective norm	A person's belief regarding the extent to which social referents or significant others support his or her performing (or not performing) the behavior

INTRODUCTION

The theory of reasoned action (TRA) and its extension, the theory of planned behavior (TPB), provide a useful framework for predicting and understanding social behavior in general and health behavior in particular.

Based on the principles of expectancy-value models of attitudes and decision-making, these theories are among the most influential and well-documented social cognitive models linking cognitive characteristics of individuals to their behavior.

HISTORICAL BACKGROUND

The Theory of Reasoned Action (TRA) was developed in 1967 (Fishbein & Ajzen, 1975). Grounded in social psychology, the theory was developed as an attempt to resolve the lack of consistency in studies aimed at examining relationships between attitudes and behavior. The main innovations introduced by the theory included the principle of compatibility and the concept of behavioral intention.

The principle of compatibility (Ajzen, 1988) states that the correspondence between attitudes and behavior will be greatest when both are measured at the same level of specificity regarding four elements: action, target, context, and time. Thus, to predict a specific behavior, directed toward a specific target, in a given context, and at a given time, researchers have to assess specific attitudes that correspond to the specific target, time, and context of the behavior.

Additionally, based on the theory of Dulany (1961) to explain awareness in verbal conditioning, Fishbein and Ajzen (1975) introduced the concept of behavioral intention as the proximal cause of behavior. Behavioral intention, or the person's motivation to engage in a behavior, was defined as the psychological construct through which attitudes influence behavior. In turn, intention to perform a behavior was defined as being determined by the attitudes toward performing the behavior and by the person's subjective norms.

In the years since its development, the TRA has been successfully applied in numerous studies, but it has received criticism as well. The main criticism was that by assuming behavior is affected directly by intention, Fishbein and Ajzen restricted the use of the TRA to behaviors that are under volitional control.

Approximately 2 decades after the TRA was introduced, the Theory of Planned Behavior (TPB) was developed by Ajzen and Fishbein (Ajzen, 1985, 1988) as a deliberate effort to overcome the above limitation. This was done by including perceptions of control regarding the performance of the behavior as an additional determinant of behavioral intention and of behavior. Perceived behavioral control was

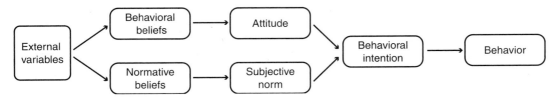

■ **Figure 6.1** Representation of the constructs in the Theory of Reasoned Action.

defined as the perception of how difficult or easy it is to perform the behavior. Its immediate determinants are control beliefs, or beliefs as to the extent to which the person has access to resources and opportunities to perform the behavior, and the perceived power of each resource or factor.

Although the TRA and the TPB are parsimonious models for predicting behavioral intention and behavior, several researchers have stressed the need to expand these theories by including a larger set of variables. The contribution of expanded models including variables such as perceived moral obligation, self-identity, affect outcomes, and past behavior or habit have been successfully tested lately (Conner & Armitage, 1998).

Finally, the latest developments stress the need to use the TRA and the TPB as the basis for designing interventions aimed at introducing behavior change (Fishbein, 1997).

The purpose of this chapter is to synthesize and discuss the main conceptual, methodological and application issues surrounding the TRA and the TPB.

DESCRIPTION OF THE THEORY OF REASONED ACTION AND THE THEORY OF PLANNED BEHAVIOR

Main Assumptions

The TRA and the TPB are both based on the assumption that individuals are guided by rational considerations regarding the implications of their actions. Thus, before engaging or not engaging in specific behaviors, individuals give careful and deliberate consideration to the information available, and then decide about their behavior. The relationships of the constructs in the TRA and TPB are presented in Figures 6-1 and 6-2 .

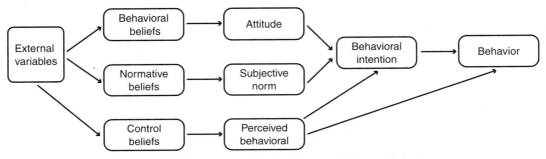

■ **Figure 6.2** Representation of the constructs in the Theory of Planned Behavior.

DEFINITION OF THE THEORIES' CONCEPTS

Behavioral Intention

Behavioral intention is the person's motivation to engage in a specific behavior. It indicates how much effort a person is willing to invest to perform such a behavior. The overall assumption underlying this concept is that the harder a person is willing to try to perform a specific behavior, the more likely that the specific behavior will indeed be performed. The determinants of behavioral intention are: attitudes, subjective norms, and perceived behavioral control (in the TPB) (Box 6-1). In general, the theories assume that the more favorable the attitude and the subjective norms held by the person, and the greater the person's perceived behavioral control, the higher the person's intention to engage in the specific behavior will be.

DETERMINANTS OF BEHAVIORAL INTENTION

Attitude.   In general, attitudes are defined as psychological tendencies expressed by evaluating a particular entity with some degree of favor or disfavor (Eagly & Chaiken, 1993). Based on the principle of compatibility, attitudes refer to the person's favorable or unfavorable evaluation of the specific behavior under study, and are assessed at the same level of specificity as the behavior.

Empirical applications of the models have repeatedly shown that the attitudes component is the most important predictor of behavioral intention (Jennings-Dozier, 1999; Powell-Cope, Lierman, Kasprzk, Young, & Benoliel, 1991; Rutter, 2000).

Subjective Norm.   Subjective norm refers to the person's subjective judgment regarding significant others' preferences and support for performing or not performing the specific behavior. The in-

---

BOX 6-1. Determinants of Behavioral Intention

Determinants of attitudes:

Attitudes are defined as a function of *behavioral beliefs*, which are perceptions regarding the consequences of the behavior, and the evaluation of those consequences.

Determinants of subjective norms:

Subjective norms are determined by normative beliefs, which are perceptions regarding significant others' support or preferences for performing or not performing the behavior,

and the person's motivation to comply with these preferences.

Determinants of perceived behavioral control:

Perceived behavioral control is determined by control beliefs, which are perceptions regarding the likelihood of having the means and opportunity to perform the behavior, and the perceived power of each one of the factors believed to be necessary to inhibit or facilitate the behavior.

clusion of subjective norms in the models imparts the social aspect to the theories (Abraham, Sheeran, & Orbell, 1998), since they stress the fact that the decisions are not taken in a social vacuum, but are influenced by the understanding and support of social referents. Subjective norms thus reflect perceptions of the social pressure exerted by significant others on the person's decisions to engage or not to engage in the behavior. Significant others are those whose opinions are important to the person (Conner & Armitage, 1998).

The concept of subjective norm was criticized as being too narrow to reflect the importance of social aspects (Conner, Martin, Silverdale, & Grogan, 1996). To overcome this criticism, several researchers have tried to differentiate injunctive and descriptive norms. Injunctive norms concern perceptions of social approval or disapproval of a behavior (i.e., subjective norms). Descriptive norms refer to perceptions of others' performance of the behavior (Povey, Conner, Sparks, James, & Shepherd, 2000a). Studies distinguishing the two types of norms found that each makes an independent significant contribution (Conner et al., 1996; DeVries, Backbier, Kok, & Dijstra, 1995).

Perceived Behavioral Control. The TPB adds perceived behavioral control as a third determinant to behavioral intention. This construct was added in an effort to expand the suitability of the TRA for behaviors that are not under complete volitional control, that is, behaviors whose performance depends not only on the person's decision but also on skills, resources, and opportunities that are not always available.

Perceived behavioral control is defined as the person's perception of how easy or difficult it is for him or her to perform the behavior (Ajzen, 1991), and is assumed to affect behavioral intention as well as behavior.

The concept has been repeatedly compared to the concept of self-efficacy (Bandura, 1982). Although, perceived behavioral control was originally conceptualized as including internal factors (e.g., abilities, skills, and compulsions), as well as external factors (e.g., time, opportunity, and resources) (Ajzen, 1985, 1988), lately, researchers have suggested conceptualizing perceived behavioral control as including only external control factors, and self-efficacy as including internal factors (Armitage & Conner, 1999; Povey, Conner, Sparks, James, & Shepherd, 2000; Sparks, Guthrie & Shepherd, 1997; Terry, 1993; Terry & O'Leary, 1995). See Box 6-2 for a comparison of the TRA and TPB models.

ADDITIONAL DETERMINANTS OF BEHAVIORAL INTENTION

Although the developers of the theories claimed that attitudes, subjective norms, and perceived behavioral control are sufficient to determine behavioral intention, they do not reject the possibility of identifying additional constructs affecting intentions to behave, on condition that they explain a considerable amount of the variance in intention (Ajzen, 1991). Indeed, several constructs have been examined lately as affecting behavioral intentions, in addition to the main constructs of the theories. These include perceived moral obligation, self-identity, past behavior and habit, affect, knowledge, and perceived susceptibility.

Perceived Moral Obligation. Perceived moral obligation refers to the person's personal beliefs about right and wrong (Schwartz & Tessler, 1972). Its addition to the models of TRA/TPB underlines the need to include internalized moral rules or personal beliefs about what one has to do, separately from the concept of beliefs about what others think one should do (i.e., subjective norm). Indeed, some studies have found that the model's overall prediction improved when moral obligation was added to at-

---

BOX 6-2. Comparison of TRA and TPB

The TRA and the TPB are both causal models in which:

1. Behavior is determined by intention to perform the behavior.
2. Intention is determined by attitude toward the behavior, subjective norm, and perceived behavioral control (in the TPB).
3. Attitude is determined by behavioral beliefs and evaluation of outcomes.
4. Subjective norms are determined by normative beliefs and motivation to comply with social referents.
5. In the TPB, perceived behavioral control is determined by control beliefs and perceived likelihood.
6. The TRA and the TPB posit that external factors, such as demographic characteristics, have no direct effect on behavioral intention, but are related to the direct antecedents of intention.

---

titudes and subjective norms (Godin et al., 1996; Kurland, 1995; Nucifora, Gallois, & Kashima, 1993; Pomazal & Jaccard, 1976; Sparks, Shepherd, & Frewer, 1995; Werner & Mendelsson, 2001).

Self-identity.   Self identity has been defined as "...the salient part of an actor's self which relates to a particular behavior" (Conner & Armitage, 1998, p. 1444), and has also been suggested as an additional predictor of behavioral intention. According to Charng and colleagues (1988), the inclusion of self-identity in the models is justified in that both the TRA and the TPB, as well as identity theory (the theoretical basis for self-identity), are based on assumptions of a rational decision-making process leading to behavior, and both see intention as a determinant of behavior.

Studies including self-identity as an additional predictor of behavior have indeed shown that it has an independent and considerable contribution to the prediction of behavior (Armitage & Conner, 2001; Sparks & Shepherd, 1992; Sparks, Shepherd, Wieringa, & Zimmermmans, 1995; Terry, Hogg, & White, 1999; Theodorakis, 1994; Theodorakis, Bagiatis, & Goudas, 1995).

Past Behavior and Habit.   The role of past behavior in intention to behave has received extensive attention during the last several years (Conner & Sparks, 1998; Eagly & Chaiken, 1993). Its inclusion in the models is based on the assumption that repetitive performance of a behavior may affect subsequent behavior as a consequence of habitual processes. While earliest studies (Bentler & Speckart, 1979; Fredricks & Dossett, 1983) suggested that past behavior impacts directly on behavior, unmediated by the components of the TPB, recent studies showed the effect of past behavior to be mediated by these constructs (Norman, Conner, & Bell, 2000; Quine & Rubin, 1997; Werner, Schatz, & Vered, 2001).

The inclusion of past behavior, when conceptualized as habit, has been criticized as conflicting with the basic assumptions of the TRA and TPB models. If habitual behaviors are characterized as "mindless" and automatic, their performance does not rely on a deliberate and evaluative decision-making process based on attitudes and intention, as stated by the theories (Aarts, Verplanken, & van Knippenberg, 1998). Sheeran, Orbell, and Trafimow (1999) recently demonstrated that the relationship between behavior and past behavior is dependent on the temporal stability of behavioral intentions—with past behavior being a significant predictor of behavior when intentions to behave are temporally stable. Conner, Sheeran, Norman, and Armitage (2000) replicated these findings.

Affect. Several researchers have stressed the need to include affective outcomes, independently of cognitive outcomes, in the models (Conner & Armitage, 1998). However, whether they should be included as predictors of intention, or as moderators between attitudes, subjective norms, perceived behavioral control, and intentions to behave, requires further theoretical and empirical clarifications (Perugini & Bagozzi, 2001).

It has been stated that the intention to perform or not to perform a behavior may be affected by the person's anticipated pleasant or unpleasant reactions associated with the performance or non-performance of the behavior. Findings regarding the contribution of including affective reactions to the TRA and the TPB remain inconclusive. While several studies demonstrated that including affective outcomes, such as anticipated regret, improved the predictive value of the models (Parker, Stradling, & Mastead, 1995; Richard, deVries, & van der Pligt, 1998; Richard, van der Pligt, & de-Vries, 1995), others failed to show their influence (Ajzen & Driver, 1992; Werner, Beeri, & Davidson, 2002).

Knowledge. Lately, several studies assessed the importance of knowledge within the framework of the TRA and TPB, and found significant relationships between level of knowledge and the intention to engage in the behavior (Bogart et al., 2000; Pearlman, Clark, Rakowski, & Ehrich, 1999; Werner et al., 2002; Werner, Schatz, & Vered, 2001).

Perceived Susceptibility. Several researchers (Norman & Conner, 1998; Oliver & Berger, 1979) noted that an important predictor for intention to behave is the person's perceptions of risk or susceptibility. Indeed, perception of susceptibility is a central concept in other cognitive models of health behavior such as the Health Belief Model (HBM) (Becker, 1974) and Protection Motivation Theory (Rogers, 1983).

Despite this criticism, few studies have included susceptibility measures as an additional determinant of behavioral intention. Norman, Conner, and Bell (1999), in a study assessing the intention to quit smoking, found that perceived behavioral control and perceived susceptibility were the main predictors of intention. Similarly, Smith and Stasson (2000), found perceived behavioral control and perceived susceptibility to be statistically significant predictors of intention to use condoms.

Additional Predictors. Additional predictors added to the models include:

- Perceived need to change (Paisley & Sparks, 1998)
- Perceived social support (Povey et al., 2000a)
- Self-schemas (Sheeran & Orbell, 2000).

The importance and role of these variables awaits further research.

APPLICATIONS OF THE THEORIES

Perhaps one of the main advantages of both the TRA and the TPB relates to the clear definitions regarding operationalization of the constructs in the models and of the relationships among them. In this section, methodological issues, such as the definition of the population to be assessed, the development of the measures to be used, and their relationships are discussed.

Definition of the Population

The first step in research in general, and in a study using the TRA or the TPB as its conceptual framework in particular, is to define the population to be assessed. Since, as already stated, the TRA and TPB are aimed at decision-making processes, it is of extreme importance for the assessed population to be motivated regarding the issues examined. This can be achieved in two different ways. The first way relies on restricting the population to those subjects for whom the topic being assessed is of relevance. For example, Quine and Rubin (1997), in a study assessing women's intentions to take hormone replacement therapy (HRT), collected information on their experiences with menopause in general from a random sample of 1,200 women aged between 38 and 58 years. However, the constructs of the TPB (i.e., women's intentions, attitudes, subjective norms, and perceived behavioral control) were assessed only for 641 women who had never taken HRT.

The second way to ensure the use of a motivated population is to provide appropriate and relevant information. For example, Norman, Conner, and Bell (2000), in a study using the TPB to assess exercise intention, provided information on the benefits of regular exercise before interviewing the participants.

Development of Appropriate Measures

This section discusses issues regarding the elicitation of salient beliefs, the conceptualization of the measures according to the principle of compatibility, scaling considerations, and the use of multiple-item constructs.

ELICITATION OF SALIENT BELIEFS

As already stated, the theories of TRA and TPB are based on the assumption that there is a relation between a person's salient beliefs about the behavior and his or her attitude to the behavior. To elicit these beliefs, the developers of the theories suggest conducting a pilot study in which semistructured interviews or focus groups are conducted, with a sample of respondents similar in their characteristics to the research population (Ajzen, 1991; Ajzen & Fishbein, 1980).

CONCEPTUALIZATION OF THE MEASURES

The level of each one of the main measures in the theories should be specified regarding the four elements stated in the principle of compatibility: action, target, context, and time (Conner & Sparks, 1998).

SCALING CONSIDERATIONS

The variables included in the theories are traditionally measured by 7-point semantic differential scales (e.g., likely–unlikely for intention to behave, or good–bad for attitudes) (Ajzen, 1991; Conner & Sparks, 1998). Although the theories do not specifically indicate whether the scales should be unipolar (i.e., from 1–7 or from 0–6) or bipolar (i.e., from –3 to +3), it is suggested that beliefs be measured by unipolar scoring and attitudes, and subjective norms by bipolar scoring (Ajzen, 1991; Gagne &

Godin, 2000). For the presentation of detailed examples of the operationalization of the measures in the models, item wording, and response format, see Conner and Sparks (1998).

THE USE OF MULTIPLE-ITEM CONSTRUCTS

Although not specifically stated, the use of multiple-item measures has been recommended, especially for the subjective norm construct, which has repeatedly proved to be the construct with the weakest statistical associations (Conner & Armitage, 1998).

Relationships Among the Constructs of the Models

Both the TRA and the TPB are expectancy-value models with the assumption that the measures of attitude, subjective norm, and perceived behavioral control should correlate well with the measure of behavioral intention. Additionally, the overall sum of the multiplicative outcome of subjective probabilities and values associated with different beliefs (i.e., Σ normative beliefs * evaluation of outcomes) should correlate well with the attitude measure; the sum of the multiplicative outcome of normative belief and motivation to comply (Σ normative beliefs * motivation to comply) should correlate well with the measure of subjective norm; and the sum of the multiplicative outcome of control beliefs and perceived power (i.e., Σ control beliefs * perceived power of each control factor) should correlate with the measure of perceived behavioral control.

The relationship among the variables in the models has been defined essentially as an additive model. As such, the influences on behavioral intention and on behavior are based on linear assumptions. However, researchers started to criticize these assumptions, and models including interaction effects are being examined (Conner & McMillan, 1999).

Research Design

Studies examining the predictors of behavioral intention are usually based on cross-sectional, correlational designs. Those examining predictors of behavior are based on longitudinal prospective designs, although only a minority are based on experimental designs (Armitage & Conner, 1999; Armitage, Conner, Loach, & Willets, 1999; Armitage, Conner, & Norman, 1999; Leone, Perugini, & Ercolani, 1999; McCaul, Sandgren, O'Neill, & Hinsz, 1993; Millstein, 1996; Norman et al., 1999; Sheeran et al., 1999; Sheeran & Orbell, 1999; Sheeran, Conner, & Norman, 2001; Terry et al., 1999).

Statistical Analysis

It has been suggested (Ajzen & Fishbein, 1980) that the correlations among all model components be examined before their overall relationships are tested. After empirical relationships among all components are established, multiple linear regression is commonly used. Studies examining expanded models of the theories (i.e., including additional predictors), usually used hierarchical regressions (Bogart et al., 2000; Fekadu & Kraft, 2002; Povey et al., 2000a; Sheeran & Orbell, 2000; Terry et al., 1999).

When multiple regression models are used, it is advisable to apply the adjusted R^2 (and not R^2) as a measure of the explained variance (Hankins, French, & Horne, 2000).

Lately, the use of structural equation modeling (SEM) for assessing the overall relationship among the variables has increased (Armitage et al., 1999; Leone et al., 1999; Levin, 1999).

SPECIFIC RESEARCH EXAMPLES

Both the TRA and the TPB have been empirically applied to health-related topics. Review the examples of how these theories have been used in actual research studies by reviewing two studies in Using Middle Range Theories 6-1 and 6-2. For a summary of the application of the theories to other health behaviors, see Table 6-1 from Conner and Sparks (1998).

The rationale for using the models of TRA and TPB for health-related issues is frequently said to be the possibility that identifying the factors affecting intention to behave will help develop educational programs and other strategies aimed at promoting behavioral change (Conner & Sparks, 1998). Since the theories assume that attitudes, subjective norms, and perceived behavioral control are affected by their respective sets of beliefs (i.e., behavioral, normative, and control beliefs), behavioral interventions should be aimed at changing the beliefs that accordingly will affect the performance of the behavior.

6-1 USING MIDDLE RANGE THEORIES

The Theory of Planned Behavior (TPB) was used as the theoretical framework for identifying the determinants of registered nurses' intentions to use opioids for pain management.

446 RNs (representing a response rate of 56%) who were members of the largest professional nursing association in Queensland, Australia participated in the study. A self-report instrument was used to assess the constructs of the TPB, as well as participants' attitudes about pain relief and opioids.

The main constructs of the TPB (i.e., attitudes, subjective norms, and perceived behavioral control) were the main independent predictors of nurses' intentions to administer opioids for analgesia. They explained almost 40% of the variation in intention. Perceived control was the strongest independent predictor, stressing the importance of control and self-efficacy for determining nurses' intentions. Overall, nurses reported positive attitudes towards opioids and their use in pain management. Subjective norms were also a significant predictor of nurses' intentions. Participants were more likely to comply with patients' requests for pain management than with physicians', other colleagues' or relatives' requests. Findings of the study based on the TPB stress the need for educational programs to improve pain management.

Source: Edwards, H. E., Nash, R. E., Najman, J. M., Yates, P. M. et al. (2001). Determinants of nurses' intention to administer opioids for pain relief. *Nursing and Health Sciences, 3,* 149–159.

6-2 USING MIDDLE RANGE THEORIES

The aim of this study was to examine nursing staff members' attitudes, subjective norms, moral obligations, and intentions to use physical restraints, using the Theory of Reasoned Action (TRA).

A correlational design was used with 303 nursing staff members from an 800-bed eldercare hospital in central Israel. Participants completed a questionnaire, including questions based on the TRA, as well as sociodemographic and professional characteristics. Regression analyses found attitudes, subjective norms, and moral considerations to be significantly related to intention to use physical restraints with older people. The constructs of the TRA explained 48% of the variance in nurses' intentions.

Findings of the study showed that the TRA was a useful framework for examining nurses' intentions to use physical restraints. Nurses' attitudes, beliefs, and expectations of significant others should be examined before implementing educational programs regarding the use of physical restraints.

Source: Werner, P., & Mendelsson, G. (2001). Nursing staff members' intentions to use physical restraints with elderly persons: Testing the theory of reasoned action. *Journal of Advanced Nursing, 35*(5),784–791.

Ajzen (nd) in a recent document published on his Web site, concluded that "...it is reasonable to target an intervention at any one of the three major predictors in the theory of planned behavior (so long as there is room for change), but that it may be safer to target predictors that account for significant variance in intention and behavior" (p. 4). Additionally, he stated that the intervention could be geared to changing the strength of the beliefs determining each one of the major predictors (i.e., behavioral, normative, and control beliefs), or their scale value or relative importance. For example, assume that when assessing a woman's intentions to perform a bone-density measurement test, the researcher found that she believed it highly unlikely that performing the test would help her detect the development of osteoporosis in its early stages, and that there was no reason for early diagnosis of osteoporosis, since it could not be treated. According to this example, interventions could be developed to change either the person's belief about the usefulness of the bone-density examination (change behavioral belief) or to change its outcome evaluation. The type of interventions designed to attain this goal could vary from group or individual educational programs to high-risk groups, such as first-degree relatives of persons suffering from osteoporosis, up to the diffusion of information and knowledge though the mass media.

Although Ajzen (nd) states that the question of which component of the beliefs to change is an empirical question, it is stated that usually more than one or two beliefs need to change before a change in attitudes can be achieved. In any case, the provision of accurate information is of extreme importance.

Although the importance of the TRA and the TPB as a basis for the development of interventions aimed at changing health behaviors has been repeatedly stressed (Armitage & Conner, 2001; Bogart et al., 2000; Conner & Armitage, 1998; Fishbein & Guinan, 1996; Norman et al., 1999; Sutton, McVey & Glanz, 1999; Werner & Mendelsson, 2001), few studies have evaluated empirically the importance of moderator variables aimed at increasing the relationship between intention and behavior. For ex-

Table 6-1. RESEARCH APPLICATIONS USING TRA/TPB

TOPIC	AUTHORS	YEAR
Smoking	Sherman	1982
	Satton	1989
Frequency of smoking	Chassin et al.	1981
	Fishbein	1982
	Budd	1986
Smoking cessation	DeVries & Kok	1986
	Martin et al.	1990
Alcohol consumption	Fishbein	1980
	Budd & Spencer	1984
Drinking behavior	Schlegal et al.	1992
Sexual behavior	Fishbein et al.	1992
Condom use	Boldero et al.	1992
	Wilson et al.	1992
	Terry et al.	1993a
Health-screening attendance	DeVellis et al.	1990
	Norman and Connor	1993
Exercise	Sejwacy	1980
	Theodorrakas et al.	1991
	Kimiecik	1992
	Yordy and Lent	1993
Breast/Testicle self exam	Young et al.	1991
	McCaul et al.	1993

Source: Conner, M., & Sparks, P. (1998). The Theory of Planned Behaviour and Health Behaviours. In M. Connor, & P. Norman (Eds.). *Predicting health behaviour: Research and practice with social cognition models.* Buckingham, UK: Open University Press.

ample, Sheeran and Orbell (2000), in a longitudinal study examining the relationship between intentions to exercise and actual behavior, found that self-schemas moderated the relationship, and that the relationship between intention and behavior was stronger for participants with stronger self-schemas regarding exercise.

Limitations of the Theories

The main limitation of the theories concerns their capacity to predict behavior. Empirical studies showed that behavioral intention and perceived behavioral control explain approximately 40% of the variance in behavior (Ajzen, 1991; Godin & Kok, 1996; Randall & Wolff, 1994; Sheeran & Orbell, 1998), suggesting that other factors should be considered. One of the main reasons for this poor predictive power may be the fact that from the time behavioral intention is assessed until the time behavior is assessed, the intention might have changed. Therefore, it has been suggested that relatively short periods be allowed to elapse between the examination of behavioral intention and the assessment of the behavior (Sheeran & Orbell, 2000). See Research Analysis 6-1 as an example of how the TRA might be applied.

An additional limitation of the theories is their tendency to rely almost exclusively on self-reported measures that might not be related to observed behavior (Armitage & Conner, 2001).

SUMMARY

Over the years, the TRA and the TPB have proved to be successful middle range theories, allowing both generalization and operationalization across a range of fields and populations in general and for nursing in particular.

Despite the theories' important contributions to the understanding of relationships between attitudes and behaviors, future research could expand our knowledge regarding theoretical, as well as methodological aspects of the models.

Theoretically, the role of additional predictors of behavioral intention should be further examined. Moreover, the role of variables mediating the effects of intentions to behave on behavioral performance should be encouraged.

6-1 RESEARCH APPLICATION

A "no shots, no school" policy has been implemented as a district-wide policy. A school nurse is trying to determine if there are ways to get more children to participate in the district-wide free immunization program. She remembers studying the theory of reasoned action in research class while at graduate nursing school. She constructs a mailed questionnaire based on the concepts contained within the middle range theory of reasoned action, receives IRB approval, and mails the survey out to all the parents in the school district who have children about to enter kindergarten next year.

By including a stamped return envelope and making a reminder call to the home 10 days after mailing, the school nurse hopes to get about a 60% return on the mailed survey. The returned data collection surveys are coded and entered into an SPSS spreadsheet.

Appropriate statistical tests are performed on the ordinal and interval level data to see if there are any correlations to the answers of parents who do not plan to get the immunizations, and factors of the survey that relate to the concepts of reasoned action and planned behavior. Depending on the results, measures will be implemented by the school nurse to increase the participation in the preschool immunization program.

Methodologically, the use of longitudinal studies examining performance-based measures of behavior, rather than self-reported measures, may help to increase the explanation of behavior. Finally, theoretically driven interventions aimed at changing behavior should be implemented.

ANALYSIS EXERCISE

Using the criteria presented in Chapter 2, critique the Theory of Reasoned Action and the Theory of Planned Behavior using the following outline. Compare your responses with the analysis done by an expert researcher who has worked with the theories in Appendix A.

Internal Criticism
1. Clarity
2. Consistency
3. Adequacy

4. Logical development
5. Level of theory development

External Criticism
1. Reality convergence
2. Utility
3. Significance
4. Discrimination
5. Scope of theory
6. Complexity

WEB RESOURCES

1. This site is maintained by Professor I. Ajzen and provides valuable information on the Theory of Planned Behavior model, with guidelines for constructing a TPB questionnaire and for designing a TPB intervention. An extensive and updated bibliography of published articles using the TPB is also provided:
   www.unix.oit.umass.edu/~aizen/tpb.html
2. Web site maintained by the University of South Florida Community and Family Health. Provides information about the originators and history of the models, key terms, and applications of health education. An annotated bibliography is also included:
   http://hsc.usf.edu/~kmbrown/TRA_TPB.htm
3. This site provides a PowerPoint presentation about an application of the TPB to nursing students' intentions to seek clinical experience, using the essential clinical behavior data:
   http://users.ipfw.edu/meyer/tpb993/index.html

REFERENCES

Aarts, H., Verplanken, B., & van Knippenberg, A. (1998). Predicting behavior from actions in the past: Repeated decision making or a matter of habit? *Journal of Applied Social Psychology, 28*(15), 1355–1374.

Abraham, C., Sheeran, P., & Orbell, S. (1998). Can social cognitive models contribute to the effectiveness of HIV-preventive behavioural interventions? A brief review of the literature and a reply to Joffe (1996, 1997) and Fife-Schaw (1997). *British Journal of Medical Psychology, 71,* 297–310.

Ajzen, I. (1985). From intentions to actions: A theory of planned behavior. In J. Kuhl, & J. Beckmann (Eds.), *Action control: From cognition to behavior*. Berlin: Springer.

Ajzen, I. (1988). *Attitudes, personality, and behaviour*. Milton Keynes, UK: Open University Press.

Ajzen, I. (1991). The Theory of Planned Behavior. *Organizational Behavior and Human Decision Processes, 50,* 179–211.

Ajzen, I. (nd). Behavioral interventions based on the Theory of Planned Behavior.
   www.unix.oit.umass.edu/~aizen/tpb.html.

Ajzen, I., & Driver, B. L. (1992). Contingent value measurement: On the nature and meaning of willingness to pay. *Journal of Consumer Psychology, 1*(4), 297–316.

Ajzen, I., & Fishbein M. (1980). *Understanding attitudes and predicting social behavior*. Englewood Cliffs, NJ: Prentice Hall.

Armitage, C.J., & Conner, M. (1999). Distinguishing perceptions of control from self-efficacy: Predicting consumption of a low-fat diet using the Theory of Planned Behavior. *Journal of Applied Psychology, 29*(1), 72–90.

Armitage, C. J., & Conner, M. (2001). Social cognitive determinants of blood donation. *Journal of Applied Psychology, 31*(7), 1431–1457.

Armitage, C. J., Conner, M., Loach, J., & Willets, D. (1999). Different perceptions of control: Applying an extended theory of planned behavior to legal and illegal drug use. *Basic and Applied Social Psychology, 21*(4), 301–316.

Armitage, C. J., Conner, M., & Norman, P. (1999). Differential effects of mood on information processing: Evidence from the theories of reasoned action and planned behavior. *European Journal of Social Psychology, 29*, 419–433.

Bandura, A. (1982). Self-efficacy mechanism in human agency. *American Psychologist, 37*, 122–147.

Becker, M. H. (1974). The health belief model and sick role behavior. *Health Education Monographs, 2*, 409–419.

Bentler, P. M., & Speckart, G. (1979). Models of attitude-behavior relations. *Psychological Review, 86*, 452–464.

Bogart, L., Cecil, H., & Pinkerton, S. (2000). Hispanic adults' beliefs, attitudes and intentions regarding the female condom. *Journal of Behavioral Medicine, 23*(2), 181–206.

Charng, H., Piliavin, J. A., & Callero, P. (1988). Role identity and reasoned action in prediction of repeated behavior. *Social Psychology Quarterly, 51*, 303–317.

Conner, M., Martin, E., Silverdale, N., & Grogan, S. (1996). Dieting in adolescence: An application of the Theory of Planned Behaviour. *British Journal of Health Psychology, 1*, 315–325.

Conner, M., & Armitage, C. J. (1998). Extending the Theory of Planned Behavior: A review and avenues for further research. *Journal of Applied Psychology, 28*(15), 1429–1464.

Conner, M., & Sparks, P. (1998). The Theory of Planned Behaviour and Health Behaviours. In M. Conner, & P. Norman (Eds.). *Predicting health behaviour: Research and practice with social cognition models*. Buckingham, UK: Open University Press.

Conner, M., & McMillan, B. (1999). Interaction effects in the theory of planned behaviour: Studying cannabis use. *British Journal of Social Psychology, 38*, 195–222.

Conner, M., Sheeran, P., Norman, P., & Armitage, C.J. (2000). Temporal stability as a moderator of relationships in the Theory of Planned Behaviour. *British Journal of Social Psychology, 39*, 469–493.

DeVries, H., Backbier, E., Kok, G., & Dijstra, M. (1995). The impact of social influence in the context of attitude, self-efficacy, intention, and previous behavior as predictors of smoking onset. *Journal of Applied Social Psychology, 25*, 237–257.

Dulany, D. E. (1961). Hypotheses and habits in verbal "operant conditioning." *Journal of Abnormal and Social Psychology, 63*, 251–263.

Eagly, A. H., & Chaiken, S. (1993). *The psychology of attitudes*. Orlando, FL: Harcourt Brace Jovanovich.

Fekadu, Z., & Kraft, P. (2002). Expanding the Theory of Planned Behaviour: The role of social norms and group identification. *Journal of Health Psychology, 7*(1), 33–43.

Fishbein, M. (1997). Predicting, understanding, and changing socially relevant behaviors: Lessons learned. In C. McGarty, & S. Haslam (Eds.), *The message of social psychology*. Oxford, UK: Blackwell.

Fishbein, M., & Ajzen, I. (1975). *Belief, attitude, intention, and behavior*. New York: Wiley.

Fishbein, M., & Guinan, M. (1996). Behavioral science and public health: A necessary partnership for HIV prevention. *Public Health Reports, 3*(1), 5–10.

Fredricks, A. J., & Dossett, D. L. (1983). Attitude-behavior relation: A comparison of the Fishbein-Ajzen and Bentler-Speckart models. *Journal of Personality and Social Psychology, 45*, 501–512.

Gagne, C., & Godin, G. (2000). The Theory of Planned Behavior: Some measurement issues concerning belief-based variables. *Journal of Applied Social Psychology, 30*(10), 2173–2193.

Godin, G., & Kok, G. (1996). The theory of planned behavior: A review of its applications to health-related behaviors. *American Journal of Health Promotion, 11*, 97–98.

Godin, G., Maticka-Tyndale, E., Adrien, A., Manson-Singer, S., Willms, D., & Cappon, C. (1996). Cross-cultural testing of three social cognitive theories: An application to condom use. *Journal of Applied Social Psychology, 26*, 1556–1586.

Hankins, M., French, D., & Horne, R. (2000). Statistical guidelines for studies of the Theory of Reasoned Action and Theory of Planned Behaviour. *Psychology and Health, 15*, 151–161.

Jennings-Dozier, K. (1999). Predicting intentions to obtain a Pap smear among African American and Latino women: Testing the Theory of Planned Behavior. *Nursing Research, 48*(4), 198–205.

Kurland, N. (1995). Ethical intentions and the theories of reasoned action and planned behavior. *Journal of Applied Psychology, 25*, 297–313.

Leone, L., Perugini, M., & Ercolani, A. (1999). A comparison of three models of attitude-behavior relationships in studying behavior domain. *European Journal of Social Psychology, 29*, 161–189.

Levin, P. F. (1999). Test of the Fishbein and Ajzen models as predictors of health care workers' glove use. *Research in Nursing & Health, 22*, 295–307.

McCaul, K. D., Sandgren, A. K., O'Neill, H. K., & Hinsz, V. B. (1993). The value of the Theory of Planned Behavior, perceived control and self-efficacy expectations for predicting health-protective behaviors. *Basic and Applied Social Psychology, 14*(2), 231–252.

Millstein, S. G. (1996). Utility of the Theories of Reasoned Action and Planned Behavior for predicting physician behavior: A prospective analysis. *Health Psychology, 5*, 398–402.

Norman, P., & Conner, M. (1998). The role of social cognition models in predicting health behaviours: Future directions. In M. Conner, & P. Norman (Eds.). *Predicting health behaviour: Research and practice with social cognition models*. Buckingham, UK: Open University Press.

Norman, P., Conner, M., & Bell, R. (1999). The Theory of Planned Behavior and smoking cessation. *Health Psychology, 18*(1), 89–94.

Norman, P., Conner, P., & Bell, R. (2000). The Theory of Planned Behaviour and exercise: Evidence for the moderating role of past behaviour. *British Journal of Health Psychology, 5*, 249–261.

Nucifora, J., Gallois, C., & Kashima, Y. (1993). Influences on condom use among undergraduates: Testing the theories of reasoned action and planned behavior. In D. J. Terrry, C. Gallois, & M. McCarmish (Eds.). *The theory of reasoned action: Its application to AIDS-preventive behaviour*. Oxford, UK: Pergamon.

Oliver, R. L., & Berger, P. K. (1979). A path analysis of preventive health care decision models. *Journal of Consumer Research, 6*, 113–122.

Paisley, C. M., & Sparks, P. (1998). Expectation of reducing fat intake: The role of perceived need within the theory of planned behaviour. *Psychology and Health, 13*, 341–353.

Parker, D., Manstead, A. S. R., & Stradling, S. G. (1995). Extending the Theory of Planned Behavior: The role of personal norm. *British Journal of Social Psychology, 34*, 127–137.

Pearlman, P., Clark, M., Rakowski, W., & Ehrich, B. (1999). Screening for breast and cervical cancers: The importance of knowledge and perceived cancer survivability. *Women and Health, 28*(4), 93–112.

Perugini, M., & Bagozzi, R. P. (2001). The role of desires and anticipated emotions in goal-directed behaviours: Broadening and deepening the theory of planned behaviour. *British Journal of Social Psychology, 40*, 79–98.

Pomazal, R., & Jaccard, J. (1976). An informational approach to altruistic behavior. *Journal of Personality and Social Psychology, 33*, 317–326.

Povey, R., Conner, M., Sparks, P., James, R., & Shepherd, R. (2000). Application of the Theory of Planned Behavior to two dietary behaviours: Roles of perceived control and self-efficacy. *British Journal of Health Psychology, 5*, 121–139.

Povey, R., Conner, M., Sparks, P., James, R., & Shepherd, R. (2000a). The Theory of Planned Behaviour and healthy eating: Examining additive and moderating effects of social influence variables. *Psychology and Health, 14*, 991–1006.

Powell-Cope, G., Lierman, L., Kasprzk, D., Young, H., & Benoliel, J. (1991). The theory of reasoned action in prediction of breast self-examination: A comparison of two studies. *Health Care of Women International, 12*(1), 51–61.

Quine, L., & Rubin, R. (1997). Attitude, subjective norm, and perceived behavioural control as predictors of women's intentions to take hormone replacement therapy. *British Journal of Health Psychology, 2*, 199–216.

Randall, D. M., & Wolff, J. A. (1994). The time interval in the intention-behavior relationship: Meta-analysis. *British Journal of Social Psychology, 33*, 405–418.

Richard, R., deVries, N., & van der Pligt, J. (1998). Anticipated regret and precautionary sexual behavior. *Journal of Applied Social Psychology, 28*, 1411–1428.

Richard, R., van der Pligt, J., & de Vries, N. (1995). Anticipated affective reactions and prevention of AIDS. *British Journal of Social Psychology, 34*, 9–21.

Rogers, R. (1983). Cognitive and physiological processes in fear appeals and attitude change: A revised theory of protection motivation. In J. T. Cacioppo, & R. E. Petty (Eds.). *Social psychophysiology: A source book*. New York: Oxford University Press.

Rutter, D. (2000). Attendance and reattendance of breast cancer screening: A prospective 3-year test of the theory of planned behavior. *British Journal of Health Psychology, 5*(1), 1–13.

Schwartz, S., & Tessler, C. (1972). A test of a model for reducing measured attitude-behavior discrepancies. *Journal of Personality and Social Psychology, 24*, 225–236.

Sheeran, P., & Orbell, S. (1998). Do intentions predict condom use in 72 studies of HIV-preventive behaviour. A critical review. *Patient Education and Counseling, 24*, 199–216.

Sheeran, P., & Orbell, S. (1999). Implementation intentions and repeated behaviour: Augmenting the predictive validity of the theory of planned behavior. *European Journal of Social Psychology, 29*, 349–369.

Sheeran, P., & Orbell, S. (2000). Self-schemas and the theory of planned behaviour. *European Journal of Social Psychology, 30*, 533–550.

Sheeran, P., Orbell, S., & Trafimow, D. (1999). Does the temporal stability of behavioral intentions moderate intention-behavior and past-behavior–future-behavior relations? *Personality and Social Psychology Bulletin, 25*(6), 721–730.

Sheeran, P., Conner, M., & Norman, P. (2001). Can the Theory of Planned Behavior explain patterns of health behavior change? *Health Psychology, 20*(1), 12–19.

Smith, B., & Stasson, M. (2000). A comparison of health behavior constructs: Social psychological predictors of

AIDS-preventive behavioral intentions. *Journal of Applied Social Psychology, 30*(3), 443–462.

Sparks, P., Guthrie, C., & Shepherd, R. (1997). The dimensional structure of the perceived behavioral control construct. *Journal of Applied Social Psychology, 27*(5), 418–438.

Sparks, P., & Shepherd, R. (1992). Self-identity and the theory of planned behavior—Assessing the role of identification with green consumerism. *Social Psychology Quarterly, 55,* 388–399.

Sparks, P., Shepherd, R., & Frewer, L. J. (1995). Assessing and structuring attitudes toward the use of gene technology in food production: The role of perceived ethical obligation. *Basic and Applied Social Psychology, 16,* 267–285.

Sparks, P., Shepherd, R., Wieringa, N., & Zimmermmanns, N. (1995). Perceived behavioural control, unrealistic optimism, and dietary change: An exploratory study. *Appetite, 24,* 243–255.

Sutton, S., McVey, D., & Glanz, A. (1999). A comparative test of the Theory of Reasoned Action and the Theory of Planned Behavior in the prediction of condom use intentions in a national sample of English young people. *Health Psychology, 18*(1), 72–81.

Terry, D. (1993). Self-efficacy expectancies and the theory of reasoned action. In D. J. Terry, C. Gallois, & M. McCamish (Eds.). *The theory of reasoned action: Its application in AIDS-preventative behavior.* Oxford, UK: Pergamon.

Terry, D., & O'Leary, J. (1995). The theory of planned behaviour: The effects of perceived behavioural control and self-efficacy. *British Journal of Social Psychology, 34,* 199–220.

Terry, D., Hogg, M., & White, K. (1999). The theory of planned behavior: Self-identity, social identity and group norms. *British Journal of Social Psychology, 38,* 225–244.

Theodorakis, Y. (1994). Planned behavior, attitude strength, role identity, and the prediction of exercise behavior. *The Sports Psychologist, 8,* 149–165.

Theodorakis, Y., Bagiatis, K., & Goudas, M. (1995). Attitudes toward teaching individuals with disabilities: Application of planned behavior theory. *Adapted Physical Activity Quarterly, 12,* 151–160.

Werner, P., Beeri, M., & Davidson, M. (2002). Family caregivers' willingness to pay for drugs indicated for the treatment of Alzheimer's disease: An economic or psychological model? *Dementia, 1*(1), 59–74.

Werner, P., & Mendelsson, G. (2001). Nursing staff members' intentions to use physical restraints with elderly persons: Testing the theory of reasoned action. *Journal of Advanced Nursing, 35*(5), 784–791.

Werner, P., Schatz, Y., & Vered, I. (2001). Predictors of women's willingness to use dual energy x-ray: Testing the Theory of Planned Behavior. The 17th World Conference of Gerontology, Vancouver, Canada.

BIBLIOGRAPHY

Abraham, C., Clift, S., & Grabowski, P. (1999). Cognitive predictors of adherence to malaria prophylaxis regimens on return from a malarious region: A prospective study. *Social Science and Medicine, 48*(11), 1641–1654.

Albarracin, D., Johnson, B. T., Fishbein, M., & Muellerleile, P. A. (2001). Theories of reasoned action and planned behavior as models of condom use: A meta analysis. *Psychological Bulletin, 127*(1), 142–161.

Aminzadeh, F., & Edwards, N. (2000). Factors associated with cane use among community dwelling older adults. *Public Health Nursing, 17*(6), 474–483 .

Aminzadeh, F., Plotnikoff, R., & Edwards, N. (1999). Development and evaluation of the cane use cognitive mediator instrument. *Nursing Research, 48*(5), 269–275.

Armitage, C. J., & Arden, M. A. (2002). Exploring discontinuity patterns in the transtheoretical model: An application of the theory of planned behavior. *British Journal of Health Psychology, 7*(1), 89–103.

Armitage, C. J., & Conner, M. (1999). Predictive validity of the theory of planned behavior: The role of questionnaire format and social desirability. *Journal of Community and Applied Social Psychology, 9*(4), 261–272.

Armitage, C. J., Conner, M., & Norman, P. (1999). Differential effects of mood on information processing: Evidence from the theories of reasoned action and planned behavior. *European Journal of Social Psychology, 29*(4), 419–433.

Armitage, C. J., & Conner, M. (1999). Distinguishing perception of control from self-efficacy: Predicting consumption of a low fat diet using the theory of planned behavior. *Journal of Applied Social Psychology, 29*(1), 72–90.

Ashing-Giwa, K. (1999). Health behavior change models and their socio-cultural relevance for breast cancer screening in African American women. *Women and Health, 28*(4), 53–71.

Astrom, A. N., & Mwangosi, I. E.(2000). Teachers intention to provide dietary counseling to Tanzanian primary schools. *American Journal of Health Behavior, 24*(4), 281–289.

Astrom, A. N., & Rise, J. (2001). Young adults intention to eat healthy food: Extending the theory of planned behavior. *Psychology and Health, 16*(2), 223–237.

Backman, D. R., Haddad, E. H., Lee, J. W., Johnston, P. K., & Hodgkin, G. E. (2002). Psychosocial predictors of healthful dietary behavior in adolescents. *Journal of Nutrition Education and Behavior, 34*(4), 184–92.

Bagozzi, R. P., Lee, K. H., & Van-Loo, M. F. (2001). Decisions to donate bone marrow: The role of attitudes and subjective norms across cultures. *Psychology and Health, 16*(1), 29–56.

Barker, J. C., Battle, R. S., Cummings, G. L., & Bancroft, K. N. (1998). Condoms and consequences: HIV\AIDS education and African American women. *Human Organization*, 57(3), 273–283.

Bebetsos, E., Chroni, S., & Theodorakis, Y. (2002). Physically active students intention and self efficacy towards healthy eating. *Psychological Reports*, 91(2), 485–495.

Becker, E. A., & Gibson, C. C. (1998). Fishbein and Ajzen's theory of reasoned action: Accurate prediction of behavior intentions for enrolling in distance education courses. *Adult Education Quarterly*, 49(1), 43–55.

Bennett, P., & Bozionelos, G. (2000). The theory of planned behavior as predictor of condom use: A narrative review. *Psychology, Health and Medicine*, 5(3), 307–326.

Bennet, P., & Clatworthy, J. (1999). Smoking cessation during pregnancy: Testing a psycho-biological model. *Psychology, Health and Medicine*, 4(3), 319–326.

Berger, J. A., & O'Brien-William, H. (1998).Clinical psychology student self reported willingness to interact with persons living with HIV–AIDS. *Education and Prevention*, 10(3), 199–214.

Bernaix, L. W. (2000). Nurses' attitudes, subjective norms, and behavioral intention toward support of breastfeeding mothers. *Journal of Human Lactation*, 16(3), 201–209.

Biddle, S. J. H., & Nigg, C. R. (2000). Theories of exercise behavior. *Intentional Journal of Sport Psychology*, 31(2), 290–304.

Bissonnette, M. M., & Contento, I. R. (2001). Adolescent perspectives and food choice behaviors in terms of the environmental impacts of food production practices: Application of a psychosocial model. *Journal of Nutrition Education*, 33(2), 72–82.

Blanchard, C. M., Courneya, K. S., Rodgers, W. M., & Murnaghan, D. M. (2002). Determinants of exercise intention and behavior in survivors of breast and prostate cancer: An application of the theory of planned behavior. *Cancer Nursing*, 25(2), 88–95.

Blue, C. L., Wilbur, J., & Marston-Scott, M. V. (2001). Exercise among blue collar workers: Application of the theory of planned behavior. *Research in Nursing and Health*, 24(6), 481–493.

Bogart, L. M., Cecil, H., & Pinkerton, S. D. (2000). Hispanic adults' beliefs, attitudes, and intention regarding the female condom. *Journal of Behavioral Medicine*, 23(2), 181–206.

Bogart, L. M., Cecil, H., & Pinkerton, S. D. (2000). Intention to use the female condom among African American adults. *Journal of Applied Social Psychology*, 30(9), 1923–1953.

Boldero, J., Moore, S., & Rosenthal, D. (1992). Intention, context, and safe sex: Australian adolescents' responses to AIDS. *Journal of Applied Social Psychology*, 22, 1374–1396.

Bosompra, K. (2001). Determinants of condom use intention of university students in Ghana: An application of the theory of reasoned action. *Social Science and Medicine*, 52(7), 1057–1069.

Bozionelos, G., & Bennett, P. (1999). The theory of planned behavior as predictor of exercise: The moderating influence of beliefs and personality variables. *Journal of Health Psychology*, 4(4), 517–529.

Brenes, G. A., Strube, M. J., & Storandt, M. (1998). An application of the theory of planned behavior to exercise among older adults. *Journal of Applied Social Psychology*, 28(24), 2274–2290.

Brewer, J. L., Blake, A. J., Rankin, S. A., & Douglass, L. W. (1999). Theory of Reasoned Action predicts milk consumption in women. *Journal of the American Dietetic Association*, 99(1), 39–44.

Brinberg, D., Axelson, M. L., & Price, S. (2000). Changing food knowledge, food choice, and dietary fiber consumption by using tailored messages. *Appetite*, 35(1), 35–43.

Bryan, A., Fisher, J. D., & Fisher, W. A. (2002). Tests of the mediational role of preparatory safer sexual behavior in the context of the theory of planned behavior. *Health Psychology*, 21(1), 71–80.

Bryan, A. D., & Rocheleau, C. A. (2002). Predicting aerobic versus resistance exercise using the theory of planned behavior. *American Journal of Health Behavior*, 26(2), 83–94.

Budd, R. (1986). Predicting cigarette use: The need to incorporate measures of salience in the theory of reasoned action. *Journal of Applied Social Psychology*, 16, 663–685.

Budd, R., & Spencer, C. (1984). Predicting undergraduates' intentions to drink. *Journal of Studies on Alcohol*, 45, 179–183.

Bunce, D., & Birdi, K. S. (1998). The theory of reasoned action and theory of planned behavior as a function of job control. *British Journal of Health Psychology*, 3(3), 265–275.

Bursey, M., & Craig, D. (2000). Attitudes, subjective norm, perceived behavioral control, and intentions related to adult smoking cessation after coronary artery bypass graft surgery. *Public Health Nursing*, 17(6), 460–467.

Carron, A. V., Hausenblas, A., & Mack, D. (1999). When a comment is much ado about little: A reply to Spence. *Journal of Sport and Exercise Psychology*, 21(4), 382–388.

Chan, D. K. S., & Cheung, S. F. (1998). An examination of premarital sexual behavior among college students in Hong Kong. *Psychology and Health*, 13(5), 805–821.

Chapados, C., Pineault, R., Tourigny, J., & Vandal, S. (2002). Perceptions of parents' participation in the care of their child undergoing day surgery: Pilot study. *Issues in Comprehensive Pediatric Nursing*, 25(1), 59–70.

Chassin, L., Corry, E., Presson, C., Othavsky, R. W., Bensenberg, M., & Sherman, S. (1981). Predicting adolescents' intentions to smoke cigarettes. *Journal of Health and Social Behavior*, 22, 445–455.

Cho, Y. H., Keller, L. R., & Cooper, M. L. (1999). Applying decision making approaches to health risk taking behavior: Progress and remaining challenges. *Journal of Mathematical Psychology, 43*(2), 261–285.

Choi, K. H., Yep, G. A., & Kumekawa, E. (1998). HIV prevention among Asian and Pacific Islander American men who have sex with men: A critical review of theoretical models and directions for future research. *AIDS Education and Prevention, 10*(3), 19–30.

Christian, J., & Armitage, C.J. (2002). Attitudes and intentions of homeless people towards service provision in South Wales. *British Journal of Social Psychology, 41*(2), 219–232.

Conner, M., & Abraham, C. (2001). Conscientiousness and the theory of planned behavior: Toward a more complete model of the antecedents of intention behavior. *Personality and Social Psychology Bulletin, 27*(11), 1547–1561.

Conner, M., Graham, S., & Moore, B. (1999). Alcohol and intention to use condoms: Applying the theory of planned behavior. *Psychology and Health, 14*(5), 795–812.

Conner, M., Norman, P., & Bell, R. (2002). The theory of planned behavior and healthy eating. *Health Psychology Association, 21*(2), 194–201.

Conner, M., Sheeran, P., Norman, P., & Armitage, C. J. (2000). Temporal stability as a moderator of relationships in the Theory of Planned Behavior. *British Journal of Social Psychology, 39*(4), 469–493.

Conner, M., Sherlock, K., & Orbell, S. (1998). Psychosocial determinants of ecstasy use in young people in the UK. *British Journal of Health Psychology, 3*(4), 295–317.

Courneya, K. S., & Friedenreich, C. M. (1999). Utility of the theory of planned behavior for understanding exercise during breast cancer treatment. *Psychooncology, 8*(2), 112–122.

Courneya, K. S., Plotnikoff, R. C., Hotz, S. B., & Birkett, N. J. (2000). Social support and the theory of planned behavior in the exercise domain. *American Journal of Health Behavior, 24*(4), 300–308.

Courneya, K. S., Blanchard, C. M., & Laing, D. M. (2001). Exercise adherence in breast cancer survivors training for a dragon boat race competition: A preliminary investigation. *Psychooncology, 10*(5), 444–452.

Courneya, K. S., Plotnikoff, R. C., Hotz, S. B., & Birkett, N. J. (2001). Predicting exercise stage transitions over two consecutive 6 month periods: A test of the theory planned behavior in a population based sample. *British Journal of Health Psychology, 6*(2), 135–150.

Crepaz, N., & Marks, G. (2002). Towards an understanding of sexual risk behavior in people living with HIV: A review of social, psychological, and medical findings. *AIDS, 16*(2), 135–149.

DeVellis, B., Blalock, S., & Sandler, R. (1990). Predicting participation in cancer screening: The role of perceived behavioral control. *Journal of Applied Social Psychology, 20,* 639–660.

DeVore, L., Fried, J. L., Dailey, J., & Qori, C. G. (2000). Dental hygiene self assessment: A key to quality care. *Journal of Dental Hygiene, 74*(4), 271–279.

DeVries, H., & Kok, G. (1986). From determinants of smoking behavior to the implications for a prevention programme. *Health Education Research, 1,* 85–94.

De-Wit, J. B. F., Stroebe, W., De-Vroome, E. M. M., & Sandfort, T. G. M. (2000). Understanding AIDS preventive behavior with casual and primary partners in homosexual men: The Theory of Planned Behavior and Information Motivation Behavioral Skills Model. *Psychology and Health, 15*(3), 325–340.

Dick, M. J., Evans, M. L., Arthurs, J. B., Barnes, J. K., Caldwell, R. S., Hutchins, S. S., & Johnson, L. K. (2002). Predicting early breastfeeding attrition. *Journal of Human Lactation, 18*(1), 21–28.

Duckett, L., Henly, S., Avery, M., Potter, S., Hills-Bonczyk, S., Hulden, R., & Savik, K. (1998). A Theory of Planned Behavior based structural model for breast feeding. *Nursing Research, 47*(6), 325–336.

Edwards, H. E., Nash, R. E., Najman, J. M., Yates, P. M., Fentiman, B. J., Dewar, A., Walsh, A. M., McDowell, J. K., & Skerman, H. M. (2001). Determination of nurses' intention to administer opioids for pain relief. *Nursing and Health Sciences, 3*(3), 149–159.

Elder, J. P., Ayala, G. X., & Harris, S. (1999). Theories and intervention approaches to health behavior change in primary care. *American Journal of Preventive Medicine, 17*(4), 275–284.

Enguidanos, S. (2001). Integrating behavior change theory into geriatric case management practice. *Home Health Care Services Quarterly, 20*(1), 67–83.

Evans, D., & Norman, P. (1998). Understanding pedestrians' road crossing decisions: An application of the theory of planned behavior. *Health Education Research, 13*(4), 481–489.

Faucher, M. A., & Carter, S. (2001). The way girls smoke: A proposed community based prevention program. *Journal of Obstetric Gynecologic and Neonatal Nursing, 30*(5), 463–471.

Faulkner, G., & Biddle, S. (2001). Predicting physical promotion in health care settings. *American Journal of Health Promotion, 16*(2), 98–106.

Fekadu, Z., & Kraft, P. (2001). Self identity in planned behavior perspective: Past behavior and its moderating effects on self identity intention relations. *Social Behavior and Personality, 29*(7), 671–685.

Fekadu, Z., & Kraft, P. (2001). Predicting intending contraception in a sample of Ethiopian female adolescents: The validity of the theory of planned behavior. *Psychology and Health, 16*(2), 207–222.

Fekadu, Z., & Kraft, P. (2002). Expanding the theory of planned behavior: The role of social norm and group identification. *Journal of Health Psychology, 7*(1), 33–43.

Fernbach, M. (2002). The impact of a media campaign on cervical screening knowledge and self efficacy. *Journal of Health Psychology, 7*(1), 85–97.

Fishbein, M. (1982). Social psychological analysis of smoking behavior. In J. R. Eiser (Ed.) *Social psychology and behavioral medicine.* New York: Wiley, 179–197.

Fishbein, M., Ajzen, I., & McArdle, J. (1980). Changing the behavior of alcoholics: effects of persuasive communication. In I. Ajzen & M. Fishbein (Eds.). *Understanding attitudes and predicting social behavior.* Englewood Cliffs, NJ: Prentice-Hall, 217–242.

Fishbein, M., Chan, D., O'Reilly, K., Schnell, D., Wood, R., Becker, C., & Cohn, D. (1992). Attitudinal and normative factors as determinants of gay men's intentions to perform AIDS-related sexual behavior: A multisite analysis. *Journal of Applied Social Psychology, 22*, 999–1011.

Flynn, B. S., Goldstein, A. O., Solomon, L. J., Bauman, K. E., Gottlieb, N. H., Cohen, J. E., Munger, M. C., & Dana, G. S. (1998). Predictors of state legislators' intention to vote for cigarette tax increases. *Preventive Medicine, 27*(2), 157–165.

Fried, J. L., DeVore, L., & Dailey, J. (2001). A study of Maryland dental hygienists' perception regarding self assessment. *Journal of Dental Hygiene, 75*(2), 121–129.

Gagne, C., & Godin, G. (2000). The theory of planned behavior: Some measurement issues concerning belief based variables. *Journal of Applied Social Psychology, 30*(10), 2173–2193.

Gagnon, M. P., & Godin, G. (2000). The impact of new antiretroviral treatments on college students' intention to use a condom with a new sexual partner. *AIDS Education and Prevention, 12*(3), 239–251.

Gantt, C. J. (2001). The theory of planned behavior and postpartum smoking relapse. *Journal of Nursing Scholarship, 33*(4), 337–341.

Godin, G., Gagne, C., Maziade, J., Moreault, L., Beaulieu, D., & Morel, S. (2001). Breast cancer: The intention to have a mammography and a clinical breast examination: Application of the theory of planned behavior. *Psychology and Health, 16*(4), 423–441.

Goksen, F. (2002). Normative vs. attitudinal consideration in breastfeeding behavior: Multifaceted social influences in a developing country context. *Social Science and Medicine, 54*(12), 1743–1753.

Goodson, P. (2002). Predictors of intention to promote family planning: A survey of Protestant seminarians in the United States. *Health Education Behavior, 29*(5), 521–541.

Hagger, M. S., Chatzisarantis, N., Biddle, S. J. H., & Orbell, S. (2001). Antecedents of children's physical activity intention and behavior: Predictive validity and longitudinal effects. *Psychology and Health, 16*(4), 391–407.

Hankins, M., French, D., & Horne, R. (2000). Statistical guidelines for studies of the theory of reasoned action and the theory of planned behavior. *Psychology and Health, 15*(2), 151–161.

Hanson, M. J. S. (1999). Cross cultural study of beliefs about smoking among teenaged females. *Western Journal of Nursing Research, 21*(5), 635–651.

Hillhouse, J. J., Turrisi, R., & Kastner, M. (2000). Modeling tanning salon behavioral tendencies using appearance motivation, self-monitoring and the Theory of Planned Behavior. *Health Education Research, 15*(4), 405–414.

Hoffmann, R. G. III., Rodriguez, J. R., & Johnson, J. H. (1999). Effectiveness of a school based program to enhance knowledge of sun exposure: Attitudes toward sun exposure and sunscreen use among children. *Children's Health Care, 28*(1), 69–86.

Humphreys, A. S., Thompson, N. J., & Miner, K.R. (1998). Assessment of breastfeeding intention using the Transtheoretical Model and the Theory of Reasoned Action. *Health Education Research, 13*(3), 331–341.

James, A. S., Tripp, M. K., Parcel, G. S., Sweeney, A., & Gritz, E. R. (2002). Psychosocial correlates of sun protective practices of preschool staff toward their student. *Health Education Research, 17*(3), 305–14.

Jemmott, J. B. 3rd., Jemmott, L. S., Hines, P. M., & Fong, G. T. (2001). The theory of planned behavior as a model of intention for fighting among African American and Latino adolescents. *Maternal and Child Health Journal, 5*(4), 253–263.

Jemmott, L. S. (2000). Saving our children: Strategies to empower African American adolescents to reduce their risk for HIV infection. *Journal of National Black-Nurses Association, 11*(1), 4–14.

Jennings-Doizer, K. (1999). Predicting intentions to obtain a Pap smear among African American and Latino women: Testing the theory of planned behavior. *Nursing Research, 48* (4), 198–205.

Jones, F., Abraham, C., Harris, P., Schulz, J., & Chrispin, C. (2001). From knowledge to action regulation: Modeling the cognitive prerequisites of sun screen use in Australian and UK samples. *Psychology and Health, 16*(2), 191–206.

Kerner, M. S., & Grossman, A. H. (1998). Attitudinal, social, and practical correlates to fitness behavior: A test of the theory of planned behavior. *Perceptual and Motor Skills, 87*(3), 1139–1154.

Kerner, M. S., Grossman, A. H., & Kurrant, A. B. (2001). The theory of planned behavior as related to intention to exercise and exercise behavior. *Perceptual and Motor Skills, 92*(3 pt 1), 721–731.

Kerner, M. S., & Kalinski, M. I. (2002). Scale construction for measuring adolescent boys' and girls' attitudes, beliefs, perception of control, and intention to engage in leisure time physical activity. *Perceptual and Motor Skills, 95*(1), 109–117.

Kimiecik, J. (1992). Predicting vigorous physical activity of corporate employees: Comparing the theories of reasoned action and planned behavior. *Journal of Sport and Exercise Psychology, 14,* 192–206.

Kloeblen-Tarver, A. S., Thompson, N. J., & Miner, K. R. (2002). Intention to breast feed: The impact of attitudes, norms, parity, and experience. *American Journal of Health Behavior, 26*(3), 182–187.

Kloeblen, A. S., Thompson, N. J., & Miner, K. R. (1999). Predicting breast feeding intention among low income pregnant women: A comparison of two theoretical models. *Health Education and Behavior, 26*(5), 675–688.

Kridli, S. A., & Libbus, K. (2002). Establishing reliability and validity of an instrument measuring Jordanian Muslim women's contraceptive beliefs. *Health Care for Women International, 23*(8), 870–881.

Legare, F., Goding, G., Guilbert, E., Laperriere, L., & Dodin, S. (2000). Determinants of the intention to adopt hormone replacement therapy among premenopausal women. *Maturitas, 34*(3), 211–218.

Levin-Pamela, F. (1999). Test of the Fishbein and Ajzen models as predictors of health care workers' glove use. *Research in Nursing and Health, 22*(4), 295–307.

Lien, N., Lytle, L. A., & Komro, K. A. (2002). Applying the Theory of Planned Behavior to fruit and vegetable consumption of young adolescents. *American Journal of Health Promotion, 16*(4), 189–197.

Lugoe, W., & Rise, J. (1999). Predicting intended condom use among Tanzanian students using the theory of planned behavior. *Journal of Health Psychology, 4*(4), 497–506.

Manfredi, C., Lacey, L. P., Warnecke, R., & Petraitis, J. (1998). Sociopsychological correlates of motivation to quit smoking among low-SES African American women. *Health Education and Behavior, 25*(3), 304–318.

Manhart, L. E., Dialmy, A., Ryan, C. A., & Mahjour, J. (2000). Sexually transmitted diseases in Morocco: Gender influences on prevention and health care seeking behavior. *Social Science and Medicine, 50*(10), 1369–1383.

Marttila, J., & Nupponen, R. (2000). Health enhancing physical activity as perceived in interviews based on the Theory of Planned Behavior. *Psychology and Health, 15*(5), 593–608.

Masalu, J. R., & Astrom, A. N. (2001). Predicting intended and self perceived sugar restriction among Tanzanian students using the theory of planned behavior. *Journal of Health Psychology, 6*(4), 435–445.

Masalu, J. R., & Astrom, A. N. (2003). The use of the theory of planned behavior to explore beliefs about sugar restriction. *American Journal of Health Behavior, 27*(1), 15–24.

Matin, G., Perez-Stable, E., Otero-Sabogal, R., & Sabogal, F. (1990). Cultural differences in attitudes towards smoking: developing messages using the theory of reasoned action, *Journal of Applied Social Psychology, 20,* 478–493.

McCarty, M. C., Hennrikus, D. J., Lando, H. A., & Vessey, J. T. (2001). Nurses' attitudes concerning the delivery of brief cessation advice to hospitalized smokers. *Preventive Medicine, 33*(6), 674–681.

McCaul, K. D., Sandgren, A., O'Neill, H., & Hinsz, V. (1993). The value of the theory of planned behavior, perceived control, and self-efficacy expectations for predicting health-protective behaviors. *Basic and Applied Social Psychology, 14,* 231–252.

McDermott, R. (1998). Adolescent HIV prevention and intervention: A prospect theory analysis. *Psychology, Health and Medicine, 3*(4), 371–385.

McGahee, T. W., Kemp, V., & Tingen, M. (2000). A theoretical model for smoking prevention studies in preteen children. *Pediatric Nursing, 26*(2), 135–138, 141.

McKinlay, A., Couston, M., & Cowan, S. (2001). Nurses' behavioral intentions towards self poisoning patients: A theory of reasoned action comparison of attitudes and subjective norms as predictive variables. *Journal of Advanced Nursing, 34*(1), 107–116.

Meyer, L. (2002). Applying the theory of planned behavior: Nursing students' intentions to seek clinical experiences using the essential clinical behavior database. *Journal of Nursing Education, 41*(3), 107–116.

More, S. M., Barling, N. R., & Hood, B. (1998). Predicting testicular and breast self examination behavior: A test of the theory of reasoned action. *Behavior Change, 15*(1), 41–49.

Mummery, W. K., Spence, J. C., & Hudec, J. C. (2000). Understanding physical activity intention in Canada school children and youth: An application of the theory of planned behavior. *Research Quarterly for Exercise and Sport, 71*(2), 116–124.

Mummery, W. K., & Wankel, L. M. (1999). Training adherence in adolescent competitive swimmers: An application of the theory of planned behavior. *Journal of Sport and Exercise Psychology, 21*(4), 313–328.

Nabi, R. L., Southwell, B., & Hornik, R. (2002). Predicting intention versus predicting behavior: Domestic violence prevention from a theory of reasoned action perspective. *Health Communication, 14*(4), 429–449.

Norman, P., Bennett, P., & Lewis, H. (1998). Understanding binge drinking among young people: An application of Theory of Planned Behavior. *Health Education Research, 13*(2), 163–169.

Norman, P., & Conner, M. (1993). The role of social cognition models in predicting attendance at health checks. *Psychology and Health, 8,* 447–462.

Norman, P., Conner, M., & Bell, R. (1999). The theory of

planned behavior and smoking cessation. *Health Psychology*, *18*(1), 89–94.

Norman, P., Conner, M., & Bell, R. (2000). The theory of planned behavior and exercise: Evidence for the moderating role of past behavior. *British Journal of Health Psychology*, *5*(3), 249–261.

O'Boyle, C. A., Henly, S. J., & Larson, E. (2001). Understanding adherence to hand hygiene recommendations: the theory of planned behavior. *American Journal of Infection Control*, *29*(6), 352–360.

Okun, M. A., Karoly, P., & Lutz, R. (2002). Clarifying the contribution of subjective norm to predicting leisure time exercise. *American Journal of Health Behavior*, *26*(4), 296–305.

Park, S., Yoo, I., & Chang, S. (2002). Relationship between the intention to repeat a papanicolaou smear test and affective response to a previous test among Korean women. *Cancer Nursing*, *25*(5), 385–390.

Payne, N., Jones, F., & Harris, P. (2002). The impact of working life on health behavior: The effect of job strain on the cognitive predictors of exercise. *Journal of Occupational Health Psychology*, *7*(4), 342–353.

Peek, M. K., Coward, R. T., Peek, C. W., & Lee, G. R. (1998). Are expectations for care related to the receipt of care? An analysis of parent care among disabled elders. *Journal of Gerontology*, *53B*(3), S127–S136.

Petrea, R. E. (2001). The theory of planned behavior: Use and application in targeting agricultural safety and health interventions. *Journal of Agricultural Safety and Health*, *7*(1), 7–19.

Poss, J. E. (1999). Developing an instrument to study the tuberculosis screening behavior of Mexican migrant farm workers. *Journal of Transcultural Nursing*, *10*(4), 306–319.

Poss, J. E. (2000). Factors associated with participation by Mexican migrant farmworkers in a tuberculosis screening program. *Nursing Research*, *49*(1), 20–28.

Poss, J. E. (2001). Developing a new model for cross cultural research: Synthesizing the Health Belief Model and the Theory of Reasoned Action. *ANS-Advances in Nursing Science*, *23*(4), 1–15.

Povey, R., Conner, M., Sparks, P., James, R., & Shepherd, R. (2000). Application of the Theory of Planned Behavior to two dietary behaviors: Roles of perceived control and self efficacy. *British Journal of Health Psychology*, *5*(2), 121–139.

Povey, R., Conner, M., Sparks, P., James, R., & Shepherd, R. (2000). The theory of planned behavior and health eating: Examining additive and moderating effects of social influence variables. *Psychology and Health*, *14*(6), 991–1006.

Quine, L., Rutter, D. R., & Arnold, L. (2001). Persuading school age cyclists to use safety helmets: Effectiveness of an intervention based on the theory of planned behavior. *British Journal of Health Psychology*, *6*(4), 327–345.

Rapaport, P., & Orbell, S. (2000). Augmenting the theory of planned behavior: Motivation to provide practical assistance and emotional support to parents. *Psychology and Health*, *15*(3), 309–324.

Reger, B., Cooper, L., Booth-Butterfield, S., Smith, H., Bauman, A., Wootan, M., Middlestadt, S., Marcus, B., & Greer, F. (2002). Wheeling Walks: A community campaign using paid media to encourage walking among sedentary older adults. *Preventive Medicine*, *35*(3), 285–292.

Rise, J., & Wilhelmsen, B. U. (1998). Prediction of adolescent intention not to drink alcohol: Theory of planned behavior. *American Journal of Health Behavior*, *22*(3), 206–217.

Rosen, C. S. (2000). Integrating stage and continuum models to explain processing messages and exercise initiation among sedentary college students. *Health Psychology*, *19*(2), 172–180.

Rosengard, C., Adler, N. E., Gurvey, J. E., Dunlop, M. B., Tschann, J. M., Millstein, S. G., & Ellen, J. M. (2001). Protective role of health values in adolescents' future intention to use condoms. *Journal of Adolescent Health*, *29*(3), 200–207.

Rutter, D. R. (2000). Attendance and reattendance for breast cancer screening: A prospective 3-year test of the Theory of Planned Behavior. *British Journal of Health Psychology*, *5*(1), 1–13.

Schlegel, R., D'Avernas, J. R., Zarma, M., & DeCourville, N. (1992). Problem drinking: A problem for the theory of reasoned action? *Journal of Applied Social Psychology*, *22*, 358–385

Sejwacz, D., Ajzen, I., & Fishbein, M. (1980). Predicting and understanding weight loss. In I. Ajzen & M. Fishbein (Eds.), *Understanding attitudes and predicting social behavior.* Englewood Cliffs, NJ: Prentice-Hall, 101–112.

Selvan, M. S., Ross, M. W., Kapadia, A. S., Mathai, R., & Hira, S. (2001). Study of perceived norms, beliefs and intended sexual behavior among higher secondary school students in India. *AIDS*, *13*(6), 779–788.

Sheeran, P., Conner, M., & Norman, P. (2001). Can the theory of planned behavior explain patterns of health behavior change? *Health Psychology*, *20*(1), 12–19.

Sheeran, P., & Orbell, S. (2000). Using implementation intention to increase attendance for cervical cancer screening. *Health Psychology*, *19*(3), 283–289.

Sheeran, P., & Taylor, S. (1999). Predicting intention to use condoms: A meta analysis and comparison of the theories reasoned action and planned behavior. *Journal of Applied Social Psychology*, *29*(8), 1624–1675.

Sherman, S., Presson, C., Chassin, L., Bensenberg, M., Corty, E., & Olshavsky, R. (1992). Smoking intension in adolescents: Direct experience and predictability. *Personality and Social Psychology Bulletin*, *8*, 376–383.

Smedslund, G. (2000). A pragmatic basis for judging models

and theories in health psychology: The axiomatic method. *Journal of Health Psychology, 5*(2), 133–149.

Smith, R. A., & Biddle, S. J. (1999). Attitudes and exercise adherence: Test of the theories of reasoned action and planned behavior. *Journal of Sports Sciences, 17*(4), 269–281.

Sneed, C. D., & Morisky, D. E. (1998). Applying the Theory of Reasoned Action to condom use among workers. *Social Behavior and Personality, 26*(4), 317–327.

Sparks, P., & Guthrie, C. A. (1998). Self identity and the theory of planned behavior: A useful addition or an unhelpful artifice? *Journal of Applied Social Psychology, 28*(5), 1393–1410.

Spence, J. C. (1999). When a note of caution in not enough: A comment on Hausenblas, Carron and Mack and theory testing in meta analysis. *Journal of Sport and Exercise Psychology, 21*(4), 376–381.

Steen, D. M., Peay, M. Y., & Owen, N. (1998). Predicting Australian adolescents' intention to minimize sun exposure. *Psychology and Health, 13*(1), 111–119.

Sultan, S., Bungener, C., & Andronikof, F. (2002). Individual psychology of risk taking behaviors in nonadherence. *Journal of Risk Research, 5*(2), 137–145.

Sutton, S. (1989). Smoking attitudes and behaviour: An application of Fishbein and Ajzen's theory of reasoned action to predicting and understanding smoking decisions. In T. Ney & A. Gale (Eds.) *Smoking and human behaviour.* Chichester, UK: Wiley, 289–312.

Sutton, S. (1998). Predicting and explaining intention and behavior: How well are we doing? *Journal of Applied Social Psychology, 28*(15), 1317–1338.

Sutton, S., McVey, D., & Glanz, A. (1999). A comparative test of the theory of reasoned action and the theory of planned behavior in the prediction of condom use intention in a national sample of English young people. *Health Psychology, 18*(1), 72–81.

Syrjala, A. M., Niskanen, M. C., & Knuuttila, M. L. (2002). The theory of reasoned action in describing tooth brushing, dental caries and diabetes adherence among diabetic patients. *Journal of Clinical Periodontology, 29*(5), 423–432.

Taylor, S. D., Bagozzi, R. P., & Gaither, C. A. (2001). Gender differences in the self regulation of hypertension. *Journal of Behavior Medicine, 24*(5), 469–487

Terry, D., Galligan, R., & Conway, V. (1993). The prediction of safe sex behaviour: The role of intentions, attitudes, norms and control beliefs. *Psychology and Health, 8,* 355–368.

Theodorakis, Y., Doganis, G., Bagiatis, K., & Gouthas, M. (1991). Preliminary study of the ability of the reasoned action model in predicting exercise behaviour of young children. *Perceptual and Motor Skills, 72,* 51–58.

Treise, D., & Weigold, M. F. (2001). AIDS public service an-nouncements: Effects of fear and repetition on predictors of condom use. *Health Marketing Quarterly, 18*(3–4), 39–61.

Trost, S., Sunders, R., & Ward, D. (2002). Determinants of physical activity in middle school children. *American Journal of Health Behavior, 26*(2), 95–102.

Trost, S., Saunders, R., & Ward, D. (2002). Determinants of physical activity in middle school children. *American Journal of Health Behavior, 26*(2), 95–102.

Trost, S., Pate, R., Dowda, M., Ward, D., Felton, G., & Saunders, R. (2002). Psychosocial correlates of physical activity in white and African American girls. *Journal of Adolescent Health, 31*(3), 226–233.

Unger, J., Rohrbach, L., Howard, P., & Ritt-Olson, A. (2001). Peer influences and susceptibility to smoking among Californian adolescents. *Substance Use and Misuse, 36*(5), 551–571.

Valois, P., Turgeon, H., Godin, G., Blondeau, D., & Cote, F. (2001). Influence of a persuasive strategy on nursing students' beliefs and attitudes toward provision of care to people living with HIV. *Journal of Nursing Education, 40*(8), 354–358.

Von-Haeften, I., Fishbein, M., Kasprzyk, D., & Montano, D. (2001). Analyzing data to obtain information to design targeted interventions. *Psychology Health and Medicine, 6*(2), 151–164.

Waiker, A., Grimshaw, J., & Armstrong, E. (2001). Salient beliefs and intentions to prescribe antibiotics for patients with a sore throat. *British Journal of Health Psychology, 6*(4), 347–360.

Werner, P., & Mendelsson, G. (2001). Nursing staff member's intention to use physical restraints with older people: Testing the theory of reasoned action. *Journal of Advanced Nursing, 35*(5), 784–791.

Wilson, D., Zenda, A., McMaster, J., & Lavelle, S. (1992). Factors predicting Wimbabwean students' intentions to use condoms, *Psychology and Health, 7,* 99–114.

Wilson, T., Dunn, D., Kraft, D., & Lisle, D. (1989). Introspection, attitude change, and attitude—behaviour consistency: The disruptive effects of explaining why we feel the way we do. In L. Berkowitz (Ed.) *Advances in experimental social psychology,* Vol. 22. New York: Academic Press, 287–343.

Yordy, G. A., & Lent, R. W. (1993). Predicting aerobic exercise participation—social cognitive, reasoned action, and planned behavior models. *Journal of Sport and Exercise Psychology, 15,* 363–374.

Young, H., Lierman, L., Powell-Cope, G., & Kasprzyk, D. (1991). Operationalizing the theory of planned behaviour. *Research in Nursing and Health, 14,* 137–144.

Yzer, M., Siero, F., & Buunk, B. (2001). Bringing up condom use and using condoms with new sexual partners: Intentional or habitual? *Psychology and Health, 16*(4), 409–421.

Middle Range Theories: Emotional

Empathy

JOANNE K. OLSON AND DIANE KUNYK

DEFINITION OF KEY TERMS

Empathy	Understanding a client's thoughts and feelings and the ability to communicate to the patient this understanding of both the patient's feelings and the reasons for those feelings
Interpersonal perception approach to empathy	Ability to know and understand another's world; to understand another person's viewpoint
Multidimensional/multiphasic approach to empathy	Ability to perceive and reason, as well as the ability to communicate an understanding of the other person's feelings and their attached meaning
Nurse-expressed empathy	Understanding what a patient is saying and feeling and communicating this understanding verbally to the patient
Patient-perceived empathy	Patient's feelings of being understood and accepted by the nurse
Patient distress	Negative emotional state resulting from unmet needs (includes anger, anxiety, and depression)
Therapeutic communication approach	Ability to go beyond merely perceiving the patient's thinking and feeling, to supportively communicating this accurate understanding to the patient

INTRODUCTION

The nurse–patient relationship is an important basis for accomplishing the goals of nursing as identified by nurse theorists, as stated in nursing social policy statements, and as described in standards for nursing practice. Empathy is one of the most essential variables in establishing and maintaining this nurse–patient relationship. Further understanding of empathy in the nurse–patient relationship is a worthwhile endeavor because, from any theoretical perspective, this relationship provides the basis for all other nurse–patient activity.

Nursing models vary in their stated goals and in the emphasis placed upon the nurse–patient relationship. Some nurse theorists view this relationship as the essence of nursing (King, 1981; Orlando, 1961; Paterson & Zderad, 1976; Peplau, 1952; Travelbee, 1971; Wiedenbach, 1963). Others accept the importance of the nurse–patient relationship but focus on other aspects of nursing or upon the interaction between metaparadigm concepts other than the nurse and the patient (Johnson, 1980; Levine, 1971; Orem, 1985; Rogers, 1970; Roy, 1976). None, however, would dispute the importance of the nurse–patient relationship as a basis for accomplishing the goals of nursing in their particular nursing model.

HISTORICAL BACKGROUND

Empathy has been described as one of the most essential and complex variables in the communication process (Forsyth, 1980; Gagan, 1983; Kalisch, 1973; La Monica, 1981; Rogers, 1957; Stetler; 1977). For the past 40 years, there has been considerable scientific interest and inquiry into this intriguing phenomenon, a characteristic at the heart of all helping relationships, and certainly essential to nurse–patient interactions. The identification of factors that are related to empathy in nurse–patient interactions is of concern to those who educate nurses, those who hire nurses, and to nurses themselves, as they strive to achieve the goals of nursing within the context of a nurse–patient relationship.

Various disciplines have been interested in describing this concept both theoretically and operationally for purposes unique to each particular discipline. In the literature of social psychology, developmental psychology, and communication, for example, there has been an attempt to understand the process of empathic helping (Archer, Diaz-Loving, Gollwitzer, Davis, & Foushee, 1981; Coke, Batson, & McDavis, 1978). The literature of counseling, psychotherapy, and health professionals reflects investigation into the phenomenon of empathy primarily because of the positive growth potential connected to therapeutic empathy (Goldstein & Michaels, 1985).

A review of the literature indicates a wide diversity in definitions and conceptualizations of empathy. Historically, however, studies about empathy and the measurement of empathy have evolved from three main conceptual viewpoints: the interpersonal perception approach (Gladstein, 1983), the therapeutic communication approach (Northouse, 1979), and an approach that is multiphased in nature (Kunyk & Olson, 2001; Olson, 1995; Sutherland, 1995; Wheeler, 1995). Figure 7-1 is a diagram representing the three conceptual views of empathy and identifying some of the authors who support each view. Each view of empathy will be further described.

Interpersonal Perception Approach

The interpersonal perception approach can be divided into two categories of empathy: cognitive or role-taking empathy, and affective or emotional empathy (Gladstein, 1983). From the interpersonal perception approach, cognitive or role-taking empathy refers to the ability to know and understand another's world, or to understand another person's viewpoint. Affective or emotional empathy is the emotional response of one individual to another's state, the ability to vicariously experience another person's feelings (Chlopan, McCain, Carbonell, & Hagen, 1985).

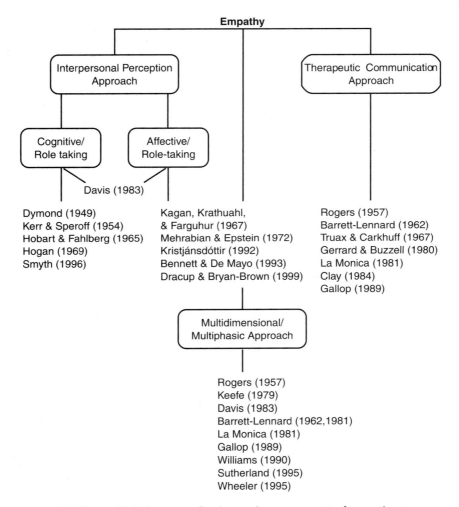

Empathy

Interpersonal Perception Approach

Therapeutic Communication Approach

Cognitive/ Role taking

Affective/ Role-taking

Davis (1983)

Dymond (1949)
Kerr & Speroff (1954)
Hobart & Fahlberg (1965)
Hogan (1969)
Smyth (1996)

Kagan, Krathuahl,
& Farguhur (1967)
Mehrabian & Epstein (1972)
Kristjánsdóttir (1992)
Bennett & De Mayo (1993)
Dracup & Bryan-Brown (1999)

Rogers (1957)
Barrett-Lennard (1962)
Truax & Carkhuff (1967)
Gerrard & Buzzell (1980)
La Monica (1981)
Clay (1984)
Gallop (1989)

Multidimensional/ Multiphasic Approach

Rogers (1957)
Keefe (1979)
Davis (1983)
Barrett-Lennard (1962,1981)
La Monica (1981)
Gallop (1989)
Williams (1990)
Sutherland (1995)
Wheeler (1995)

■ **Figure 7.1** Conceptualization and measurement of empathy.

The majority of empathy measures have their roots in the cognitive approach to empathy. These include the Dymond (1949) Rating Test of Insight and Empathy, the Kerr and Speroff Empathy Test (1954), Hobart and Fahlberg's (1965) measurement of empathy, and the Hogan Empathy Scale (1969). The Questionnaire Measure of Emotional Empathy (Mehrabian & Epstein, 1972) and the Affective Sensitivity Scale (Kagan, Krathwohl, & Farquhar, 1967) are measures of the emotional aspect of empathy. Davis (1983) used a multidimensional approach to measure both the cognitive role-taking and the vicarious arousal or emotional aspects of empathy.

Therapeutic Communication Approach

Therapeutic empathy is conceptualized as the ability of the helper to go beyond merely perceiving the patient's thinking and feeling to supportively communicating this accurate understanding to the patient (Northouse, 1979). Therapeutic empathy could also be referred to as expressed empathy.

Carl Rogers (1957) suggested that expressed empathy was one of the core conditions in a helping relationship. Without this communicative aspect (expressed empathy) of empathy, the goals of a therapeutic relationship may not be fully realized. Stetler (1977) concurred when she suggested that verbal communication is essential because a helper's knowledge of the feelings and experiences of the other is of little value unless successfully communicated.

A number of reviews have been conducted which have summarized the literature about efforts to measure the effects of empathy (Chlopan et al., 1985; Gurman, 1977; Hornblow, 1980; Lambert, De Julio, & Stein, 1978; Patterson, 1984). There is general agreement that the earliest attempts to operationalize the concepts of client-centered therapy (Rogers, 1957) were by Barrett-Lennard (1962) and Truax and Carkhuff (1967). Several other more recent instruments in the category of therapeutic communication of empathy include the LaMonica Empathy Construct Rating Scale (1981), the Behavioral Test of Interpersonal Skills (BTIS) (Gerrard & Buzzell, 1980), an empathic interaction skills schedule (Clay, 1984) and the Staff–Patient Interaction Response Scale (SPIRS) (Gallop, 1989).

Multidimensional/Multiphasic Approach

In some models, cognitive, affective, and therapeutic aspects of empathy have been combined, resulting in a more comprehensive definition of empathy (Barrett-Lennard, 1981; Davis, 1983; Elliot, Filipovich, Harrigan, Gaynor, Reimschuessel, & Zapadaka, 1982; Keefe, 1979; Rogers, 1957). Rogers described empathy as having three components: affective (sensitivity), cognitive, and communicative (helper's response); Barrett-Lennard (1981) spoke of a three-phased empathy cycle: empathic resonation, expressed empathy, and perceived empathy. The third phase, perceived empathy, is described by Rogers, Glendlin, and Kiesler (1967) and others. They suggest that a patient's perception of a helper's empathy is an essential part of a therapeutic relationship; if a patient does not perceive empathy, a positive outcome is not likely. Sutherland's (1995) qualitative research resulted in a four-stage conceptualization of empathy. These stages include identification, introjection, nursing intervention, and patient response. This view of empathy is unique in its inclusion of nurse intervention and patient response as phases in the empathy process.

The Barrett-Lennard Relationship Inventory (BLRI) (Barrett-Lennard, 1962), and the SPIRS (Gallop, 1989) could be classified in the multidimensional category of empathy. They measure empathy as a process made up of phases.

DEFINITION OF THEORY CONCEPTS

The proliferation of literature on empathy in the past 10 years proves it to be a concept of interest to nursing. While nurse authors do not agree on a single definition, the concept is developing more depth and breadth. A conceptual analysis on the recent nursing literature revealed that there are five common conceptualizations of empathy. These include empathy as a human trait, empathy as a professional state, empathy as a communication process, empathy as caring, and empathy as a special relationship (Kunyk & Olson, 2001).

When empathy is considered a human trait, it involves an innate, natural ability. This form of empathy can be identified, reinforced, and refined but it cannot be taught. Nurse authors who view empathy as a professional state say that empathy is a learned skill, consisting of cognitive and behavioral components used to transmit understanding of the patient's reality back to him or her. From this perspective, empathy is a learned phenomenon whereby the nurse cognitively selects the best response.

Some authors consider empathy an exceptional form of a communication process. In this process, the patient is accurately understood and this understanding is communicated back to him/her. The process is not predetermined or rote, but a learned skill applied uniquely to each nurse–patient interaction. When empathy is seen as caring, the nurse is compelled to act because of the experience of understanding the patient. Nursing intervention is the outcome of the empathic process rather than understanding the client. In the conceptualization of empathy as a special relationship, a long-term reciprocal relationship develops between the nurse and the patient that resembles a special friendship.

In the middle range theory developed by Olson (Olson & Hanchett, 1997), other empathy-related definitions are key. These include nurse-expressed empathy, patient-perceived empathy, and patient distress. Nurse-expressed empathy is defined as understanding what a patient is saying and feeling, and communicating this understanding verbally to the patient. A patient's feeling of being understood and accepted by the nurse is the definition of patient-perceived empathy. Finally, patient distress is a negative emotional state that results from unmet needs (includes anger, anxiety, and depression).

DESCRIPTION OF OLSON'S THEORY OF THE EMPATHIC PROCESS

Olson deductively developed a middle range theory of the empathic process from Orlando's more abstract model of nursing (Orlando, 1961, 1972). This model was selected for several reasons. Orlando's model specifically describes nursing as a relationship between a nurse and a patient. She also describes a process of verification in a therapeutic encounter that could be likened to expressed empathy, the communicative component of empathy. This process of verification of the meaning of observations with the patient is said to be one of three crucial elements in a process discipline. Nurses must have their perceptions validated or corrected for understanding of another's experience. A final reason for selecting Orlando's model is that it addresses nursing outcomes. Specifically, she speaks of patient distress as an outcome measure of nursing care.

Orlando's model of nursing provides a global perspective but is too general and abstract to allow for testing. Using a deductive process, a set of propositions was derived from the model. The middle range theory development process involved outlining the relational statements in Orlando's model and identifying the propositions of the middle range theory. Finally, the connections of Orlando's relational statements to propositions of the middle range theory were identified. Three relevant relational statements in Orlando's model were selected for further theory development:

1. There will be greater improvement in patient behavior and more effective nursing care when nurses use the disciplined professional response than when they use automatic personal response.
2. When a nurse assesses a patient's immediate needs, immediate experiences, and immediate resultant behaviors, nursing care is more effective in decreasing distress and helplessness and increasing comfort.

3. There will be greater improvement in patient outcomes when nurses have accurate perceptions of patient needs and when these accurate perceptions are shared verbally with patients.

From Orlando's relational statements, three middle range theory propositions were developed using the following logic:

Given that:

1. Nurses' accurate perceptions lead to better patient outcomes, and
2. Nurse assessments lead to decreased patient distress, and

Assuming that:

1. Nurse assessment must be based on accurate perceptions to decrease distress, and
2. Nurses' accurate perceptions (verbally shared with patients) equal empathy,

Then (middle range theory propositions):

1. Nurse-expressed empathy (accurate perceptions verbally shared with patients) leads to decreased patient distress, and
2. If accurate perceptions are verbally shared with patients (nurse-expressed empathy), the patient experiences greater perceived empathy (feelings of being understood and accepted by the nurse), and
3. Patient-perceived empathy leads to lower patient distress.

In Figure 7-2, the structure of the middle range theory is diagrammed. Concepts from Orlando's model and concepts and propositions of the middle range theory are included.

A nurse's verbal empathy relates to what Orlando refers to as a nurse's sharing of accurate perceptions with a patient. Nurses do not achieve therapeutic levels of empathy automatically; becoming empathic with patients requires an empathic attitude and the skills necessary to convey this caring to a patient. This is part of the disciplined professional response to which Orlando refers. Though Orlando has not specifically alluded to the development of empathy skills in her discussion of a disciplined professional response, the professional response described would be difficult to achieve without high levels of empathy.

When a nurse assesses a patient's immediate needs and immediate experiences (as described in Orlando's proposition number two), that nurse is exploring the patient's thoughts and feelings, and this is part of being empathic. In Orlando's proposition number three, there is reference to nurses having accurate perception of patient needs. The middle range theory, therefore, addresses the patient's perception of nurse empathy and the patient's feelings of being understood, in addition to the nurse's verbal expressions of empathy. These feelings of being understood, as described in the middle range theory, are linked theoretically to what is referred to in Orlando's proposition number two as decreased distress, decreased helplessness, and increased comfort.

APPLICATIONS OF THE THEORY

Olson's middle range theory of the empathic process offers a structure from which to study the relationships among nurse-expressed empathy, patient-perceived empathy, and patient outcomes. This middle range theory provides a basis from which nurse researchers could conceptualize various other

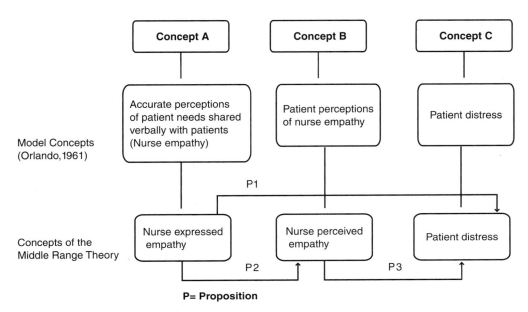

Figure 7.2 Middle range theory: Relationship between nurse-expressed empathy, patient-perceived empathy, and patient distress.

ways of examining the empathic process. The process involves three concepts that could be explored further in future research.

The first concept is nurse-expressed empathy. Given that the theory is based on the idea of a disciplined professional response, researchers interested in nursing education and continuing professional competence may want to explore factors that contribute to the development of a disciplined professional response: nurse-expressed empathy. These factors could include variables such as age, educational background, and clinical experience.

A second concept in the theory is patient-perceived empathy. Other researchers may want to explore factors related to various levels of patient-perceived empathy. For example, how does patient-perceived empathy vary across cultures, patient age, and experience, or in situations where clients are experiencing pain, mental health issues, or cognitive impairment?

The final concept of the theory is that of patient outcome. Though one patient outcome (patient distress) was selected for use in this middle range theory, other measures of patient outcome could be substituted for patient distress without significantly modifying the model. This would allow the theory to be used in multiple client situations and health care settings. For example, researchers might consider studying the relationship between nurse-expressed empathy, patient-perceived empathy, and patient satisfaction with nursing care. Using specific populations of patients, for example, people living with cancer, AIDS, or dementia, other researchers may be interested in determining the relationships among nurse-expressed empathy, patient-perceived empathy, and distress.

This theory is about the very intimate relationship that forms between a nurse and a patient. Therefore, this theory will mainly have implications for nursing education and practice rather than at the more macro level such as public health policy.

The published research in Using Middle Range Theories 7-1 examined the effect of nurse-expressed empathy on patients' perceptions of empathy and their level of distress. Table 7-1 presents a description of the empathy instruments used to develop Olson's theory of the empathy process.

7-1 USING MIDDLE RANGE THEORIES

A descriptive, correlational study investigated relationships between nurse-expressed empathy and two patient outcomes: patient-perceived empathy and patient distress. The sample consisted of 140 subjects: 70 registered nurses and 70 patients for whom they were caring. Fifty percent of eligible nurses on medical-surgical units in large urban hospitals were invited to participate in the study. For each nurse-subject who participated, one patient-subject was randomly selected from those for whom the nurse had cared during a day shift. Each nurse-subject completed two measures of nurse-expressed empathy: the Staff Patient Interpersonal Relationship Scale (SPIRS) and the Behavioral Test of Interpersonal Skills (BTIS). Each patient-subject completed the Profile of Mood States (POMS) and the Multiple Affect Adjective Checklist (MAACL), instruments that measure components of distress (anxiety, depression, and anger), and the Barrett-Lennard Relationship Inventory (BLRI), a measure of patient-perceived empathy.

Hypotheses included the following:

1. There will be a negative relationship between multiple measures of nurse-expressed empathy and the multiple measures of patient distress.
2. There will be a positive relationship between multiple measures of nurse-expressed empathy and patient-perceived empathy.
3. There will be a negative relationship between patient-perceived empathy and multiple measures of patient distress.

Hypotheses were tested using canonical correlation, multiple regression, and Pearson Product Moment correlations.

Using the BTIS as a measure of nurse-expressed empathy, there was a negative relationship between nurse-expressed empathy and patient distress ($r = -.31$ to $-.71$, $p \leq 0.001$–0.01); a positive relationship between nurse-expressed empathy and patient-perceived empathy ($r = .24$ to $.47$, $p \leq 0.01$ – 0.05); and a negative relationship between patient-perceived empathy and patient distress ($r = -.32$ to $-.71$, $p \leq 0.001$–0.01). The main importance of this study is that it was one of the first studies of its kind to behaviorally measure nurses' empathy skills and link these actual behaviors to patient outcomes. The findings demonstrated a connection between nurse-expressed empathy and patient outcomes, and lend support to continued efforts to develop empathic communication skills in nursing students and practicing nurses.

Olson, J. K. (1995). Relationships between nurse-expressed empathy, patient-perceived empathy, and patient distress. *Image: Journal of Nursing Scholarship, 27*, 317–322.

Table 7-1. EMPATHY INSTRUMENTS USED TO DEVELOP OLSON'S THEORY OF THE EMPATHIC PROCESS

INSTRUMENT NAME	AUTHOR	RESPONSE/FORMAT	DESCRIPTION
Barrett-Lennard Relationship Inventory (BLRI)	Barrett-Lennard	Written	16 statements descriptive of either an empathic or nonempathic clinician
Behavioral Test of Interpersonal Skills (BTIS)	Gerrard & Buzzell	Audiotaped or video-taped verbal responses	28 common patient and health professional situations played by actors and actresses and recorded on videotape
Staff–Patient Interaction Response Scale (SPIRS)	Gallop	Written	A series of hypothetical patient situations, with five possible patient statements per situation that require a written response

INSTRUMENTS USED IN EMPIRICAL TESTING

Instruments designed to operationalize the empathy construct have been derived from a variety of theoretical basis and disciplines. The resulting measures of empathy are quite different and each samples a different domain of the multidimensional construct of empathy. In Table 7-2, the instruments used to develop this middle range theory are described.

Some measures can be labeled objective (external, independent reports of actual counseling sessions), while others are subjective in nature (counselor's or client's perceptions of the counseling sessions) (Feldstein & Gladstein, 1980). Few available measures of empathy are behavioral measurements (measuring helper's actual verbal or written responses to clients). The various scales are all designed

Table 7-2. EXAMPLES OF EMPATHY INSTRUMENTS

CATEGORY	EXAMPLES
Interpersonal perception approach Cognitive approach	Dymond Rating Test of Insight & Empathy Kerr & Speroff Empathy Test Hobart & Fahlberg Hogan Empathy Scale
Affective/Emotional approach	Questionnaire Measure of Emotional Empathy Affective Sensitivity Scale
Therapeutic communication approach	LaMonica Empathy Construct Rating Scale (ECRS) Behavioral Test of Interpersonal Skills (BTIS) Staff–Patient Interaction Response Scale (SPIRS)
Multidimensional/Multiphasic approach	Barrett-Lennard Relationship Inventory (BLRI) Staff–Patient Interaction Response Scale (SPIRS)

to measure empathy, but some researchers suggest that the tools may be tapping different empathic aspects, or that they are assessing qualities related to but different from empathy. Kurtz & Grummon (1972) suggest that the various tools are measuring different aspects of the same construct because they found no statistically significant relationships among six commonly used empathy scales. Hackney (1978) commented that too much attention has been put on measuring empathic communication skill and not enough on the empathic experience. Barrett-Lennard (1981) argues that each phase of the empathy cycle requires its own unique measurement.

7-1 RESEARCH APPLICATION

In Canada, faith community nursing has recently emerged as a subspecialty of community health nursing (Clark & Olson, 2000). Minimal research has been conducted to describe the practice, determine required educational background, or to determine health outcomes related to this developing type of nursing practice. More information is needed about the qualities and educational preparation necssary for practice within a setting where nursing is practiced in a faith community ministry team. Though baccalaureate nursing education is often sufficient to prepare a nurse for practice in this specialized setting, many are taking additional preparation both in nursing and in areas such as clinical pastoral education. Clinical pastoral education (CPE) for faith community nurses involves clinically based learning that combines theological and nursing knowledge in reflective practice within a faith community. Using the Olson model, a research study could be designed to determine whether clinical pastoral education after baccalaureate nursing education increases nurses' levels of empathy and patient-perceived empathy. A nurse researcher may want an answer to the following questions:

1. What differences exist in the levels of faith community nurse-expressed empathy for nurses who have taken CPE as compared to those who have not?
2. What differences exist in the levels of patient-perceived empathy for clients of faith community nurses who have taken CPE as compared to clients of faith community nurses who have not had the same preparation?

The nature of the questions directs the researcher to a comparative research study. The nurse researcher would locate two groups of faith community nurses: those who have taken CPE preparation and those who have not. The researcher would administer the Behavioral Test of Interpersonal Skills (BTIS) to faith community nurses in the two groups. In addition, faith community clients with whom the two groups of faith community nurses are working would be assessed for patient-perceived empathy, using the Barrett-Lennard Relationship Inventory (BLRI). Comparisons could be made between the two groups of nurses to determine differences in levels of nurse-expressed empathy. Comparisons could also be made between the two groups of clients to determine differences in levels of patient-perceived empathy. Data analysis would follow to statistically determine if significant differences exist between the two groups of nurses regarding nurse-expressed empathy levels, and between the two groups of clients for patient-perceived empathy levels. Findings could help us understand whether CPE contributes to a nurse's ability to interact empathically with clients with whom nurses work in the faith community setting.

Much of the confusion about empathy measurement results from studying only a part or parts of a complex phenomenon by reducing it to quantifiable elements. While this approach is consistent with reductionism, it is inconsistent with a holistic, philosophical perspective that is perhaps needed in the study of empathy. Stewart (1956) argued that empathy cannot be studied by using traditional scientific, psychological methods; by inserting the outsider's objective measurement, we destroy what we are trying to measure. Major methodological strengths in empathy research in the 1980s included a multidimensional approach to the measurement of empathy and a consideration of the extent to which empathy is situationally determined (Barrett-Lennard, 1981; Davis, 1983; Gallop, 1989; Gallop, Lancee, & Garfinkel, 1989).

In addition to the overall measurement concern, some have questioned the validity of some tools used to measure empathy (Gladstein, 1983). This critique primarily centered on the use of independent raters, problems concerning the material rated, the training of the raters, and the fact that there are inconsistencies between stated empathy definitions and actual measures of empathy (Chinsky & Rappoport, 1970; Feldstein & Gladstein, 1980; Fridman & Stone, 1978; Gagan, 1983; Gormally & Hill, 1974; Hill & King, 1976).

All types of empathy tools have received some criticism. Chinsky and Rappaport (1970) argued against the use of objective measures of empathy because the data collected from such tools as Truax's Accurate Empathy Scale do not use client's responses. These scales measure empathy from the therapist's viewpoint and may reflect a quality other than what the scale is attempting to measure. There has also been criticism of the self-rated tools (helpers rate their own empathy) such as the Hogan Empathy Scale, because these tools carry the potential for inherent bias in that they rely on a cognitive understanding of empathy rather than measuring the subject's empathic ability (Gagan, 1983). It has been suggested that studies be designed so that the results of empathy ratings by external observers are compared with perceptions of patients and objective therapeutic outcomes (Jarski, Gjerde, Bratton, Brown, & Matthes, 1985). It has also been suggested that the most valid measure of empathic ability assesses perceptions of the client (BLRI), but even these tools raise validity questions. In Forsyth's (1979) study, patients seemed to perceive all nurses as empathic. The dependent, passive nature of the client's role could contribute to this phenomenon. There exists the possibility that a hospitalized patient may not be able to evaluate his or her caregivers objectively (Gagan, 1983).

The measurement of empathy has perhaps been the major methodological problem in the research in this area. Additional instruments that behaviorally measure and improve nurses' expressed empathy skills need to be developed for use in educational and clinical settings. These measures need to be easy to administer and clinically relevant to specific areas in which nurses work. In addition, instruments that are designed to specifically measure patient outcomes that are possibly related to nurses' empathy skills might be developed.

SUMMARY

Empathy is an important concept for nursing, as evidenced by the plethora of literature referred to in this chapter. The concept has a long history outside of and within nursing, yet it continues to be of interest to nursing today (Kunyk & Olson, 2001). The middle range theory described in this chapter has conceptualized empathy as a three-step process. Nurses who conceptualize empathy as a communication process could use this middle range theory to gain further understanding about the antecedents and the outcomes related to empathy.

ANALYSIS EXERCISE

Using the criteria presented in Chapter 2, critique Olson's Theory of the Empathic Process. Compare your conclusions about the theory with those found in Appendix A. A nurse scholar who has worked with the theory completed the analysis found in the Appendix.

Internal Criticism
1. Clarity
2. Consistency
3. Adequacy

4. Logical development
5. Level of theory development

External Criticism
1. Reality convergence
2. Utility
3. Significance
4. Discrimination
5. Scope of theory
6. Complexity

WEB RESOURCES

1. Sigma Theta Tau International Nursing Honor Society of Nursing, Virginia Henderson International Nursing Library. Type in "empathy" in the search engine box under library search: *http://www.stti.iupui.edu/library/*.
2. This site contains various on-line nursing journals with full-text articles on empathy: *http://www.sci.lib.uci.edu/HSG/Nursing. html#NN3*.
3. The Association for Clinical Pastoral Education, Inc. This is a multicultural, multifaith organization devoted to providing education and improving the quality of ministry and pastoral care offered by spiritual caregivers of all faiths through the clinical educational methods of Clinical Pastoral Education: *http://www.acpe.edu*.
4. The Canadian Association for Pastoral Practice and Education. This is a Canadian national multifaith organization that is committed to the professional education, certification, and support of people involved in pastoral care and pastoral counseling: *http://www.cappe.org/englishhome.html*.
5. Parish Nursing Education at Marquette University, Milwaukee, Wisconsin. Marquette University is one of many programs that prepare

nurses for practice within faith communities: *http://www.mu.edu/dept/nursing/parish.html*.
6. Parish Nursing Education at McMaster University, Hamilton, Ontario, Canada. McMaster University is one of several Canadian programs that prepare nurses for practice within faith communities:*http://www.mcmaster.ca/divinity/ parishnursing.html*.

REFERENCES

Archer, R., Diaz-Loving, R., Gollwitzer, R., Davis, M., & Foushee, H. (1981). The role of dispositional empathy and social evaluation in the empathic mediation of helping. *Journal of Personality and Social Psychology, 40,* 786–796.

Barrett-Lennard, G. (1962). Dimensions of therapist response as causal factors in therapeutic change. *Psychological Monographs, 76* (43, Whole No. 562).

Barrett-Lennard, G. (1981). The empathy cycle: Refinement of a nuclear concept. *Journal of Counseling Psychology, 28* (2), 91–99.

Bennett, J., & De Mayo, M. (1993). Caring in the time of AIDS: The importance of empathy. *The Nursing Administration Quarterly, 17,* 46–60.

Chinsky, J., & Rappaport, J. (1970). Brief critique of the meaning and reliability of "accurate empathy" ratings. *Psychological Bulletin, 73,* 379–382.

Chlopan, B., McCain, M., Carbonell, J., & Hagen, R. (1985). Empathy: Review of available measure. *Journal of Personality and Social Psychology, 48*(3), 635–653.

Clark, M., & Olson, J. (2000). *Nursing within a faith community: Promoting health in times of transition.* Thousand Oaks, CA: Sage.

Clay, M. (1984). Development of an empathic interaction skills schedule in a nursing context. *Journal of Advanced Nursing, 9,* 343–350.

Coke, J., Batson, C., & McDavis, K. (1978). Empathic mediation of helping: A two-stage model. *Journal of Personality and Social Psychology, 36,* 752–766.

Davis, M. (1983). Measuring individual differences in empathy: Evidence for a multidimensional approach. *Journal of Personality and Social Psychology, 44,* 113–126.

Dracup, K., & Bryan-Brown, C. W. (1999). Empathy: A challenge for critical care. *American Journal of Critical Care, 8,* 204–206.

Dymond, F. (1949). A scale for the measurement of empathic ability. *The Journal of Consulting Psychology, 13,* 127–133.

Elliott, R., Filipovich, H., Harrigan, L., Gaynor, J., Reimschuessel, C., & Zapadaka, J. (1982). Measuring response empathy: The development of a multicomponent rating scale. *Journal of Counseling Psychology, 29,* 379–387.

Feldstein, J., & Gladstein, G. (1980). A comparison of the construct validities of four measures of empathy. *Measurement and Evaluation in Guidance, 13,* 49–57.

Forsyth, G. (1979). Exploration of empathy in nurse-client interaction. *Advances in Nursing Science, 1,* 53–61.

Forsyth, G. (1980). Analysis of the concept of empathy: Illustration of one approach. *Advances in Nursing Science, 2*(2), 33–42.

Fridman, M., & Stone, S. (1978). Effect of training, stimulus context, and mode of stimulus presentation on empathy ratings. *Journal of Counseling Psychology, 25,* 131–136.

Gagan, J. (1983). Methodological notes on empathy. *Advances in Nursing Science, 5*(2), 65–72.

Gallop, R. (1989). The influence of diagnostic labeling on the expressed empathy of nursing staff. Unpublished doctoral dissertation, University of Toronto, Toronto, ON.

Gallop, R., Lancee, W., & Garfinkel, P. (1989). How nursing staff respond to the label "borderline personality disorder." *Hospital and Community Psychiatry, 40*(8), 7–18.

Gerrard, B., & Buzzell, M. (1980). *The user's manual for the Behavioral Test of Interpersonal Skills for Health Professionals.* Reston, VA: Reston Publishing.

Gladstein, G. (1983). Understanding empathy: Integrating counseling, developmental, and social psychology perspectives. *Journal of Counseling Psychology, 30,* 467–482.

Goldstein, A., & Michaels, G. (1985). *Empathy: Development, training, and consequences.* Hillsdale, NJ: Lawrence Earlbaum Associates.

Gormally, J., & Hill, C. (1974). Guidelines for research on Carkhuff's training model. *Journal of Counseling Psychology, 21,* 539–547.

Gurman, A. (1977). The patient's perception of the therapeutic relationship. In A. Gurman & A. Razen (Eds.), *Effective psychotherapy: A handbook of research* (pp. 503–543). Oxford, UK: Pergamon Press.

Hackney, H. (1978). The evolution of empathy. *Personnel and Guidance Journal, 57,* 14–18.

Hill, C., & King, J. (1976). Perceptions of empathy as a function of the measuring instrument. *Journal of Counseling Psychology, 23,* 155–157.

Hobart, C., & Fahlberg, N. (1965). The measurement of empathy. *American Journal of Sociology, 70,* 595–603.

Hogan, R. (1969). Development of an empathy scale. *Journal of Consulting and Clinical Psychology, 33,* 307–316.

Hornblow, A. (1980). The study of empathy. *The New Zealand Psychologist, 9,* 19–28.

Jarski, R. W., Gjerde, C. L., Bratton, B., Brown, D. D., & Matthes, S. S. (1985). A comparison of four empathy instruments in simulated patient-medical student interactions. *Journal of Medical Education, 60,* 545–551.

Johnson, D. (1980). The behavioral system model for nursing. In J. P. Riehl & C. Roy (Eds.), *Conceptual models for nursing practice* (2nd ed.). New York: Appleton-Century-Crofts.

Kagan, N., Krathwohl, D., & Farquhar, W. (1967). *Studies in human interaction.* East Lansing, MI: Educational Publication Services, College of Education, Michigan State University.

Kalisch, B. (1973). What is empathy? *American Journal of Nursing, 73* (9), 1548–1552.

Keefe, T. (1979). The development of empathic skill. *Journal of Education for Social Work, 15,* 30–37.

Kerr, W., & Speroff, B. (1954). Validation and evaluation of the empathy test. *Journal of General Psychology, 50,* 369–376.

King, I. (1981). *A theory for nursing: Systems, concepts, process.* New York: John Wiley & Sons.

Kristjánsdóttir, G. (1992). Empathy: A therapeutic phenomenon in nursing. *Journal of Clinical Nursing, 1,* 131–140.

Kunyk, D., & Olson, J. (2001). Clarification of conceptualizations of empathy. *Journal of Advanced Nursing, 35*(3), 317–325.

Kurtz, R., & Grummon, D. (1972). Different approaches to the measurement of therapist empathy and their relationship to therapy outcomes. *Journal of Counselling Psychology, 39,* 106–115.

Lambert, M., De Julio, S., & Stein, D. (1978). Therapist interpersonal skills. *Psychological Bulletin, 83,* 467–489.

La Monica, E. (1981). Construct validity of an empathy instrument. *Research in Nursing and Health, 4*(4), 389–400.

Levine, M. (1971). Holistic nursing. *Nursing Clinics of North America, 6*(2), 253–264.

Mehrabian, A., & Epstein, N. (1972). A measure of emotional empathy. *Journal of Personality, 40,* 525–543.

Northouse, P. (1979). Interpersonal trust and empathy in nurse–nurse relationships. *Nursing Research, 28*(6), 365.

Olson, J. K. (1995). Relationships between nurse-expressed empathy, patient-perceived empathy, and patient distress. *Image: Journal of Nursing Scholarship, 27,* 317–322.

Olson, J., & Hanchett, E. (1997). Nurse-expressed empathy, patient-perceived empathy and patient distress. *Image: Journal of Nursing Scholarship, 29,* 73–76.

Orem, D. (1985). *Nursing: Concepts of practice* (3rd ed.). Toronto: McGraw-Hill.

Orlando, I. (1961). The dynamic nurse-patient relationship. New York: G. P. Putnam's Sons.

Orlando, I. (1972). *The discipline and teaching of nursing process.* New York: G. P. Putnam's Sons.

Paterson, J., & Zderad, L. (1976). *Humanistic nursing.* New York: John Wiley & Sons.

Patterson, C. (1984). Empathy, warmth, and genuineness in psychotherapy: A review of reviews. *Psychotherapy, 21,* 431–438.

Peplau, H. (1952). *Interpersonal relationships in nursing: A conceptual frame of reference for psychodynamic nursing.* New York: G. P. Putnam.

Rogers, C. (1957). The necessary and sufficient conditions of therapeutic personality change. *Journal of Consulting Psychology, 21,* 95–103.

Rogers, M. (1970). *An introduction to the theoretical basis of nursing.* Philadelphia: F. A. Davis.

Rogers, C., Glendlin, E. T., & Kiesler, D. J. (1967). *The therapeutic relationship and its impact: A study of psychotherapy with schizophrenics.* Madison, WI: University of Wisconsin Press.

Roy, C. (1976). *Introduction to nursing: An adaptation model.* Englewood Cliffs, NJ: Prentice-Hall.

Smyth, T. (1996). Reinstating the person in the professional: Reflections on empathy and aesthetic experience. *Journal of Advanced Nursing, 24,* 932–937.

Stetler, C. (1977). Relationship of perceived empathy to nurses' communication. *Nursing Research, 26*(6), 432–438.

Stewart, D. (1956). *Preface to empathy.* New York: Philosophical Library.

Sutherland, J. A. (1995). Historical concept analysis of empathy. *Issues in Mental Health Nursing, 16,* 555–566.

Travelbee, J. (1971). *Interpersonal aspects of nursing.* (2nd ed.). Philadelphia: F. A. Davis.

Truax, C., & Carkhuff, R. (1967). *Toward effective counseling and psychotherapy.* Chicago, IL: Aldine.

Wheeler, K. (1995). Development of the perception of empathy inventory. *The International Journal of Psychiatric Research, 1,* 281–289.

Wiedenbach, E. (1963). The helping art of nursing. *American Journal of Nursing, 63*(11), 54–57.

Chronic Sorrow

GEORGENE GASKILL EAKES

DEFINITION OF KEY TERMS

Chronic sorrow	Periodic recurrence of permanent, pervasive sadness or other grief-related feelings associated with ongoing disparity resulting from a loss experience
Disparity	A gap between the current reality and the desired as a result of a loss experience
External management methods	Interventions provided by professionals to assist individuals to cope with chronic sorrow
Internal management methods	Positive personal coping strategies used to deal with the periodic episodes of chronic sorrow
Loss experience	A significant loss, either actual or symbolic, that may be ongoing, with no predictable end, or a more circumscribed single-loss event
Trigger event	A situation, circumstance, or condition that brings the negative disparity resulting from the loss into focus, or exacerbates the disparity

INTRODUCTION

The middle range theory of chronic sorrow, first documented in the literature in 1998 by Eakes, Burke and Hainsworth, offers a framework for explaining how individuals may respond to both ongoing and single-loss events. Moreover, the theoretical model of chronic sorrow provides an alternative way of viewing the experience of grief. The theory of chronic sorrow was inductively derived and subsequently validated from an extensive review of the literature, and from data gathered through 10 qualitative research studies conducted by members of the Nursing Consortium for Research on Chronic Sorrow (NCRCS). Using the Burke/NCRCS Chronic Sorrow Questionnaire (adapted from a guide developed by Burke [1989]) as an interview guide, these nurse researchers interviewed 196 individuals, who shared their loss experiences as people with chronic conditions, as family caregivers of the chronically ill or disabled, or as bereaved family members.

HISTORICAL BACKGROUND

The term "chronic sorrow" was introduced into the literature 40 years ago to characterize the recurring episodes of grief experienced by parents of children with disabilities (Olshansky, 1962). This recurring sadness appeared to persist throughout the lives of these parents, although its intensity varied from time to time, from situation to situation, and from one family member to another. Rather than viewing this phenomenon as pathological, Olshansky described chronic sorrow as a normal response to an ongoing loss situation. Professionals were encouraged to recognize the presence of this phenomenon when working with the parent of a disabled child and to support parents' expressions of feelings. Although the term gained wide use in the professional literature, almost 2 decades passed before there was any documented research on chronic sorrow.

Initial research conducted in the 1980s validated the occurrence of chronic sorrow among parents of disabled young children. Several investigators suggested that the never-ending nature of the loss of the "perfect" child prevented resolution of grief (Burke, 1989; Damrosch & Perry, 1989; Fraley, 1986; Kratochvil & Devereux, 1988; Wikler, Wasow, & Hatfield, 1981). Moreover, it was this inability to bring closure to the loss experience that was thought to precipitate periodic episodes of re-grief, labeled as chronic sorrow. These early studies refined and operationalized the definition of chronic sorrow as a pervasive sadness that was permanent, periodic, and progressive in nature.

More recent research supports the fact that chronic sorrow is a common experience among family caregivers (Burke, Eakes, & Hainsworth, 1999; Clubb, 1991; Copley & Bodensteiner, 1987; Doornbos, 1997; Eakes, 1995; Eakes, Burke, Hainsworth, & Lindgren, 1993; Fraley, 1990; Golden, 1994; Hainsworth, 1995; Hainsworth, Busch, Eakes, & Burke, 1995; Hobdell & Deatrick, 1996; Hummel & Eastman, 1991; Johsonius, 1996; Kearny & Griffin, 2001; Krafft & Krafft, 1998; Lindgren, 1996; Lowes & Lyne, 2000; Mallow & Bechtel, 1999; Northington, 2000; Phillips, 1991; Rosenberg, 1998; Seideman & Kleine, 1995; Shumaker, 1995). The caregivers studied represent parents of young children with various disabilities, spouses of individuals diagnosed with chronic illnesses, and parents of adult children with debilitating conditions.

The NCRCS, established in 1989 (Eakes, Hainsworth, Lindgren, & Burke, 1991), expanded research on chronic sorrow and explored the relevance of the concept of chronic sorrow among individuals experiencing a variety of loss situations. This group of nurse researchers not only conducted research on chronic sorrow among family caregivers, but also investigated individuals affected with chronic conditions and bereaved individuals. Among those diagnosed with a chronic condition, 83% evidenced chronic sorrow (Burke, 1992; Eakes, 1993; Hainsworth, 1994; Hainsworth, Burke, Lindgren, & Eakes, 1993; Hainsworth, Eakes, & Burke, 1994; Lindgren, 1996). The NCRCS also conducted research studies designed to investigate the occurrence of chronic sorrow among individuals who had experienced a single-loss event rather than an ongoing loss. Toward this end, people who had experienced the death of a significant other a minimum of 2 years before the study were interviewed. This time lapse was to allow for acute grief to subside. Findings revealed that a vast majority (97%) of those interviewed evidenced chronic sorrow (Eakes, Burke, & Hainsworth, 1999). These findings lead to further modification of the defining characteristics of chronic sorrow, recognizing that it was ongoing disparity associated with the loss, rather than the ongoing nature of the loss experience, as originally thought, that was the antecedent to chronic sorrow. Consequently, chronic sorrow was redefined as permanent, periodic, recurrence of pervasive sadness, or other grief-related feelings associated with ongoing disparity resulting from significant loss (Eakes et al., 1998). The necessary antecedent event is involvement in an experience of significant loss. This loss may be ongoing in nature, with no predictable end, such as the birth of a disabled child or a diagnosis of a debilitating illness, or it may be more circumscribed, such as the death of a loved one. Disparity is created by a loss/situation when an individual's current reality differs markedly from the idealized, or when a gap exists between the desired and the actual. This lack of closure sets the stage for grief to be periodically re-experienced. That is, the chronic sorrow experience is cyclical and continues as long as the disparity created by the loss remains.

DESCRIPTION OF THE THEORY OF CHRONIC SORROW

The middle range theory of chronic sorrow (Eakes et al., 1998) was inductively derived and validated through the qualitative studies described above, as well as through a critical review of existing literature (Figure 8-1). Based on these findings, chronic sorrow was reconceptualized and is now defined as "the periodic recurrence of permanent, pervasive sadness or other grief-related feelings associated with ongoing disparity resulting from a loss experience" (Eakes et al., 1998, p. 180, 1999). Moreover, chronic sorrow is characterized as pervasive, permanent, periodic, and potentially progressive in nature and continues to be viewed as a normal response to loss. Indeed, the theory of chronic sorrow purports that the periodic return of grief among individuals and caregivers whose anticipated life course has been interrupted continues throughout one's lifetime, as long as the disparity created by the loss remains (Lindgren, Burke, Hainesworth, & Eakes).

The middle range theory of chronic sorrow provides a framework for understanding the reactions of individuals to various loss situations and offers a new way of viewing the experience of bereavement. Although chronic sorrow is viewed as a normal response to the ongoing disparity or void created by significant loss, it is important to note that normalization of the experience in no way diminishes the validity or the intensity of the feelings experienced. At times, feelings can be intense and distressing for the individual experiencing chronic sorrow

The Development of Chronic Sorrow

Involvement in an experience of significant loss is the necessary antecedent to the development of chronic sorrow. As stated earlier this may be a loss with no predictable end, such as the birth of a disabled child or diagnosis of a chronic illness or a more clearly defined loss event such as the death of a loved one. The second antecedent to chronic sorrow is ongoing disparity resulting from the loss. That is, a gap exists between the desired and the actual reality. The lack of closure associated with ongoing disparity sets the stage for chronic sorrow, with the loss experienced in bits and pieces over time. The defining characteristics of chronic sorrow, borne out by the research, are pervasiveness, permanence, periodicity and the potential for progressivity. As graphically represented in the theoretical model of chronic sorrow (see Figure 8-1), the experience of chronic sorrow may occur at any point across the life span.

Trigger Events

Trigger events, also referred to as milestones, are those situations or circumstances that bring the disparity created by the loss into focus, thereby triggering the grief-related feelings associated with chronic sorrow. Triggers of chronic sorrow vary depending on the nature of the loss experience. For

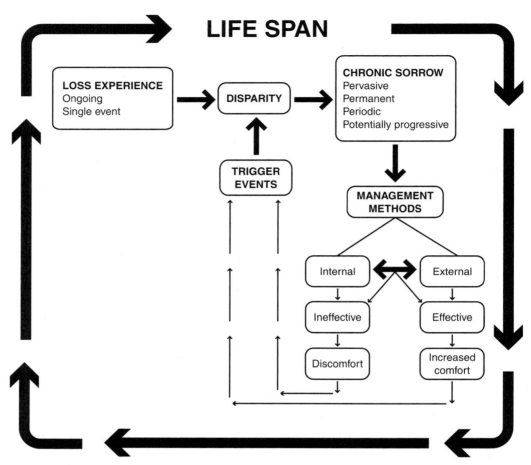

■ **Figure 8.1** Theoretical model of chronic sorrow. Source: Eakes, G. G., Burke, M. L., & Hainsworth, M. A. (1998). Middle range theory of chronic sorrow. *Image: Journal of Nursing Scholarship, 30*(2), 179–184.

affected individuals, chronic sorrow is most commonly triggered when individuals confront disparity with established norms, whether, social, developmental, or personal in nature (Burke et al., 1999; Eakes, 1993; Eakes et al., 1993; Hainsworth, 1994). For example, a trigger may exist when someone diagnosed with a chronic illness is unable to engage in an activity that they once enjoyed due to exacerbation of their condition.

The most frequent trigger of chronic sorrow among parents of young children with disabilities is disparity associated with developmental milestones (Burke, 1989; Clubb, 1991; Damrosch & Perry, 1989; Fraley, 1986, 1990; Golden, 1994; Hummel & Eastman, 1991; Kafft & Krafft, 1998; Mallow & Bechtel, 1999; Olshansky, 1962; Phillips, 1991; Seideman & Kleine, 1995; Shumaker, 1995; Wikler et al., 1981).

The chronic sorrow of other family caregivers is often triggered by crises associated with management of the family member's illness and by recognition of the never-ending nature of the caregiving activities (Burke et al, 1999; Eakes, 1995; Eakes et al., 1993; Hainsworth, 1995; Hainsworth et al., 1995; Lindgren, 1996).

The chronic sorrow experience of bereaved individuals is triggered by those situations and circumstances that magnify the "presence of the absence" of the deceased, such as anniversaries and other special occasions (Eakes et al., 1998, p. 182). Also, changes in roles and responsibilities necessitated by the death of a loved one may trigger chronic sorrow.

Management Methods

Another key element of the theoretical model of chronic sorrow is management methods. This term is used to refer to both personal coping strategies used by individuals during the chronic sorrow experience (internal) as well as supportive interventions provided by helping professionals (external). As depicted in the theoretical model, effective internal and external management methods lead to increased comfort and may serve to extend the time between episodes of chronic sorrow.

INTERNAL MANAGEMENT

Effective internal management strategies used by those with chronic sorrow are consistent across the various loss situations. Action-oriented strategies that increase feelings of control are most frequently used to cope with the recurrence grief-related feelings of chronic sorrow (Burke, 1989; Eakes, 1993, 1995; Hainsworth et al., 1994; Hainsworth, 1995; Hainsworth et al., 1995; Lindgren, 1996). Examples of action-oriented coping include continuing to pursue involvement in interests and activities, gathering information specific to one's loss experience, and seeking out respite opportunities. Cognitive and interpersonal are other types of internal management strategies identified as helpful in dealing with the chronic sorrow. Cognitive strategies include adopting a "can do" attitude and focusing on the positive elements of one's life (Burke, 1989; Eakes, 1993, 1995; Hainsworth et al., 1994, 1995; Hainsworth, 1995). Interpersonal ways of coping include talking with someone close or a trusted professional and interacting with others in a similar situation such as in a support group (Burke, 1989; Eakes, 1993, 1995; Fraley, 1990; Hainsworth et al., 1994, 1995; Hainsworth, 1995; Wikler et al., 1981).

EXTERNAL MANAGEMENT

Interventions provided by health care professionals, referred to as external management methods, must be based upon the premise that chronic sorrow is a normal response to a significant loss situation. As long as disparity created by a loss experience remains, one can anticipate that the individual will likely experience chronic sorrow. Indeed, normalization of the periodic re-grief of chronic sorrow is basic to all other interventions. It is important for professionals to recognize that individuals who have experienced a significant loss may evidence the periodic recurrence of grief-related feelings, defined as chronic sorrow. Armed with this awareness, anticipatory guidance may be provided regarding the situations and circumstances likely to trigger episodes of chronic sorrow. Personal coping mechanisms (internal management methods) can be assessed, strengthened, and supported.

Additionally, specific interventions provided by health care professionals, categorized as roles, have been helpful for those experiencing chronic sorrow (Burke, 1989; Copley & Bodensteiner, 1987; Eakes, 1993, 1995; Eakes et al., 1993; Fraley, 1990; Hainsworth, 1995; Hainsworth et al., 1995; Hummel & Eastman, 1991; Wikler et al., 1981). Family caregivers with chronic sorrow derive the most benefit from professional interventions labeled as the role of "teacher/expert." More specifically, these actions include providing situation-specific information in a manner that can be easily understood and giving practical tips for managing caregiving responsibilities (Burke, 1989; Clubb, 1991; Eakes, 1995; Fraley, 1990; Hainsworth, 1995; Hainsworth et al., 1995; Hummel & Eastman, 1991; Warda, 1992; Wikler et al., 1981). Actions associated with the professional role of "empathetic presence," characterized by taking time to listen, offering support, focusing on feelings, and recognizing uniqueness of each individual, are also helpful to those who were in a caregiver role (Burke, 1989; Clubb, 1991; Eakes, 1995; Fraley, 1990; Hainsworth, 1995; Hummel & Eastman, 1991; Olshansky, 1962; Phillips, 1991; Teel, 1991; Warda, 1992).

For those individuals affected with a chronic or life-threatening condition, as well as bereaved persons, the professional role of "empathetic presence" discussed above is perceived as most helpful in dealing with the periodic episodes of chronic sorrow. In addition, the complementary role of "caring professional", evidenced by sensitivity, respectfulness, nonjudgmental acceptance, and intervention associated with the role of "teacher/expert" are described as beneficial (Burke, 1989; Eakes, 1993; Eakes et al., 1993; Hainsworth et al., 1995).

APPLICATIONS OF THE THEORY

Chronic sorrow has research applications among a variety of populations and across a myriad of loss situations. Identifying the presence of chronic sorrow among family caregivers alerts professionals to potential triggers of the recurrent grief, and leads to the identification and reinforcement of effective coping mechanisms for those experiencing chronic sorrow. See Using Middle Range Theories 8-1 and 8-2 for examples.

 8-1 USING MIDDLE RANGE THEORIES

This researcher explored the experience of chronic sorrow among African-American caregivers of school-age children diagnosed with sickle cell disease (SCD). Findings revealed that the process of chronic sorrow was initially triggered by a diagnosis of SCD. Subsequent resurgence of chronic sorrow was triggered by both internal and external events. Internal triggers were found to relate to future-oriented thoughts, including thoughts of the child's death. External factors triggering episodes of chronic sorrow were associated with consequences of the illness itself, as well as concerns about costs of health care and education. Significant others, spirituality, and the strength exhibited by the child with SCD were the primary sources of support for those caregivers studied. The researcher concluded that caregivers of children with

8-1 USING MIDDLE RANGE THEORIES

(Continued)

SCD engage in a process of readjusting and redefining reality. Thus, the cyclic nature of chronic sorrow they experience assists in the individuals' growth and adjustment. Nurses were encouraged to recognize the existence of chronic sorrow among this population of caregivers so that supportive interventions could be provided.

This study supports the need for reconceptualization of existing grief theories. Indeed, these findings question the expectation purported in traditional grief theories that closure is an expected outcome of the grieving process.

Northington, L. (2000). Chronic sorrow in caregivers of school age children with sickle cell disease: A grounded theory approach. *Issues in Comprehensive Pediatric Nursing*, 23, 141–154.

INSTRUMENTS USED IN EMPIRICAL TESTING

Historically, research on chronic sorrow has employed qualitative methods with open-ended interview guides, used with study participants both in face-to-face and in telephone interviews. The Burke/NCRCS Chronic Sorrow Questionnaire (Burke, 1989; Eakes, 1993, 1995), with versions adapted for individuals affected with chronic conditions, for family caregivers, and for bereaved individuals, has been used for the majority of studies documented in the literature. This interview guide is com-

8-2 USING MIDDLE RANGE THEORIES

Researchers interviewed 34 bereaved individuals who had experienced the death of a loved one. A minimum of 2 years had lapsed since the death occurred, allowing acute grief to subside, with a range from 2 to more than 20 years. The Burke/NCRCS Chronic Sorrow Questionnaire (Bereaved Individual Version), revised from Burke's (1989) original interview guide, was used to gather data about both recurrence of feelings associated with the loss and the triggers of those periodic episodes of re-grief. Findings revealed that 97% of the subjects experienced chronic sorrow. Moreover, common triggers were those situations and circumstances that brought into focus disparity with social norms—parents without children, children without parents, wives without husbands, and husbands without wives. Additionally, memories often associated with anniversaries and special occasions triggered recurrence of the grief-related feelings of chronic sorrow. Normalization of the periodic episodes of chronic sorrow through caring and empathetic professional roles was found to be beneficial to those with chronic sorrow.

Eakes, G., Burke, M., & Hainsworth, M. (1999). Chronic sorrow: The experiences of bereaved individuals. *Illness, Crisis & Loss*, 7(2), 172–182.

prised of 10 open-ended questions that explore feelings experienced at the time of the loss, and whether or not they have been re-experienced. Moreover, questions focus on circumstances or situations that trigger recurrence of the grief-related feeling and identification of effective coping mechanisms. See Research Application 8-1.

SUMMARY

Chronic sorrow has gained increased attention in the past decade, based in large part on the research endeavors of the NCRCS. Additionally, increased awareness of the changing nature of grief associated with significant losses, whether ongoing in nature or single loss events, has spurred interest in this phenomenon. The newly established theory of chronic sorrow provides a framework for understanding and working with individuals who have experienced significant loss. Specifically, situations and circumstances that trigger chronic sorrow are identified, and management methods deemed helpful to those experiencing chronic sorrow are described. Moreover, the theoretical model of chronic sorrow, along with the recently constructed Burke/Eakes Chronic Sorrow Assessment Tool, will facilitate further expansion of research on chronic sorrow and provide opportunities for testing of the theory. The need for exploration of cultural variations in the experience of chronic sorrow has virtually been ignored and must be addressed in future research. Additionally, relevance of the theory of chronic sorrow to types of loss experiences not yet studied (i.e., divorce, abuse) needs to be investigated.

The middle range theory of chronic sorrow has widespread application for nurses and others who strive to better understand individuals' responses to loss and to define effective interventions for those

---

8 -1 RESEARCH APPLICATION

In 2001, two of the original members of the Nursing Consortium for Research on Chronic Sorrow undertook the development of a quantitative assessment tool (Eakes & Burke, 2002). Questions for the instrument were developed based on the theoretical model and findings from the qualitative studies previously conducted by members of the NCRCS and other researchers. Face and content validity were established by using Lynn's (1986) methodology for establishing validity of an instrument. Once face and content validity of the Burke/Eakes Chronic Sorrow Assessment Tool were established, test–retest reliability studies were conducted. Subjects participating in this aspect of instrument development represented each of the populations previously studied (family caregivers, affected individuals, and bereaved persons). Test–retest correlations for items 4 through 9 (the first three questions assess demographic data) were at acceptable levels, ranging from .72 to .93. Questions 10 and 11 allow for little variability in responses, and the restricted response range resulted in more marginal test–retest correlations on these items (.62 and .56, respectively).

See Appendix B for a sample of the assessment tool.

experiencing chronic sorrow. Although chronic sorrow is viewed as a normal response to ongoing disparity resulting from a loss, recognition of the periodic re-grief characteristic of chronic sorrow and provision of supportive interventions can provide an increased level of comfort for those experiencing it.

ANALYSIS EXERCISE

Using the criteria presented in Chapter 2, critique the theory, Chronic Sorrow. Compare your conclusions about the theory with those found in Appendix A. A nurse who has worked with the theory completed the analysis found in the Appendix.

Internal Criticism
1. Clarity
2. Consistency
3. Adequacy

4. Logical development
5. Level of theory development

External Criticism
1. Reality convergence
2. Utility
3. Significance
4. Discrimination
5. Scope of theory
6. Complexity

WEB RESOURCES

1. This site has a nursing theory page, including nursing text and book reviews, plus a variety of nursing-related topics:
www.enursescribe.com
2. This site contains links to a variety on nursing-related Web pages. It has pages on nurse theorists and a special section called Other Nursing Resources:
www.healthsci.clayton.edu

REFERENCES

Burke, M. L. (1989). Chronic sorrow in mothers of school-age children with a myelomeningocele disability (Doctoral dissertation, Boston University, 1989). *Dissertation Abstracts International, 50,* 233–234B.

Burke, M. L., Eakes, G. G., & Hainsworth, M.A. (1999). Milestones of chronic sorrow: Perspectives of affected individuals and family caregivers. *Journal of Family Nursing, 5*(4), 374–387.

Burke, M. L., Hainsworth, M. A., Eakes, G. G., & Lindgren, C. L. (1992). Current knowledge and research on

chronic sorrow: A foundation for inquiry. *Death Studies, 16,* 231–245.

Clubb, R. L. (1991). Chronic sorrow: Adaptation patterns of parents with chronically ill children. *Pediatric Nursing, 17,* 462–466.

Copley, M. F., & Bodensteiner, J. B. (1987). Chronic sorrow in families of disabled children. *Journal of Child Neurology, 2,* 67–70.

Damrosch, S. P., & Perry, L. A. (1989). Self-reported adjustment, chronic sorrow, and coping of parents of children with Down syndrome. *Nursing Research, 38,* 25–30.

Doornbos, M. M. (1997). The problems and coping methods of caregivers of young adults with mental illness. *Journal of Psychosocial Nursing, 35,* (9), 22–26.

Eakes, G. G. (1993). Chronic sorrow: A response to living with cancer. *Oncology Nursing Forum, 20,* 1327–1334.

Eakes, G. G. (1995). Chronic sorrow: The lived experience of parents of chronically mentally ill individuals. *Archives of Psychiatric Nursing, IX,* 77–84.

Eakes, G. G., & Burke, M. L. (2002). Development and validation of the Burke/Eakes chronic sorrow assessment tool. Unpublished raw data. EakesG@mail.ecu.edu.

Eakes, G. G., Burke, M. L., & Hainsworth, M. A. (1999). Chronic sorrow: The lived experience of bereaved individuals. *Illness, Crisis, and Loss, 7*(1), 172–182.

Eakes, G. G., Burke, M. L., & Hainsworth, M. A. (1998). Middle range theory of chronic sorrow. *Image: Journal of Nursing Scholarship, 30*(2), 179–184.

Eakes, G. G., Burke, M. L., Hainsworth, M. A., & Lindgren, C. L. (1993). Chronic sorrow: An examination of nursing roles. In S. G. Funk, E. M. Tornquist, M. T. Champagne, & R. A. Wiese (Eds.). *Key aspects of caring for the chronically ill: Hospital and home* (pp. 231–236). New York: Springer Publishing.

Eakes, G. G., Hainsworth, M. E., Lindgren, C. L., & Burke, M. L. (1991). Establishing a long-distance research consortium. *Nursing Connections, 4,* 51–57.

Fraley, A. M. (1986). Chronic sorrow in parents of premature children. *Children's Health Care, 15,* 114–118.

Fraley, A. M. (1990). Chronic sorrow: A parental response. *Journal of Pediatric Nursing, 5,* 268–273.

Golden, B. (1994). *The presence of chronic sorrow in mothers of children with cerebral palsy.* Unpublished master's thesis, Arizona State University, Tempe.

Hainsworth, M. A. (1994). Living with multiple sclerosis: The experience of chronic sorrow. *Journal of Neuroscience Nursing, 26,* 237–240.

Hainsworth, M. A. (1995). Chronic sorrow in spouse caregivers of individuals with multiple sclerosis: A case study. *Journal of Gerontological Nursing, 21,* 29–33.

Hainsworth, M. A., Burke, M. L., Lindgren, C. L., & Eakes, G. G. (1993). Chronic sorrow in multiple sclerosis: A case study. *Home Healthcare Nurse, 11,* 9–13.

Hainsworth, M. A., Busch, P. V., Eakes, G. G., & Burke, M. L. (1995). Chronic sorrow in women with chronically mentally disabled husbands. *Journal of the American Psychiatric Association, 1*(4), 120–124.

Hainsworth, M. A., Eakes, G. G., & Burke, M. L. (1994). Coping with chronic sorrow. *Issues in Mental Health Nursing, 15,* 59–66.

Hobdell, E., & Deatrick, J. (1996). Chronic sorrow: A content analysis of parental differences. *Journal of Genetic Counseling. 5*(2), 57–68.

Hummel, P. A., & Eastman, D. L. (1991). Do parents of premature infants suffer chronic sorrow? *Neonatal Network, 10,* 59–65.

Johnsonius, J. (1996). Lived experiences that reflect embodied themes of chronic sorrow: A phenomenological pilot study. *Journal of Nursing Science, 1*(5/6), 165–173.

Keamey, P., & Griffin, T., (2001). Between joy and sorrow: Being a parent of a child with a developmental disability. *Journal of Advanced Nursing, 34*(5), 582–592.

Krafft, S. K., & Krafft, L. J. (1998). Chronic sorrow: Parents' lived experience. *Holistic Nursing Practice, 13*(1), 59–67.

Kratochvil, M. S., & Devereaux, S. A. (1988). Counseling needs of parents of handicapped children. *Social Casework, 68,* 420–426.

Lindgren, C. L. (1996). Chronic sorrow in persons with Parkinson's and their spouses. *Scholarly Inquiry for Nursing Practice, 10,* 351–367.

Lindgren, C. L., Burke, M. L., Hainsworth, M. A., & Eakes,

G. G. (1992). Chronic sorrow: A lifespan concept. *Scholarly Inquiry for Nursing Practice, 6,* 27–40.

Lowes, L. L., & Lyne, P. (2000). Chronic sorrow in parents of children with newly diagnosed diabetes: A review of the literature and discussion of the implications for nursing practice. *Journal of Advanced Nursing, 32*(1), 41–48.

Lynn, M. (1986). Determination and quantification of content validity. *Nursing Research, 35*(6), 382–385.

Mallow, G. E., & Bechtel, G. A. (1999). Chronic sorrow: The experience of parents with children who are developmentally disabled. *Journal of Psychosocial Nursing, 37*(7), 31–35.

Northington, L. (2000). Chronic sorrow in caregivers of school age children with sickle cell disease: A grounded theory approach. *Issues in Comprehensive Pediatric Nursing, 23,* 141–154.

Olshansky, S. (1962). Chronic sorrow: A response to having a mentally defective child. *Social Casework, 43,* 191–193.

Phillips, M. (1991). Chronic sorrow in mothers of chronically ill and disabled children. *Issues in Comprehensive Pediatric Nursing, 14,* 111–120.

Rosenberg, C. J. (1998). Faculty-student mentoring. A father's chronic sorrow: A daughter's perspective. *Journal of Holistic Nursing, 16*(3), 399–404.

Seideman, R. Y., & Kleine, P. F. (1995). A theory of transformed parenting: Parenting a child with developmental delay/mental retardation. *Nursing Research, 44,* 38–44.

Shumaker, D. (1995). *Chronic sorrow in mothers of children with cystic fibrosis.* Unpublished master's thesis, University of Tennessee, Memphis.

Teel, C. S. (1991). Chronic sorrow: Analysis of the concept. *Journal of Advanced Nursing, 16,* 1322.

Warda, M. (1992). The family and chronic sorrow: Role theory approach. *Journal of Pediatric Nursing, 7,* 205–210.

Wikler, L. M., Wasow, M., & Hatfield, E. (1981). Chronic sorrow revisited: Parents vs. professional depiction of the adjustment of parents of mentally retarded children. *American Journal of Orthopsychiatry, 51,* 63–70.

BIBLIOGRAPHY

Burke, M. L., Eakes, G. G., & Hainsworth, M.A. (1999). Milestones of chronic sorrow: Perspectives of affected individuals and family caregivers. *Journal of Family Nursing, 5*(4), 374–387.

Burke, M. L., Hainsworth, M. A., Eakes, G. G., & Lindgren, C. L. (1992). Current knowledge and research on chronic sorrow: A foundation for inquiry. *Death Studies, 16,* 231–245.

Chang G. Y. (1999). Room with no flowers. *Clinical Nurse Specialist, 13*(6), 276.

Hainsworth, M. A., Burke, M. L., Lindgren, C. L., & Eakes, G. G. (1993). Chronic sorrow in multiple sclerosis: A case study. *Home Healthcare Nurse, 11*, 9–13.

Hayes, M. (2001). A phenomenological study of chronic sorrow in people with type I diabetes. *Practical Diabetes International, 18*(2), 65–69.

Hobdell, E., & Deatrick, J. (1996). Chronic sorrow: A content analysis of parental differences. *Journal of Genetic Counseling. 5*(2), 57–68.

Johnsonius, J. (1996). Lived experiences that reflect embodied themes of chronic sorrow: A phenomenological pilot study. *Journal of Nursing Science, 1*(5/6), 165–173.

Keamey, P., & Griffin, T., (2001). Between joy and sorrow: Being a parent of a child with a developmental disability. *Journal of Advanced Nursing, 34*(5), 582–592.

Langridge, P. (2002). Reduction of chronic sorrow: A health promotion role for children's community nurses? *Journal of Child Health Care, 6*(3), 157–170.

Lichtenstein, B., Laska, M., & Clair, J. M. (2002). Chronic sorrow in the HIV-positive patient: Issues of race, gender, and social support. *AIDS Patient Care & Stds, 16*(1), 27–38.

Lindgren, C. L., Burke, M. L., Hainsworth, M. A., & Eakes, G. G. (1992). Chronic sorrow: A lifespan concept. *Scholarly Inquiry for Nursing Practice, 6*, 27–40.

Martin, K., & Elder, S. (1993). Pathways through grief: A model of the process. In J. D. Morgan (Ed.). *Personal care in an impersonal world: A multidimensional look at bereavement.* (pp. 73–86). Amityville, NY: Baywood Publishing Company, Inc.

Nehfing, W. (2001). The child with a chronic condition.... commentary on ......*Journal of Child & Family Nursing. 4*(3), 203–204.

Stephenson, J. S., & Murphy, D. (1986). Existential grief: The special case of the chronically ill and disabled. *Death Studies, 10*, 135–145.

Middle Range Theories: Social

Social Support

MARJORIE A. SCHAFFER

DEFINITION OF KEY TERMS

Appraisal support	Affirmation from statements or actions made by another (Kahn & Antonucci, 1980)
Emotional support	Experience of feeling liked, admired, respected, or loved (Norbeck, Lindsey, & Carrieri, 1981)
Formal support	Help from professionals, paraprofessionals, or other service providers from structured community organizations (may be paid or unpaid assistance)
Informal support	Help provided through a person's "lay" social network, such as from family members and friends
Informational support	Knowledge provided to another during a time of stress that assists in problem solving (House, 1981)
Instrumental support	Tangible aid, goods, or services (House, 1981)
Negative support	Interactions that cause stress or are more demanding than helpful (Coyne & DeLongis, 1986)
Perceived support	Generalized appraisal that individuals are cared for and valued, have others available to them, and are satisfied with relationships (Heller, Swindle, & Dusenbury, 1986)
Social network	Structure of the interactive process of persons who give and receive help and protection (Langford, Bowsher, Maloney, & Lillis, 1997)
Social support	(1) An exchange of resources that the provider and recipient perceive to enhance the recipient's well-being (Shumaker & Brownwell, 1984); (2) "A well-intentioned action that is given willingly to a person with whom there is a personal relationship and that produces an immediate or delayed positive response in the recipient" (Hupcey, 1998b, p. 313)

INTRODUCTION

Social support is a middle range theory that addresses structure and interaction in relationships. Related midlevel theories include social exchange, social comparison, coping, attribution, social learning, and social competence theories (Stewart, 1993). Theorists and researchers have experienced challenges in conceptualizing, defining, and measuring social support (Hupcey, 1998a). Disagreement exists about the dimensionality of social support (Bloom, 1990). Some authors give credence to one broad factor (Brown, 1986), while others view social support as multidimensional, with several categories or components (Barrera, 1986; Wandersman, Wandersman, & Kahn, 1980). In addition, there is a need to distinguish between social support and social network, because a social network can contribute to both stress and support (Hutchinson, 1999).

Social support theory is important for middle range theory development in nursing, because social support impacts health status, health behavior, and use of health services (Stewart, 1993). As health professionals, nurses often have access to clients' social networks. Through communication with clients and their family members, nurses can intervene to promote or strengthen social support. The literature identifies many positive consequences of social support, including health-promoting behaviors, personal competence, coping, a sense of well-being, self-worth, and decreased anxiety and depression (Langford et al., 1997). Research on social support interventions can provide nurses with knowledge about the most effective strategies for strengthening social support for clients, which contributes to improved health status.

HISTORICAL BACKGROUND

Cassel (1974), one of the early social support theorists, introduced the term "social support." Based on animal studies, he theorized that strengthening social supports could improve the health of humans. Studies in the early 1970s suggested that social support mediates the negative effects of stress (Roberts, 1984). The "buffer" theory and attachment theory have been the basis for considerable research on the relationship of social support and health (Callaghan & Morrissey, 1993). The buffer theory suggests that social support protects persons from life stressors (Cassel, 1976; Cobb, 1976). The attachment theory holds that the ability to form socially supportive relationships is related to the secure attachments formed in childhood (Bowlby, 1971). In the mid 1970s to early 1980s, the literature most often described social support in concrete terms, such as an interaction, person, or relationship (Veiel & Baumann, 1992). In recent years, the term has been used more abstractly, to include perceptions, quality and quantity of support, behaviors, and social systems.

The analysis and testing of social support theory has gained multidisciplinary interest and is prominent in nursing and social–psychological literature. For nurses, social support can connect family assessment, patient needs, and health outcomes (Hupcey, 1998b). Nurses have focused on the client–environment interaction for specific social support situations, such as transition to parenthood, bereavement, and vulnerable children and families (Stewart, 1993).

DEFINITION OF THEORY CONCEPTS

Developers of social support theory have organized definitions of social support by a variety of component labels: aspects, categories, constructs, defining attributes, dimensions, interpersonal transactions, subconcepts, taxonomies, and types (Table 9-1). The variety of definitions of social support provided by theorists illustrates the lack of consensus about the nature of social support. This lack of consensus contributes to complexity in evaluating social support interventions and outcomes, comparing research findings, and developing social support theory.

Although multidimensional definitions predominate, positive interaction or helpful behavior is shared by all social support definitions (Rook & Dooley, 1985). In addition, most social support theories have the assumption that support is given and received by members of a social network, leading to social integration or a feeling of belonging (Diamond, 1985; Norbeck & Tilden, 1988). Recipients perceive that social support facilitates coping with stressors in their lives (Pierce, Sarason, & Sarason, 1990). Shumaker and Brownell (1984) defined social support as an exchange of resources that the provider or recipient perceives to enhance the recipient's well-being. Social support can be structural, focusing on who provides the support, or functional, emphasizing the act of providing social support activities (Callaghan & Morrissey, 1993; Norwood, 1996). In addition, there are many characteristics that influence the quality and adequacy of social support, such as the stability, direction, and source of support (Stewart, 1989a). Social networks can be described by the number and categories of persons who provide social support: family members, close friends, neighbors, coworkers, and professionals (Tardy, 1985).

Emotional, Informational, Instrumental, and Appraisal Support

Researchers have often used the conceptualization of social support created by House (1981) and confirmed by others (Barrera, 1986; Tilden, & Weinert, 1987). The four theoretical constructs or defining attributes, as labeled by House, are emotional, informational, instrumental, and appraisal support. These four attributes include all possible actions of social support (Langford et al., 1997). Emotional support involves the experience of feeling liked, admired, respected, or loved (Norbeck, 1981). Tangible aid, goods, or services define instrumental support (House, 1981). Providing information during a time of stress is informational support (House, 1981). Appraisal support affirms one's actions or statements (Kahn & Antonucci, 1980).

Two examples from nursing practice illustrate the meaning of emotional, informational, instrumental, and appraisal support. In the first example, a public health nurse can strengthen social support through a comprehensive home visitation program for young mothers (Olds et al., 1999). Through referral to an early childhood parenting program, a young mother can develop friendships with other mothers in the group and receive emotional support from others who are experiencing similar life events. Instrumental support is provided when the pubic health nurse links a young mother to community resources that can provide assistance with child care, education, health care, and financial needs. The public health nurse provides informational support by teaching the young mother about child growth and development. Appraisal support occurs as the young mother engages in positive self-assessment of her parenting abilities based on feedback from the nurse.

In a second example, Ragsdale, Yarbrough, and Lasher (1993) developed a social support protocol for clients who have had a cerebral vascular accident (CVA). By including specific social support interventions on the care plan, nurses can assist a client with a CVA and his wife meet their needs for social support. The nursing care plan can guide nurses to help the wife of the CVA client provide emotional support to her husband by maintaining a positive attitude and listening to her husband when he expresses frustration. The wife can provide tangible assistance or instrumental support when she acts

Table 9-1. THEORETICAL MULTIDIMENSIONAL DEFINITIONS OF SOCIAL SUPPORT

LABEL	SUPPORT COMPONENTS
Aspects (Cohen, 1992)	Social networks Perceived support Supportive behaviors
Categories (Hupcey, 1998a)	Types of support provided Recipients' perceptions Intentions/Behaviors of provider of support Reciprocal support Social networks
Constructs (Vaux, 1988)	Support network resources Support incidents Support behaviors Support appraisals Support or network orientation
Defining attributes (House, 1981)	Emotional support Informational support Instrumental support Appraisal support
Dimensions (Cutrona, 1990)	Emotional Esteem (appraisal) Tangible (instrumental) Information Social integration
Interpersonal transactions (Kahn, 1979)	Affect—feeling liked or loved Affirmation—of behavior, perceptions, and views Affect—feeling respected or admired Aid—material or symbolic
Subconcepts (Barrera, 1981)	Material aid Physical assistance Intimate interaction Guidance Feedback Social participation
Taxonomies (Laireiter & Baumann, 1992)	Social integration Network resources Supportive climate and environment Received and enacted support Perception of being supported
Types (Wortman, 1984)	Expression of positive affect Expression of agreement Encouragement of open expression of feelings Offer of advice and information Provision of material aid Network of reciprocal help and mutual obligation

as an interpreter for professional caregivers or helps with suctioning. Nurses can strengthen the ability of the spouse of the CVA client to provide social support to her husband by giving information about how to care for her husband. Nurses can offer appraisal support to the wife, encouraging her and making positive comments about the effectiveness of her caregiving actions.

Negative Social Support

Although often viewed as implying a positive influence, social support may contribute negatively to well-being. The social support activity alone may not be as important as the recipient's perception of the support (perceived support). The perception of or the satisfaction with the support is likely to influence the outcome of the support activity (Heller et al., 1986). The support activity could actually be unrecognized or perceived negatively by the recipient. Negative social support is perceived as unhelpful and may undermine self-esteem. Characteristics of negative social support include stressful or conflicted social networks, misguided or absent support, inappropriate advice, avoidance, and disagreement (Stewart, 1993). Moreover, costs to the provider of social support such as overload, over commitment, and stressful emotional involvement may occur (Coyne & DeLongis, 1986; La Gaipa, 1990).

In a discussion of the "darker side" of social support, Tilden and Galyen (1987) recommended that the costs of relationships should be addressed in future social support research. They described how social exchange and equity theories explain the costs that may be incurred in social relationships. Social exchanges include both rewards and costs; people behave in ways that maximize their rewards and reduce their costs. The balance of rewards and costs is likely to influence both perceptions and effects of social support. Equity theory addresses this imbalance and suggests that unequal or nonreciprocal social exchanges contribute to stress. Four subdimensions that could be measured to capture the effects of negative aspects of social support are cost, conflict, reciprocity, and equity (Tilden & Galyen, 1987).

DESCRIPTION OF THE THEORY OF SOCIAL SUPPORT

The various definitions of social support range from encompassing too little by focusing only on structural or functional aspects, to addressing too many characteristics of social support, which contributes to an ambiguous definition. Hupcey (1998b) conducted a concept analysis of social support, based on an examination of 200 studies published from 1978 to 1996, in which social support was one of the variables. Most studies did not include a specific reference to a theoretical definition, and researchers who defined social support often did not use a definition that addressed the interactional nature of social support. According to Hupcey, the four structural factors that help to define social support are precondition, characteristic, outcome, and boundary. The precondition of the provider who perceives a need for social support and is motivated to take action precedes the act of social support. The social support action must be well intentioned and given willingly toward a particular person (characteristic). The outcome is a positive response or change in the recipient. Actions are not considered social support if an organization, the community, or a professional provides them, or if actions have a negative intent or are given grudgingly (boundary). Hupcey (1998b) states that the boundaries of social support help to differentiate it from related concepts. These four structural factors are integrated into Hupcey's definition of social support: "a well-intentioned action that is given willingly to a person with whom there is a personal relationship and that produces an immediate or delayed positive response in the recipient." (p. 313)

Other descriptions of social support in the literature are not consistent with the boundary limitation of personal relationship described by Hupcey. Shumaker and Brownell (1984) stated that acts of social support might also occur during Internet interactions and calling in to radio talk shows or crisis hotlines. Rook & Dooley (1985) described how social support can be viewed as an environmental or an individual variable. Gottlieb (1978) included environmental action among four classes of helping behaviors. From an ecological perspective, community environments can enhance the likelihood of social support exchanges. Although not included as providers of social support in Hupcey's definition, professionals can intervene to strengthen existing social support networks for clients or choose to provide social support when it is lacking. Many researchers have included professionals when measuring sources of social support. The controversy seems to be about how broad or narrow to focus the definition; a consensus on the definition of social support continues to be elusive.

A number of variables affect the social support that is given and received or experienced. These include perceptions of the need and availability for support, timing, motivation for providing support, duration, direction, life stage, and the source of support. In addition, social network, social embeddedness, and social climate are viewed as antecedent variables to social support (Langford et al., 1997).

Perceptions of the Need for and Availability of Support

The provider of the social support first recognizes another's need for social support before determining the response to the need. If there is a mismatch in the provider's and recipient's perceptions of the need for support or the type of support that is provided, the recipient may not consider the support to be helpful (Dunkel-Schetter & Bennett, 1990; Dunkel-Schetter & Skokan, 1990). The recipient's recognition, desire, and request for the support will influence the perceived helpfulness of the support (Krishnamsamy, 1996). Providers of support may assume that the recipient who is experiencing stress needs support. If this assumption is inaccurate, the act of support could result in feelings of dependency, inadequacy, and lower self-esteem (Dunkel-Schetter, Blasband, Feinstein, & Herbert, 1992). Research data suggest that the perception of the availability of support is more important for health and well-being than the actual receiving of the support (Cohen, Gottlieb, & Underwood, 2001).

Timing

Timing is also important, because the support needs of the recipient can change relative to the recipient's appraisal of the situation over time (Jacobson, 1986; Tilden, 1986). The social support provided and the perceived adequacy of the social support vary over time and situations (Norwood, 1996). Social support can be viewed as a contingency rather than a fixed resource, because it is a dynamic process influenced by personal characteristics and situations. Examples of changes affecting both the giving and receiving of social support are: (a) the ongoing nature of relationships from a historical perspective; (b) expectations of support based on an assessment of the potential for support from the network; and (c) personal coping skills that range from extreme independence to wanting as much support as could be provided (Lackner, Goldenberg, Arrizza, & Tjosvold, 1994).

Motivation for Providing Support

Motivation for providing social support can affect the quality of the support provided. A sense of obligation on the part of the provider may decrease the recipient's satisfaction with the support (Hupcey, 1998a). Providers of social support are likely to consider the recipient's responsibility and effort relative to the needed support and the costs to the provider that result from the act of support (Jung, 1988). The provider's previous experiences with providing support and previous interactions with the intended recipient will also influence choices of support actions (Hupcey, 1998a).

Duration, Direction, and Life Stage

Duration of the support, referring to length of time or stability of the support, is a consideration for the chronically ill and persons who experience long-term loss (Cohen & Syme, 1985). The long-term effects of stressors on individuals may require ongoing support, as well as support from sources outside the usual social networks. For example, in a longitudinal study of the perceived support and support sources of older women with heart failure, the women identified paid helpers as sources of support at a later time in progression of their illness (Friedman, 1997). If persons requiring care for chronic illness can remain in their community setting, social support from paid caregivers can supplement the available support from informal networks.

The direction of support may be unidirectional or bidirectional. Bidirectional support is characterized by mutuality and reciprocity (Stewart, 1993). Professional support is usually unidirectional. In family and intimate relationships, the roles of "helper" and "helpee" may alternate (Clark, 1983; Rook & Dooley, 1985). Reciprocity in social support is likely to reduce feelings of burden and strain in providers and inadequacy and lack of control in recipients (Albrecht & Adelman, 1987).

The provision and receiving of social support vary over the life span. Some life stages offer more capability for providing social support, while other life stages require more receiving than giving of social support. Social support needs are greater during times of change and additional stress, such as during the birth of a child or with the loss of strength and function associated with aging. Vaux (1988) identified social support resources, social support needs related to growth and development issues, and typical sources of stress for family life-cycle stages from infancy to late adulthood.

Sources of Social Support

Individuals are much less likely to identify professionals as sources of support, compared to family members and friends (Hupcey & Morse, 1997; Schaffer & Lia-Hoagberg, 1997). Professionals, who provide formal support, can intervene to enhance the existing social support resources of clients or can act as surrogates to provide support not currently available in the client's social network (Norbeck, 1988). To enhance informal and formal sources of support, professionals can develop and strengthen relationships with personal support networks, mutual aid groups, neighborhood support systems, volunteer programs, and community resources (Froland, Pancoast, Chapman, & Kimboko, 1981).

Nurses may be a source of support for caregivers of family members by facilitating tangible assistance to families (such as provision of transportation, respite care, and caregiving activities), through mobilization of the client's existing social support network, or by linking the client to relevant community resources. Nurses can provide informational support through giving the client knowledge about self-care practices or educating members of the client's network. Finding ways to expand the support network may decrease caregiver burden and increase available emotional and appraisal support for the client. However, assessing the quality of the social support is also important. Research shows there's a negative relationship between the quality of social support and caregiver burden (Vrabec, 1997). In particular, the amount of conflict in the relationship can result in negative social support that contributes to stress rather than well-being.

Newsom, Bookwala, and Schulz (1997) compared differences in formal and informal support sources in a study that described the social support needs and relationships of older adults in nursing homes, residential care facilities, and congregate apartments. The high degree of instrumental support available in institutional settings is provided primarily by professional and nonprofessional paid staff. These formal support sources may also provide a sizeable amount of emotional support for older adults who have physical and cognitive challenges, because paid staff are more often available for older adults in group residences (Pearlman & Crown, 1992). Newsom et al. (1997) discussed four differences in the formal social support provided by paid staff compared to the informal social support provided by family and friends: (1) Older adults do not have a choice among staff members for their interactions or when interactions occur; (2) They may experience discomfort in receiving personal care from someone they do not know well; (3) The relationship may still be labeled as a professional relationship, although companionship and emotional support is provided by paid staff; and (4) The relationship is characterized by less reciprocity than would probably occur with informal sources of support.

Social Network, Social Embeddedness, and Social Climate

The size of the social network is sometimes considered to be an indicator of social support. Key sources of support, including immediate family members and close friends, are distinguished from sources viewed as less important—other relatives, coworkers, church and community members, and professional caregivers (Griffith, 1985). However, a large social network does not necessarily guarantee that a large amount of support is present (Kahn & Antonucci, 1980). The quality of the relationships and availability of persons in the social network, as well as the number of persons in the network, contribute to the enacted social support.

A variety of network members can better provide the range of needed social support actions. For example, in one study, persons with a cancer diagnosis perceived spouses or partners as helpful for their physical presence, while friends provided practical help (Dakof & Taylor, 1990). In another study with cancer patients, informational support was perceived as helpful from experts but not from friends or families (Dunkel-Schetter, 1984).

Social embeddedness refers to a person's connectedness with others in his or her social network (Barrera, 1986). The strength of the connections contributes to the ability to obtain social support from the network. A favorable social climate can create an atmosphere that promotes acts of social support and the perception of help and protection by the recipient. An available and high-quality social network and the strength and quality of connectedness, or social embeddedness, contribute to a positive social climate in which social supportive behaviors occur (Langford et al., 1997).

The Relationship of Social Support and Health

Heller, Swindle, and Dusenbury (1986) posited that two facets of social support, esteem-enhancing appraisal and stress-related, interpersonal transactions, have an effect on health outcomes. They hypothesized that the appraisal or perception of the social interaction is health protective, rather than the social interaction or support activity itself. Esteem-enhancing appraisal results from an assessment of how one is viewed by others. In stress-related interpersonal transactions, network members provide tangible assistance, which facilitates coping (Figure 9-1).

Cohen, Gottlieb, and Underwood (2001) described two models that explain how social support influences health. The stress-buffering model holds that social support contributes to health-promoting

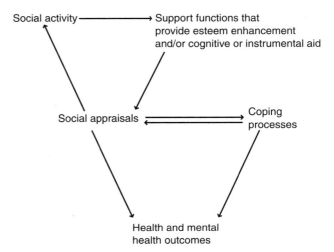

■ Figure 9.1 Hypothesized relationships between facets of social support, coping, and health outcomes. From Heller, K., Swindle, R.W., & Dusenbery, L. (1986). Component social support processes: Comments and integration. *Journal of Continuing and Clinical Psychology, 54*(4), 466–470. Copyright © 1986 by the American Psychological Association. Reprinted with permission.

behaviors in persons who are experiencing stress. Rather than choosing behaviors that may be harmful to health, the support resources strengthen an individual's perceived ability to cope with a stressful situation (Thoits, 1986). These beliefs lead to a calmer psychological and physiological response to the stressful situation and can decrease negative behavioral responses. In this case, an individual is more likely to have an adaptive response to the stressful situation, thus avoiding a maladaptive response with a greater potential for negative health effects.

The main effect model, the second model described by Cohen et al. (2001), suggests that social support directly impacts psychological and physical health, whether or not an individual is experiencing a stressful situation. Integration into a social network, as contrasted to isolation, can provide social control and peer pressure to engage in health-promoting behaviors and lead to positive psychological states, such as a sense of predictability, stability, purpose, belonging, and security (Cassel, 1976; Hammer, 1981; Thoits, 1983). In addition, social networks can provide multiple sources of information about health care services and may also provide informal health care that prevents progression of illness (Cohen et al., 2001).

Norbeck (1981) proposed a model for using social support as a nursing intervention to improve health outcomes. The social support environment of the client is assessed by determining the need for social support compared to the available social support. An assessment of inadequate social support necessitates developing an intervention plan to increase social support. Possible interventions can focus on strengthening the client's existing social support structure or function or providing direct support during a crisis. According to this nursing process model, adequate social support will result in a positive health outcome; inadequate social support without intervention will result in a negative health outcome.

APPLICATIONS OF THE THEORY

Clinical Applications

Nurses have the knowledge and expertise to assess the interpersonal and social environments of clients, implement health promotion strategies, and facilitate clients in initiating self-care practices

(Tilden, 1985). From a prevention perspective, social support can be viewed as "social inoculation" (Pilisuk, 1982). Through "network therapy," nurses can assess social support adequacy, use existing social support measures, determine the roles of professionals and nonprofessional providers of social support to move clients to increasing independence, and organize and evaluate community support groups (Roberts, 1984).

One example of preventive support is comprehensive home visitation for vulnerable young mothers provided by public health nurses (Olds et al., 1999). Nurses provided regular home visits to young mothers beginning during their pregnancy and continuing until their children were 2 years of age. The purposes of the visits were to improve pregnancy outcomes, to promote children's healthy development, and to improve the financial self-sufficiency of participating families. Nurses both provided formal support and strengthened informal sources of support. Evaluation of the long-term outcomes through two randomized clinical trials demonstrated an increase in positive self-care practices and child well-being for the mothers who participated in the program.

Additional clinical application examples are described in Table 9-2. Examples are provided for the five social support intervention levels suggested by Stewart (1989b): individual, dyadic, groups, community, and social system. Interventions at these levels include strengthening available social support and providing direct social support with the goal of improving health status. Table 9-2 provides a summary of the level of intervention based on Stewart's framework, social support intervention examples with the relevant social support theoretical constructs (emotional, informational, instrumental, and appraisal support), and desired health outcomes.

Research Applications

Researchers have explored a great variety of nursing practice issues from a social support perspective. Topics include social support and chronic illness, social support for persons who are grieving, the relationship of social support to acute chest complaints, social support for new mothers in stressful situations, and administrative support for nurses. Researchers have also investigated how social support interacts with other variables, such as pain and loneliness, to predict depression. The majority of studies focus on the individual or family level experience of social support. Few researchers have investigated social support from a community or systems perspective. See the Bibliography at the end of the chapter for citations on social support research on issues relevant to nursing.

MEASURES OF SOCIAL SUPPORT

Although a great number of social support measures have been developed in several disciplines, many measures do not have adequate reliability and validity testing, and many are situation-specific rather than general measures of social support. Available measures address (a) interconnectedness in a social network; (b) received support, based on a person's report of support that was provided; and (c) perceived support, which is support a person believes to be available to them (Sarason, Sarason, & Pierce, 1990). Researchers have primarily developed situation-specific measures of social support for groups who encounter a common stressor event, such as pregnancy or chronic illness (Stewart, 1993). Of 21 social support instruments reviewed by Stewart (1998a), only four were applicable on a general level.

Five measures of social support developed by nurse researchers are described in Table 9-3. The selected instruments represent both general and specific measures of social support and have been psy-

text continues on p. 193

Table 9-2. CLINICAL APPLICATION: SOCIAL SUPPORT INTERVENTIONS

INTERVENTION LEVEL	SITUATION	SOCIAL SUPPORT INTERVENTIONS	DESIRED HEALTH OUTCOMES
Individual—Modify how individual seeks or perceives support provided by others	A pregnant woman is placed on bed rest for a high-risk pregnancy. She has a 2-year-old son and her husband works long hours. She views her husband as her primary source of social support and does not know how she will manage getting the assistance she needs during her confinement to bed rest. She is receiving care through a hospital-based home care agency that provides nursing care to perinatal clients.	Assess her available components and sources of social support. Educate her about the importance of bed rest for her pregnancy and describe the kind of support she will need (*informational support*). Counsel her about the need to seek social support from other sources during a time of increased stress and need (*appraisal support*). Listen to the client's concerns about her husband's potential reactions to asking the client's mother to assist with household tasks and child care (*emotional support*). The client arranges for help with childcare from her mother and several neighborhood families (*instrumental support*).	Reduced family stress Positive coping strategies Healthy infant
Dyadic—Strengthen support from a key network member or introduce outsider to provide support	A 35-year-old woman is having a mastectomy for breast cancer. She states she has a very close relationship with her husband but has not talked with him about how the surgery will affect their sexual relationship.	Assess her available sources of support for talking about her specific concern. Reassure her that this is a common concern that is difficult for couples to discuss (*appraisal support*). Give her information about a program that provides a visitor who has had a breast cancer experience and suggest that referral for couples' counseling is an option (*informational support*). Following a meeting with the visitor from the volunteer program, the client discusses her concerns with her husband and is reassured by his response (*emotional support*).	Maintenance of healthy self-concept Positive couple relationship Reduced complications

(Continues)

Table 9-2. CLINICAL APPLICATION: SOCIAL SUPPORT INTERVENTIONS (Continued)

INTERVENTION LEVEL	SITUATION	SOCIAL SUPPORT INTERVENTIONS	DESIRED HEALTH OUTCOMES
Group—Enlarge existing informal network, improve skills of natural helpers, refer to or create support groups	A 45-year-old man has MS and recently became wheelchair dependent. His wife has returned to full-time work. The couple has two teenagers. Case management is provided through a home health agency. The wife has become increasingly frustrated with trying to manage her work demands and the needs of her husband.	Assess the family's social support components and sources of family, extended family, friend, community, and professional support. Suggest that a support group for persons with MS and their families could be helpful in providing them with understanding and practical ideas for their situation (*informational support*). Because a local support group does not exist, work with a community service agency to develop a support group (*instrumental support*). The family participates in a local support group (*emotional support*). Reevaluate the current nursing services. Provide additional services needed to reduce the wife's workload (*instrumental support*).	Reduced caregiver stress level Effective family functioning Increased community resources through provision of a support group for clients with MS and their family members
Community—Promote social support and social network frequency of interaction in neighborhoods, organizations, and communities	Elderly residents in an urban, ethnically diverse, low-income neighborhood are more isolated in the winter. A Block Nurse program has been recently established to address the health care needs of this population. A high percentage of the clients served by the program have diabetes.	Survey a sample of the neighborhood elderly population to determine health concerns and social support needs. Consult and collaborate with a foot-care nurse to offer a foot-care program in a community clinic, as well as through home visits. During the clinic and home visits, assess the social support needs of the elderly persons. Educate them about foot care and community resources that can offer them assistance with house cleaning and maintenance (*instrumental support and informational support*).	Reduction in complications from diabetes in elderly population in neighborhood Elderly residents stay in their own homes for a longer time period Reduction in health care costs for nursing home care

INTERVENTION LEVEL	SITUATION	SOCIAL SUPPORT INTERVENTIONS	DESIRED HEALTH OUTCOMES
		Collaborate with a local faith-based organization to extend their visitation ministry to isolated elderly persons in the neighborhood for the purpose of increasing their social interaction (*emotional support and appraisal support*).	
Systems—Promote policy and structural changes to increase social support in environments and/or remove barriers to social support (in schools, municipalities, hospitals)	The percentage of children who are overweight in an elementary school population has increased. The cafeteria serves highly processed food. The school breakfast program includes sugared cereals.	Educate parents and school staff/administrators about the health concern and collaborate with them to develop a plan to respond to the problem (*informational support*). Use social marketing in the school setting (posters, announcements, bulletins) to increase awareness of the problem and provide classroom education about health behaviors that influence body mass (*informational support*). Contribute to development of policy for more nutritional food choices in the breakfast and lunch program (*instrumental support*). Create a peer support program to encourage positive change in health behavior patterns, such as nutritional food choices and physical activity (*appraisal support*).	Increase in attractive, nutritious food choices and a reduction in the amount of processed food in meals served at the school. Increase in knowledge about the contribution of food choices and exercise to Body Mass Index (BMI) among school children Increase in percentage of children with a normal BMI

Table 9-3. SELECTED SOCIAL SUPPORT INSTRUMENTS DEVELOPED BY NURSE RESEARCHERS

INSTRUMENT	SOCIAL SUPPORT COMPONENTS	DESCRIPTION	SAMPLE ITEM
Interpersonal Relationships Inventory (IPRI) (Tilden, Nelson, & May, 1990)	Social support Reciprocity Conflict	39 items (13 for each subscale) 5-point agree/disagree scale Subscales used separately Internal consistency and test–retest reliability Construct validity for social support and conflict subscales	Someone believes in me (support). I let others know I care (reciprocity). Wish people were more sensitive (conflict).
Norbeck Social Support Questionnaire (NSSQ) (Norbeck, Lindsey, & Carrieri, 1981, 1983)	Affect Affirmation Aid Loss Duration of relationship Frequency of contact	Identify persons in network 5-point scale on extent of support provided for 9 questions Internal consistency and test–retest reliability Construct validity	How much does this person make you feel liked or loved?
Perceived Resource Questionnaire (PRQ-85) (Weinert, 1988, 1990)	Intimacy Social integration Nurturance Worth Assistance	Part 1—Identifies resources and satisfaction with help Part 2—25 items on perceived social support; 7-point agree/disagree scale Internal consistency reliability—Part 2 Construct validity—Part 2	If I need advice, there is someone who would assist me to work out a plan for dealing with the situation.
Support Behaviors Inventory (SBI) (Brown, 1986)	Perceived degree of experiential support during pregnancy—satisfaction with partner support and satisfaction with other support	11 items on shortened version 6-point satisfied/dissatisfied scale Internal consistency reliability for total support score on shortened version	Tolerates my ups and downs and unusual behaviors
Social Support in Chronic Illness Survey (SSCII) (Hilbert, 1990)	Intimate interaction Guidance Feedback Maternal aid Behavioral assistance Positive social interaction	38 items 6-point satisfied/dissatisfied scale Internal consistency reliability Content validity	Commented favorably when (s)he noticed me doing something that the health team recommended

chometrically analyzed. The Interpersonal Relationships Inventory (IPRI), the Norbeck Social Support Questionnaire (NSSQ), and the Perceived Resource Questionnaire (PRQ-85) are general measures of social support, which are applicable to any clinical setting where clients have the capacity to respond to a self-report instrument. None of the instruments are applicable to young children. The Support Behaviors Inventory (SBI) is specific for support during pregnancy, and the Social Support in Chronic Illness Survey (SSCII) is specific to social support for persons who are experiencing chronic illness.

The IPRI includes subscales that address reciprocal interaction and conflict in relationships, in addition to social support (Tilden, Nelson, & May, 1990). The inclusion of the reciprocity and conflict subscales can potentially capture the fuller context of relationships, unlike most social support measures. The social support items are consistent with perceived availability of support and the enactment of helping behaviors by members of a person's social network.

On the NSSQ, respondents make a list of up to 24 persons who are important to them. Respondents are given a list of suggested categories to help them identify persons in their social network. Then, each person in the social network is rated on how much social support is provided on several social support components. Although perceived negative aspects of relationships are not addressed, the NSSQ does include an item on loss of persons in the social network and the extent of support that was provided by persons who are no longer available (Norbeck, Lindsey, & Carrieri, 1981, 1983).

Originally designed in 1981, the PRQ has undergone extensive psychometric evaluation (Brandt & Weinert, 1981; Weinert, 1987, 1988). Based on instrument testing with a variety of populations, the authors revised Parts 1 and 2. The nurturance items were extended to include adults as well as younger persons.

Brown (1986) developed the SBI specifically for social support during pregnancy. Although the items were based on the components of emotional, material, informational, and appraisal support, a factor analysis resulted in the identification of one dimension of social support in a sample of pregnant couples. This finding led Brown to question the multidimensional nature of social support. About one half of the original 45 items in the instrument-development stage applied specifically to social support during pregnancy, while the remainder were applicable to general social support situations. Through theoretical analysis, Brown selected 11 items for a shortened version of the SBI. Respondents rate their satisfaction with social support from partners and others for each of the 11 items.

Hilbert (1990) created the SSCII in response to the lack of a social support measure specific to chronic illness. She included items from other measures and added items based on the literature and interviews with myocardial infarction clients. The original 45 items were reduced to 38 items, as a result of a content analysis for relevance to the purpose of the instrument. The finalized instrument includes 29 general social support items and 9 items specific to chronic illness.

A six-item general measure of social support (not included in Table 9-3), the Social Support Questionnaire (SSQ6), developed by psychologists (Sarason, Sarason, Shearing, & Pierce, 1987) may be of interest to nurse researchers who are looking for a brief and convenient measure of social support. For each item, the respondent identifies the number of persons available in time of need related to a situation, as well as the satisfaction with the perceived available support, on a six-point scale. Through psychometric evaluation that also involved comparison with other measures of social support, Sarason et al. (1987) determined that the SSQ6 is psychometrically sound and can substitute for the SSQ, the original 27-item instrument. The authors determined the items on the six-item scale were conceptually consistent with the affective component of social support but not with instrumental support. An example of one of the items is "Whom can you count on to console you when you are very upset?" They hypothesized that peoples' perceptions about the availability of others to help in times of need may be the most important social support component in relationship to health outcomes.

Most measures of social support are self-reports. Newsom et al. (1997) discussed the challenge of measuring social support for the cognitively impaired. They suggested that proxy and observational measures of social support may be an alternative strategy for determining the adequacy of social support for persons who cannot provide an accurate self-report. Proxies, such as nursing home staff and primary caregivers, can provide information about social network contacts and interactions. Observational methods include recording interaction behaviors and videotaping. A coding system can be used to label the source of the support, the type of support, the recipient response, and other characteristics of the support interaction.

QUALITATIVE METHODS

Some researchers have used qualitative approaches for investigating social support, although quantitative measures appear to be predominant. In Finland, nurse researchers asked one open-ended question to explore perceptions of social support after the death of a spouse: "What helped you cope with your grief?" (Kaunonen, Tarkka, Paunonen, & Laippla, 1999). The researchers used content analysis to classify the data by the structure of social relationships and the social support functions of aid, affirmation, and affect in relationships (Kahn, 1979).

Lugton (1997) used a strategy called social contact analysis, in addition to interview data, to explore the social support experienced by women treated for breast cancer. Participants drew their social networks, with self at center, using shorter lines for closer relationships and arrows to indicate whether the relationship involved support, strain, or both. The researcher then asked participants to describe how professional and informal persons in the social network had responded to the illness of the participant in supportive and nonsupportive ways. Types of support that facilitated adjustment were emotional support, companionship, practical help, opportunities for confiding, experiential support (from others who had experienced breast cancer), and sexual identity support. See Using Middle Range Theories 9-1 and 9-2 for two examples of how social support has been used in research.

CHALLENGES TO SOCIAL SUPPORT THEORY DEVELOPMENT AND RESEARCH

Future efforts in social support theory development and research need to move from a description of the relationship of social support and health outcomes to the investigation of interactional characteristics, negative aspects, gender and cultural contexts, causal relationships in social support, and effective social support interventions. In particular, multilevel interventions that address both interpersonal support and community-level environmental support could contribute to knowledge about cost-effective social support strategies for improving the health status of populations.

Because researchers have used a variety of definitions of social support and have measured different aspects of social support, it is difficult to compare study results (Heitzmann & Kaplan, 1988; Roberts, 1984). Hupcey (1998b) commented that many other concepts, such as marital status and frequency of contact, have often been included in definitions of social support. What is missing in many studies is a focus on the interactional nature of social support. To determine effectiveness of social support, an understanding of the perceptions of the providers of social support as well as those of the recipient merits further exploration (Hupcey, 1998b). The reciprocity of social support is an interactional variable that can contribute to understanding effective social support interventions.

9-1 USING MIDDLE RANGE THEORIES

Adequate social support during pregnancy can mediate the stress of changes related to pregnancy. For pregnant women, social support can contribute to a healthy response to pregnancy if the support encourages women to seek prenatal care and maintain healthy behaviors during the pregnancy, resulting in improved birth outcomes. This study investigated the relationship of social support provided by the partner and others to the adequacy of prenatal care and the prenatal health behaviors of low-income women. Social support was operationalized using the components of affect, affirmation, aid, and loss (Kahn, 1979; Norbeck, Lindsey, & Carrieri, 1981). The researcher added two pregnancy-specific questions to the Norbeck Social Support Questionnaire: (1) How much does this person talk with you about your pregnancy, and (2) How much does this person give you information that helps you with your pregnancy? The sample included 101 low-income women, ages 18 to 35, from five urban prenatal clinics. Adequacy of prenatal care was determined using Kotelchuck's Adequacy of Prenatal Care Index (1994). Schaffer developed the Prenatal Health Questionnaire (PHQ) to measure behaviors known to contribute to a healthy pregnancy: participation in prenatal education, healthy food choices, and avoidance of tobacco, alcohol, and illegal drugs. Pearson's *r* correlation coefficient was used to determine the relationship of social support variables (source and component of social support) to adequacy of prenatal care and prenatal health behaviors. Social support from the partner was positively related to prenatal care adequacy, while social support from others was positively related to healthy prenatal behaviors. Both sources of support were important, but for different health outcomes. The women in the sample infrequently identified professionals as sources of support in comparison with others from their informal social network. Nurses can provide informational support to the partners and other network members of low-income women to enhance the emotional, instrumental, informational, and appraisal support available in the women's social networks. Social support actions can encourage healthy self-care practices in low-income pregnant women.

Schaffer, M. A., & Lia-Hoagberg, B. (1997). Effects of social support on prenatal care and health behaviors of low-income women. *Journal of Obstetric, Gynecologic, and Neonatal Nursing, 26*(4), 433–440.

Middle range social support theory development could be enhanced by greater exploration of the negative effects of informal social support. Many social support measures do not include negative aspects of relationships (Krishnasamy, 1996; Stewart, 1993). In a review of 50 studies on social support and caregiver burden, Vrabec (1997) recommended further examination of the amount of conflict in the social support network as a predictor of caregiver burden. The IPRI is one of the few measures that attempts to encompass the full context of relationships through inclusion of reciprocity and conflict subscales (Tilden et al., 1990).

Few authors have discussed the impact of culture in regard to social support theory and measurement. Ducharme, Stevens, and Rowat (1994) acknowledged that few measures consider the personal and contextual factors that can influence social support interactions, such as culture and gender. Higgins and Dicharry (1991) evaluated the Personal Resources Inventory Part 2 (PRQ) for its applicability to Navajo women. They found that 10 of the 25 items were not applicable to Navajo culture. The 10 items were considered too personal because in the Navajo culture family problems and feelings are

9-2 USING MIDDLE RANGE THEORIES

This study addressed the structure, function, and nature of social support. The researchers explored how caregivers of relatives with Alzheimer's disease used formal and informal support. A multidimensional definition of social support was used through the administration of the reciprocity and conflict subscales from the Interpersonal Relationships Inventory (Tilden, Nelson, & May, 1990), in addition to measures of informal and formal support developed by the researchers. The informal support measure included seven items that addressed tangible, emotional, and informational support on a 4-point scale of frequency of support. Participants also rated their satisfaction for each informal support item. Formal support was determined by the number and usefulness of formal services provided by structured organizations. The researchers explored characteristics of support sources such as the gender and kinship (adult children or spouses) of the caregivers. The researchers wished to determine whether formal support would substitute for or supplement the informal support based on gender and kinship. The sample, recruited from health and social service agencies in Quebec, consisted of 193 daughters, wives, and husbands who lived with their family member with Alzheimer's disease. Multivariate analyses of variances (MANOVAs) were used to determine differences in support variables among caregiver groups. The researchers used *t*-tests to investigate gender and kinship hypotheses. Gender differences emerged in the use of and response to informal support, while there were kinship differences regarding formal support. In comparison to husbands, wives experienced less satisfaction and a greater level of conflict in situations of less informal support. The researchers commented that women might be socialized to expect more from their informal sources of support. Regarding formal sources of support, the frequency of formal services seemed more important to spouses than to daughters. The researchers found that the support provided by the informal network was not reduced when formal agencies were also providing support. The formal support did not substitute for the informal support. This study demonstrates the importance of exploring social support source characteristics, such as gender and kinship. It is important that the researchers explored negative aspects of social support through use of the conflict subscale of the IPRI. To understand the full context of social support, middle range theory development must also consider the relationship of negative social support actions to health outcomes.

Cossette, S., Levesque, L., & Laurin, L. (1995). Informal and formal support for caregivers of a demented relative: Do gender and kinship make a difference? *Research in Nursing and Health, 18,* 437–451.

not discussed with others. Different cultural groups may vary in perceptions of the number of persons they consider to be a part of their social network, as well as the relative importance of the different components of social support. Expectations for independence and help may differ. Some types of assistance could be expected and appreciated by one culture and be interpreted as shameful by another culture. The meaning of social support across cultures needs further exploration. In addition, males are a neglected population in social support research (Langford et al., 1997). Qualitative research approaches could be useful for discovering meanings of social support across cultures.

Causality in social support research needs further exploration. Researchers have conducted many descriptive and correlational studies that link social support to positive health outcomes, but few studies substantiate causal links (Callaghan & Morrissey, 1993). The impact of health status on how people seek and receive support has been explored less often than the effects of social support on health status (Stewart, 1993). Changes in health status are likely to influence the amount of and components of social support that are needed. With increased stress resulting from threats to health, social support actions can facilitate coping. Moreover, the balance of reciprocity in relationships and the amount of conflict present may change in response to health status changes. One question suggested by Cohen et al. (2001) for future study is whether persons with chronic illness decrease their provision of support, resulting in an imbalance in the social network (reciprocity).

To further develop understanding of the linkages of social support to health outcomes, theoretically based social support interventions need to be tested in controlled intervention trials in varied settings and age groups (Ducharme et al., 1994). Cohen et al. (2001) suggested that more intervention research should be conducted on promising interventions, such as support groups and support provided in dyads (partner or peer support). In addition, research on interventions that focus on strengthening the social support environments at a community or systems level can develop knowledge about how to use social support to improve the health status of populations. Multilevel interventions may be the most effective. Rook and Dooley (1985) described two categorical approaches to social support interventions—individual and environmental. Individual interventions are used to change how a person perceives or seeks support, while an environmental approach targets the community to improve the social support climate. Social support is likely to be maximized with the implementation of both approaches. Research methods used to test the effectiveness of social support interventions need to be tailored to the intervention level. Measures for any level should include the potential negative aspects of social support in the person's interactions and environment, which, if not considered, can confound the interpretation of study findings. Evaluation of social support interventions at the individual, dyadic, and group levels is likely to focus on the perceptions of social support actions and available support. Evaluation of social support interventions at the community and systems levels emphasizes analysis of social support available in networks and the environment. The impact of a nurse-initiated program on social support for a group is described in Research Application 9-1.

9-1 RESEARCH APPLICATION

A nurse researcher is evaluating the effectiveness of a parish nursing program to strengthen the social support available to many elderly individuals who live alone in the surrounding low-income, urban community. The goals of the program are to connect elderly residents with needed health care services and make it possible for them to continue living safely in their homes. The program includes bimonthly group meetings of seniors at the church for informational and emotional support, and an outreach program in which congregational members make regular visits and phone calls to elderly residents in the neighborhood who wish to participate in the program. Both program components can strengthen instrumental support by connecting residents to community organizations that provide services needed by the residents, such as health care and home maintenance.

(Continued)

(Continued) **9-1 RESEARCH APPLICATION**

The researcher administers Part 2 of the Personal Resource Questionnaire (PRQ-85) to program participants at the time of initial enrollment, and 6 months later to determine any changes in level of perceived social support. In addition, the researcher conducts a focus group with the senior group meeting at the church. Several open-ended questions are used to explore participants' social support experiences related to appraisal, emotional, informational, and instrumental support. For elderly residents who are in the outreach program, the researcher interviews a sample of participants in their homes to collect data on changes in health status and use of health care and community services.

SUMMARY

Social support theory is important to nurses because it can explain and suggest nursing interventions to improve health outcomes. Nurses and others from psychosocial disciplines have contributed to the development of social support theory and measures. Although a great variety of social support measures have been developed, many are for specific situations. There is a lack of consensus on the definition of social support. Authors disagree on the dimensionality of social support. A major concern is the omission of considering potential negative aspects of social support. The next step for expanding social support theory is knowledge development about effective multilevel social support interventions.

ANALYSIS EXERCISE

The chapter on social support provides several constructs with which to view the phenomenon. Using the criteria presented in Chapter 2, critique the body of knowledge presented in this chapter. You will be using each criterion in a manner different from its use when applied to one specific theory. Specific questions related to the use of each criterion in this new context follow. Compare your conclusions about the constructs across theories with those found in Appendix A. A nurse scholar who has worked with this phenomenon completed the analysis found in the Appendix.

Internal Criticism
1. Clarity (Do we have theories of social support that are clear?)
2. Consistency (Is there consistency in approach, i.e., terms, interpretations, principles, and methods, across theories?)

3. Adequacy (How adequate is the body of theories in accounting for social support?)
4. Level of theory development (At what level of development are the social support theories?)

External Criticism
1. Reality convergence (Do these theories reflect "real world" nursing experiences of social support?)
2. Utility (How useful are present theories when applied in practice and research?)
3. Significance (Do the theories reflect issues essential to nursing?)
4. Discrimination (Do the theories help distinguish social support from other interpersonal processes?)
5. Scope of theory (What seems to be the scope of the theories?)
6. Complexity (As a group, how would you judge the complexity of social support theories?)

WEB RESOURCES

1. Jane S. Norbeck's Web page includes ordering information for the Norbeck Social Support Questionnaire (NSSQ). The NSSQ was revised in 1995 to be compatible with Microsoft Windows for data entry and analysis. Her web page can be reached at:
http://nurseweb.ucsf.edu/www/ffnorb.htm
2. RAND is a nonprofit institute that helps improve policy and decision-making through research and analysis. This site includes a brief, self-administered social support survey (18 items) with four subscales that was developed for the Medical Outcomes Study (MOS). The subscales include emotional/informational support, tangible support, affectionate support, and positive social interaction. Scoring instructions are available. This site can be accessed at: *http://www.rand.org/health/surveys/mos.descrip.html*
3. This site lists social support items on the Berlin Social Support Scales (BSSS), developed for coping with cancer-surgery settings. Listed scales include Perceived Available Support, Need for Support, Support Seeking, Actually Received Support (provider), Actually Received Support (recipient), and Protective Buffering (provider and recipient). Access this site at: *http://userpage.fu-berlin.de/~health/soc_e.htm*

REFERENCES

Albrecht, T., & Adelman, M. (1987). Communication networks as structures of social support. In T. Albrecht, & M. Adelman (Eds.), *Communicating social support* (pp. 40–61). Newbury Park, CA: Sage.

Barrera, M. (1981). Social support in the adjustment of pregnant adolescents: Assessment issues. In B. Gottlieb (Ed.), *Social networks and social support* (pp. 69–96). Beverly Hills, CA: Sage.

Barrera, Jr., M. (1986). Distinctions between social support concepts, measures, and models. *American Journal of Community Psychology, 14*(4), 413–445.

Bloom, J. R. (1990). The relationship of social support and health. *Social Science and Medicine, 39*(5), 635–637.

Bowlby, J. (1971). *Attachment.* London: Pelican.

Brandt, P. A., & Weinert, C. (1981). The PRQ—A social support measure. *Nursing Research, 30*(5), 277–280.

Brown, M. A. (1986). Social support during pregnancy: A unidimensional or multidimensional concept? *Nursing Research, 35*(1), 4–9.

Callaghan, P., & Morrissey, J. (1993). Social support and health: A review. *Journal of Advanced Nursing, 18*, 203–210.

Cassel, J. (1974). Psychosocial process and "stress": Theoretical perspectives. *International Journal of Health Services, 4*(3), 471–482.

Cassel, J. (1976). The contribution of the social environment to host resistance. *American Journal of Epidemiology, 104*(2), 107–123.

Clark, J. S. (1983). Reactions to aid in communal and exchange relationships. In J. D. Fisher, D. Nadler, & B. M. DePaulo (Eds.), *New directions in helping: Vol 1. Recipient reactions to aid* (pp. 281–305). New York: Academic Press.

Cobb, S. (1976). Social support as a moderator of life stress. *Psychosomatic Medicine, 38*, 300–314.

Cohen, S. (1992). Stress, social support, and disorder. In H. O. Veiel & U. Baumann (Eds.), *The meaning and measurement of social support* (pp.109–204). New York: Hemisphere Publishing Corporation.

Cohen, S., Gottlieb, B. H., & Underwood, L. G. (2001). Social relationships and health: Challenges for measurement and intervention. *Advances in Mind–Body Medicine, 17*, 129–141.

Cohen, S., & Syme, S. L. (1985). Issues in the study and application of social support. In S. Cohen & S. L. Syme (Eds.), *Social support and health* (pp. 3–32). New York: Academic Press.

Cossette, S., Levesque, L., & Laurin, L. (1995). Informal and formal support for caregivers of a demented relative: Do gender and kinship make a difference? *Research in Nursing and Health, 18*, 437–451.

Coyne, J. C., & DeLongis, A. (1986). Going beyond social support: The role of social relationships in adaptation. *Journal of Consulting and Clinical Psychology, 54*, 454–460.

Cutrona, C. E. (1990). Stress and social support: In search of optimal matching. *Journal of Social and Clinical Psychology, 9*(1), 3–14.

Dakof, G., & Taylor, S. (1990). Victim's perception of social support: What is helpful from whom? *Journal of Personality and Social Psychology, 58*(1), 80–89.

Diamond, M. (1985). A review and critique of the concepts of social support. In R. A. O'Brien (Ed.), *Social support and health: New directions for theory and research* (pp. 1–32). Rochester, NY: University of Rochester Press.

Ducharme, F., Stevens, B., & Rowat, K. (1994). Social support: Conceptual and methodological issues for research in mental health nursing. *Issues in Mental Health Nursing, 15*, 373–392.

Dunkel-Schetter, C. (1984). Social support and cancer:

Findings based on patient interviews and their implications. *Journal of Social Issues, 40*(4), 77–98.

Dunkel-Schetter, C., & Bennett, T. L. (1990). Differentiating the cognitive and behavioral aspects of social support. In B. R. Sarason, I. G. Sarason, & G. R. Pierce (Eds.), *Social support: An interactional view* (pp. 267–296). New York: Wiley.

Dunkel-Schetter, C., Blasband, D., Feinstein, L., & Herbert, T. (1992). Elements of supportive interactions. When are attempts to help effective? In S. Spacapan & S. Oskamp, (Eds.), *Helping and being helped* (pp. 83–114). New York: Academic Press.

Dunkel-Schetter, C., & Skokan, L. A. (1990). Determinants of social support provision in personal relationships. *Journal of Social and Personal Relationships, 7*(4), 437–450.

Friedman, M. M. (1997). Social support sources among older women with heart failure: Continuity versus loss over time. *Research in Nursing and Health, 20,* 319–327.

Froland, C., Pancoast, D., Chapman, D., & Kimboko, P. (1981). *Helping networks and human services.* Beverly Hills, CA: Sage.

Gottlieb, B. H. (1978). The development and application of a classification scheme of informal helping networks. *Canadian Journal of Behavioral Science, 10,* 105–115.

Griffith, J. (1985). Social support providers: Who are they? Where are they met? And the relationships of network characteristics to psychological distress. *Basic and Applied Social Psychology, 6*(1), 41–60.

Hammer, M. (1981). "Core" and "extended" social networks in relation to health and illness. *Social Science and Medicine, 17,* 405–411.

Heitzmann, C. A., & Kaplan, R. M. (1988). Assessment of methods for measuring social support. *Health Psychology, 7*(1), 75–109.

Heller, K., Swindle, R. W., & Dusenbury, L. (1986). Component social support processes: Comments and integration. *Journal of Consulting and Clinical Psychology, 54*(4), 466–470.

Hilbert, G. A. (1990). Measuring social support in chronic illness. In O. L. Strickland & C. F. Waltz (Eds.), *Measurement of nursing outcomes,* Vol. 4 (pp. 79–95). New York: Springer Publishing Company.

Higgins, P. G., & Dicharry, E. K. (1991). Measurement issues addressing social support with Navajo women. *Western Journal of Nursing Research, 13*(2), 242–255.

House, J. S. (1981). Work stress and social support. Englewood Cliffs, NJ: Prentice Hall.

Hupcey, J. E. (1998a). Clarifying the social support theory–research linkage. *Journal of Advanced Nursing, 27*(6), 1231–1241.

Hupcey, J. E. (1998b). Social support: Assessing conceptual coherence. *Qualitative Health Research, 8*(3), 304–318.

Hupcey, J. E., & Morse, J. M. (1997). Can a professional relationship be considered social support? *Nursing Outlook, 45,* 270–276.

Hutchinson, C. (1999). Social support: Factors to consider when designing studies that measure social support. *Journal of Advanced Nursing, 29*(6), 1520–1526.

Jacobson, D. E. (1986). Types and timing of social support. *Journal of Health and Social Behavior, 27,* 250–264.

Jung, J. (1988). Social support providers: Why do they help? *Basic and Applied Social Psychology, 9,* 231–240.

Kahn, R. L. (1979). Aging and social support. In M. W. Riley (Ed.), *Aging from birth to death: Interdisciplinary perspectives* (pp. 77–91). Boulder, CO: Westview Press.

Kahn, R. L., & Antonucci, T. C. (1980). Convoys over the life course: Attachment, roles, and social support. In P. B. Baltes & G. Brim (Eds.), *Life span development and behavior.* (Vol. 3) (pp. 253–283). New York: Academic Press.

Kaunonen, M., Tarkka, M., Paunonen, M., & Laippala, P. (1999). Grief and social support after the death of a spouse. *Journal of Advanced Nursing, 30*(6), 1304–1311.

Kotelchuck, M. (1994). An evaluation of the Kessner Adequacy of Prenatal Care Utilization Index. *American Journal of Public Health, 84*(9), 1414–1420.

Krishnasamy, M. (1996). Social support and the patient with cancer: A consideration of the literature. *Journal of Advanced Nursing, 23*(4), 757–762.

La Gaipa, J. J. (1990). The negative effects of informal support systems. In S. Duck (Ed.), *Personal relationships and social support* (pp. 122–139). London: Sage.

Lackner, S., Goldenberg, S., Arrizza, G., & Tjosvold, I. (1994). The contingency of social support. *Qualitative Health Research, 4*(2), 224–243.

Laireiter, A., & Baumann, U. (1992). Network structures and support functions theoretical and empirical analyses. In H. O. Veiel & U. Baumann (Eds.), *The meaning and measurement of social support* (pp. 33–55). London: Hemisphere Publishing Corporation.

Langford, C. P. H., Bowsher, J., Maloney, J. P., & Lillis, P. (1997). Social support: A conceptual analysis. *Journal of Advanced Nursing, 25*(1), 95–100.

Lugton, J. (1997). The nature of social support as experienced by women treated for breast cancer. *Journal of Advanced Nursing, 25*(6), 1184–1191.

Newsom, J. T., Bookwala, J., & Schulz, R. (1997). Social support measurement in group residences for older adults. *Journal of Mental Health and Aging, 3*(1), 47–66.

Norbeck, J. S. (1981). Social support: A model for clinical research and application. *Advances in Nursing Science, 3*(4), 43–59.

Norbeck, J. S. (1988). Social support. *Annual Review of Nursing Research, 6*, 85–109.

Norbeck, J. S., Lindsey, A. M., & Carrieri, V. L. (1981). The development of an instrument to measure social support. *Nursing Research, 30*(5), 264–269.

Norbeck, J. S., Lindsey, A. M., & Carrieri, V. L. (1983). Further development of the Norbeck social support questionnaire: Normative data and validity testing. *Nursing Research, 32*(1), 4–9.

Norbeck, J. S., & Tilden, V. P. (1988). International research in social support: Theoretical and methodological issues. *Journal of Advanced Nursing, 13*, 173–178.

Norwood, S. L. (1996). The social support Apgar: Instrument development and testing. *Research in Nursing and Health, 19*, 143–152.

Olds, D. L., Henderson, C. R., Kitzman, H. J., Echenrode, J. J., Cole, R. E., & Tatelbaum, R. C. (1999). Prenatal and infancy home visitation by nurses: Recent findings. *Future of Children, 9*(1), 44–65.

Pearlman, D. N., & Crown, W. H. (1992). Alternative sources of social support and their impacts on institutional risk. *The Gerontologist, 32*, 527–535.

Pierce, G. R., Sarason, B. R., & Sarason, I. G. (1990). Integrating social support perspectives: Working models, personal relationships, and situational factors. In S. Duck (Ed.), *Personal relationships and social support* (pp. 173–189). London: Sage.

Pilisuk, M. (1982). Delivery of social support: The social inoculation. *American Journal of Orthopsychiatry, 52*, 20–31.

Ragsdale, D., Yarbrough, S., & Lasher, A. T. (1993). Using social support theory to care for CVA patients. *Rehabilitation Nursing, 18*(3), 154–172.

Roberts, S. J. (1984). Social support—meaning, measurement, and relevance to community health nursing practice. *Public Health Nursing, 1*(3), 158–167.

Rook, K. S., & Dooley, D. (1985). Applying social support research: Theoretical problems and future directions. *Journal of Social Issues, 41*(1), 5–28.

Sarason, I. G., Sarason, B. R., Shearin, E. N., & Pierce, G. R. (1987). A brief measure of social support: Practical and theoretical implications. *Journal of Social and Personal Relationships, 4*, 497–510.

Sarason, B. R., Sarason, I. G., & Pierce, G. R. (1990). *Social support: An interactional view.* New York: John Wiley.

Schaffer, M. A., & Lia-Hoagberg, B. (1997). Effects of social support on prenatal care and health behaviors of low-income women. *Journal of Obstetric, Gynecologic, and Neonatal Nursing, 26*(4), 433–440.

Shumaker, S. A., & Brownell, A. (1984). Toward a theory of social support: Closing conceptual gaps. *Journal of Social Issues, 40*(4), 11–36.

Stewart, M. J. (1993). *Integrating social support in nursing.* Newbury Park, CA: Sage.

Stewart, M. J. (1989a). Social support instruments created by nurse investigators. *Nursing Research, 38*(5), 268–275.

Stewart, M. J. (1989b). Social support intervention studies: A review and prospectus of nursing contributions. *International Journal of Nursing Studies, 26*(2), 93–114.

Tardy, C. H. (1985). Social support measurement. *American Journal of Community Psychology, 13*(2), 187–202.

Thoits, P. A. (1983). Multiple identities and psychosocial well-being: A reformation and test of the social isolation hypothesis. *American Sociological Review, 48*, 174–187.

Thoits, P. A. (1986). Social support as coping assistance. *Journal of Consulting and Clinical Psychology, 54*(4), 416–423.

Tilden, V. P. (1985). Issues of conceptualization and measurement of social support in construction of nursing theory. *Research in Nursing and Health, 81*, 199–206.

Tilden, V. P. (1986). New perspectives on social support. *The Nurse Practitioner, 11*, 60–61.

Tilden, V. P., & Galyen, R. D. (1987). Cost and conflict: The darker side of social support. *Western Journal of Nursing Research, 9*(1), 9–18.

Tilden, V. P., Nelson, C. A., & May, B. A. (1990). The IPR inventory: Development and psychometric characteristics. *Nursing Research, 39*(6), 337–343.

Tilden, V. P., & Weinert, S. C. (1987). Social support and the chronically ill individual. *Nursing Clinics of North America, 22*(3), 613–620.

Vaux, A. (1988). *Social support—theory, research, and intervention.* New York: Praeger.

Veiel, H. O., & Baumann, U. (1992). The many meanings of social support. In H. O. Veiel & U. Baumann (Eds.), *The meaning and measurement of social support* (pp. 1–9). New York: Hemisphere.

Vrabec, N. J. (1997). Literature review of social support and caregiver burden, 1980 to 1985. *Image: Journal of Nursing Scholarship, 29*(4), 383–388.

Wandersman, L., Wandersman, A., & Kahn, S. (1980). Social support in the transition to parenthood. *Journal of Community Psychology, 8*, 332–342.

Weinert, C. (1987). A social support measure: PRQ85. *Nursing Research, 36*(5), 273–277.

Weinert, C. (1988). Measuring social support: Revision and further development of the personal resource questionnaire. In O. L. Strickland & C. F. Waltz (Eds.), *Measurement of nursing outcomes*, Vol. 1 (pp. 309–327). New York: Springer Publishing Company.

Wortman, C. B., & Dunkel-Schetter, C. (1987). Conceptual and methodological issues in the study of social support. In A. Baum & J. E. Singer (Eds.), *Handbook of psychology and health* (pp. 63–108). Hillsdale, NJ: Lawrence Erlbaum Associates.

BIBLIOGRAPHY

Blixen, C., & Kippes, C. (1999). Depression, social support, and quality of life in older adults with osteoarthritis. *Image: Journal of Nursing Scholarship, 31*(3), 221–226.

Bolla, C. D., De Joseph, J. Norbeck, J., & Smith, R. (1996). Social support as road map and vehicle: An analysis of data from focus group interviews with a group of African American women. *Public Health Nursing, 13*(5), 331–336.

Christopher, S. E., Bauman, K. E., & Veness-Meehan, K. (2000). Perceived stress, social support, and affectionate behaviors of adolescent mothers with infants in neonatal intensive care. *Journal of Pediatric Health Care, 14*, 288–296.

Cossette, S., Levesque, L., & Laurin, L. (1995). Informal and formal support for caregivers of a demented relative: Do gender and kinship make a difference? *Research in Nursing and Health, 18*, 437–451.

Friedman, M. M. (1997). Social support sources among older women with heart failure: Continuity versus loss over time. *Research in Nursing and Health, 20*, 319–327.

Hagerty, B. M., & Williams, R. A. (1999). The effects of sense of belonging, social support, conflict, and loneliness on depression. *Nursing Research, 48*(4), 215–219.

Hubbard, P., Muhlenkamp, A. F., & Brown, N. (1984). The relationship between social support and self-care practices. *Nursing Research, 33*(5), 266–270.

Hudson, A. L., & Morris, R. I. (1994). Perceptions of social support of African Americans with acquired immunodeficiency syndrome. *Journal of National Black Nurses Association, 7*(1), 36–49.

Ihlenfeld, J. T. (1996). Nurses' perceptions of administrative social support. *Issues in Mental Health Nursing, 17*, 469–477.

Kaunonen, M., Tarkka, M., Paunonen, M., & Laippala, P. (1999). Grief and social support after the death of a spouse. *Journal of Advanced Nursing, 30*(6), 1304–1311.

Lugton, J. (1997). The nature of social support as experienced by women treated for breast cancer. *Journal of Advanced Nursing, 25*(6), 1184–1191.

Mahon, N. E., Yarcheski, A., & Yarcheski, T. J. (1998). Social support and positive health practices in young adults: Loneliness as a mediating variable. *Clinical Nursing Research, 7*(3), 292–309.

McVeigh, C. A. (2000). Investigating the relationship between satisfaction with social support and functional status after childbirth. *MCN, The American Journal of Maternal/Child Nursing, 25*(1), 25–30.

Norbeck, J. S., De Joseph, J. F., & Smith, R. T. (1996). A randomized trial of an empirically derived social support intervention to prevent low birthweight. *Social Science and Medicine, 43*, 947–954.

Ostergren, P. O., Hanson, B. S., Isacsson, S. O., & Tejler, L. (1991). Social network, social support and acute chest complaints among young and middle-aged patients in an emergency department—a case control study. *Social Science and Medicine, 33*(3), 257–267.

Reece, S. M. (1993). Social support and the early maternal experience of primiparas over 35. *Maternal-Child Nursing Journal, 21*(3), 91–98.

Roberts, B. L., Matecjyck, M., & Anthony, M. (1996). The effects of social support on the relationship of functional limitations and pain to depression. *Arthritis Care and Research, 9*(1), 67–73.

Schaffer, M. A., & Lia-Hoagberg, B. (1997). Effects of social support on prenatal care and health behaviors of low-income women. *Journal of Obstetric, Gynecologic, and Neonatal Nursing, 26*(4), 433–440.

Tarkka, M., & Paunonen, M. (1996). Social support provided by nurses to recent mothers on a maternity ward. *Journal of Advanced Nursing, 23*(6), 1202–1206.

Interpersonal Relations

SANDRA J. PETERSON

DEFINITION OF KEY TERMS

Communication	A skill necessary to understand the nurse–patient relationship. Comprises "spoken language, rational and nonrational expressions of wishes, needs, and desires, and the body gesture" (Peplau, 1991, p. 289)
Interpersonal relations	Any process that occurs between two people. The interpersonal processes between nurse and patient are identified as the core of nursing (Forchuk, 1993).
Nursing situation	What occurs between the nurse and the patient; thus, the interaction of the individual thoughts, feelings, and actions of both
Observation	A skill necessary to understand the nurse–patient relationship. Its aim, "as an interpersonal process, is the identification, clarification, and verification of impressions about the interactive drama, of the pushes and pulls in the relationship between nurse and patient as they occur" (Peplau, 1991, p. 263).
Personality	"...Pattern that is relatively stable and that characterizes persisting situations in the life of an individual.... total assets and liabilities that determine an individual action" (Peplau, 1991, pp. 164–165). Nurses attempt to provide experiences for patients that promote personality development.
Phases of nurse–patient relationship	Four overlapping but generally sequential aspects of the relationship identified as orientation, identification, exploitation, and resolution
Psychobiological experiences	Factors that influence the functioning of personalities, providing energy that is converted into constructive or destructive behavior. The primary source of this energy is anxiety.

Psychological tasks	"Tasks encountered in the process of learning to live with people as an aspect of formation and development of personality and as an aspect of the tasks demanded of nurses in their relations with patients" (Peplau, 1991, p. 159). For example: counting on others, delaying satisfaction, identifying self, participating with others
Recording	Methods used to create documents of nurse–patient interactions, primarily for the purpose of student learning
Roles in nursing	Set of functions that nurses use in the context of nurse–patient situations as a means of helping the patient, identified as stranger, resource person, teacher, leader, surrogate, and counselor.

INTRODUCTION

"When the history of nursing theory comes to be written few names will be seen to have been more influential than that of Hildegard Peplau" (Welch, 1995, p. 53). Peplau, who developed the Theory of Interpersonal Relations, is identified as the first contemporary nurse theorist (McKenna, 1997). Sills (1978) credits Peplau with clarifying the relationships between nursing theory, practice, and research. "Theory was used to guide nursing practice. Theory was tested in the real world of practice" (Sills, 1978, p. 122).

Though Peplau entitled her work a conceptual frame of reference, she often referred to it as a theory (Peplau, 1992, p. 13). Peplau produced a testable theory, identifying her work as a "source of hypotheses that may be examined with profit in all nursing situations" (Peplau, 1991, p. ix). The Theory of Interpersonal Relations is currently labeled a middle range theory (Armstrong & Kelly, 1995; Fawcett, 2000; O'Toole & Welt, 1989). Peplau, herself, defined the scope of her theory as in the middle range. She referred to it as "a partial theory for the practice of nursing as an interpersonal process" (Peplau, 1991, p. 261).

> Concepts contained within interpersonal relations theory are primarily relevant as [descriptions] of the personal behavior of nurse and patient in nursing situations and of psychological phenomena. Obviously, then for the practice of nursing, a more comprehensive scope of theoretical constructs is needed. (Peplau, 1992, p. 13)

Initially developed with a focus on phenomena of most concern to psychiatric nurses, the Theory of Interpersonal Relations is applicable to all nurses (Peplau, 1964, 1992). Peplau (1997, p. 163) claimed that "the nurse–patient relationship is the primary human contact that is central in a fundamental way to providing nursing care." The stated purpose of her theory is the improvement of nurses' relations with patients. This is achieved through the nurse's understanding of his or her own behavior, helping others identify personally experienced difficulties, and applying principles of human relations to the problems that arise in the context of relationships (Peplau, 1991, p. xi). This process results in a nursing situation in which both the patient and the nurse learn and grow. A growth-producing relationship with others is a goal that transcends any particular nursing specialty, and, in her description of the theory, Peplau (1952, 1991) used examples of patients with a variety of health issues (e.g., a woman diagnosed with lymphosarcoma, a child having surgery on his hand to correct a congenital problem, a woman in labor, and a man with a coronary occlusion).

HISTORICAL BACKGROUND

What makes Peplau's Theory of Interpersonal Relations so remarkable is that it was conceived during a period in nursing's history when nurses had little or no independent role or investment in the development of nursing theory. Peplau was educated and began her nursing practice, as described in her own words, at a time when "we were absolutely not allowed to talk to a patient, because if we did we might say the wrong thing" (Welch, 1995, p. 54). It was not until the late 1930s, while working as a staff nurse at Mount Sinai Hospital, New York, that she discovered "there was more to nursing than just this doing activity, because there we were allowed to talk to the patients" (Welch, 1995, p. 54). In the 1940s, Peplau found psychiatric nursing still focused on activities, such as helping patients with tasks of daily living, which included cleaning patients' rooms and doing patients' laundry (Peplau, 1985, p. 31). It was out of her desire to be more useful to patients that the idea of interpersonal relations theory was developed.

Peplau used both deductive and inductive methods in her theory development work (Reed, 1995). Deductively, she integrated ideas from a number of theories into her theory of interpersonal relations. She was influenced by the work of Sigmund Freud, particularly his interest in unconscious motivation. Harry S. Sullivan's theory of interpersonal relations also contributed to her thinking about interpersonal processes in nursing. For example, she refers to his concepts of anxiety, self-system, and modes of experiencing. She also incorporated into her theory elements from developmental psychology and learning theory (Armstrong & Kelly, 1995; Lego, 1980), and the ideas of the humanistic psychologists, Abraham Maslow, Rollo May, and Carl Rogers (Gastmans, 1998).

Peplau defined her inductive approach both in general and specific terms. The inductive approach for concept naming that she described included several steps:

1. Observing behaviors for which no explanatory concepts are available
2. Seeking to repeat those observations in others, under similar conditions
3. Noting regularities concerning the nature of the data being observed
4. Naming the phenomena (Peplau, 1989, p. 28).

These steps would be followed by further observation that more clearly defined the phenomenon and allowed for testing with additional patients. "Eventually, useful interventions would be derived from the explanation of the phenomenon and the effects of these interventions upon it also tested" (Peplau, 1969, p. 28).

Peplau's specific inductive process of theory development used data from student–patient interactions. "I just happened to hit upon the notion of sitting students down with one patient for a long time and then study what they did with patients" (Peplau, 1985, p. 31). It was from these observations that psychotherapy by nurses in the context of the interpersonal relationship emerged.

Her theory of interpersonal relations, first appearing in 1952 in the book, *Interpersonal Relations in Nursing*, has been published unchanged several times. During the 1950s and 1960s, her theory was used and tested in the challenging environment of state psychiatric hospitals. Some of this work is reported in *Basic Principles of Patient Counseling*, published in 1964 by Smith, Kline and French (Sills, 1978, p. 124). In 4 decades since its inception, interpersonal theory has been expanded by Peplau and by other nurse scientists (Peplau, 1991, p. vi). For example, work on therapeutic milieu, crisis, and family therapy has been based on Peplau's theory. Sills (1978) conducted a review of three major nursing journals from 1972 to 1977 (one published for the first time in 1963). She identified 93 citations of Peplau's work and concluded that "it [is] remarkable that twenty-five years after the publication of *Interpersonal Relations in Nursing* that it, with no revisions, is still found useful. And ...that utilization increases" (Sills, 1978, p. 125).

DEFINITION OF THEORY CONCEPTS

Though not specified when the theory was developed in 1952, Peplau addresses each domain of the traditional metaparadigm of nursing. Her definitions of these major domain concepts are useful in understanding the rather complex Theory of Interpersonal Relations.

Nursing

The foundation of her theory is her definition of nursing. Perhaps what is unique, but not unexpectedly so, is the primacy of the nurse–patient relationship in her definition. She defines nursing as an interpersonal process, intended to be therapeutic. It "is a human relationship between an individual who is sick or in need of health services" (Peplau, 1991, pp. 5–6) and a nurse who has appropriate preparation to respond to the need. The use of technical procedures in nursing is acknowledged but relegated to a secondary role. Her most frequently quoted definition is:

> Nursing is a significant, therapeutic, interpersonal process. It functions co-operatively with other human processes that make health possible for individuals in communities.... Nursing is an educative instrument, a maturing force, that aims to promote forward movement of personality in the direction of creative, constructive, productive, personal, and community living. (Peplau, 1952, p. 16)

Persons

In her theory, Peplau includes as components two persons: the nurse and client, or more often, patient (O'Toole & Welt, 1989; Peplau, 1992). Peplau (1952) initially defined Man as:

> An organism that lives in an unstable equilibrium (i.e., physiological, psychological, and social fluidity) and life is the process of striving in the direction of stable equilibrium, i.e., a fixed pattern that is never reached except in death. (p. 82)

Forchuk (1991, p. 55) revised that definition, omitting the terms "organism" and "equilibrium" because they represent a more "mechanical, closed-system perspective" that is inconsistent with Peplau's view of humans as growth-seeking. A person is a relational being experiencing "interacting expectations, conceptions, wishes, and desires, as well as feelings when ... in situations with other persons" (O'Toole & Welt, 1989, p. 5). This perspective of persons as relational beings is fundamental to the theory.

NURSE

The nurse is identified as a professional with definable expertise (Peplau, 1992). This expertise should include the ability to "identify human problems that confront patients, the degrees of skill used to meet situations, and be able to develop with patients the kind of relationships that will be conducive to improvement in skill" (Peplau, 1991, p. xiii). The nurse also possesses "a unique blend of ideals, values, integrity, and commitment to the well-being of others" (Peplau, 1988, p. 10).

PATIENT

The patient is defined first as a person, deserving of "all of the humane considerations: respect, dignity, privacy, confidentiality, and ethical care" (Peplau, 1992, p. 14), but a person who has problems that now require the services of a nurse. Ideally, the patient participates actively in the nurse–patient relationship (O'Toole & Welt, 1989, p. 57).

Health

Peplau (1952, pp. 12–13) provided a definition of health in her initial description of the theory. "It [health] is a word symbol that implies forward movement of personality and other human processes in the direction of creative, constructive, productive, personal, and community living." In addition she identified two processes that are necessary for health: (a) biological, for instance absorption and elimination and (b) social, which promotes physical, emotional, and social well-being.

Environment

Peplau focused on the issue of environment as milieu, using the term to describe a therapeutic environment (O'Toole & Welt, 1989, p. 78). The milieu comprises structured (e.g., ward government) and unstructured components. The unstructured components consist of the complex relationships between patients, staff, visitors, and other patients, which is often neglected and yet has a significant impact on patient outcomes. Milieu ideally involves the creation of an atmosphere conducive to recovery.

DESCRIPTION OF THE THEORY OF INTERPERSONAL RELATIONS

Peplau implied a philosophical foundation to her Theory of Interpersonal Relations and provided two basic assumptions, which have been expanded by others, using the initial publication of the theory as the primary source. Peplau did not label the propositional statements in her theory as such; instead, they are integrated into her discussion of the components of the theory.

Philosophical Foundations

There are some different perspectives on the nature of the philosophical underpinnings of Peplau's Theory of Interpersonal Relations in Nursing. Sellers (1991) labels the theory:

> ...a mechanistic, deterministic, persistence ontological view; an epistemology that is consistent with the totality paradigm, with its emphasis on a received view of knowledge and logical positivism; and an axiology that values stability, traditionalism, and nursing's close alignment with medicine. (p. 158)

Sellers did not support these conclusions with examples from the theory. Because the complexity of Peplau's theory makes it difficult to categorize, it is not surprising that others have considered it from a different philosophical perspective.

More recently, existential phenomenology has been identified as the philosophical foundation of Peplau's theory (Gastmans, 1998). Consistent with phenomenology, observation of patients as a fundamental task of nursing, is seen as contextual and value laden. It requires openness to and involvement with patients' existential situations. "Nursing has a human interpretive character" (Gastmans, 1998, Phenomenology and Nursing Science, para. 5) with the nurse–patient relationship at its core. Interpretations are meaning-seeking activities that arise from a caring relationship between nurse and patient.

These perspectives of nursing are themes found in Peplau's writings. She identifies observation of patients as an essential component of an interpersonal process that is therapeutic and educational for patients (Peplau, 1991, p. 309). Peplau (1992) also believes understanding of the patient best comes from observations of the patient's immediate situation, and that participant observation is the preferred form of making observations. This participation with the patient is described as respectful, communicating positive interest and nonjudgmental regard (Peplau, 1991). Peplau uses the term "professional closeness" (Peplau, 1969) to summarize these characteristics that allow the nurse to communicate care when participating with patients. The importance of values is acknowledged by Peplau, as evidenced by her belief that the nurse's self-knowledge of feelings, attitudes, and behaviors is fundamental to understanding the client's situation (Peplau, 1991).

Though most of Peplau's philosophy is imbedded in her writings, she does delineate six "beliefs about patients" (Peplau, 1964, pp. 30–35). She identifies these as her "philosophy about patients and their care," attributed primarily to psychiatric nurses but applicable to all patients:

1. All behavior is purposeful, has meaning, and can be understood.
2. The nurse must observe what is going on; she must interpret what is observed, and then she must decide action on the basis of her interpretations.
3. The nurse meets the needs of the patient.
4. The nurse–patient interaction—the verbal and nonverbal exchanges in the nursing situation—can influence recovery.
5. The personality of the patient is somehow involved in his illness.
6. The nurse must be alert to the possibility that all patients experience anxiety.

Assumptions

In the initial publication of her theory, Peplau (1952) listed two guiding assumptions, emphasizing the importance of the nurse's own growth and development in establishing helpful interpersonal relationships with patients. Others have expanded that list through personal correspondence with Peplau and through review of her writings. Table 10-1 provides a list of the assumptions of the Theory of Interpersonal Relations.

These thirteen assumptions serve to illustrate the complexity of Peplau's Theory of Interpersonal Relations.

Theory Description With Propositional Statements

The core of the theory, the relationship between nurse and patient, is comprised of phases, fulfilled through roles, influenced by psychobiological experiences, and requires attending to certain psychological tasks. Peplau also identified methods that can help the nurse to develop understanding of the nurse–patient relationship. The description of the theory uses the same sequence of content as Peplau (1952, 1991) did in her seminal work, *Interpersonal Relations in Nursing*.

COMPRISED OF PHASES

Peplau (1991) initially defined four phases of the nurse–patient relationship as orientation, identification, exploitation, and resolution. Forchuk (1991) later reconceptualized these into three phases, with the working phase replacing the identification and exploitation phases. These phases are considered overlapping and interlocking, with each phase possessing characteristic functions. They are experienced in every nursing situation.

Phase of Orientation. There are four functions that nurses use during orientation:

- *Provide the resources* of specific, needed information to help the patient understand the problem and the health care situation
- *Serve as a counselor* to encourage the patient to express thoughts and feelings related to the problem situation
- *Act as surrogate* to family members so that the patient can reenact and examine relevant issues from previous relationships
- *Use technical expertise* to attend to concerns or issues that require the use of professional devices.

These nursing functions help the patient to address the needs experienced during the phase of orientation.

The patient needs to recognize and understand the extent of the difficulty and the help that is needed to address it. Orienting the patient to the nature of the problem is a complex task, requiring the nurse to act as both a resource person and a counselor. As a resource person, the nurse provides specific information about the problem confronting the patient, and helps the patient see the personal relevance of the information. As a counselor, the nurse encourages the patient to be actively involved in identifying and assessing the problem.

Table 10-1. ASSUMPTIONS OF THE THEORY OF INTERPERSONAL RELATIONS

SOURCE	ASSUMPTIONS
Identified by Peplau (1952)	1. "The kind of person each nurse becomes makes a substantial difference in what each patient will learn as he is nursed throughout his experience with illness." (p. xii) 2. "Fostering personality development in the direction of maturity is a function of nursing and nursing education; it requires the use of principles and methods that permit and guide the process of grappling with everyday interpersonal problems or difficulties." (p. xii)
Based on correspondence with Peplau (Forchuk, 1993)	3. Nursing can claim as its uniqueness, the responses of clients to the circumstances of their illnesses or health problems. 4. Because illness provides an opportunity for learning and growth, nurses can assist clients to further develop their intellectual and interpersonal competencies, during the illness experience, by gearing nursing practices to evolving such competencies through nurse-client interactions. (p. 6).
Inferred from Peplau's writings (Forchuk, 1993)	5. Psychodynamic nursing crosses all specialty areas of nursing. It is not synonymous with psychiatric nursing because every nurse–client relationship is an interpersonal situation in which recurring difficulties of everyday life arise (summarized from Peplau, 1952). 6. Difficulties in interpersonal relations recur in varying intensities throughout the life of everyone (Peplau, 1952, p. xiv). 7. The need to harness energy that derives from tension and anxiety connected to felt needs to positive means for defining, understanding, and meeting productively the problem at hand is a universal need (Peplau, 1952, p. 26). 8. All human behavior is purposeful and goal-seeking in terms of feelings of satisfaction and/or security (Peplau, 1952, p. 26). 9. The interaction of nurse and client is fruitful when a method of communication that identifies and uses common meanings is at work in the situation (Peplau, 1952, p. 284). 10. The meaning of behavior to the client is the only relevant basis on which nurses can determine needs to be met (Peplau, 1952, p. 226). 11. Each client will behave, during crisis, in a way that has worked in relation to crises faced in the past (Peplau, 1952, p. 255).
Inferred from Peplau's writings (Sellers, 1991)	12. The function of personality is to grow and to develop. Nursing is a process that seeks to facilitate development of personality by aiding individuals to use those compelling forces and experiences that influence personality in ways that ensure maximum productivity (p. 73). 13. Because illness is an event that is experienced along with feelings that derive from older experiences but are re-enacted in the relationship of nurse to patient, the nurse–patient relationship is an opportunity for nurses to help patients to complete the unfinished psychological tasks of childhood to some degree (p. 59).

The patient also needs to recognize and use the professional services offered. The nurse serves as a resource person to help the patient identify the range and limitations of available services. It is important for the patient to know what he or she can expect from the nurse. It is equally important that the patient understands the limitations in the health care environment, both situational (i.e., related to the routines) and cultural (i.e., related to the standards of conduct).

For the patient to move successfully to the next phase in the nurse–patient relationship, he or she must harness the energy from the tension and anxiety created by felt needs in a constructive fashion, to define, understand, and resolve the problem. The counseling role of the nurse is vital in dealing with patient's anxiety. The nurse must understand the meaning of the situation to the patient and be alert to evidence of anxiety manifested by apathy, dependency, or overaggressiveness. Anxiety can escalate to terror or panic if the patient fails to deal with it. As a resource person, the nurse helps the patient understand the meaning of the anxiety-promoting events he or she is experiencing in the health care environment. In the counseling role, the nurse encourages the expression of expectations and feelings by responding unconditionally to the patient. This response communicates to the patient that the focus of the relationship is on his or her needs, not those of the nurse. Through nondirective listening, the nurse encourages the patient to focus on the problem and express related feelings, without offering advice, reassurance, suggestions, or persuasions. This establishes the foundation for the work of the next phase of the relationship.

Phase of Identification. This phase begins after the patient has, to a degree, clarified first impressions and arrived at some understanding of what the situation has to offer. At this time, the patient can selectively begin to identify with some of the individuals who are offering help in one of three ways: with interdependence/participation, independence/isolation, or dependence/helplessness. This identification is based on the degree to which the patient believes the nurse will be helpful and on the nature of his or her past relationships.

The patient who responds interdependently feels more powerful, and identifies with and expresses the attitudes of cheerfulness, optimism, and problem-solving that he or she perceives in the nurse. Under these conditions, the patient may express feelings that are not normally considered acceptable (e.g., helplessness or self-centeredness). These expressions are seen as potentially growth-producing if the nurse accepts the feelings and continues to meet the needs of the patient.

Not all patients can identify with the nurse offering help because of the influence of earlier negative relationships with others. This experience often leads to a response that is independent or isolative. At this time, the nurse in the surrogate family member role may provide the patient with the opportunity to have new and more positive relational experiences.

Other patients may identify with the nurse too quickly, resulting in an overly dependent response to the nurse. These patients want all their needs to be met by others, with no expectations placed on them. This common response limits the possibility of growth through the experience.

It is important for the nurse to consider the phenomenon of leadership during the identification phase. The nurse attempts to provide opportunities for the patient to assume responsibility in the situation that promotes more constructive rather than imitative learning. The patient is encouraged to develop the skills to perceive, focus, and interpret cues in the situation, and then respond appropriately, independent of the nurse.

Phase of Exploitation. During this phase, the patient feels comfortable enough to take full advantage of the services being offered and to experience full value from the relationship with the nurse. Varying degrees of dependence and self-directedness are manifested by vacillation between the states.

Ideally, the patient begins to identify and orient to new goals beyond solving the immediate problem; for example, in the case of a hospitalized patient, the goal of functioning at home.

Phase of Resolution. As old needs are met, they are replaced by new goals that began to be formulated while the patient used the services provided by the nurse. It is hoped that the patient will experience a sense of security and release that occurs because help was received in the time of need. This security is accompanied by less reliance on and decreasing identification with helping persons, and increasing reliance on self to deal with the problem. This is the result of a nurse–patient relationship that is characterized during all phases by:

- An unconditional, patient-focused, and ongoing relationship that provides for the patient's needs
- A recognition of and appropriate response to cues that indicate the patient's desire and readiness to grow
- A shift of power from nurse to patient as patient assumes responsibility for achieving new goals (Peplau, 1991, pp. 40–41).

FULFILLED THROUGH NURSING ROLES

The roles of nursing are defined by nurses, endorsed by patients, influenced by society, and promoted by the professional literature. Peplau identified the roles that she considered most relevant to nurse–patient situations, and delineated principles for the successful fulfilling of those roles. The roles she identified were stranger, resource person, teacher, leader, surrogate, and counselor. Table 10-2 lists principles related to each role.

INFLUENCED BY PSYCHOBIOLOGICAL EXPERIENCES

The psychobiological experiences of needs, frustration, conflict, and anxiety influence the functioning of personalities. These experiences are also sources of energy that can result in both constructive and destructive actions. It is through understanding these experiences that individuals can learn to become more productive human beings (Peplau, 1991).

Needs. Though Peplau identifies needs as both physiological and psychological, her emphasis is on those that are psychological in nature. Security, new experiences, affection, recognition, and mastery are identified as psychological needs.

Needs create tension, which individuals strive to reduce through the expenditure of energy (behavior). Behavior is directed at meeting the uppermost need, which may leave other needs unrecognized. Underactivity and overactivity are ineffective ways of meeting unrecognized needs. Unmet needs, if persistent, can lead to ever-increasing tension or anxiety. When immediate needs are met, others emerge, some of which may be more consistent with promoting health (e.g., recovery and personality development).

Frustration. Frustration occurs when fulfillment of a need or pursuit of a goal is blocked. The primary goal identified by Peplau (1991) is the need for a "feeling of satisfaction and/or security"(p. 86). "Three interacting factors seem to determine the effects of frustration: 1) the degree, 2) the need that is not met, 3) the personality of the individual [e.g. frustration tolerance]" (Peplau, 1991, p. 94).

Frustration can be manifested as aggression and/or anxiety. Direct expression of aggression occurs when the source is identified and is the recipient of its expression; indirect expression of aggression

Table 10-2. ROLES IN NURSING

ROLE	PRINCIPLE	COMMENTS
Stranger	1. "Respect and positive interest accorded a stranger is at first nonpersonal and includes the same ordinary courtesies that are accorded a new guest who has been brought into any situation" (p. 44).	1. The patient is accepted as he/she is and related to as a capable individual, unless there is evidence to the contrary.
	2. "In communicating with a new patient, who is also a stranger, try to say whatever it is that you wish the patient to hear" (p. 46).	2. Inappropriate casual comments by the nurse can interfere with the development of the relationship.
	3. In a home, "accommodate to the direction of activity in the situation as [the nurse] finds it, await the development of good feeling, and then orient the family of the purpose of the visit and the services offered in a simple manner" (pp. 46–47).	3. Developing rapport promotes the establishment of identification with the nurse and the relationship can proceed to address the problems confronting the patient.
Resource person	1. "A resource person provides specific answers to questions usually formulated with relation to a larger problem" (p. 47).	1. The level of functioning, psychological readiness, psychological atmosphere, and the relevance of the question are determinants of the nature of the nurse's response to the questions. The goal of the response is constructive learning.
Teacher	1. "Teaching always proceeds from what the patient knows and it develops around his interest in wanting and being able to use additional medical information" (p. 48).	1. The nurse needs to attempt to develop learning situations that enable the patient to learn through experience.
Leader	1. A goal to pursue is "democratic leadership in nursing situations, [which] implies that the patient will be permitted to be an active participant in designing nursing plans for him" (p. 50).	1. This also assists the patient to learn problem solving.
	2. To promote democratic leadership the nurse needs "to be able to sit at the bedside of any patient, observe, and gather evidence on the way the patient views the situation confronting him, visualize what is happening inside the patient, as well as observe what is going on between them in the interpersonal relations" (p. 50).	2. This allows the nurse to recognize when the patient is overvaluing the nurse.

(Continued)

Table 10-2. ROLES IN NURSING (Continued)

ROLE	PRINCIPLE	COMMENTS
Surrogate	1. "A nurse helps the patient to learn that there are likenesses and differences between people by being herself" (p. 53).	1. This requires that the nurse is aware of how he/she behaves in relationships with others.
	2. "The nurse and patient relationship moves on a continuum" (p. 55).	2. The nurse attempts to move the relationship in the direction of chronological age appropriate relationships.
	3. "Surrogate roles are determined by psychological age factors that operate by reason of arrests in development, feelings that have been reactivated on the basis of illness, or demands made by individuals in a situation" (p. 55).	3. The patient psychologically substitutes the nurse for an individual from his/her past. This substitution affects the nursing situation.
	4. "...ways of responding, which do not impose goals that the nurse has in mind about how patients should feel, aid the patient in becoming aware of what is actually felt during the experience" (p. 56).	4. By not imposing goals on the patient the nurse frees him or her to make those judgments. This becomes a growth-producing experience.
	5. "Permitting the patient to re-experience older feelings in new situations of helplessness, but with professional acceptance and attention that provokes personality development, requires a relationship in which the nurse recognizes and responds in a variety of surrogate roles" (p. 57).	5. As the patient deals constructively with these feelings, the nurse may need to assume new surrogate roles that are based on greater patient autonomy.
	6. The nurse needs to consider the "perception of the role in which the patient casts the nurse, identification of the difficulty that is being worked through, and sustaining a working relationship that develops awareness in the patient of how he feels [about] nursing skills" (pp. 57–58).	6. This allows the nurse to develop learning experiences with patients making use of the nurse–patient relationship.
Counselor	1. "All counseling functions in nursing are determined by the purpose of all nurse–patient relationships, namely the promotion of experiences leading to health" (p. 61).	1. The functions include assisting the patient to recognize the conditions necessary for health, providing those when possible, helping the patient identify ongoing threats to health, and using the nurse–patient relationship to promote learning.
	2. "Counseling in nursing has to do with helping the patient to remember and to understand fully what is happening to him in the present situation" (p. 64).	2. This enables the experience to be integrated rather than dissociated from other life experiences.

(Continued)

Table 10-2. ROLES IN NURSING (Continued)

ROLE	PRINCIPLE	COMMENTS
	3. Helping a patient to become aware of real feelings related to an event in an immediate way is a counseling function (p. 67).	3. Feelings not acknowledged will be pushed into the unconscious and can function to distort other feeling experiences and relationships.
	4. "Observation [and listening] precedes interpretation of the collected data" (p. 64).	4. By using nondirective and nonmoralizing listening, the patient can discover aspects of self previously unknown, a process that is quite therapeutic.

Source: Peplau, H. E. (1991). *Interpersonal relations in nursing: A conceptual frame of reference for psychodynamic nursing.* New York: Springer.

occurs when the recipient only resembles the original source. The intensity of the expression varies, based on the degree to which the recipient resembles the original source. The greater the resemblance, the higher the intensity is. More intense aggression results in a threat to the goals of safety or security and can be directed at self or others.

Anxiety is a result of repeated frustrations that are perceived as failure to accomplish goals. Because the experience of anxiety is difficult to tolerate, the individual defends self from it by: (1) modifying the goal to one for which success is more likely; (2) giving up on the goal, with the possibility of dissociation of feelings occurring; and/or (3) adopting fixed responses (e.g., stereotyping, delusions).

The nurse may discover that his or her goals and those of the patient are not mutual. In fact, the nurse's goals may be perceived as an obstacle by the patient. It is important for the nurse and patient to communicate to clarify goals and arrive at some mutually acceptable ones.

Conflict. Another issue that the nurse and patient deal with in their interpersonal relationship is conflicting goals. Conflicting goals are often unrecognized and are expressed in the behavioral responses of hesitation, tension, vacillation, or complete blocking.

Blocking occurs when approaching a goal is completely incompatible with avoiding another one (approach–avoidance conflict). The most common example is the desire to go home (approaching goal) that coexists with the desire to not leave the perceived safety of the hospital (avoiding goal). Fear results and intensifies when approaching a goal for which there is a conflicting goal of avoiding. This fear can express itself as withdrawal or avoidance. If the fear is external to the patient and can be identified, the nurse can act as a resource person by providing information and experiences to reduce the strength of avoidance. If the source of the fear cannot be identified, it is referred to as anxiety and is likely an internal conflict that is more difficult to resolve.

Individuals often are required to make choices between two desirable goals (approach–approach conflict). This is manifested with slightly different behavioral responses; for example, ignoring the feelings about the desired goals or keeping them from conscious awareness. The nurse is most helpful by fulfilling the counselor role in this situation. Listening in a way that encourages the expression of feelings allows the individual to recognize the factors that influence the choice to be made.

Unexplained Discomfort/Anxiety. As previously noted, anxiety or "unexplained discomfort," as Peplau sometimes referred to it, can occur when there are unmet needs, obstacles to goals, or conflicting goals. Anxiety is often associated with guilt, doubt, fears, and obsessions. Both patients and nurses experience this feeling state, which influences behavior productively or destructively through the energy it produces.

Peplau (1991) identifies two principles that nurses can use to help patients use anxiety productively:

1. "When anxiety is held within tolerable limits it can be a functionally effective element in interpersonal relations" (p. 127).
2. As anxiety increases in severity, there is a narrowing of perceptual awareness.

Mild anxiety can manifest itself as restlessness, sleeplessness, hostility, misunderstanding, repeated questioning, seeking attention, or reassurance. This level of anxiety also creates a felt need that can serve as a source of motivation for personality growth. If the nurse provides the help needed, the patient can begin to identify and deal with the anxiety-producing situation. In contrast to mild anxiety, severe anxiety can be crippling and incapacitating. The patient cannot collaborate with the nurse, and useful learning cannot take place. The nurse helps reduce the anxiety to a more manageable and useful level by his or her presence, as someone who will listen and provide for the patient's physical needs.

The ability of the nurse to be helpful to the patient during the experiences of anxiety is predicated on his or her self-understanding. "If a nurse has developed ability to undergo tension and stress, in order to identify a difficulty that she feels and to take steps that lead to a course of action based on evidence of what is involved, she will be able to help patients to do likewise" (Peplau, 1991, p. 135). Peplau (1991) summarized the responsibility of the nurse in assisting the patient experiencing anxiety in the form of a "hypothesis":

> Nurses face the task of developing experiences with patients that aid them to discriminate aspects of a total experience, to understand what is happening in their relations with nurses, and to develop ways that convert tension and anxiety into purposeful action. (p. 130)

REQUIRES ATTENDING TO CERTAIN PSYCHOLOGICAL TASKS

Psychological tasks are those related to learning to live with others. Peplau addresses the tasks of:

- Learning to count on others
- Learning to delay satisfaction
- Identifying oneself
- Developing skills in participation.

These tasks occur not only as an aspect of the development of personality, but also as features of nurse–patient relationships. During this relationship, the nurse has the opportunity to help patients develop in areas of task deficit. To provide this assistance, the nurse uses the previously discussed roles and understanding of the previously examined psychobiological experiences. Additionally, to understand his or her own personality and the patient's, the nurse needs to appreciate the "dynamic interaction that occurs in early infancy and childhood as personality is undergoing formation" (Peplau, 1991, p. 162).

Peplau (1991, p. 166) based her conceptualizations of psychological tasks on the works of Sigmund Freud and Richard Havighurst:

> The infant's biological functioning and the need for acculturation set up certain require-
> ments or psychological tasks, which every infant and child must undergo with relative
> success in order to develop a sound basis for mature functioning of personality as an
> adult (Peplau, 1991, p. 165).

The acculturation processes of children are general in nature and include both family members' and surrogates' expressions of feelings, attitudes, and ideas.

Counting on Others. This is the first psychological task of the infant. Initially, comfort and discomfort are the only feeling states experienced. If the caregiver (mother) appreciates the feelings of discomfort being communicated, responds unconditionally, and in a way consistent with the infant's biological make-up, the infant learns to rely on the caregiver for help. Thus, dependency is learned in an unambiguous fashion. Healthy dependence is not the only possible outcome of a mother's response to the child's needs. If there is maternal rejection and/or overprotection, an ongoing need for dependency may develop. An individual's longing for dependency operates as a persistent need, resulting from a denial that help is needed or would be useful, or a belief that others will be able to identify and meet needs without his or her attempts to communicate them.

The nurse encounters varying degrees of both healthy dependency and dependency longings in nursing situations.

> Nurses have two responsibilities in their relations with patients who express longings for
> dependence: (1) to help the patient to learn that nurses can be counted on for help when
> needed; ... (2) to aid the patient to become aware of his wants and to improve his ways of
> expressing what those wants are. (Peplau, 1991, p. 181)

There are a number of positive consequences of having needs met. The patient experiences a feeling of self-worth and, as a result, begins to collaborate with the nurse in his or her growth. As needs are met, new, more mature ones can emerge.

Delaying Satisfaction. The socialization of a child includes the lesson of deferring to the wishes of others and delaying gratification of his or her own wishes, a lesson dependent on having already learned that those being deferred to are also those who can also be counted upon. According to Peplau (1991), this lesson takes place primarily during the process of toilet training. A rigorous and rigid form of training may inhibit the child's natural desire to explore this newly developing skill (i.e., producing feces) and can result in a sense of powerlessness. By contrast,

> Every child will learn to accept interference [with his/her own wishes] as inevitable, rea-
> sonable, perhaps useful life experience, if personality is not threatened and if anxiety and
> conflict are not generated through the use of mother love as a barter in the learning
> process. (Peplau, 1991, pp. 193–194)

During the toilet training experience, the child has three possible responses: (1) adapt his or her needs to those of family, and gradually learn to behave in a way consistent with family members with whom he or she identifies; (2) give up feelings of power and comply with others' demands; or (3) refuse to give up power, becoming defiant and resistant. The latter two responses result in distorted relations with others and unresolved personality issues that persist into adulthood. The nurse may note these issues manifested in patients who are exploitive and manipulative, those who hoard and withhold, being unable to share (including the inability to share feelings), and those who alter their responses to others in a way that indicates a lack of stability and consistency in personality structure.

To respond in growth-producing ways to patients exhibiting these behaviors, nurses need insight into their own character traits and the ways they relate to others. With this insight, a nurse can modify his or her own behavior, a process that, once learned, can be used to help others modify their behaviors. Peplau (1991, p. 206) also identifies additional principles that are consistent with healthy toilet training and general socialization activities that help the nurse establish rapport with the patient:

- Show unconditional interest and acceptance.
- Encourage expression of needs and feelings.
- Provide times in which demands are met and times in which they are not met.
- Promote participation in decision making so patients can become more self-directing.
- Allow for some "hoarding," which reinforces feelings of security.
- Encourage sharing, which can only occur when there is freedom from coercion.

When rapport between the nurse and patient has been developed, a rapport that allows them to "understand each other's preconceptions and expectations, it is possible for the nurse anticipatorily to suggest interferences and delays in meeting needs and requests" (Peplau, 1991, p. 206).

Identifying Oneself. Self identity or concept of self enhances or distorts relationships with others, a fact that is true for both the patient and the nurse. This sense of self develops initially through a child's interactions with adults as he or she learns to rely on others and to delay gratification in relation to needs. The way the child is appraised during these interactions results in three possible views of self: (1) *a sense of competency* to identify wants and needs, communicate them to others, and receive needed assistance; (2) *a sense of helplessness and dependence* on others to provide what is needed, and a belief that this helplessness will produce a sense of safety (because making no demands will result in not being deserted); and (3) *a sense of distrust* in others as a source of assistance that results in independently taking what is needed.

This appraisal by others and its significance to the child intensifies during the genital phase of psychosocial development. During this phase, the child discovers, explores, and finds pleasure in his or her genitalia. Ideally, the child is also introduced to other experiences that provide pleasure and is allowed the freedom of make decisions about their pursuit. If this does not occur, and, instead, the child is coerced into certain activities and blocked from others, he or she will experience frustration.

> When a child needs to focus all of his activities in the direction of getting and sustaining approval, or avoiding anxiety connected with disapproval, from parents or surrogates, his concept of self cannot expand beyond what works and is acceptable to the adults upon whom he must count for feelings of safety or security (Peplau, 1991, p. 219).

These concepts of self are established in childhood but can be reinforced or modified by experiences with others throughout life.

The nurse can provide experiences that help the patient develop a concept of self that facilitates the establishment of interdependent relationships with others. To provide the appropriate experiences, the nurse needs to understand the patient's self-perception. Peplau (1992) suggests a number of activities that help the nurse understand a patient's self concept:

- Consider own response to patient as a source of information about the patient's perceptions of self and situation confronting him or her.

- Develop self-awareness of own habits (e.g., regarding cleanliness) and how they are expressed in the nursing situation.
- Identify patient's patterns of feeling expressions and other behavioral responses as he or she encounters situational challenges.
- Consider patient's specific responses to the nursing situation as indicators of needs to be met.

In addition, the nurse can be helpful to the patient by:

- Being value neutral, "...providing merely conditions and acting as a sounding board against which the patient may air his views and give full expression to his feelings in a nonjudgmental relationship" (Peplau, 1991, p. 226).
- Communicating hope and acceptance.
- Avoiding the problematic responses of praise, blame, and indifference.

The nurse who exhibits these characteristics can enhance the patient's whole concept of self and, as a result of this enhanced self-concept, the patient will experience more interdependent and mutually productive relationships with others.

Participating with Others. When individuals participate in making decisions that affect them, they are more likely to understand the decisions, be involved in implementing them, and appreciate the contributions of others to the ultimate decision. The task of learning to participate with others initially occurs during what Sullivan refers to as the "juvenile era," (ages 6–9 years). This task of participating with others comprises the abilities to (a) *compromise*, arbitrate, make personal concessions; (b) *compete*, express rivalry, struggle with peers; and (c) *cooperate,* subordinate individual wishes to achieve mutually beneficial goals. The process of developing these skills is influenced by the appraisals of parents and peers. Children will act out in their relationships the lessons about self and others that those appraisals taught.

Following the juvenile era is what Sullivan calls "preadolescence" (ages 8½–12 years). During this time, the abilities to participate with others are consolidated in a process referred to as consensual validation. The view of self becomes more consistent with the views of peers and a more realistic perspective of life and one's role in it develops. It is also at this time that a child begins to be able to care for and accept others, occurring to the degree that he or she cares for and accepts self.

In the therapeutic interpersonal relationship, the nurse attempts to encourage participation with others through collaboration with the patient in addressing his or her problems. This participatory approach serves to improve the patient's skills in meeting problems. Peplau (1991) describes a three-step process:

1. Assist the patient to identify the problem.
2. Collaborate to "achieve a decision on what is possible, what can be done, and then move into other items that have been mentioned and other *possible courses of action* that can be taken in behalf of and with the co-operation of the patient" (p. 248).
3. Encourage patient to try out what has been proposed.

As part of the process of identifying the problem, the nurse will need to assess the patient's attitude, because attitude will affect the way the patient attempts to solve the problem. The two most common attitudes are overconcern or underconcern. If overconcerned, the patient may attempt to arrive at a solution too quickly, and the solution will be inadequate. If underconcerned, the patient may not invest sufficient energy in its solution, and the solution will be superficial.

In formulating a possible solution to the problem, the nurse needs to allow the patient to determine the pace for working through it. Time pressures are often communicated by the nurse in the form of suggestions about what is wrong, and advice as to what needs to be done, leading to premature and ineffective solutions. "The process for recognition and solutions of a problem, like the processes of self-renewal, self-repair, self-awareness, arise within the individual" (Peplau, 1991, p. 251).

Nurses can help patients to experience the process of problem solving and to develop the skills needed to actively participate in a solution. The inability to participate with others in problem solving comes with negative consequences. "Ineffective participation in life impedes the development of a democratic society in which all are free to grow, to change, to mature, and to design a way of life that ensures productive relations among people" (Peplau, 1991, p. 147).

NURSING METHODS USED TO UNDERSTAND INTERPERSONAL PROCESSES

Observation, communication, and recording are three basic skills that are "valuable to the use of nursing as an interpersonal process that is therapeutic and educative for patients" (Peplau, 1991, p. 309). Peplau considered these three operations as integral to the nursing process.

Observation. "The aim of observation in nursing, when it is viewed as an interpersonal process, is the identification, clarification, and verification of impressions about the interactive drama, of the pushes and pulls in the relationship between nurse and patient, as they occur" (Peplau, 1991, p. 263). Observation as described by Peplau comprises four components:

1. Intuitive impressions
2. Hypothesis statements
3. Organized observations
4. Judgment formations.

Intuitive impressions are hunches or generalizations about what is occurring in an experience. They are an important component of understanding the problems of patients. Impressions are the foundation for the development of hypotheses, and it is hypotheses that provide a means of reducing the risk of prematurely concentrating on details of the situation. Concentrating on details is more likely to lead to rationalization than to understanding of what has been observed. When the impressions or generalizations are formulated as a hypothesis, they serve to provide a useful focus to the observations. The nurse proceeds to gather evidence related to the hypotheses (units of experience), providing both elaboration of the whole impression and differentiation of the details.

Peplau (1991) provides a classification of types of observer-observed relationships that the nurse can use to gather evidence:

- Spectator. The patient is unaware of being observed. The nurse generally is engaged in another activity while observing the patient.
- Interviewer. The patient is aware of being observed as he or she responds to the situation or to the directive or nondirective questioning of the nurse. The nurse frequently takes notes while observing as an interviewer.
- Collector. The nurse uses records and reports created by others as a way of determining what has happened in a particular situation. Observations made using this approach can help form partial impressions.

- Participant. "The nurse engages in ordinary activities connected with nursing a patient and at the same time observes the relationship between the patient and herself" (Peplau, 1991, p. 274). The patient is aware that nursing care is being given but is unaware that his or her responses are being observed.

Participant observation is further described as composed of three foci: the nurse, the patient, and the relations (Peplau, 1997, p. 162). During participant observation, in addition to noting the behaviors of the patient, the nurse is required to undergo self-scrutiny, observing and analyzing his or her own behavior. By attending to that behavior, the nurse can evaluate its usefulness in the relationship and modify it if appropriate.

The observations need to be organized. Organization helps provide focus to the multiplicity and complexity of the observations of human behavior in interpersonal relationships. Peplau (1991) suggests hypotheses and the phases of the nurse–patient relationship as two approaches to organizing observations. This organization of observations made through participant observation is the basis of all nursing judgments in practice. "Observation and understanding of what is observed are essential operations for making judgments and for designing experiences with patients that aid them in the solution of their problems" (Peplau, 1991, p. 289).

There are two types of judgments that occur during a therapeutic relationship with a patient: judgments in practice and judgments in fact. The judgments in practice, based on interpretation of observations, are more situationally specific. The judgments in fact, based on objective data, are less situationally specific. Judgments in practice exist when:

- Situations demand a decision as to what action a nurse should take.
- Even though policies exist as a guide to nursing action, nurses need to make appropriate choices between alternative actions.
- Choices depend upon the interpretation of facts.

Judgments in fact occur when:

- The facts further limit choices.
- The facts identify the possibilities and limitations of actions.

Communication. One of the basic tools of nursing is communication, requiring "awareness of means of communication; spoken language, rational and nonrational expressions of wishes, needs, and desires, and the body gesture" (Peplau, 1991, p. 289). Use of words or verbal communication can convey facts, focus on every day events, and provide interpretations. Spoken language can reveal personal realities or express hidden meanings, but it can also avoid conveying anything meaningful.

There are two main principles for effective verbal communication: clarity and continuity. Clarity occurs when there is a common frame of reference or when specific efforts are made to arrive at mutual understanding. "Clarity is promoted when the meaning to the patient is expressed and talked over and a new view is expanded in awareness" (Peplau, 1991, p. 291). Continuity occurs when the connections between ideas and the related feelings, events, or themes expressed through the ideas is made evident. "Continuity is promoted when the nurse is able to pick up threads of conversation [that occur over time]...and when she aids the patient to focus and to expand these threads" (Peplau, 1991, p. 293).

Following up on what patients say communicates that what they said is important and that as individuals they are worthwhile.

In the process of promoting clarity and continuity in communication, nurses need to understand more than what the patient communicates directly. The nurse must also be able to interpret symbols to arrive at the hidden meanings of patients' indirect communications. Self-awareness is one of the primary conditions for achieving this understanding.

> Consciousness of meaning and use of words requires awareness of self. Ability to recognize meaning and the actions implied in words, or concepts, or principles, and to relate them to everyday nursing practices improves practices at the same time leading to sounder personality organization. (Peplau, 1991, pp. 297–298)

For a nurse, this awareness enables him or her to express congruence in the use of words, their relevance, and related actions.

> Awareness is also the primary distinction between rational and nonrational expressions. *Rational* attitudes and communication are those of which the participant is aware, recognizing connections between the meaning of an idea and the actions related to it, or between the behavior expressed and the traits of character of the individual whose behavior is being studied. *Nonrational* attitudes and communications are governed by traits of character of which the subject is unaware; they often govern behavior that occurs automatically, without recognition of underlying relationships. (Peplau, 1991, p. 298. Used by permission.)

Rational expressions more likely occur when individuals see themselves rather than others as a source of personal security, and when they are oriented toward the future in the context of the present rather than the past.

Nonrational expressions communicate in more ambiguous and indirect ways than do rational expressions. Longings, hopes, and fears are often conveyed in a disguised form. Myths, dreams, rituals, and folk tales are examples of culturally shared nonrational communication. Nonrational expressions can also be specific to an individual. In either case, the nurse attempts to interpret the meaning of the language by considering the symbols being used. Interestingly, Peplau provided interpretations of dreams for her friends and colleagues (Spray, 1999).

In addition to the spoken word, gestures can be considered either rational or nonrational expressions. "The body as a whole, as well as parts of it, act as expressional instruments that communicate to others the feelings, wishes, and aspirations of an individual" (Peplau, 1991, p. 304). Underactivity and overactivity are examples of whole body gestures. Hand gestures (e.g., clenched fist) and facial grimaces (e.g., biting a lip) are examples of more specific gestures. The nurse's responsibility is to observe gestures and to attempt to understand both what he or she and the patient are communicating to each other. Arriving at understanding or meaning is a complicated and ongoing process of observation and communication.

Recording. Peplau focuses primarily on recording for the purpose of student learning. In addition to charting in medical records, students need additional forms for recording what has occurred between student and patient. These additional recordings provide a means of examining the relationship for insight into the student nurse's own behavior and the ways in which the patients responded. They also can help the student develop skills in observation by using hypotheses and units of observation as a structure for the recording. How useful the recording is to the student's development of interpersonal skills is dependent in part on the exactness of the wording of the recording. To produce an exact record, Peplau suggests recall but also "wire recordings," "television and motion pictures," and the use of another student to observe and document the interaction between the student nurse and the patient. The ultimate goal of recordings, as well as observation and communication, is nurse–patient relationships that result in improved health outcomes for the patient.

APPLICATIONS OF THE THEORY

Peplau is frequently cited in the nursing literature, though the majority of the literature focuses on applications to practice rather than use in nursing research. Sills (1978) found 93 references to Peplau's theory in articles published in three journals: 43 were published in *American Journal of Nursing* (1952–1977); 27 were published in *Nursing Outlook* (1952–1977); and 23 were published in *Perspectives of Psychiatric Care* (1963–1977). A search of the CINAHL database found 69 publications from 1988 through 2002 related to Peplau's Theory of Interpersonal Relations. Articles published in Spain, Italy, Great Britain, Slovenia, and China were among those cited. The articles focused on the life and works of Peplau, her theory, her theory applied to research, and most commonly, her theory used in practice.

Lego (1980) found similar rates of publication. Of the 166 papers (1952–1979) reviewed with a clinical focus on the one-to-one nurse–patient relationship, students or colleagues of Peplau wrote 78. Most of the work reviewed and analyzed demonstrated little or no linkage to the work of other nursing scientists. If literature was cited, it was most often from other disciplines.

Three types of papers on the one-to-one nurse–patient relationship were identified:

1. *Care or case study,* in which the author describes a difficult patient situation, discusses the nursing interventions used, and shares his or her learning from the situation.
2. *Concept presentation,* in which the author reviews the relevant literature, provides operational definition, uses vignettes to illustrate the concept, and recommends nursing interventions.
3. *Hypothesis testing,* in which the author makes an empirical observation of a clinical phenomenon, generates a hypothesis that is supported through further investigation, and draws conclusions that can be used to guide practice (Lego, 1980, pp. 80–81).

The volume of literature on Peplau's theory reflects its popularity with practicing nurses, particularly those practicing psychiatric–mental health nursing. Surveys of psychiatric nurses in Canada and the United States have found more than half of them claiming to use Peplau's theory in their practices (Forchuk, 1993, p. 28). Some recent examples of applications to practice include use of the theory: (a) in development of relationships in the community (McCann & Baker, 2001); (b) with patients diagnosed with multiple sclerosis (McGuinness & Peters, 1999); (c) in body image care (Price, 1998); (d) with individuals who have problems with alcohol (Buswell, 1997); (e) with families (Forchuk & Dorsay, 1995); (f) with stroke patients (Jones, 1995); (g) with an individual with AIDS (Hall, 1994), and (h) in case management (Forchuk et al., 1989).

Peplau's contributions to nursing are not limited to the content of her theory. She is credited with promoting the "scholarship of nursing practice" (Reed, 1996), integrating nursing practice with the ongoing development of nursing's knowledge base.

> Peplau introduced an approach to knowledge development that was anchored in nursing practice, and in the science and art of the nurse-patient interaction. Development and testing of explanations through the interpersonal process between patient and nurse was done for therapeutic purposes. ...it can be seen that this interpersonal process is also a strategy for generating nursing knowledge, which can then be examined further and refined through research. (Reed, 1996, Used with permission.)

This approach to converting practice knowledge into general nursing knowledge involves a three-step process:

1. *Observation of fundamental units.* The nurse generally assumes the role of participant observer, focusing on relevant units of observation. The units are defined as those that are useful to patients, understandable to all involved in the study, measurable to allow for objective and reliable categorization, and satisfactory to allow for comparison with other data (Peplau, 1991, pp. 270–271).
2. *Peeling out theoretical explanations.* The nurse applies knowledge from practice and relevant theories to interpret what has been observed. The interpretations become hypotheses that are "validated with the patient and tested for their meaningfulness and usefulness in the context of the nurse–patient relationship" (Reed, 1996, Step 2: Peeling Out Theoretical Explanations, para. 2).
3. *Transforming energy and transforming knowledge.* The nurse uses theoretical knowledge in interactions with patients as a means of transforming knowledge that is theoretical into knowledge that is practical. The critical test of this nursing knowledge is not whether it is consistent with theoretical perspectives but whether it can be used constructively by and with the patient.

These steps initiate what Reed (1996, Cycle of Inquiry, para. 1) refers to as a cycle of inquiry in which "nursing knowledge that is generated through practice is further refined through research" and then used to enhance nursing practice.

Though Peplau's theory has had a significant impact on nursing practice and has influenced nursing's research methodology, it has not generated a large number of research studies. It is surprising, given the theory's popularity as a topic in clinically-based articles and nursing texts, that there is so little empirical testing of Peplau's theory of the nurse–patient relationship. Forchuk is the major exception. She is acknowledged as having the most extensive and sustained research agenda of Peplau's theory (Young, Taylor, & Renpenning, 2001), as Table 10-3 illustrates.

Forchuk and her colleagues' work has focused on the factors that influence the development of a therapeutic nurse–client relationship. Using Middle Range Theories 10-1 provides a description of one of their published studies.

Consistent with the few research studies of Peplau's theory, only a limited number of instruments have been identified as applicable to the Theory of Interpersonal Relations. Instrument development to study the nurse–patient relationship began in the 1960s and continued into the late 1980s. Table 10-4 provides an overview of those instruments.

This limited number of instruments and quantitative studies of Peplau's theory of interpersonal relations may be explained in part by the phenomenological nature of the theory (Haber, 2000) and in part by its complexity.

"Optimistically, legitimatization of practice-derived theory in the 1990s will make theory-testing and hypothesis-generating qualitative research related to Peplau's model a priority for nurse researchers in the new millennium" (Haber, 2000, pp. 59–60). Peplau and others have suggested re-

Table 10-3. EXAMPLES OF RESEARCH ON INTERPERSONAL RELATIONS

CITATION	FOCUS
Vogelsang, J. (1990). Continued contact with a familiar nurse affects women's perceptions of the ambulatory surgical experience: A qualitative design. *Journal of Post Anesthesia Nursing, 5*(5) 315–320.	Impact of familiar nurse working with ambulatory surgical patients from preadmission through discharge
Forchuk, C. (1992). The orientation phase of the nurse–client relationship: How long does it take? *Perspectives in Psychiatric Care, 28*(4), 7–10.	The length of the orientation phase of patients diagnosed with depression or schizophrenia in a community health program
Forchuk, C. (1994). The orientation phase of the nurse–client relationship: Testing Peplau's theory. *Journal of Advanced Nursing, 20*(3), 532–537.	Patient and nurse intrapersonal factors (e.g., preconceptions) that influence the development of a therapeutic relationship during the orientation phase
Forchuk, C. (1995). Development of nurse–client relationships: What helps. *Journal of American Psychiatric Nurses Association, 1*(5), 146–151.	Factors (e.g., length of previous hospitalizations, age of nurse and patient, and amount of meeting time) that influence progress of a therapeutic relationship during the orientation phase
Morrison, E. G., Shealy, A. H., Kowalski, C., LaMont, J., & Range, B. A. (1996). Workroles of staff nurses in psychiatric settings. *Nursing Science Quarterly, 9*(1),17–21.	Role behaviors of psychiatric staff nurses in interactions with adult, child, and adolescent psychiatric patients as compared to those conceptualized by Peplau
Forchuk, C., Westfall, J., Martin, M., Bamber-Azzapardi, W., Kosterewa-Tolman, D., & Hux, M. (1998). Factors influencing movement of chronic psychiatric patients from the orientation to the working phase of the nurse–client relationship of an inpatient unit. *Perspectives in Psychiatric Care, 34*(1), 36–44.	Factors that influence movement from the orientation to working phase of the nurse–client relationship
Jacobson, G. (1999). Parenting processes: A descriptive explanatory study using Peplau's theory. *Nursing Science Quarterly, 12*, 240–244.	Qualities that were considered examples of positive parenting by recently graduated high school students
Middleton, J., Steward, N., & Richardson, J. (1999). Caregiver distress related to disruptive behaviors on special care units versus traditional long-care units. *Journal of Gerontological Nursing, 2*(3), 11–19.	Perceptions of formal caregivers on units for dementia patients in long-term care facility
Williams, C., & Tappen, R. (1999). Can we create a therapeutic relationship with nursing home residents in the later stages of Alzheimer's disease? *Journal of Psychosocial Nursing, 37*(3), 28–35.	Behaviors exhibited by patients diagnosed with Alzheimer's disease during one-to-one interactions over a 16-week period
Edwards, K. (2000). Service users and mental health nursing. *Journal of Psychiatric & Mental Health Nursing, 7*, 555–565.	Views and perceived needs of users of mental health services in the context of the role that users see nurses fulfilling as identified by the users themselves

(Continued)

Table 10-3. EXAMPLES OF RESEARCH ON INTERPERSONAL RELATIONS (*Continued*)

CITATION	FOCUS
Forchuk, C., Westfall, J., Martin, M., Bamber-Azzapardi, W., Kosterewa-Tolman, D., & Hux, M. (2000). The developing nurse–client relationship: Nurses' perceptions. *Journal of Psychiatric & Mental Health Nursing, 6*(1), 3–10.	Perspectives of nurses in a tertiary care hospital on the nature and progression of the nurse–client relationship, and the factors that facilitate or interfere with the development of the relationship
Forchuk, C., & Reynolds, W. (2001). Clients' reflections on relationships with nurses: Comparisons from Canada and Scotland. *Journal of Psychiatric & Mental Health Nursing, 8*(1), 45–51.	Comparison of what clients from Canada and Scotland want and do not want in relationships with nurses
Kai, J., and Crosland, A. (2002). People with enduring health problems described the importance of communication, continuity of care, and stigma. *Evidence-Based Nursing, 5*(3), 93(1).	Significance of therapeutic relationships in maintaining contacts with primary care and mental health services for individuals with chronic mental illness

search needs or questions for this new millennium. Peplau (1964) identified the following questions for nurses in general hospital settings:

- How do nurses distinguish between a demand and a need of a patient?
- What is the language behavior during the nurse–patient exchange in the general hospital?
- How do patients develop sufficient flexibility to incorporate body image changes into views of self after major surgery or major life experiences? What nursing interventions are most helpful to patients during this process?

Lego (1980) recommended questions for further study of psychiatric nursing:

1. How does the practice of psychiatric nursing through the one-to-one relationship differ from the practice of one-to-one relationships with psychiatrist and patient, psychologist and patient, or social worker and patient?
2. What exactly does or should take place in the one-to-one relationship? Can this process be measured?
3. Are certain patients susceptible to change while others are not?

 10-1 USING MIDDLE RANGE THEORIES

The researchers using qualitative methods studied the factors that influenced movement of nurse–patient dyads from Peplau's orientation phase to working phase. The three questions that this study was designed to answer were:

1. What seems to help the movement from the orientation to working phase?
2. What seems to hamper the movement from the orientation to the working phase?
3. What is the nature of the therapeutic relationship in the working phase?

(Continued) **10-1 USING MIDDLE RANGE THEORIES**

The sample consisted of 10 newly formed nurse–client dyads, with clients admitted to either admission or long-term care units at a tertiary care psychiatric hospital in Canada. The clients were diagnosed with schizophrenia or major mood disorders. Data were collected, using audiotaped unstructured interviews of clients. The open-ended questions focused on the clients' perceptions of what was occurring in the nurse–client relationship. Determination of movement into the working phase of the relationship was made by mutual agreement of the client, nurse, and researcher. Interviews were transcribed, using Martin v2 software for coding and development of themes. The nurse researchers arrived at consensus to identify the themes.

Seven of the 10 dyads reached the working phase of the nurse–patient relationship during the one year of the study. "...availability, consistency, and trust in the nurse were perceived to be important factors moving relationships from the orientation to the working phase" (Factors That Helped Movement from Orientation to Working Phase, para. 6). The factors that were identified as barriers to movement to the working phase of the relationship were lack of availability, sense of distance/inequity, differences in realities/values, and mutual withdrawal. The clients in the working phase described feelings of closeness, genuine liking, and trust of the nurses. The nurses were described as safe, dependable, interested, sociable and friendly (but not a friend). In general, nursing behaviors were found to have an impact on the development of a working relationship with clients.

Forchuk, C., Westwell, J., Martin, M., Azzapardi, W., Kosterewa-Tolman, D., & Hux, M. (1998). Factors influencing movement of chronic psychiatric patients from the orientation to the working phase of the nurse-client relationship on an inpatient unit. *Perspectives in Psychiatric Care, 34*(1), 36ff. Retrieved September 23, 2002 from *http://web1.infotrac.gale-group.library.bethel.edu/itw/infomark.*

4. What kind of educational and experiential background should the nurse have? What variables affect success? What is success?
5. How does the one-to-one relationship fit into the current and the future health care delivery system (pp. 81–82)?

Perhaps the most fundamental and pervasive question that researchers of the nurse–patient relationship can ask and attempt to answer is, "What aspects of the nurse–patient relationship contribute to the welfare and well-being of patients?" (Caris-Verhallen, Kerkstra, & Bensing, 1997). The promotion of the welfare of patients is core to all nursing theories, but for Peplau the means of achieving that goal focus on the attributes and behaviors of both the nurse and the patient and in the dynamic interaction that occurs between the two of them.

One of the attributes of nurses, cited by Peplau (1991, p. 135) as helpful to patients experiencing anxiety, is self-knowledge. Research Application 10-1 is designed to examine the relationship between nurses' self-knowledge and the relief of patient's anxiety.

TABLE 10-4. INSTRUMENTS USED TO TEST THEORY OF INTERPERSONAL RELATIONS

INSTRUMENT	REFERENCE	DESCRIPTION
Social Interaction Inventory	Methven, D., & Schlotfeldt, R. (1962). The social interaction inventory. *Nursing Research, 11*(2), 83–88.	Inventory comprised of 30 common nurse–patient situations in which the stress faced by the patient and his/her family is identified. For each situation, responses representing five different types are given (i.e., expression of concern that encourages verbalization; expression of sympathy and giving reassurance; inquiry into tangential aspects of the situation; explanations, justifications or defense of nurse's point of view; rejection or denunciation of patient's need). Validity described.
Therapeutic Behavior Scale	Spring, R., & Turk, H. (1962). A therapeutic behavior scale. *Nursing Research, 11*(4), 214–218.	Tool to rate nurses' responses to patients as therapeutic or nontherapeutic in relation to approach, level, topic, focus, and consistency. Validity and reliability data included.
Facilitative Level of a Therapeutic Relationship	Aiken, L., & Aiken, J. (1973). A systematic approach to the evaluation of interpersonal relationships. *American Journal of Nursing, 73*, 863–867.	Tool to evaluate the implementation of the five core dimensions (empathetic understanding, positive regard, genuineness, concreteness, and self-exploration) using a 5-point scale of descriptors of nurse's or patient's behaviors. No data on validity or reliability included.
Working Alliance Inventory (WAI)	Horvath, A. O., & Greenberg, L. (1986). The development of the Working Alliance Inventory. In L. Greenberg & W. Pinsof, (Eds.), *Psychotherapeutic process: A research handbook* (pp. 529–556). New York: Guilford Press.	36-item instrument, with parallel forms for client and therapist to self-report sense of bonding and tasks and goals of the developing therapeutic relationship. Validity and reliability data included.
Relationship Form	Forchuk, C., & Brown, B. (1989). Establishing a nurse–client relationship. *Journal of Psychosocial Nursing, 27*(2), 30–34.	7-point analog scale of the stages of the nurse–patient relationship, using brief descriptions of both the nurse's and client's roles at each stage. Validity and reliability data provided.

SUMMARY

Peplau is acknowledged as the first theorist of the modern era of nursing. Her theory of interpersonal relations in nursing focuses on the stages experienced, the nursing roles used, and the issues addressed in the context of the nurse–patient relationship. Though Peplau's work has not attracted the attention of nurse researchers that it would seem to warrant, her theory of interpersonal relations is widely taught in schools of nursing and extensively used in practice. In the nursing profession, the primacy

10-1 RESEARCH APPLICATION

A research study was designed to answer the question: Is there a relationship between the self-knowledge of psychiatric clinical nurse specialists serving as therapists in out-patient settings and relief of symptoms of patients diagnosed with anxiety disorders? Twenty nurse–patient dyads are recruited from four hospital-based clinics and four community-based, freestanding clinics in a metropolitan setting. To be included as a dyad, the nurse needs to be a master's-prepared psychiatric clinical nurse specialist with at least 1 year of experience, and the patient needs to have a DSM-IV diagnosis of anxiety disorder and not being treated with psychotropic medications. In addition, the nurse and patient need to have had no more than one therapy session before enrolling in the study.

Each patient completes the self-administered Behavior and Symptom Identification Scale (BASIS-32) at the onset of the study. The next four sessions between nurse and patient are audiotaped. From the audiotape, a randomly selected 15-minute segment is transcribed. After all four transcriptions are completed, the nurse rates his or her responses as provided on the transcript, using the Therapeutic Behavior Scale (TBS). Concurrently, psychiatric clinical nurse specialists in similar positions in an adjacent state rate the responses on the transcripts, using the TBS. The effectiveness scores on the TBS are used to calculate a Pearson's Perfect Product Moment Coefficient. This coefficient is used to operationalize the nurse's self-knowledge in the nurse–patient relationship. After the fourth session with the nurse, the patient retakes the self-administered Behavior and Symptom Identification Scale (BASIS-32). The difference between the overall mean scores on the first and second tests is calculated to operationalize relief from symptoms. Simple linear regression is used for statistical analysis.

To help interpret the findings, semistructured interviews of nurses and patients are conducted within 1 week following their fourth session. The researcher asks the nurse to describe himself or herself as therapist, and to evaluate effectiveness with the patient, discussing the factors that contributed to that level of success. The researcher asks the patient to describe any changes in symptoms and functioning during the period of the four sessions with the nurse, to discuss what contributed to those changes, and to provide a description of the nurse therapist. Findings may indicate if a relationship exists between the nurse's self-knowledge of the nurse–patient relationship, and the relief of symptoms experienced by patients diagnosed with anxiety disorders.

of the nurse–patient relationship is still recognized, and Peplau's phenomenological approach to theory development is still valued. Peplau was able to pull together "loose, ambiguous data and put them into systematic terms that that could be tested, applied, and integrated into the practice of psychiatric nursing" (Lego, 1980, p. 68). Research on the theory of interpersonal relations, because of its complexity, is not a simple undertaking, yet further testing of Peplau's theory could make significant contributions to nursing's body of knowledge.

ANALYSIS EXERCISE

Using the criteria presented in Chapter 2, critique the Theory of Interpersonal Relations. Compare your conclusions about the theory with those found in Appendix A. A nurse scholar who has worked with the theory completed the analysis found in the Appendix.

Internal Criticism

1. Clarity
2. Consistency
3. Adequacy

4. Logical development
5. Level of theory development

External Criticism

1. Reality convergence
2. Utility
3. Significance
4. Discrimination
5. Scope of theory
6. Complexity

WEB RESOURCES

1. This is the primary site for Peplau's work. The site provides a brief biography of Peplau, but is mostly devoted to bibliographies of work about and by Peplau. In addition to the traditional list of journal articles and books authored by Peplau, it includes lists of papers and speeches, audiotapes, and videotapes. It also provides E-mail links to Cheryl Forchuk and two of her colleagues at University of Western Ontario. It can be accessed at: *http://publish.uwo.ca/%7Ecforchuk/peplau/hpcb.html*
2. NurseScribe maintains a nursing theory page that identifies Peplau as one of the early nurse theorists. It provides a brief overview of the theory and links to two other sites devoted to Peplau. The major feature of the site is a direct link to Medline/PubMed, which identifies 71 citations of her work. It can be reached at: *http://www.enursescribe.com/nurse_theorists.htm*

REFERENCES

Armstrong, M. E., & Kelly, A. E. (1995). More than the sum of their parts: Martha Rogers and Hildegard Peplau. *Archives of Psychiatric Nursing, 9*(1), 40–44.

Buswell, C. (1997). A model approach to care of a patient with alcohol problems...Peplau's model. *Nursing Times, 93*(3), 34–35.

Caris-Verhallen, W., Kerkstra, A., & Bensing, J. (1997). The role of communication in nursing care for elderly peo-

ple: A review of the literature. *Journal of Advanced Nursing, 25,* 915–933.

Fawcett, J. (2000). *Analysis and evaluation of contemporary nursing knowledge: Nursing models and theories.* Philadelphia: F. A. Davis.

Forchuk, C. (1991). Peplau's theory: Concepts and their relations. *Nursing Science Quarterly, 4*(2), 54–60.

Forchuk, C. (1993). *Hildegarde E. Peplau: Interpersonal nursing theory.* Newbury Park, CA: Sage.

Forchuk, C., Beaton, S., Crawford, L., Ide, L., Voorberg, N., & Bethune, J. (1989). Incorporating Peplau's theory and case management. *Journal of Psychosocial Nursing, 27*(2), 35–38.

Forchuk, C., & Dorsay, J. P. (1995). Hildegard Peplau meets family systems nursing: Innovation in theory-based practice. *Journal of Advanced Nursing, 21*(1), 110–115. Retrieved July, 24, 2002 from *http://gateway1.ovid.com/ovidweb.cgi*

Gastmans, C. (1998). Interpersonal relations in nursing: A philosophical-ethical analysis of the work of Hildegard E. Peplau. *Journal of Advanced Nursing, 28,* 1312–1319. Retrieved August 1, 2002 from *http://gateway1.ovid.com/ovidweb.cgi*

Haber, J. (2000). Hildegard E. Peplau: The psychiatric nursing legacy of a legend. *Journal of the American Psychiatric Nurses, 6*(2), 56–62.

Hall, K. (1994). Peplau's model of nursing: Caring for a man with AIDS. *British Journal of Nursing, 11,* 418–422.

Jones, A. (1995). Utilizing Peplau's psychodynamic theory for stroke patient care. *Journal of Clinical Nursing, 4*(1), 49–54. Retrieved September 19, 2002 from *http://gateway1.ovid.com/ovidweb.cgi*

Lego, S. (1980). The one-to-one nurse-patient relationship. *Perspectives in Psychiatric Care, 18*(2), 67–89.

McCann, T., & Baker, H. (2001). Mutual relating: Developing interpersonal relationships in the community. *Jour-*

nal of Advanced Nursing, 34, 530–537. Retrieved September 19, 2002 from *http://gateway1.ovid.com/ovidweb.cgi*

McGuinness, S. D., & Peters, S. (1999). The diagnosis of multiple sclerosis: Peplau's interpersonal relations model. *Rehabilitation Nursing, 24*(1), 30–33.

McKenna, H. (1997). *Nursing theories and models.* London: Routledge.

O'Toole, A. W., & Welt, S. R. (1989). *Interpersonal theory in nursing practice: Selected works of Hildegard E. Peplau.* New York: Springer.

Peplau, H. E. (1952). *Interpersonal relations in nursing.* New York: G. P. Putnam's Sons.

Peplau, H. E. (1964). Psychiatric nursing skills and the general hospital patient. *Nursing Forum, 3*(2), 28–37.

Peplau, H. E. (1969). Professional closeness...as a special kind of involvement with a patient, client or family group. *Nursing Forum, 8,* 343–360.

Peplau, H. E. (1985). Help the public maintain mental health. *Nursing Success Today, 2*(5), 30–34.

Peplau, H. E. (1988). The art and science of nursing: Similarities, differences and relations. *Nursing Science Quarterly, 1,* 8–15.

Peplau, H. E. (1989). Theory: The professional dimension. In A. W. O'Toole & S. R. Welt (Eds.), *Interpersonal theory in nursing practice: Selected works of Hildegard E. Peplau* (pp. 21–30). New York: Springer.

Peplau, H. E. (1991). *Interpersonal relations in nursing: A conceptual frame of reference for psychodynamic nursing.* New York: Springer.

Peplau, H. E. (1992). Interpersonal relations: A theoretical framework for application in nursing practice. *Nursing Science Quarterly, 5*(1), 13–18.

Peplau, H. E. (1997). Peplau's theory of interpersonal relations. *Nursing Science Quarterly, 10*(4), 162–167.

Price, B. (1998). Explorations in body image care: Peplau and practice knowledge. *Journal of Psychiatric & Mental Health Nursing, 5*(3), 179–186.

Reed, P. G. (1995). A treatise on nursing knowledge development for the 21st century: Beyond postmodernism [Electronic version]. *Advances in Nursing Science, 17*(3), 70–84.

Reed, P. G. (1996). Transforming practice knowledge into nursing knowledge—A revisionist analysis of Peplau. *Image—the Journal of Nursing Scholarship, 28,* 29–33. Retrieved September 19, 2002 from *http://gateway1.ovid.com/ovidweb.cgi*

Sellers, S. C. (1991). *A philosophical analysis of conceptual models of nursing.* Unpublished doctoral dissertation, Iowa State University, Ames.

Sills, G. M. (1978). Hildegard E. Peplau: Leader, practitioner, academician, scholar, and theorist. *Perspectives in Psychiatric Care, 16*(3), 122–128.

Spray, L. (1999). Living interpersonal theory: The Hildegard Peplau-Suzanne Lego Letters, March 1998–March 1999.

Perspectives in Psychiatric Care, 35(4), 24ff. Retrieved September 18, 2002 from *http://web5.infotrac.galegroup.com.*

Welch, M. (1995). Hildegard Peplau in a conversation with Mark Welch. Part I. *Nursing Inquiry, 2*(1), 53–56.

Young, A., Taylor, S. G., & Renpenning, K. (2001). *Connections: Nursing research, theory, and practice.* St. Louis: Mosby.

BIBLIOGRAPHY

Selected Works by Peplau

Peplau, H. E. (1984). Help the public maintain mental health (Interview). *Nursing Success, 2*(5), 30–34.

Peplau, H. E. (1986). The nurse as counsellor. *Journal of American College Health, 35*(11), 11–14.

Peplau, H. E. (1987). Interpersonal constructs for nursing practice. *Nurse Education Today, 7*(5), 201–208.

Peplau, H. E. (1989). Future directions in psychiatric nursing from the perspective of history. *Journal of Psychosocial Nursing, 27*(2), 18–21, 25–28, 39–40.

Peplau, H. E. (1994). Quality of life: An interpersonal perspective. *Nursing Science Quarterly, 7*(1), 10–15.

Peplau, H. E. (1995). Some unresolved issues in era of biopsychosocial nursing. *Journal of American Psychiatric Nurses Association, 1*(3), 92–96.

Peplau, H. E. (1996). Fundamental and special—the dilemma of psychiatric mental nursing—commentary. *Archives of Psychiatric Nursing, 10*(4), 162–167.

Selected Works on Peplau's Theory

Armstrong, M. A., & Kelly, A. E. (1993). Enhancing staff nurses' interpersonal skills: Theory to practice. *Clinical Nurse Specialist, 7*(6), 313–317.

Barker, P. J., Reynolds, W., & Stevens, C. (1997). The human science basis of psychiatric nursing theory and practice. *Journal of Advanced Nursing, 25,* 660–667.

Beeber, L., Anderson, C. A., & Sills, G. M. (1990). Peplau's theory in practice. *Nursing Science, 3*(1), 6–8.

Beeber, L. S. (1998). Treating depression through the therapeutic nurse-patient relationship. *Nursing Clinics of North America, 33*(1), 153–157.

Comley, A. L. (1994). A comparative analysis of Orem's self-care model and Peplau's interpersonal theory. *Journal of Advanced Nursing, 20*(4), 755–760.

Feely, M. (1997). Using Peplau's theory in nurse-client relations. *International Nursing Review, 44*(4), 115–120.

Forchuk, C. (1991). A comparison of the works of Peplau and Orlando. *Archives of Psychiatric Nursing, 5*(1), 38–45.

Forchuk, C. (1991). Conceptualizing the environment of the individual with chronic mental illness. *Issues in Mental Health Nursing, 12,* 159–170.

Forchuk, C. (1994). Preconceptions in the nurse-client relationship. *Journal of Psychiatric & Mental Health Nursing, 1*(3), 145–149.

Fowler, J. (1994). A welcome focus on a key relationship: Using Peplau's model in palliative care. *Professional Nurse, 10*(3), 194–197.

Fowler, J. (1995). Taking theory into practice: Using Peplau's model in the care of a patient. *Professional Nurse, 10*(4), 226–230.

Greg, D. E. (1978). Hildegard E. Peplau: Her contributions. *Perspectives in Psychiatric Care, 16*(3), 118–121.

Martin, M. L., Forchuk, C., Santopinto, M., & Butcher, H. K. (1992). Alternative approaches to nursing practice: Application of Peplau, Rogers, and Parse. *Nursing Science Quarterly, 5*(2) 80–85.

Schroder, P. J. (1979). Nursing intervention with patients with thought disorders. *Perspectives in Psychiatric Care, 17*(1), 32–39.

Middle Range Theories: Integrative

Modeling and Role-Modeling

ELLEN D. SCHULTZ

DEFINITION OF KEY TERMS

GENERAL TERMS

Facilitation	Through the interactive process of facilitation, the nurse assists the client to identify, develop, and mobilize personal strengths. The nurse does not effect the outcomes for the client, but, rather, helps the client move toward holistic health.
Modeling	Modeling is the process used by the nurse to develop an accurate understanding of the client's perceptions and environment. The nurse seeks to understand the client's world from the perspective and framework of the client.
Nursing	Nursing is a holistic, interactive, and interpersonal process. The nurse nurtures the client's strengths and facilitates the client's self care, with the goal of achieving optimum health.
Nurturance	Nurturance integrates the client's affective, cognitive and physiological processes to assist the client toward holistic health. To nurture, the nurse must understand the client's model of the world.
Role-modeling	In role-modeling, the nurse uses purposeful interventions, based on nursing science, that are unique to the client, to assist the client toward holistic health.
Unconditional acceptance	The individual is accepted as a unique and worthwhile human being.

TERMS RELATED TO PERSONS

Adaptation	Adaptation is the "process by which an individual responds to external and internal stressors in a health and growth-directed manner" (Erickson, Tomlin, & Swain, 1983, p. 252).

DEFINITION OF KEY TERMS

Affiliated-individuation	Affiliated-individuation is an inherent need to be dependent on support systems, while maintaining a sense of autonomy and separateness from those systems.
Environment	The client's environment includes internal and external stressors, as well as internal and external resources. The theorists see the environment in "the social subsystems as the interaction between self and other both cultural and individual" (Erickson, 2002a, p. 452).
Health	Health is a "state of physical, mental and social well-being not merely the absence of disease or infirmity. Additionally, it connotes a state of equilibrium within each of the various subsystems of a holistic person" (Erickson, Tomlin, & Swain, 1983, p. 253).
Holism	"The interaction of the multiple subsystems and the inherent bases creates holism. Holism implies that the whole is greater than the sum of the parts" (Erickson, Tomlin, & Swain, 1983, p. 45). There is a blending of the unconscious and conscious.
Inherent endowment	Inherent endowment includes both the genetic makeup of the person and the inherent characteristics that can result from birth and/or disease, influencing the person's health status.
Lifetime growth and development	Persons change throughout their lifetime, responding to an inherent desire to fulfill their potential in the areas of basic needs and psychological and cognitive stages.
Person	"Human beings are holistic persons who have multiple interacting subsystems" including the biophysical, cognitive, psychological, and social subsystems (Erickson, Tomlin, & Swain, 1983, p. 44). Intersecting and permeating these subsystems are the genetic base and spiritual drive.
Self-care knowledge	Each person knows, at some level, what interferes with or what promotes his or her own health and development.

DEFINITION OF KEY TERMS

Self-care resources   These include both internal and external resources that can be mobilized to promote holistic health.

Self-care action   Clients demonstrate self-care action when they develop and use self-care knowledge and self-care resources. "Through self-care action the individual mobilizes internal resources and acquires additional resources that will help the individual gain, maintain and promote optimal level of holistic health" (Erickson, Tomlin, & Swain, 1983, p. 48).

Stressor   A stressor is a stimulus experienced by the individual as a challenge that mounts an adaptive response.

INTRODUCTION

Modeling and Role-Modeling (MRM) is a theory and paradigm for nursing that serves as a foundation for nursing research, education, and practice. It is among the theories "most commonly used by holistic nurses" (Frisch, 2000, p. 176). As a theory that is strongly tied to nursing practice, it is a positive response to the criticism cited by Fawcett (1995, p. 519) that many models and theories are "invented by scholars and academics" and, therefore, may have little relevance for nursing practice.

Chapter 1 of this text describes the hierarchy of nursing knowledge and the classification of nursing theories as grand, middle range, or practice theories. While MRM is included here among the middle range theories, consensus has not been established on this classification. Tomey and Alligood (1998) classified MRM as a middle range theory, yet McEwen and Wills (2002) consider MRM to be a grand theory, and categorized it as one of the interactive process theories. One system for classifying theory is to consider the scope of the theory. A grand theory includes the nursing metaparadigm concepts of nursing, health, environment, and person, all of which are addressed in MRM. This chapter on MRM is appropriately included in this text because it presents, as components of the grand theory, a number of the middle range concepts that have developed from MRM theory. These concepts are best understood within the context of the grand theory.

Modeling and Role-Modeling is a client-centered nursing theory that places the client's perceptions, or model of the world, at the center of the nurse–client interaction. The theory integrates concepts from several interdisciplinary theories, including psychosocial development (Erikson, 1968), cognitive development (Piaget, 1952), basic human needs (Maslow, 1968), and stress adaptation (Selye, 1976; Engel, 1962). These concepts are linked to those unique to MRM theory. Through the processes of modeling and role-modeling, the nurse facilitates and nurtures the client to achieve high-level, holistic wellness.

HISTORICAL BACKGROUND

Modeling and Role-Modeling is a theory "born in practice," as described by Dickoff, James, and Weidenback (1968). "...Using nursing practice as a basis for theory development promotes not only a broader view of reality but also an increased relevance of theory to practice" (McClosky & Grace, 1994, p. 78). Through observations made in clinical practice in a variety of nursing settings, Helen Erickson became aware of the nurse's role as a healer. Based on a combination of insights gleaned through personal experience, clinical practice, and discussions with her father-in-law, renowned psychotherapist, Milton Erickson, Helen Erickson began, in the mid-1970s, to formulate the ideals that later became MRM theory (Keegan & Dossey, 1998).

During her student experience in both a baccalaureate completion program and a graduate education, Erickson began describing the theoretical components of the theory. Challenged by her colleagues, Mary Ann Swain and Evelyn Tomlin, Erickson refined the concepts and their linkages. Erickson began testing components of the theory as a graduate student, beginning with research on the Adaptive Potential Assessment Model (Erickson, 2002b; Erickson & Swain, 1982), followed by additional testing of this concept (Barnfather, Swain & Erickson, 1989) and the concept of self-care resources (Erickson & Swain, 1990).

The process of articulating and researching MRM concepts and the effects of MRM interventions led the way to the publication of *Modeling and Role-Modeling: A Theory and Paradigm for Nursing* (Erickson, Tomlin, & Swain, 1983). This text made the theory more accessible to nurses, thus promoting the use of MRM in practice, education, and research.

Modeling and Role-Modeling serves as a foundation for nursing education. Metropolitan State University, St. Paul, Minnesota uses MRM as the theoretical foundation for the baccalaureate completion program and teaches the theory in the graduate program. Humboldt State University, Arcata, California has also selected MRM as the conceptual framework for the nursing program. Other schools that have incorporated MRM into their nursing programs are The College of St. Catherine, Minneapolis; Foo Yin College of Nursing and Medical Technology, Taiwan; the University of Texas at Austin; and the University of Michigan (Erickson, 2002a). MRM can also be used as a framework for academic advising (Schultz, 1998).

Nurses in many settings who have been exposed to MRM either through the literature or as students in MRM-based programs have introduced the concepts into their practice environments, both informally and in structured ways. For example, nurses on a surgical unit at the University of Michigan developed and implemented an assessment tool that is based on MRM (Campbell, Finch, Allport, Erickson, & Swain, 1985; Finch, 1990; Walsh, VandenBosch, & Boehm, 1989); the nurses on the vascular surgery unit use MRM as their practice framework (University of Michigan, 2002); and MRM has been used as the theoretical foundation for the nursing practice model at Brigham and Women's Hospital in Boston, MA and the University of Pittsburgh hospitals. Baker (1999) developed a psycho-educational program based on MRM for parents of children with attention-deficit hyperactivity disorder. MRM has also been the theoretical foundation for the practice of school nursing (Barnfather, 1991).

The Society for the Advancement of Modeling and Role-Modeling was established to advance the development and application of the theory. It promoted the study and integration of the theoretical propositions and philosophical underpinnings, developed a support network, disseminated knowledge and information and promoted the improvement of holistic health (Bylaws, 2000). The society has sponsored biennial conferences since 1986.

Since the development of the theory, Erickson has conducted research, consulted with schools of nursing and health care institutions, authored several articles, presented papers, and supervised graduate students' research in MRM. Several dissertations completed at the University of Michigan in the late 1980s and at the University of Texas at Austin in the 1990s, under the advisement of Helen Erickson, implement MRM as the theoretical foundation for research. MRM concepts continue to be tested. Examples of MRM-based research are described elsewhere in this chapter.

DEFINITION OF THEORY CONCEPTS

Modeling and Role-Modeling theory is described in terms of its theoretical bases, including how people are alike and how they are different, a philosophy of nursing, and a paradigm for the practice of nursing. To define the major concepts of the theory, they can be categorized into concepts that relate to nursing and those that relate to persons.

Concepts Related to Nursing

Erickson has identified and described several concepts that relate to the discipline of nursing. They include nursing, facilitation, nurturance, unconditional acceptance, modeling, and role-modeling.

NURSING

Modeling and Role-Modeling emphasizes the holistic, interpersonal nature of nursing. Nursing is described as an interactive process that nurtures client strengths to "enable development, release and channeling of resources for coping with one's circumstances and environment. The goal is to achieve a state of perceived optimal health and contentment" (Erickson, Tomlin, & Swain, 1983, p. 49). In the process of assisting clients to achieve holistic health, the nurse must nurture the client, facilitate, not effect, the adaptive process, and accept the client unconditionally.

FACILITATION

Through the activities of facilitation, the nurse assists the client to identify, develop, and mobilize personal strengths as he or she moves toward health. The nurse does not produce the outcomes for the client, but, rather, "aids the client in meeting his or her own needs so that he or she may have the necessary resources" for coping with stressors, growth, development, and self-actualization (Erickson, 1990, p. 13).

NURTURANCE

In the process of nurturance, the nurse promotes the integration of the client's affective, cognitive, and physiologic processes as the client moves toward holistic health. For nurturance to occur, the nurse must seek to understand and support the client's model of the world and appreciate the value of the client's self-care knowledge. This understanding can be used to develop nursing interventions that are unique to the client.

UNCONDITIONAL ACCEPTANCE

The nurse accepts the client as a "unique, worthwhile, important individual with no strings attached" (Erickson, Tomlin, & Swain, 1983, p. 255). Empathy is used to communicate nonjudgmental respect with the client.

MODELING

Modeling is a central concept in the theory because understanding the client's viewpoint is the foundation for implementing the nursing process. Modeling is defined as "the process the nurse uses as she develops an image and understanding of the client's world—an image and understanding developed within the client's framework and from the client's perspective" (Erickson, Tomlin, & Swain, 1983, p. 95). The nurse suspends his or her judgment to fully understand the client's perspective.

Both the art and science of nursing are reflected in modeling. The art is demonstrated through the use of therapeutic communication to develop an accurate picture of the client's situation. The science is demonstrated in the data aggregation and analysis based on scientific principles and the concepts from the theory.

ROLE-MODELING

"Role-modeling is the facilitation of the individual in attaining, maintaining, or promoting health through purposeful interventions" (Erickson, Tomlin, & Swain, 1983, p. 95). Role-modeling can occur only after the nurse accurately understands the client's worldview. The art of role-modeling is demonstrated by planning and implementing nursing interventions that are based on the client's model of the world and are, therefore, unique. The science of role-modeling is demonstrated through planning theory-based interventions.

Concepts That Relate to Persons

In describing the concepts that relate to person, Erickson has included concepts formulated for the theory and others that rely on borrowed theories from other disciplines. While nursing seeks to develop "distinctive knowledge" related to the discipline of nursing, the linking of borrowed theory with nursing theory is appropriate if there is congruence between the worldviews of the two (Villarruel, Bishop, Simpson, Jemmott, & Fawcett, 2001). Concepts that have been described in MRM theory that relate to persons include person, health, environment, ways the people are alike, and ways in which they differ.

PERSON

The individual is viewed as holistic, having multiple interacting subsystems. These dynamic subsystems are the biological, cognitive, psychological, and social subsystems. The person's genetic makeup and spiritual drive permeate and intersect the subsystems. When caring for the person, the nurse does not focus on one subsystem but on the integrated, dynamic relationships among the subsystems of the person. His or her internal model of the world determines the person's perceptions and interpretations of the environment.

HEALTH

Health is a "state of physical, mental and social well-being, not merely the absence of disease or infirmity. Additionally, it connotes a state of equilibrium within each of the various subsystems of a holistic person" (Erickson, Tomlin, & Swain, 1983, p. 253). A goal of nursing is to facilitate the client's achievement of perceived optimal health.

ENVIRONMENT

The concept of environment was not defined in Erickson's original work but has been described in later publications. The concept includes the client's internal and external stressors, as well as internal and external resources. "The theorists see environment in the social subsystems as the interaction between self and others both cultural and individual" (Erickson, 2002a, p. 452). The importance of the interpersonal environment is emphasized in the theory.

HOW PEOPLE ARE ALIKE

While recognizing the uniqueness of persons, MRM identifies ways in which people are alike: they are holistic, they experience lifetime growth and development, and have a need for affiliated-individuation. In understanding how people are alike and how they are different, Erickson synthesizes a number of interdisciplinary theories identified below.

Holism. "The interaction of the multiple subsystems and the inherent bases create holism" (Erickson, Tomlin & Swain, 1983, p. 45). Dynamic relationships exist among mind, body, emotion, and spirit. Figure 11-1 shows the holistic model. The figure demonstrates the integration of biophysical, psychosocial, cognitive, and social aspects of the person. Both the genetic base and the spiritual drive permeate all of these aspects. While identified as separate parts, the figure shows that the multiple subsystems are integrated. They interact and function as a total unit.

Lifetime Growth: Basic Needs. People are alike in that they all have basic needs. MRM theory incorporates Maslow's (1968) hierarchy of needs as the framework for understanding basic need satisfaction. Individuals have an inherent desire to fulfill one's potential. Holistic growth is impeded when basic needs are unmet. Consistent with the concept of modeling, the theory supports the view that "all human beings have basic needs that can be satisfied, but only from within the framework of the individual" (Erickson, Tomlin, & Swain, 1983, p. 58).

Lifetime Development. People are also alike because they mature and develop over their lifetimes. The theoretical support for psychosocial development comes from the work of Erik Erikson (1968). As individuals move through the eight developmental stages, they resolve the tasks or crisis of that stage. Resolution of the developmental stage results in the acquisition of lasting strengths and virtues.

Piaget's (1952) theory provides the framework for understanding how people are alike in their cognitive development. Individuals progress through a series of stages in which the ability to think and reason becomes more complex.

Affiliated-Individuation. "Individuals have an instinctual need for affiliated-individuation. They need to be able to be dependent on support systems while simultaneously maintaining independence from these support systems" (Erickson, Tomlin, & Swain, 1983, p. 47). The need for affiliation motivates individuals to seek support. As the need for affiliation is met through supportive contacts, an "af-

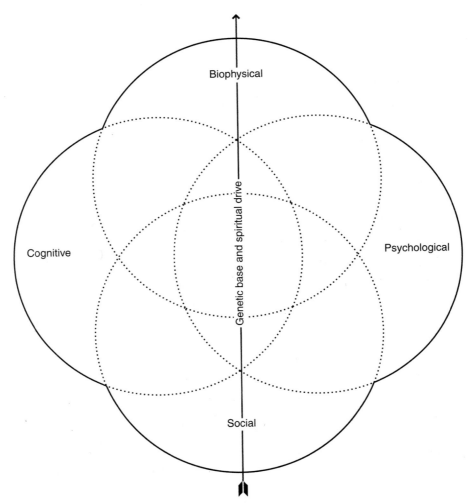

■ Figure 11.1 Model of the holistic person.

filiative resource" is developed. A healthy sense of individuation is developed as individuals make independent choices, feel good about themselves, and feel esteem from others (Acton, 1997).

HOW PEOPLE ARE DIFFERENT

Although people are alike in that they are holistic and share a common process of growth and development, each person is unique. MRM theory identifies these unique aspects of people as the inherent endowment, the ability to adapt, and one's personal model of the world.

Inherent Endowment. A person's inherent endowment comprises both the genetic base and inherent characteristics. The genetic base determines, to some extent, how a person progresses through

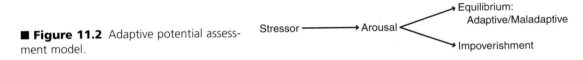

■ **Figure 11.2** Adaptive potential assessment model.

the developmental processes and responds to stressors. Inherent characteristics also influence health and growth and development. These characteristics include "malformation, brain damage, or other physiological states secondary to birth, prenatal disease, sicknesses, or other factors" (Erickson, Tomlin, & Swain, 1983, p. 75).

Adaptation. People differ in the ability to adapt. Adaptation is defined as the "process by which an individual responds to external and internal stressors in a health and growth-directed manner" (Erickson, Tomlin, & Swain, 1983, p. 252). Within MRM theory, adaptation is approached from an integrated perspective. Theoretical support for the physiological response to stressors comes from the work of Selye (1976), particularly the general adaptation syndrome. The psychosocial perspective is supported by Engel's (1962) research on the human response to stressors.

Erickson conceptualized a biophysical-psychosocial model, the adaptive potential assessment model (APAM), that identifies states of coping that "reflect an individual's potential to mobilize self-care resources." In Erickson's model, stress states are distinguished from nonstress states. When a stimulus is experienced as a challenge, it is a stressor; when experienced as threatening, it is a distressor and leads to a maladaptive response (Barnfather, Swain, & Erickson, 1989; Erickson & Swain, 1982; Erickson, Tomlin, & Swain, 1983).

Three categories are identified in the adaptive potential assessment model: arousal, equilibrium, and impoverishment. As shown in Figure 11-2, the experience of a stressor leads to a state of arousal. Arousal may be experienced by feelings of tenseness and anxiousness, accompanied by elevations in blood pressure, pulse rate, respirations, and motor-sensory behavior. From arousal, the person may move to a state of equilibrium or impoverishment. In a state of impoverishment, the individual experiences marked feelings of tension and anxiety, with feelings of fatigue, sadness, or depression. In addition to elevated pulse, respiration, blood pressure, and motor-sensory behavior, there is an elevation in verbal anxiety. Equilibrium may be adaptive or maladaptive. In adaptive equilibrium, the individual has normal vital signs and sensory-motor behavior, expresses hope, has low or absent feelings of tenseness, fatigue, sadness, and depression. In a state of maladaptive equilibrium, one may appear to be coping with stressors, but at the expense of draining energy from another subsystem (Erickson, Tomlin, & Swain, 1983).

Each state is associated with different coping potentials or different abilities to mobilize coping resources. Movement among the states, either to equilibrium or impoverishment, depends on both the ability to mobilize resources and the presence of new stressors. Figure 11-3 shows the relationship among the APAM states. Nursing interventions are directed toward assisting the client to mobilize resources (Erickson, Tomlin, & Swain, 1983).

Person's Model of the World—Self-Care Knowledge, Resources, and Action. Each person has a unique worldview. Nurses use the process of modeling to develop an understanding of how the person perceives the world from his or her own perspective. One aspect of this "model of the world" that relates to health is self-care knowledge. Each person knows, at some level, what interferes with and what promotes his or her own health and development. This self-care knowledge makes the client the primary source of information in nurse–client interactions. There are two ad-

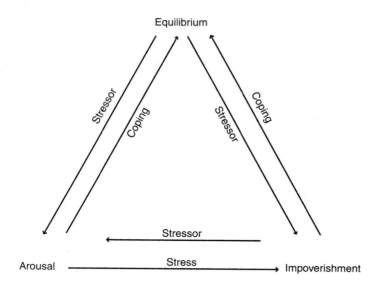

■ **Figure 11.3** Dynamic relationships among states of the adaptive potential assessment model.

ditional self-care concepts related to self-care knowledge. Self-care resources include both internal and external resources that can be mobilized to promote holistic health. Finally, self-care action is the "development and utilization" of self-care knowledge and self-care resources. Activities include both the acquisition of additional resources and the mobilization of self-care resources toward the goal of achieving optimal holistic health. Nursing intervention can assist the client in acquiring and mobilizing resources (Erickson, Tomlin, & Swain, 1983).

DESCRIPTION OF THE THEORY OF MODELING AND ROLE-MODELING

Theoretical Linkages

Modeling and Role-Modeling theory draws on concepts from several theorists. Each theorist places emphasis on one aspect of the person. However, Erickson's creation of a holistic nursing theory explains the dynamic relationships among basic need satisfaction, growth, developmental processes, loss, grief, and adaptation. The functional relationships among these concepts leads to theoretical linkages. Relationships exist between/among:

- Need satisfaction and developmental task resolution
- Need satisfaction and adaptive potential
- Need satisfaction, object attachment and loss, grief, growth, and development
- Developmental residue and self-care resources (Erickson, 1990, 2002)

Figure 11-4 shows the relationships among MRM concepts. For example, the figure demonstrates possible outcomes resulting from basic need deficits. Unmet basic needs will interfere with the growth

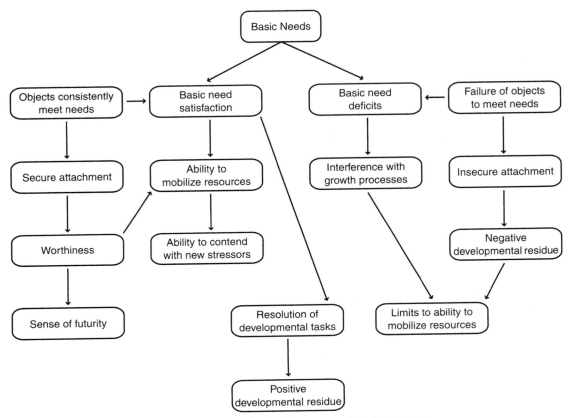

■ Figure 11.4 Relationships among MRM concepts.

process which, in turn, limits the person's ability to mobilize resources to adapt to stressors. However, when basic needs are satisfied, the person is able to mobilize resources to contend with new stressors. The figure further demonstrates the relationship between basic needs and attachment. When an object consistently meets one's needs, secure attachments form, leading to a sense of worthiness and the ability to mobilize resources. On the other hand, when objects fail to meet one's needs, insecure attachments form, limiting the ability to mobilize resources to deal with stressors. While the concepts presented in the theory, when viewed individually, may seem simple, the interactions among the factors demonstrate the complexity of the theory.

From these theoretical linkages, Erickson identified 13 propositions that can be used to predict outcomes, direct the planning of nursing care, and evaluate care:

1. Individual's ability to contend with new stressors is directly related to the ability to mobilize resources needed.
2. Individual's ability to mobilize resources is directly related to his or her need deficits and assets.
3. Distressors are related to unmet basic needs; stressors are related to unmet growth needs.

4. Objects that repeatedly facilitate the individual in need satisfaction take on significance for the individual. When this occurs, attachment to the object results.
5. Secure attachment produces feelings of worthiness.
6. Feelings of worthiness result in a sense of futurity.
7. Real, threatened, or perceived loss of the attachment object results in the grief process.
8. Basic-need deficits coexist with the grief process.
9. An adequate alternative object must be perceived available for the individual to resolve the grief process.
10. Prolonged grief due to an unavailable or inadequate object results in morbid grief.
11. Unmet basic and growth needs interfere with growth processes.
12. Repeated satisfaction of basic needs is prerequisite to working through developmental tasks and resolution of related developmental crises.
13. Morbid grief is always related to need deficits. (Erickson, 1990, p. 28)

Paradigm for Nursing Practice

The practice paradigm of MRM is presented within the framework of the nursing process, emphasizing the importance of both the interactive, interpersonal nature of nursing and the theoretical and scientific bases of nursing practice. Nursing care begins by determining the client's model of the world and then focusing on the most immediate concerns expressed by the client. The practice paradigm directs data collection, data aggregation, analysis, and synthesis, and provides a framework for planning nursing interventions. Critical thinking is required to implement these activities.

Consistent with the concept of modeling, the client is viewed as the primary data source. Other data sources are included as well, and the nurse looks for congruence between data received from the client and that received from significant others and health care professionals. Data are collected and organized in the following categories:

- Description of the situation—to develop an overview of the client's perspective of the situation
- Expectations—to determine the client's expectations for the future
- Resource potential—to determine internal and external resources available to the client
- Goals and life tasks—to determine developmental status and personal model of the world (Erickson, Tomlin, & Swain, 1983)

The use of standardized nursing interventions is not consistent with modeling and role-modeling beliefs. The theory does provide general aims of interventions that are associated with the principles of the theory and facilitate the planning of systematic interventions. These are to build trust, promote client's positive orientation, promote client's control, affirm and promote client's strengths, and set mutual goals that are health-directed. Table 11-1 shows the aims of intervention and the MRM principle associated with each intervention. *Modeling and Role-Modeling: A Theory and Paradigm for Nursing* (Erickson, Tomlin, & Swain, 1983) provides specific examples of how the aims of interventions can be linked to basic need satisfaction. In the implementation of nursing interventions, the goal is to carry out one intervention that reflects each aim during every contact with the client. A single intervention can meet more than one of the general aims of intervention.

Table 11-1. RELATIONSHIP BETWEEN AIMS OF INTERVENTION AND MRM PRINCIPLES

AIM	PRINCIPLE
Build trust	The nursing process requires that a trusting and functional relationship exist between nurse and client.
Promote client's positive orientation	Affiliated-individuation is dependent on the individual's perceiving that he or she is an acceptable, respectable, and worthwhile human being.
Promote client's control	Human development is dependent on the individual's perceiving that he or she has some control over his or her life, while concurrently sensing a state of affiliation.
Affirm and promote client's strengths	There is an innate drive toward holistic health that is facilitated by consistent and systematic nurturance.
Set mutual goals that are health-directed	Human growth is dependent on satisfaction of basic needs and facilitated by growth-need satisfaction.

Erickson, H. C., Tomlin, E. M., & Swain, M. A. (1983). *Modeling and role-modeling: A theory and paradigm for nursing* (p. 170). Englewood Cliffs, NJ: Prentice-Hall, Inc.

APPLICATIONS OF THE THEORY

Modeling and Role-Modeling has been the theoretical foundation for numerous published research studies, master's theses, and doctoral dissertations. Many studies test the middle range concepts found in MRM theory or explore the relationships between or among concepts. The concepts are clearly defined and are used consistently. The relationships among the concepts are complex and have provided the stimulus for several studies.

Affiliated-Individuation

Acton (1997) tested the concept of affiliated-individuation to determine its ability to be a mediator between stress and the burden of caregivers, and caregiver satisfaction with family caregivers of adults with dementia. Acton and Miller (1996) investigated the effects of a theory-based, support-group intervention on affiliated-individuation with a group of caregivers of adults with dementia. This study is summarized in the example found in Using Middle Range Theories 11-1.

Adaptive Potential Assessment Model

The adaptive potential assessment model (APAM) was first tested by Erickson (1976). Erickson and Swain (1982) studied the model to statistically validate the three categories of the APAM, arousal, equilibrium, and impoverishment, and to determine whether a relationship existed between the categories and length of hospital stay. Further testing of the validity of the model was conducted by Barnfather, Swain, and Erickson (1989) to determine if subjects could be classified into the three adaptive states, as a measure of ability to mobilize coping resources. Barnfather (1987) applied the adaptive potential

11-1   USING MIDDLE RANGE THEORIES

The researchers studied the effects of a support group intervention on affiliated-individuation (AI) in caregivers of persons with dementia. AI was viewed as a self-care resource to help caregivers deal with the stressors associated with their caregiving roles. Twenty-six caregivers were placed in intervention groups of 6 to 7 per group for one year. The support group interventions were based on MRM's five aims of intervention. AI was measured using subscales of the Basic Needs Satisfaction Inventory (BNSI). Data collection consisted of semistructured interviews and participant completion of BNSI and demographic questionnaires. Qualitative data were analyzed for essential meaning. Multivariate analysis of variance was used to analyze the quantitative data. Data analysis indicated that the needs associated with AI were facilitated through the intervention of the support group. In addition, the theoretical definition of AI was supported through this research, and it provided support for the linkage between AI and coping as proposed by MRM theory.

Acton, G. J., & Miller, E. W. (1996). Affiliated-individuation in caregivers of adults with dementia. *Issues in Mental Health Nursing, 17*, 245–260.

assessment model to healthy subjects to test the relationship between basic need satisfaction and the ability to mobilize coping resources. In another study, Barnfather (1993) conducted additional testing of the model and the relationship between basic need status and adaptive potential with male students experiencing stress. Research on perceived stress as one of the predictors of health is reported in the example in Using Middle Range Theories 11-2.

Health/Well-being

Research conducted by Irvin and Acton (1996) tested a model of caregiver stress mediation to determine if perceived support and self worth had a mediating effect on well-being. Acton and Malathum (2000) studied the relationship between basic need satisfaction and health-promoting behavior and determined the best predictors of health-promoting self-care behavior.

Self-Care Resources/Actions

Erickson and Swain (1990) conducted a nursing intervention study with hypertensive clients to determine the efficacy of modeling and role-modeling based interventions directed toward mobilizing self-care resources. Irvin (1993), identifying social support, self-worth and hope as self-care resources, studied the relationships among these resources and caregiver stress. Using hope as a self-care resource, Irvin and Acton (1997) studied stress mediation in women caregivers, testing ways that stress and well-being were affected by self-care resources.

Research by Baas (1992) identified the predictor variables related to self-care resources on life satisfaction in persons following myocardial infarction. The concept of self-care resources was also studied in its relationship to quality of life (Bass, Fontana, & Bhat, 1997). The researchers conducted an

11-2   USING MIDDLE RANGE THEORIES

The purpose of this study was to examine predictors of health in undereducated adults, using constructs from Modeling and Role-Modeling theory, psychosocial resources, perceived stress, and health. Subjects studied were 171 individuals without a 12th-grade education, who were enrolled in an adult education program.

Four variables were measured. Psychosocial development was measured using the Modified Eriksonian Psychological Stage Inventory (MEPSI); basic need satisfaction was measured with the Basic Need Satisfaction Inventory (BNSI); subjects were asked to rate their level and frequency of stress and a measure of perceived stress; and health was assessed using the Positive Health Index. Structural equation modeling and latent variables were used to test the relationships among the variables in the model developed by the researchers. This model design reflected the theoretical linkages proposed in MRM theory.

The researchers found that "psychosocial development and basic need satisfaction had significant direct effects on health, with the expected positive signs," with psychosocial development having the strongest direct effect on health (Barnfather & Ronis, 2000, p. 62). No significant relationship between health and perceived stress was found in the study. The researchers recommended that therapeutic nursing interventions "include strengthening psychosocial resources and focusing in the client's perceived needs..." (Barnfather & Ronis, 2000, p. 63). This research supported the theoretical linkages delineated in MRM theory.

Barnfather, J. S., & Ronis, D. L. (2000). Test of a model of psychosocial resources, stress and health among undereducated adults. *Research in Nursing and Health, 23,* 55–66.

exploratory pilot study with individuals diagnosed with heart failure to determine potential differences among the groups in measures of self-care needs, resources, and quality of life.

The purpose of Rosehow's (1992) research was to identify self-care actions perceived as significant for persons 6 months after myocardial infarction. Preferences and rankings of self-care actions were also identified.

A new concept, perceived enactment of autonomy (PEA), was developed, based on the concept of self-care (Baas, Curl, Hertz, & Robinson, 1994; Hertz, 1991). Perceived enactment of autonomy is conceptually defined as a state of sensing and recognizing the ability to freely choose behaviors and courses of action on one's own behalf and in accordance with one's own needs and goals" (Hertz, 1995, p. 269). Additional testing on the concept is underway with a group of elders (Hertz, 2002).

Other Studies

Additional studies, not related to the categories of concepts included above, employed MRM as the theoretical foundation. Examples of the concepts researched are comfort (Kennedy, 1991), compassionate visiting (Holl, 1992), psychophysiological processes of stress (Kline, 1988), uncertainty, spiritual well-being, and psychological adjustment to illness (Landis, 1991), unmet needs of persons with chronic mental illness (Perese, 1997), and psychological development and coping ability (Miller, 1986).

INSTRUMENTS USED IN EMPIRICAL TESTING

Several instruments have been developed to test MRM theory. Two instruments were developed relating to the developmental processes of individuals. Darling-Fisher and Leidy (1988) developed the Modified Erikson Psychosocial Stage Inventory. This tool is designed to measure Erikson's eight stages of the life cycle in adults. The Basic Need Satisfaction Inventory (BNSI) was developed and tested by Leidy (1994). The purpose of the BNSI is to "operationalize Maslow's construct of need satisfaction and for testing many of his theoretical propositions" (p. 293). Each item on the BNSI reflects one of Maslow's five basic needs. Both of these tools are relevant to MRM-based research because of the integration of psychosocial development and basic needs into the theory.

Hertz (1991) designed an instrument, the Hertz Perceived Enactment of Autonomy Scale (HPEAS) to measure the concept, perceived enactment of autonomy, and its attributes: individuality, self-direction and voluntariness (PEA). The concept of PEA is the potential for self-care action and "links self care knowledge, resources and actions..." (Baas et al., 1994, p. 151). Erickson (1996) developed an instrument to measure the bonding-attachment process related to need satisfaction in teenage mothers. The Robinson Self-Appraisal Inventory was developed as a self-reporting instrument to measure the concept of denial (Robinson, 1991). The Health-Promoting Lifestyle Profile II, although not developed from MRM theory, has been used to measure health-promoting self-care behavior in MRM research seeking to study self-care resources (Walker, Sechrist & Pender, 1995). Research Application 11-1 describes how this concept could be used in a study. However, Baas (1992) developed an instrument based on MRM theory to measure self-care resources, Self-Care Resource Inventory. This tool provides three scores: resources available, resources needed, and the difference in resources. Table 11-2 lists instruments commonly used in MRM research.

11-1   RESEARCH APPLICATION

A school nurse, working with a support group for pregnant teenage girls, is concerned about their health-promoting, or self-care behavior. Based on the MRM proposition that one's ability to mobilize self-care resources is related to need deficits and assets, the nurse is interested in examining the relationship between the girls' basic needs satisfaction and their health-promoting behaviors. A random sample of the 30 teenagers is selected from the 23 high schools located in the nurse's county.

The girls in the study are asked to complete the Basic Needs Satisfaction Inventory (Leidy, 1994) that measures need satisfaction, the Health-Promoting Lifestyle Profile II (Walker, Sechrist & Pender, 1995), used to measure self-promoting self-care behavior, and a demographic questionnaire. Statistical analysis will reveal correlations between the subscales of the Basic Need Satisfaction Inventory and the Health-Promoting Lifestyle Profile. In addition, regression analysis may be used to determine the ability to predict self-care behaviors from basic need subscales (Acton & Malathum, 2000).

Table 11-2.   INSTRUMENTS COMMONLY USED IN MRM RESEARCH

INSTRUMENT	VARIABLE(S) MEASURED	SOURCE
Basic Need Satisfaction Inventory	Basic-need satisfaction based on Maslow's five basic needs	Leidy, 1994
Health-Promoting Lifestyle Profile II	Health-promoting, self-care behavior	Walker, Sechrist, & Pender, 1995
Modified Erikson Psychosocial Stage Inventory	Erikson's eight stages of the life cycle in adults	Darling-Fisher & Leidy, 1988
Perceived Enactment of Autonomy Scale	Potential for self-care action Perceived enactment of autonomy and its attributes: individuality, self-direction, voluntariness	Hertz, 1991
Robinson Self-Appraisal Inventory	Self-reported denial	Robinson, 1991
Self-Care Resource Inventory	Self-care resources	Baas, 1992

SUMMARY

Modeling and Role-Modeling is a nursing theory and paradigm for nursing practice. MRM synthesizes theories of development, basic needs, stress, and loss, and explains interrelationships among these concepts. These concepts are linked to several concepts specific to MRM theory, such as holism, adaptation, affiliated-individuation, nurturance, facilitation, self-care, and unconditional acceptance. At the heart of the theory is modeling, the process of "stepping into" and understanding the client's thoughts, feelings, and needs. The nurse uses role-modeling to design scientifically based nursing interventions, developed within the understanding of the client's model of the world, to help the client move toward perceived optimal health. MRM serves as a framework for nursing research, education and practice.

ANALYSIS EXERCISE

Using the criteria presented in Chapter 2, critique the theory Modeling and Role-Modeling. Compare your conclusions about the theory with those found in Appendix A.

Internal Criticism
1. Clarity
2. Consistency
3. Adequacy
4. Logical development
5. Level of theory development

External Criticism
1. Reality convergence
2. Utility
3. Significance
4. Discrimination
5. Scope of theory
6. Complexity

WEB RESOURCES

1. The Society for the Advancement of Modeling and Role-Modeling sponsors a site that provides an overview of MRM theory, a description of the society, a reference list, and directions for accessing the society listserve: *http://www.mrmnursingtheory.org*
2. MRM resources are available on the Sigma Theta Tau Nursing Honor Society Virginia Henderson Library. Select Library Search, then type Modeling and Role-Modeling in the search box: *http://www.stti.iupui.edu/library/*
3. MRM is listed on several university nursing theory pages. These sites refer to MRM theory and provide a link to the MRM site but offer only limited information about the theory:
http:// www.ualberta.ca/~jrnorris/nt/theory.html
http://www.healthsci.clayton.edu/eichelberger/nursing.htm
http://www.valdosta.edu/nursing/nursing_theory.html

REFERENCES

Acton, G. J. (1997). Affiliated-individuation as a mediator of stress and burden in caregivers of adults with dementia. *Journal of Holistic Nursing, 15*(4), 336–357.

Acton, G. J., & Malathum, P. (2000). Basic need status and health-promoting self-care behavior in adults. *Western Journal of Nursing Research, 22*(7), 796–811.

Acton, G. J., & Miller, E. W. (1996). Affiliated-individuation in caregivers of adults with dementia. *Issues in Mental Health Nursing, 17*, 245–260.

Baas, L. S. (1992). The relationship among self-care knowledge, self-care resources, activity level and life satisfaction in persons three to six months after myocardial infarction. *Dissertation Abstracts International, 53*, 04B.

Baas, L. S., Curl, E. D., Hertz, J. E., & Robinson, K. R. (1994). Innovative approaches to theory-based measurement: Modeling and role-modeling research. In Chinn, (Ed.). *Advanced Methods of Inquiry in Nursing.* Gaithersburg, MD: Aspen Publication.

Baas, L. S., Fontana, J. A., & Bhat, G. (1997). Relationships between self-care resources and quality of life of persons with heart failure: A comparison of treatment groups. *Progress in Cardiovascular Nursing, 12*(1), 25–38.

Baker, C. (1999). From chaos to order: A nursing-based psycho-educational program for parents of children with attention-deficit hyperactivity disorder. *Canadian Journal of Nursing Research, 31*(2), 7–15.

Barnfather, J. S. (1987). Mobilizing coping resources related to basic need status in healthy, young adults. *Dissertation Abstracts International, 49*, 02B.

Barnfather, J. S. (1991). Restructuring the role of school nursing in health promotion. *Public Health Nursing, 8*(4), 234–238.

Barnfather, J. S. (1993). Testing a theoretical proposition for modeling and role-modeling: Basic need and adaptive potential status. *Issues in Mental Health Nursing, 14*, 1–18.

Barnfather, J. S., & Ronis, D. L. (2000). Test of a model of psychosocial resources, stress, and health among under-educated adults. *Research in Nursing and Health, 23*, 55–66.

Barnfather, J. S., Swain, M. A., & Erickson, H. C. (1984). Evaluation of two assessment techniques for adaptation to stress. *Nursing Science Quarterly, 2*(4), 172–182.

Barnfather, J. S., Swain, M. A., & Erickson, H. C. (1989). Construct validity of an aspect of the coping process: Potential adaptation to stress. *Issues in Mental Health Nursing, 10*, 23–40.

Bylaws. (2000). Society for the Advancement of Modeling and Role Modeling. Retrieved August 6, 2003 from *www.mrmnursingtheory.org/Bylaws.htm*

Campbell, J., Finch, D., Allport, C., Erickson, H., & Swain, M. A. (1985). A theoretical approach to nursing assessment. *Journal of Advanced Nursing, 10*, 111–115.

Darling-Fisher, C. S., & Leidy, N. K. (1988). Measuring Eriksonian development in the adult: The modified Erikson psychosocial stage inventory. *Psychological Reports, 62*, 747–754.

Dickoff, J., James, P., & Weidenback, E. (1968). Theory in a practice discipline: Practice oriented theory. *Nursing Research, 5*, 415–435.

Engel, G. S. (1962). *Psychological development in health and disease.* Philadelphia: W. B. Saunders.

Erickson, H. C. (1976). Identification of state of coping utilizing physiological and psychological data. Unpublished master's thesis, University of Michigan—Ann Arbor, Michigan.

Erickson, H. C. (1989). *Looking at patient's needs through new eyes: Modeling and role-modeling.* Unpublished manuscript.

Erickson, H. C. (1990). Theory based practice. *Modeling and Role-Modeling: Theory, Practice and Research 1*(1), 1–27.

Erickson, H. C., & Swain, M. A. (1982). A model for assessing potential adaptation to stress. *Research in Nursing and Health, 5*, 93–101.

Erickson, H. C., & Swain, M. A. (1990). Mobilizing self-care resources: A nursing intervention for hypertension. *Issues in Mental Health Nursing, 11*, 217–235.

Erickson, H. C., Tomlin, E. M., & Swain, M. A. (1983). *Modeling and role-modeling: A theory and paradigm for nursing.* Englewood Cliffs, NJ: Prentice-Hall, Inc.

Erickson, M. E. (2002a). Modeling and role-modeling. In A. M. Tomey & M. R. Alligood (Eds.), *Nursing theorists and their work.* St. Louis: Mosby, Inc.

Erickson, M. E. (2002b). Modeling and role-modeling theory in nursing practice. In M. R. Alligood & A. M. Tomey (Eds.), *Nursing theory utilization & application,* 2nd ed., St. Louis: Mosby, Inc.

Erickson, M. E. (1996). Relationships among support, needs satisfaction and maternal attachment in adolescent mothers. Unpublished doctoral dissertation, University of Texas, Austin.

Erikson, E. (1968). *Identity, youth and crisis.* New York, NY: Norton.

Fawcett, J. (1995). *Analysis and evaluation of conceptual models of nursing,* 3rd Ed. Philadelphia: F. A. Davis Company.

Finch, D. A. (1990). Testing a theoretically based nursing assessment. *Modeling and role-modeling: Theory, practice and research, 1*(1), 203–213.

Frisch, N. C. (2000). Nursing theory in holistic nursing practice. In B. M. Dossey, L. Keegan, & C. E. Guzzetta (Eds.), *Holistic nursing: A handbook for practice,* 3rd ed., Gaithersburg, MA: Aspen Publishers.

Hertz, J. E. (1991). The perceived enactment of autonomy scale: Measuring the potential for self-care action in the elderly. *Dissertation Abstracts International, 52,* 04B.

Hertz, J. E. (1995). Conceptualization of perceived enactment of autonomy in the elderly. *Issues in Mental Health Nursing, 17,* 261–273.

Hertz, J.E. (2002, April). *A triangulated study of relationships among self-care resources, perceived autonomy, and health in community dwelling older adults.* Paper presented at the Ninth Biennial Conference, Society for the Advancement of Modeling and Role Modeling, Camp Buckner, Marble Falls, TX.

Holl, R. M. (1992). The effects of role-modeled visiting in comparison to restricted visiting on the well-being of clients who had open heart surgery and their significant family members in the critical care unit. *Dissertation Abstracts International, 53,* 08B.

Irvin, B. L. (1993). Social support, self-worth, and hope as self-care resources for coping with caregiver stress. *Dissertation Abstracts International, 53,* 06B.

Irvin, B. L., & Acton, G. J. (1996). Stress mediation in caregivers of cognitively impaired adults: Theoretical model testing. *Nursing Research. 45*(3), 160–166.

Irvin, B. L., & Acton, G. J. (1997). Stress, hope, and well-being of women caring for family members with Alzheimer's disease. *Holistic Nursing Practice, 11*(2) 69–79.

Keegan, L., & Dossey, B. M. (1998). *Profile of nurse healers.* Albany, NY: Delmar Publishers.

Kennedy, G. T. (1991). A nursing investigation of comfort and comforting care of the acutely ill patient. *Dissertation Abstracts International, 52,* 12B.

Kline, N. W. (1988). Psychophysiological processes of stress in people with a chronic physical illness. *Dissertation Abstracts International, 49,* 06B.

Landis, B. J. (1991). Uncertainty, spiritual well-being, and psychosocial adjustment to chronic illness. *Dissertation Abstracts International, 52,* 08B.

Leidy, N. K. (1994). Operationalizing Maslow's theory: Development and testing of the basic need satisfaction inventory. *Issues in Mental Health Nursing, 15,* 277–295.

Maslow, A. H. (1968). *Toward a psychology of being.* New York, NY: Van Norstrand Reinhold.

McClosky, J., & Grace, H. (1994). *Current issues in nursing,* 4th Ed., St. Louis: C.V. Mosby Company.

McEwin, M., & Wills, E. (2002). *Theoretical basis for nursing.* Philadelphia: Lippincott Williams & Wilkins.

Miller, S. H. (1986). The relationships between psychosocial development and coping ability among disabled teenagers. *Dissertation Abstracts International, 47,* 10B.

Perese, E. F. (1997). Unmet need of persons with chronic mental illnesses: Relationship to their adaptation to community living. *Issues in Mental Health Nursing, 18,* 19–34.

Piaget, J. (1952). *The origins of intelligence in children.* New York: International Universities Press, Inc.

Robinson, K. R. (1992). Developing a scale to measure responses of clients with actual or potential myocardial infarctions. *Dissertation Abstracts International, 53,* 12B.

Rosehow, D. J. (1992). Multidimensional scaling analysis of self-care actions for reintegrating holistic health after myocardial infarction. *Dissertation Abstracts International, 53,* 04B.

Schultz. E. D. (1998). Academic advising from a nursing theory perspective. *Nurse Educator, 23*(2), 22–25.

Selye, H. (1976). *The stress of life.* New York, NY: McGraw-Hill.

Tomey, A. M., & Alligood, M. R. (1998). *Nursing theorists and their work* (4th ed.). Philadelphia: F. A. Davis.

University of Michigan, 5B Vascular Surgery Unit. Retrieved July 1, 2002, from *http://www.med.umich.edu/nursing/5b.htm.*

Villarruel, A. M., Bishop, T. L., Simpson, E. M., Jemmott, L. S., & Fawcett, J. (2001). Borrowed theories, shared theories, and the advancement of nursing knowledge. *Nursing Science Quarterly, 14*(2), 158–163.

Walker, S. N., Sechrist, K., & Pender, N. (1995). *The health-promoting lifestyle profile II.* Omaha: University of Nebraska Medical Center, College of Nursing.

Walsh, K. K., VandenBosch, T. M., & Boehm, S. (1989). Modeling and role-modeling: Integrating theory into practice. *Journal of Advanced Nursing, 14*, 755–761.

BIBLIOGRAPHY

Acton, G. J., Irvin, B. L., Jensen, B. A., Hopkins, B. A., & Miller, E. W. (1997). Explicating middle-range theory through methodological diversity. *Advances in Nursing Science, 19*(3), 78–86.

Baldwin, C. M. (1996). Perceptions of hope: Loved experiences of elementary school children in an urban setting. *Journal of Multicultural Nursing and Health, 2*(3) 41–45.

Barnfather, J. S., & Erickson, H. C. (1989). Construct validity of an aspect of the coping process: Potential adaptation to stress. *Issues in Mental Health Nursing, 10*, 23–40.

Erickson, M. E. (1996). Factors that influence the mother-infant dyad relationships and infant well-being. *Issues in Mental Health Nursing, 18*, 185–200.

Kinney, C. K. (1990). Facilitating growth and development: A paradigm case for modeling and role-modeling. *Issues in Mental Health Nursing, 11*, 375–395.

Rogers, S. (1996). Facilitative affiliation: Nurse-client interactions that enhance healing. *Issues in Mental Health Nursing, 17*, 171–184.

Comfort

KATHARINE KOLCABA

DEFINITION OF KEY TERMS

Comfort	The immediate experience of being strengthened by having needs for relief, ease, and transcendence addressed in four contexts (physical, psychospiritual, sociocultural, and environmental); much more than the absence of pain or other physical discomforts
Comfort Care	A philosophy of health care that addresses physical (including homeostatic mechanisms as well as sensations), psychospiritual, sociocultural, and environmental comfort needs of patients. Comfort Care has three components: (1) an appropriate and timely intervention; (2) a mode of delivery that projects caring and empathy; and (3) the intent to comfort.
Comfort measures	Interventions intentionally designed to enhance patients' or families' comfort
Comfort needs	Patients' or families' desire for or deficit in relief/ease/transcendence in physical, psychospiritual, sociocultural, and environmental contexts of human experience
Health-seeking behaviors (HSB)	Behaviors in which patients or families engage consciously or subconsciously, moving them toward well-being; HSBs can be internal, external, or dying peacefully
Institutional integrity	The quality or state of health care organizations as complete, whole, sound, upright, professional, and ethical providers of health care
Intervening variables	Positive or negative factors over which nurses or institutions have little control, but which affect the direction and success of Comfort Care plans or comfort studies. Examples are presence or absence of social support, poverty, positive prognosis, concurrent medical or psychological conditions, and health habits.

INTRODUCTION

The concept of comfort has had an historic and consistent association with nursing. Nurses traditionally provide comfort to patients and their families through interventions that, in this theory, are called comfort measures. The Theory of Comfort, also called Comfort Care, explicates a philosophy of care whereby holistic comfort needs of patients and families are identified and addressed. Planning and assessment account for intervening variables. The desired and immediate outcome is enhanced comfort, an altruistic and patient-centered goal. In addition, enhanced comfort is related to subsequent desirable outcomes, such as higher patient function, quicker discharge, fewer readmissions, increased satisfaction with care, and stronger cost–benefit ratios for the institution. These subsequent outcomes provide additional rationale for health care teams to adopt Comfort Care as a unifying framework for care delivery.

HISTORICAL BACKGROUND

Florence Nightingale was perhaps the first health care worker to recognize that comfort was essential for patients. She said, "It must never be lost sight of what observation is for. It is not for the sake of piling up miscellaneous information or curious facts, but for the sake of saving life and increasing health and comfort" (Nightingale, 1859, p. 70). In this quote, Nightingale seems to imply that the relationship between health and comfort is dependent, and that both are equally important.

At the beginning of the 20th century, the term comfort was used in a general sense, much as Nightingale had used it, and comfort was highly valued in nursing. For example, Aikens (1908) stated there was nothing regarding the comfort of patients that was too insignificant for nurses to attend to. Patients' comfort was the nurse's first and last consideration, and a good nurse was one who made patients comfortable. Moreover, the ability to provide comfort determined, to a large degree, the nurse's skill and character. In 1926, Harmer stated that nursing care was concerned with providing a "general atmosphere of comfort" and that personal care of patients included attention to "happiness, comfort, and ease, physical and mental" (p. 25). (In addition, nurses were to attend to their patients' rest and sleep, nutrition, cleanliness, and elimination.) Goodnow, in her book, *The Technic of Nursing* (1935), devoted a chapter to 'The Patient's Comfort.' She wrote, "The nurse was judged by the ability to make her [sic] patient comfortable. Comfort was both physical and mental, and a nurse's responsibility did not end with physical care" (p. 95).

At this time, nurses believed that the provision of comfort was their unique mission. Comfort was especially important because curative medical strategies were not yet developed. Enhancing patient comfort was seen as a positive nursing goal that also was nurturing, and, in most cases, should entail an improvement from a previous state or condition. Comfort resulted from physical, emotional, and environmental interventions, but orders for specific comfort measures were under the physician's authority. Some common "comfort orders" in this period were for poultices, heat, and positioning of the bed (McIlveen & Morse, 1995).

Although emotional care was not one of the specified roles of nurses, physical comfort measures were intended to bring about mental comfort of patients, indicating that physical and mental comfort were closely related. In early nursing texts, the meaning of comfort was implicit, hidden in context, complex, and general. Many semantic variations, such as "comforting," "in comfort," and "comfortable," were used and the term could be in the form of a verb, noun, adjective, or adverb. Comfort also referred to the process of comforting, such as "The nurse comforted the patient" or the *outcome* of comfort, such as "The patient was comforted by the nurse."

Since that early time, the meaning and importance of comfort have undergone changes that parallel developments in health care. From its general meaning and significant worth in nursing at the beginning of the 20th century, comfort evolved to a less important nursing goal, with a connotation more specific to the physical sense. In the 1950s, as analgesics became popular for pain control, few additional treatments for comfort were described (McIlveen & Morse, 1995). At this time, nurses took responsibility for patients' feelings, although nurses were told to refrain from discussing patients' medical conditions with them.

Physical comfort became one of many strategies for promoting health and was secondary to other goals, such as prevention of complications. By the 1970s, nurses' autonomy increased, and they could implement comfort measures without a doctor's order. But without doctors' orders for comfort, the motivation and recognition for enhancing patient comfort also diminished (McIlveen & Morse, 1995). As the use of technology intensified, many traditional comfort measures were relegated to minor significance, were viewed as simple to administer, or were implemented by assistive personnel. Because anyone could provide comfort, it was no longer a specialized nursing goal or included in definitions of "skilled" care. The term remained undefined in the discipline, but now comfort was narrowly interpreted, written about rarely, and, of course, not measured.

The 1980s saw many advances in medicine, and cures often resulted from surgery, antibiotics, radiation therapy, and chemotherapy. Narcotics were used for treating severe pain. Another trend that began to emerge in the 1980s was a focus on the comfort of the family; families were considered legitimate recipients of care and comfort measures (McIlveen & Morse, 1995). The relationship between the comfort of the patient and the comfort of the family was implied.

During the 1980s, nurses promoted *self*-care, and comfort was a minor goal. Indeed, comfort was the *main* goal of nursing only when patients were terminally ill, an observation that supported Glaser and Strauss' earlier suggestion that the goal of nursing reverted to comfort when there were no available cures (1965). Also, where nursing settings were less under the control of technology, such as hospice and long-term care, comfort was more important as a nursing goal. McIlveen & Morse (1995) suggested that this trend had broad implications for nursing in the 21st century, because demographics would shift to large numbers of elders who may wish for less technology and more comfort in their last years of life.

In nursing literature, the connection between strengthening patients for rehabilitation and their comfort was implied throughout nursing's history. Nightingale (1859) had claimed that patients who were kept comfortable by nurses would be in a better position to regain health. In 1926, Harmer noted a link between nursing comfort and the dictionary definition, which included the component of strengthening. The linking of comfort, especially emotional comfort, to strength continued to be implied in the nursing literature through the 1980s (McIlveen & Morse, 1995). For example, an early case study in a popular journal described how the nurse came to recognize that the patient's strength and courage to fight disease were derived from comforting visits by his mother (Oerlemans, 1972). According to Paterson and Zderad (1976, 1988), nurses helped their psychiatric patients achieve comfort, which these authors defined as "more being," to facilitate their function at highest possible levels.

DEFINITION OF THEORY CONCEPTS

When a concept is germane to a discipline, as comfort is, but it has not yet been specifically defined, a concept analysis is necessary. Thus, in 1988, this task was undertaken by Kolcaba. It began with a study of several contemporary dictionaries, each of which contained between six and eight definitions of comfort. Those meanings were compared to usages found in an extensive literature search in the journals of several disciplines (nursing, medicine, theology, ergonomics, psychology, and psychiatry). From ergonomics came the insight that comfort of persons, for example, in their workplace or their cars, was important for optimum function or productivity (Kolcaba & Kolcaba, 1991).

Also consulted were nursing textbooks, nursing history books, and the Oxford English Dictionary (OED), which traces the origins and evolution of English words. In 1988, the nursing diagnosis for altered comfort was limited to specific physical discomforts such as pain, nausea, and itching. In nursing textbooks, comfort was discussed in terms of pain management. But the origins of comfort supported its later association with strengthening, because the concept itself came from the Latin word *confortare*, meaning "to strengthen greatly." Those obsolete meanings of comfort, not included in modern dictionaries, were still appropriate for nursing. From the OED, the following definitions of comfort were given: (a) strengthening; encouragement, incitement, aid, succor, support and (b) physical refreshment or sustenance; refreshing or invigorating influence (Kolcaba & Kolcaba, 1991). These meanings, plus the link to optimum function in the ergonomic literature, provide theoretical significance for comfort in nursing.

From the above process, which took 2 years, three technical senses of comfort were derived and labeled relief, ease, and renewal. *Relief* was defined as the experience of a patient who has had a specific comfort need addressed; its theoretical background was consistent with Orlando's (1961, 1990) need-based philosophy of nursing. *Ease* was defined as a state of calm or contentment; its theoretical background was enriched by the writings of Henderson (1978) about essential human requirements. *Renewal* was defined as the state in which one rises above problems or pain. Later, the term renewal was changed to *transcendence*, a term already used in the nursing literature by Paterson and Zderad (1976, 1988).

[Author's note: Publishing this part of the concept analysis (Kolcaba & Kolcaba, 1991) took 1 year because the language was rather complicated. The analysis was comprehensive, but not particularly welcomed by American journals. Hence, this first article actually was published at the same time as the second article, described below.]

After presenting these senses or types of comfort at a research conference, audience feedback was so provocative that, in the middle of the night, Kolcaba awoke with the idea that the types of comfort (relief, ease, and renewal) occurred physically and mentally. She sketched out a preliminary grid with **relief**, **ease**, and **renewal** across the top and **physical** and **mental** down the side. Thus, there were six cells in this first grid. After presenting this preliminary grid to colleagues and professors at Case Western Reserve University (where she was a doctoral student), Kolcaba was advised that her "physical" and "mental" categories were not holistic, and to go back to the literature to discover how holism was conceptualized for nursing.

Doing so took another year. Four contexts of holistic experience were derived from the literature, labeled physical, psychospiritual, social, and environmental (Kolcaba, 1991). *Physical comfort* pertained to bodily sensations and homeostatic mechanisms. *Psychospiritual comfort* pertained to the internal awareness of self, including esteem, sexuality, and meaning in one's life; it also encompassed one's relationship to a higher order or being. *Social comfort* pertained to interpersonal, family, and societal relationships (later this term was changed to *sociocultural comfort* and the idea of family and cultural traditions was added to the definition). *Environmental comfort* pertained to the external background of human experience; it encompassed light, noise, ambience, color, temperature, and natural versus synthetic elements.

When the three types of comfort were juxtaposed with the four contexts of experience, a 12-cell grid, or taxonomic structure (TS), was created, as illustrated in Figure 12-1 (Kolcaba, 1991). The grid depicted the attributes of comfort, and was helpful for deriving the technical definition of *comfort* (provided at the beginning of this chapter): *the immediate experience of being strengthened by having needs for relief, ease, and transcendence met in four contexts (physical, psychospiritual, sociocultural, and environmental* (Kolcaba, 1992). This grid has been useful for assessing comfort needs, planning interventions to address those needs, informally evaluating the effectiveness of those interventions to enhance comfort, and measuring patients' comfort for research and practice.

DESCRIPTION OF THE THEORY OF COMFORT

Assumptions

Assumptions are a theorist's point of view about reality, set forth so future readers know where the theorist is "coming from." Kolcaba's (1994) assumptions are:

- Human beings have holistic responses to complex stimuli.
- Comfort is a desirable holistic outcome that is germane to the discipline of nursing.
- Human beings strive to meet, or to have met, their basic comfort needs. It is an active endeavor.
- Comfort is more than the absence of pain, anxiety, and other physical discomfort.

	Relief	Ease	Transcendence
Physical			
Psychospiritual			
Environmental			
Sociocultural			

■ **Figure 12.1** Taxonomic structure of comfort.

Concepts

Concepts are ideas that make up the building blocks of specific theories. The concepts for the middle range Theory of Comfort are those listed and defined at the beginning of this chapter: comfort needs, comfort measures (interventions), intervening variables, enhanced comfort, HSBs, and institutional integrity. Consistent with middle range theories, these concepts are at a low level of abstraction (easily defined and measured) and are limited in number. All of the above concepts are relative to patients and families; the term *family* encompasses significant others as determined by the patient. Kolcaba also has applied her theory to nurses' comfort, which is especially relevant to recruitment and retention (Kolcaba, 2003).

Figure 12-2 is a diagram showing three levels of abstraction, from highest (at the top of the diagram) to lowest (at the bottom of the diagram)—a depiction called a substruction. This particular figure served as the organizing framework for Kolcaba's study of women going through radiation therapy, discussed later in this chapter. Such diagrams are helpful for planning research studies and are used in many of Kolcaba's articles and on her Web site (Kolcaba, 1997, on-line).

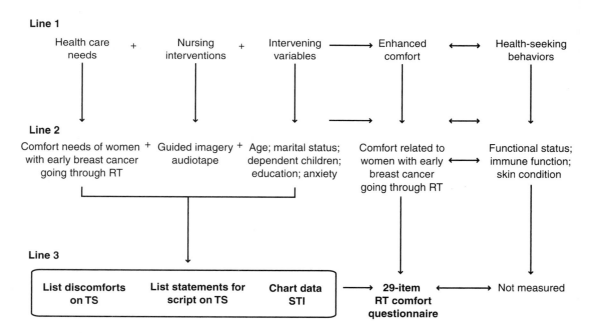

Note: **Bold type** indicates operational variables measured in this study.

■ **Figure 12.2** Theoretical framework for breast cancer radiation therapy (RT) study. Source: Kolcaba, K., & Fox, C. (1999). The effects of guided imagery on comfort of women with early stage breast cancer undergoing radiation therapy. *Oncology Nursing Forum, 26*(1), 67–72.

Propositions

Propositions are relational statements that link concepts together. At the *middle range level* (see Fig. 12-2, Line 1), the following basic propositions of Comfort Theory link those respective variables (Kolcaba, 2001):

1. Nurses identify comfort needs of patients and their family members, especially those needs that have not been met by existing support systems.
2. Nurses design interventions to address those needs.
3. Intervening variables are taken into account in designing the interventions and determining their probability for success.
4. When interventions are effective, and delivered in a caring manner, the immediate outcome of enhanced comfort is attained and the interventions can be called comfort measures. *Comfort Care* entails all of these components.
5. Patients and nurses agree upon desirable and realistic health-seeking behaviors (HSBs).
6. If enhanced comfort is achieved, patients and family members are strengthened to engage in HSBs, which further enhances comfort.
7. When patients and family members engage in HSBs as result of being strengthened by Comfort Care, nurses, families, and patients are more satisfied with health care and demonstrate better health-related outcomes.
8. When patients, families, and nurses are satisfied with health care in a specific institution, public acknowledgment about the institutions' contributions to health in the United States will help those institutions remain viable and flourishing.

Comfort Theory can be adapted to any patient setting or age group, whether in the home, hospital, or community. For research or practice, the concepts can be further defined at a lower level of abstraction, in terms of specific patient populations. Such a level of abstraction is sometimes called the *practice level* (see Fig. 12-2, Line 2). The lowest level of abstraction states how each concept will be measured or put into practice. This level is called the *operational level* (see Fig. 12-2, Line 3).

APPLICATIONS OF THE THEORY

All or parts of Comfort Theory can be tested for research. The first part of the theory, which entails propositions 1 through 4, is the most frequently tested portion to date. Here, the effectiveness of a holistic intervention (targeted to the 12 cells in the taxonomic structure) for enhancing comfort (in a specific patient population) over time would be tested. Some holistic interventions that are congruent with the theory are guided imagery, progressive muscle relaxation, meditation, music or art therapy, massage, and therapeutic touch.

In an experimental design, patients meeting inclusion criteria are randomly assigned to a treatment group or a comparison group. Researchers use the General Comfort Questionnaire (GCQ) as a starting point, removing items that are not relevant to their research setting or questions, and adding items that are relevant. They can plot all items on the taxonomic structure, making sure that the content domain of comfort is evenly represented. Similar numbers of positive and negative items are constructed, unless patients are cognitively frail. In that case, primarily positive items are used (Cohen & Mount, 1992).

Kolcaba usually uses three measurement points, the first being baseline measures of the selected outcomes. Her preferred test statistic is Repeated Measures Multivariate Analysis of Variance (RM MANOVA), or, if using a covariate, Multivariate of Analysis of Covariates (MANCOVA). These are good statistics for comfort research because they capture the interaction between time and the intervention (group assignment) and they have strong power (fewer subjects needed). Accounting for the impact of the interaction between time and the intervention (in other words, does the intervention increase comfort over time?) is congruent with Comfort Theory because, although comfort is not a stable state, a trend for increased comfort over time can be demonstrated, given an effective and consistently applied intervention (comfort measure).

The second part of the Theory is represented by Proposition 6, relating comfort to selected HSBs. While not tested as often as the first part of the theory, the second part provides rationale for *why* nurses and other health care providers should focus on patient comfort, beyond altruistic reasons. Because HSBs include internal and external behaviors, almost any outcome that is deemed important in a given research setting can be classified as an HSB. The task for the investigator is to justify the choice of HSBs and discuss reasons that patients would want to engage in those HSBs, whether consciously or unconsciously.

Research with patients near end of life and their family members is in its infancy. Comfort is consistently stated as a desired outcome in hospice standards of care, which makes Comfort Theory particularly cogent for research with patients near end of life. Making it even more applicable for hospice or palliative research is Schlotfeldt's (1975) inclusion of Peaceful Death as an HSB. Sometimes, a peaceful death is the most realistic outcome in a particular situation, and Scholtfeldt's elevating Peaceful Death to an HSB is an example of how her thinking was "ahead of her time." However, recruitment and data collection with patients near end of life is fraught with difficulties. For these reasons, Kolcaba currently is working on an instrument to measure comfort behaviors, which data collectors could use to rate a patient's *apparent* comfort. While not as desirable as actually asking a patient about his or her comfort, the instrument will fill a gap in data collection from frail or cognitively limited patients.

The third part of Comfort Theory is represented by Propositions 7 and 8, relating patients' comfort and their engagement in HSBs to Institutional Integrity (InI). This part of the theory is relatively new, having been published in 2001 (Kolcaba). The concept of InI was added to the theory to provide direction for outcomes research that would support the discipline of nursing. Comfort and Patient Satisfaction currently are among the few positive outcomes being used for this type of research. Kolcaba believes that future research will show that these two positive outcomes are highly correlated. Because institutions are driven by market competition to produce high patient-satisfaction scores, those same institutions will be interested to know that patient comfort is a strong predictor of patient satisfaction, as well as other positive outcomes, such as shorter lengths of stay, better responses to rehabilitation programs, and fewer hospital readmissions.

Perhaps because nursing outcomes research is a newer science, data thus far have largely focused on "absence of" adverse events related to hospitalization, such as new decubiti, medication errors, nosocomial infections, pneumonia, and death. Surely, patients and their family members want and need more from their hospital stays than freedom from adverse events. They want to get well, avoid future hospitalizations, understand their new health regimen, be treated with respect and care, return to previous levels of function, and, yes, be comforted by their nurses when necessary. Positive outcomes brought about by sufficiently supported and motivated nurses, would create "value added" benefits in contemporary health care situations.

The research examples shown in Using Middle Range Theories 12-1 and 12-2 are published studies that tested the effectiveness of holistic interventions in promoting comfort in specific populations.

12-1 USING MIDDLE RANGE THEORIES

For her dissertation study, Kolcaba developed a Guided Imagery (GI) audiotape for women with breast cancer who were undergoing conservative treatment. Breast-conserving therapy consisted of lumpectomy and radiation therapy (RT). The research question was: Will women who receive GI while going through RT for early-stage breast cancer have greater comfort over time compared to a control group? (see Figure 12-2.)

The audiotape medium facilitated the delivery of the same holistic message over and over to all women in the treatment group. In the script for GI, positive statements were directed to every cell in the taxonomic structure of comfort known to be important for this population. Input for construction of the audiotape and design of the study was received from the RT nurses, technicians, and physicians.

The instruments used in this study were the Radiation Therapy Comfort Questionnaire (RTCQ) and four visual analog scales (Total Comfort, Relief, Ease, and Transcendence). The development and psychometric performance of these instruments are discussed in the section "Instruments Used in Empirical Testing." During the pilot test for the methods, the women were asked specifically if there was anything left out of the questionnaire, anything that was forgotten or awkward in the audiotape, and if the instruments were easy to use. When everyone was satisfied with the protocol, the study began.

Nurses told the women about the study during their first appointment in the RT department. When the patients first heard about the study, about half the women burst into tears; the other half wanted to enroll. The nurses faxed the names and phone numbers of those who wanted to enroll to the data collectors, and the intake visit took place before the women's simulation visit. The women in the treatment group were asked to listen to the tape every day, in their own homes, with tape players that the study provided. They indicated in journals and during interviews that they complied with this request diligently for the first 3 weeks of RT, after which, some tired of the audiotape. When this occurred, they were encouraged to continue listening to the music side of the tape, which would reinforce recall of the guided imagery script. In this way, the script could be internalized.

Three complete data sets were collected (3 visits for each woman) on 53 women, which took a year after IRB approvals were obtained. RM MANOVA was used to test the hypotheses. Alpha was set at .10 because the intervention had no risks and the higher alpha reduced Type II error (Lipsey, 1990).

Results. This study was a test of the new Comfort Theory, as well as a test of the guided imagery intervention and the ability to show quantitative differences in the complex phenomenon of patient comfort. Analysis of group differences at baseline on demographic data and comfort revealed that the groups were similar for all baseline variables. This was the desired result for Time 1 data. The result of the MANOVA, which analyzed data from all three time points, was that the groups were significantly different on comfort at Times 2 and 3 (p = .07), a second desired result. Then two posttests were conducted. The first was to determine which group had higher comfort (the treatment group did) and the second was to

(Continued)

(Continued) **USING MIDDLE RANGE THEORIES**

perform a trend analysis, looking at the "slopes" of the comfort data for both groups. This analysis revealed a linear slope over time, meaning that differences between the groups increased steadily over time. A simplified picture of the trend analysis for this study is in Figure 12-3. All of these results confirmed the efficacy of guided imagery, and supported the Theory of Comfort.

Kolcaba, K., & Fox, C. (1999). The effects of guided imagery on comfort of women with early stage breast cancer undergoing radiation therapy. *Oncology Nursing Forum, 26*(1), 67–72.

INSTRUMENTS USED IN EMPIRICAL TESTING

General Comfort Questionnaire (GCQ)

If researchers want to conduct a comfort study and need to construct a comfort instrument for a unique population, they can use and adapt the General Comfort Questionnaire (GCQ). Detailed instructions for doing so are on the Web (Kolcaba, 1997, on-line), and some psychometric properties of the GCQ are discussed here. (A full discussion of how the instrument was developed is in Kolcaba, 1992, 2003.)

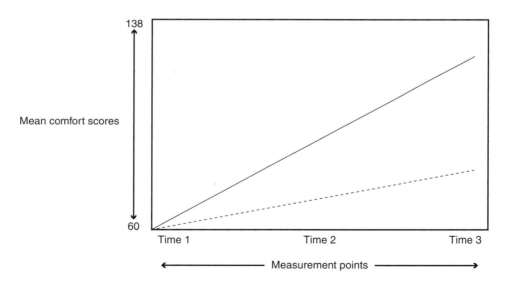

Treatment group= solid line
Comparison group= dotted line

■ **Figure 12.3** Trend analysis for breast cancer study. Source: Kolcaba, K., & Fox, C. (1999). The effects of guided imagery on comfort of women with early stage breast cancer undergoing radiation therapy. *Oncology Nursing Forum, 26*(1), 67–72.

12-2 USING MIDDLE RANGE THEORIES

The purpose of this study was to test the effectiveness of audiotaped cognitive strategies for improving comfort related to bladder function. The research question was: Will the group practicing cognitive strategies have higher *comfort* related to bladder function and better actual *bladder function* compared to the control group over time?

A substructed diagram similar to the radiation therapy diagram was used to organize the study. Following this diagram, the known comfort needs of this population were targeted, with the cognitive strategies recorded on a new audiotape. The taxonomic structure was used as a guide to cover the domain of comfort with the recorded statements. Possible covariates (intervening variables) were age, gender, and particulars of bladder health history. To measure comfort in this population, the taxonomic structure was used to develop the Urinary Incontinence and Frequency Comfort Questionnaire (UIFCQ), which was pilot-tested before using it in this study. The health-seeking behavior that was measured was improved bladder function, operationalized by number of incontinent episodes, number of toileting trips, and the Bladder Function Questionnaire (researcher developed).

Most of the methods from the breast cancer study (described previously) were replicated (because of their success), including having persons in the treatment group listen to the tape daily, having three data collection points, and using the same method of data analaysis.

Results indicated that the treatment group had more comfort and improved bladder function over time compared with the comparison group. In addition, a crossover component was added when those in the original comparison group listened to the audiotape for 3 weeks, after which data were collected again from both groups. A significant improvement in bladder function was found in the crossover group, and their comfort had increased to the level of the treatment group after 3 weeks of the intervention.

Another interesting finding was that the UIFCQ predicted which participants (n = 17, or 90% of the treatment group) would demonstrate improvement in incontinence. Because comfort was a strong predictor of benefit from treatment for incontinence and frequency, these findings also supported the middle range Theory of Comfort (Dowd, Kolcaba, & Steiner, 2000).

Dowd, T., Kolcaba, K., & Steiner, R. (2000). Using cognitive strategies to enhance bladder control and comfort. *Holistic Nursing Practice, 14*(2), 91–103.

As with the other comfort questionnaires available, the GCQ began with the taxonomic structure. For each cell, an equal number of positive and negative items were created. The GCQ contains two positive and two negative items for each of the 12 cells in the taxonomic structure, resulting in 48 items. The researcher's own experience with patient comfort and findings from a thorough literature review about the population are used to write these items. A four-response, Likert-type scale was used for the pilot test, although subsequent questionnaires have six responses, which increases sensitivity of the instrument. An even number of responses also forces the responder to choose one side of the comfort fence or the other.

The GCQ was pilot-tested both in the community (N = 30) and in several types of hospital units (N = 226). Results of this first instrumentation study were encouraging, because the Cronbach's alpha was .88, high for a new instrument. (Perhaps working from a theoretically driven map of the content domain accounts for this result.) Factor analysis, using Principal Components Analysis extracted 13 factors with eigenvalues above 1.0. The 13th factor had only one item and was collapsed into one of the other factors that was semantically similar, producing 12 factors consistent with the TS. In addition, factors clumped together in three subscales on the scree plot and semantically were similar to the types of comfort (Relief, Ease, and Transcendence). This factor structure accounted for 63.4% of the variance in the 48 items (Kolcaba, 1992).

Reliabilities for the subscales (factors) ranged from .66 to .80, which were lower than for the whole GCQ (.88). This is because lower numbers of items generally decrease reliability scores. The GCQ revealed significant sensitivity in expected directions between several groups (construct validity). Findings were that (a) the community group had higher comfort than the hospital group, and (b) people with higher comfort demonstrated a higher correlation with their own estimates of progress in rehabilitation.

When researchers adapt the GCQ to fit their population, they can use the psychometric properties and description of the instrumentation study (above) to support their choice of a comfort instrument. If they wish, they can shorten the number of items and remove whole subscales that are not relevant. However, with each of those strategies, reliability scores may decrease. It is important, therefore, to pilot-test adapted instruments with at least 10 subjects who are characteristic of those in the proposed study. A Cronbach's alpha of at least .70 is desirable for a new instrument. A copy of the GCQ is found in Appendix B.

Radiation Therapy Comfort Questionnaire (RTCQ)

To adapt the GCQ to women with breast cancer, items that were not relevant for radiation therapy were deleted. The literature identified critical comfort needs specific to this population. From this list of needs, positive and negative items were developed to complete and balance the questionnaire for this population.

A consideration when developing the Radiation Therapy Comfort Questionnaire (RTCQ) was the length of time it would take for the women to answer it. The nurses thought, and it was later confirmed, that many research participants would choose to complete the questionnaires in the Radiation Therapy (RT) department rather than in their homes. The design of the study was to administer all questionnaires immediately before radiation therapy. A 48-item questionnaire was deemed too long by the RT staff, and considered too stressful for the women. So, for this study, a 26-item RTCQ was pilot-tested. The instrument performed fairly well in the final study, with a Cronbach's alpha of .76 (n = 53, 26 items). This instrument is available online (Kolcaba, 1997).

Visual Analog Scales (VAS)

For the radiation therapy study, VASs were developed to measure the three subscales of comfort (Relief, Ease, and Transcendence). Each VAS was a 10-centimeter vertical line, anchored at the bottom with "strongly disagree" and at the top with "strongly agree." Stems for the VASs were, "I have many discomforts right now" (Relief); "I am feeling at ease right now" (Ease); and "I am feeling motivated, determined, and strengthened right now" (Transcendence). Higher scores, after reverse coding "Relief," meant higher comfort. The VASs were developed, in part, to begin establishing concurrent validity for comfort questionnaires. Concurrent validity is the extent to which a measure correlates with another simultaneously obtained measure of the same trait or state (Goodwin & Goodwin, 1991). There were no other measures available for comfort. Secondly, it was possible that VASs could measure patient comfort more efficiently than the longer questionnaire.

While the statistical performance of the RTCQ was adequate, the performance of the VASs was mixed and required more involved secondary analyses. Hence, these scales were discussed in a second article (Kolcaba & Steiner, 2000). Findings were that the Total Comfort (TC) Line was not sensitive to differences in comfort over time. The scores for Summed Comfort Subscales (Relief, Ease, and Transcendence) provided data that approached significance (p = .17) and seemed to be more sensitive to individual perceptions of comfort than the Total Comfort line (Kolcaba & Steiner, 2000). However, in clinical settings, asking a patient to rate his or her comfort from 0 to 10, with 10 being high comfort, will result in meaningful conversations about detractors from comfort, so that nurses will know how to proceed with comfort care.

Correlations between the VASs and the RTCQ supported preliminary concurrent validity between the two measures of comfort. Data were skewed to the right because most women indicated on the VASs relatively high comfort (7.3 on scale of 1–10, with 10 being high comfort) and in a rather narrow range (standard deviation 1.58). Thus, nonparametric measures of association were performed. Pair-wise correlations between the RTCQ and the VAS for Total Comfort revealed moderate correlations at each of the three time points: Time 1 = .31, p = .02; Time 2 = .31, p = .02; and Time 3 = .44, p = .00 and the conclusion was that there was moderate concurrent validity between the two comfort instruments (Kolcaba & Steiner, 2000).

Urinary Incontinence and Frequency Comfort Questionnaire (UIFCQ)

For the comfort study with persons with urinary incontinence, the Urinary Incontinence and Frequency Comfort Questionnaire (UIFCQ) was adapted from the GCQ and contained 23 positive and negative items specific to the experience of living with UI. A six-response, Likert-type format, ranging from "strongly agree" to "strongly disagree," was used. After reverse coding negative items, higher scores indicated higher comfort. 31 women and 9 men participated in this study. The Cronbach's alpha averaged .82 across the four measurement points, indicating good reliability. The instrument was sensitive to changes in comfort over time (p = .01) (Dowd, Kolcaba, & Steiner, 2000). It is available online (Kolcaba, 1997).

Hospice Comfort Questionnaire (HCQ): Family and Patient

For this population, the GCQ was adapted again to create a 49-item questionnaire. Family members were asked to rate their own comfort, not that of their patient. The adapted instruments were tested in two phases (Novak, Kolcaba, Steiner, & Dowd, 2001). In phase I of the study, patient and family-member questionnaires had a Likert scale with response set of six, ranging from "strongly agree" to "strongly disagree," and higher scores indicated higher comfort. Each questionnaire took about 12 minutes for patients to complete and usually less time for family members. Approximately equal numbers of positive and negative items were created for the family members' end-of-life questionnaire, and items were worded more simply, with less alternating between positive and negative orientation. This adaptation was necessary because of decreased mental agility in dying patients (Cohen & Mount, 1992).

For phase II of the study, patient and caregiver questionnaires were reduced to a four-item, Likert response set, because of concerns of the data collectors that six responses were too confusing. However, results showed that the instrument in Phase I (six responses) had the strongest psychometric properties for both family members and patients. Cronbach's alpha for the family-member questionnaire was .89 (N=38) and for the patient questionnaire was .83 (N = 48) (Novak et al., 2001).

In spite of these high reliability scores, nurse researchers working with this population a few years later thought that 49 items were too many, and they asked a panel of experts to prioritize the items. From that list, 24 of the highest items were plotted on the taxonomic structure and balanced over the content domain. The result was a 24-item HCQ. All of these instruments are available on Kolcaba's Web site (Kolcaba, 1997, on-line).

Comfort Behaviors Checklist (CBC)

Many nurses who want to do comfort studies have asked about measuring comfort in patients who can't use the traditional comfort questionnaires, the VASs, or rate their comfort from 0 to 10. These patients might be young children or infants, or they might be mentally disabled, brain-injured, heavily sedated, or

Table 12-1. PSYCHOMETRIC PROPERTIES OF OTHER QUANTITATIVE COMFORT INSTRUMENTS

NAME OF INSTRUMENT	RELIABILITY	# ITEMS	# SUBJECTS	STRUCTURE ANALYSIS?	REFERENCE
Maternal Comfort Assessment Tool (observer rating)	Inter-rater: 89%	7	40	NA	Andrews & Chrzanowski, 1990
Dementia Comfort Checklist (observer rating)	Correlation coefficient r .88	9	82	NA	Hurley, Volicer, Hanrahan, & Volicer, 1992
The Comfort Scale (Distress in Pediatric Intensive Care Units)	Inter-rater: .84 Int. Consis: .90	8 and VAS	50	Correlations between 8 dimensions	Ambuel, Hamlett, Marx, & Blumer, 1992
Physical Bedrest Comfort Measure (patient rating)	Cronbach's Alpha .73	19	30	No (not enough subjects)	Hogan-Miller, Rustad, Sendelbach, & Goldenberg, 1995
Radiation Therapy Comfort (position of bed)	Significant difference between groups	1 VAS	17	No	Cox, 1996
Comfort Questionnaire (dehydration/hydration at end of life)	NA	1 4-point Likert scale	31	No	Vullo-Navich et al., 1998
Infant Comfort Behaviour (Pain)	Kappa .63–.93	6 and VAS	158	LISREL	Van Dijk et al., 2000

unconscious. Therefore, the Comfort Behavior Checklist (CBC) was developed, on which a nurse or data collector rates the patient's comfort based on observable behaviors. It contains 30 observations with possible responses of Not Applicable, No, Somewhat, Moderate, and Strong (Kolcaba, 1997, on-line).

Because scoring of the CBC results in a percent out of 100, a deviation of 20 percentage points between raters for each subject is considered clinically and empirically unreliable. Conversely, a deviation between raters of 10 percentage points for each subject is considered to be acceptable, and of 5 percentage points is a demonstration of very strong inter-rater consistency. Distributions of the differences in ratings in 39 data sets were as follows: (a) 36 data sets revealed a 10-point difference or less between rater 1 and rater 2 for each subject (p = .92; alpha .95); and (b) 31 data sets revealed a 5-point difference or less between rater 1 and rater 2 for each subject (p = .80; alpha .95). These findings indicate strong inter-rater consistency. However, when correlated with patients' responses on the traditional comfort questionnaire, low correlations were revealed, averaging a Cronbach's alpha of .14 over three time points. These disappointing findings seem to indicate that the interior life or feelings of human beings cannot be fully appreciated until they are asked. The stoic demeanors of the long-term care residents, which appeared to indicate comfort, masked many complex and interrelated feelings about their own comfort. However, in the absence of the ability to verbalize specific feelings about comfort, or a general comfort rating, the CBC (see Appendix B) is, perhaps, better than no comfort assessment at all. Table 12-1 provides a listing of comfort instruments developed by other researchers.

Research Application 12-1 provides a model of how the theory can be used and tested in practice.

12-1   RESEARCH APPLICATION

Jim, 75 years old, is apprehensive about his upcoming knee surgery. He is afraid of a general anesthetic, pain, blood loss, loss of mobility, and loss of dignity and independence during the procedure and in the postoperative period. All of these separate fears seem rather minor when considered objectively and separately. However, when Jim, sitting in the waiting room, experiences them simultaneously, they create panic. "This is MY body, MY surgery, MY unknowns. **I'm** going under the knife!" Jim's whole-person response is greater or stronger than if he thought only about immobility at one time, blood loss at another time, etc.

A study could be designed where the receptionist gives Jim a brief comfort questionnaire to complete along with his other forms. (Remember that high comfort scores indicate a high degree of comfort.) From the description of his fears, we would expect Jim's *total comfort score* to be quite *low* at Time 1. Then a perioperative nurse begins working with him, senses his panic, and takes his vital signs (blood pressure, pulse, and respirations are high). He is demonstrating a fight-or-flight response and really would just like to leave.

The nurse talks with Jim about alternatives to general anesthesia and about patient-controlled analgesia after surgery. The nurse talks about exercises to strengthen the knee and about minimal blood loss usually associated with his surgery. The nurse assures Jim that the surgeon will carefully drape him, and that the anesthetist will maintain constant supervision

(continued)

12-1   RESEARCH APPLICATION

(Continued)

over Jim during the entire procedure. Most reassuring, perhaps, is the fact that Jim's nurse will accompany him into the operating room and will stay with him. The nurse fully understands how he feels about his personal dignity and will be his advocate. This is called "usual care" in a research study.

The nurse can see that Jim is calming down. Jim completes the comfort questionnaire again (Time 2, after usual care) and vital signs are improved. Then the nurse begins a guided imagery (GI) exercise with Jim. Jim is asked to close his eyes, picture himself in a favorite place, relax his body incrementally, and then imagine the surgery in the most positive ways, as suggested by the nurse. "You will feel no pain upon awaking, you will barely have any bleeding," etc. When Jim completes the GI, he is fully relaxed and confident. He completes a third comfort questionnaire (Time 3), and his vital signs are even better.

The nurse quickly adds up Jim's three comfort scores at each time point (Time 1, Time 2, and Time 3) and notices that his comfort scores improved considerably at each time point. "Well, the usual care improved Jim's comfort but not as much as the guided imagery. And it is interesting that his vital signs improved with each time point, although there was a bigger change between Time 2 and Time 3...could increased comfort be related to improved vital signs?" The Theory of Comfort posits that the immediate outcome of comfort is related to the subsequent outcome of improved vital signs. Other subsequent outcomes of interest might be postoperative bleeding or pain. All of these are health-seeking behaviors (HSBs).

In this study, the nurse wanted to know if usual care and GI (a holistic intervention) increased Jim's comfort, a holistic outcome. To demonstrate that patient comfort is important not only for the nurse but for the hospital, the nurse also wanted to know if comfort was related to other outcomes that may be considered more significant clinically. Other HSBs might be his adherence to a rehabilitation regimen, return to previous functional level, healing of the surgical site, and amount of pain medication. Furthermore, an example of an institutional outcome would be Jim's score on his patient satisfaction survey; an exciting finding would be that his score was higher than a similar patient who did not have the GI intervention. [Of course, the design of this study would be much stronger with both an experimental (receives GI) and comparison group (usual care), each consisting of a large number of patients undergoing a similar surgery.]

In this way, concepts such as comfort gain importance when they are related to other concepts. Nurses and other members of the health team have rationale for taking the time to enhance patient comfort, in addition to the altruistic reason from which nurses usually are motivated. And nurses can demonstrate that GI improves patient outcomes—a quality improvement issue.

ANALYSIS EXERCISE

Using the criteria presented in Chapter 2, critique the Theory of Comfort. Compare your conclusion about the theory with those found in Appendix A. A nurse scholar who has worked with the theory completed the analysis found in the Appendix

Internal Criticism
1. Clarity
2. Consistency
3. Adequacy

4. Logical development
5. Level of theory development

External Criticism
1. Reality convergence
2. Utility
3. Significance
4. Discrimination
5. Scope of theory
6. Complexity

SUMMARY

The Theory of Comfort provides a framework for research in any setting where patients' comfort is valued. The theory has been used to test the effectiveness of specific holistic interventions for increasing comfort, to demonstrate the correlation between comfort and subsequent HSBs, and to relate HSBs to desirable institutional outcomes. It is important as a framework for interdisciplinary care and research because the focus is on the unifying and positive outcome of patient comfort. It also provides an ethical perspective for decision-making in difficult health care situations. As such, Comfort Theory has been used in many health care specialties, both nationally and internationally.

WEB RESOURCES

Currently, the only Internet resource about the outcome of patient comfort is Kolcaba's. On her Web page, references instrumental in the development of this theory are listed. A few minor Internet resources (in the area of psychology and religion) refer to comfort, but they don't define it or give instructions for measuring it: *www.uakron.edu/comfort*

REFERENCES

Aikens, C. (1908). Making the patient comfortable. *Canadian Nurse and Hospital Review, 4*(9), 422–424.

Ambuel, B., Hamlett, K., Marx, C., & Blumer, J. (1992). Assessing distress in pediatric intensive care environments: The COMFORT scale. *Journal of Pediatric Psychology, 17*(1), 95–109.

Andrews, C., & Chrzanowski, M. (1990). Maternal position, labor, and comfort. *Applied Nursing Research, 3*(1), 7–13.

Cohen, S., & Mount, B. (1992). Quality of life in terminal illness: Defining and measuring subjective well-being in the dying. *Journal of Palliative Care, 8*(3), 40–45.

Cox, J. (1996). Assessing patient comfort in radiation therapy. *Radiation Therapist, 5*(2), 119–125.

Dowd, T., Kolcaba, K., & Steiner, R. (2000). Using cognitive strategies to enhance bladder control and comfort. *Holistic Nursing Practice, 14*(2), 91–103.

Glaser, C., & Strauss, A. (1965). *Awareness of dying.* Chicago: Aldine.

Goodnow, M. (1935). *The technic of nursing.* Philadelphia: W.B. Saunders.

Goodwin, L., & Goodwin, W. (1991). Focus on psychometrics: Estimating construct validity. *Research in Nursing and Health, 14*, 235–243.

Harmer, B. (1926). *Methods and principles of teaching the principles and practice of nursing.* New York: MacMillan.

Henderson, V. (1978). *Principles and practice of nursing.* New York: Macmillan.

Hogan-Miller, E., Rustad, D., Sendelbach, S., & Goldenberg, I. (1995). Effects of three methods of femoral site immobilization on bleeding and comfort after coronary angiogram. *American Journal of Critical Care, 4*(2), 143–148.

Hurley, A., Volicer, B., Hanrahan, S., & Volicer, L. (1992).

Assessment of discomfort in advanced Alzheimer patient. *Research in Nursing & Health, 15*, 369–377.

Kolcaba, K. (1991). A taxonomic structure for the concept comfort. *Image: Journal of Nursing Scholarship, 23*(4), 237–239.

Kolcaba, K. (1992). Holistic comfort: Operationalizing the construct as a nurse-sensitive outcome. *Advances in Nursing Science, 15*(1), 1–10.

Kolcaba, K. (1994). A theory of holistic comfort for nursing. *Journal of Advanced Nursing,19*, 1178–1184.

Kolcaba, K. (1997). The Comfort Line. [On-line]. Available: *http://www.uakron.edu/comfort/*. [Copyright, 1997, and updated continuously]

Kolcaba, K. (2001). Evolution of the mid range theory of comfort for outcomes research. *Nursing Outlook, 49*(2), 86–92.

Kolcaba, K. (2003). *Comfort Theory and practice: A vision for holistic health care and research.* New York: Springer.

Kolcaba, K., & Kolcaba, R. (1991). An analysis of the concept of comfort. *Journal of Advanced Nursing, 16*, 1301–1310.

Kolcaba, K., & Fox, C. (1999). The effects of guided imagery on comfort of women with early stage breast cancer undergoing radiation therapy. *Oncology Nursing Forum, 26*(1), 67–72.

Kolcaba, K., & Steiner, R. (2000). Empirical evidence for the nature of holistic comfort. *Journal of Holistic Nursing, 18*(1), 46–62.

Lipsey, M. (1990). Design sensitivity. Newbury Park, CA: Sage.

McIlveen, K., & Morse, J. (1995). The role of comfort in nursing care: 1900–1980. *Clinical Nursing Research, 4*(2), 127–148.

Nightingale, F. (1859). *Notes on nursing.* London, Great Britain: Harrison.

Novak, B., Kolcaba, K., Steiner, R., & Dowd, T. (2001). Measuring comfort in caregivers and patients during late end-of-life care. *American Journal of Hospice & Palliative Care, 18*(3), 170–180.

Oerlemans, M. (1972). Eli. *American Journal of Nursing, 72*, 1440–1441.

Orlando, I. (1961/1990). *The dynamic nurse-patient relationship.* New York: National League for Nursing.

Paterson, J., & Zderad, L. (1976/1988). *Humanistic nursing.* New York: National League for Nursing.

Schlotfeldt, R. (1975). The need for a conceptual framework. In P. Verhonic (Ed.) *Nursing research* (pp. 3–25). Boston: Little & Brown.

Stevens, J. (1992). *Applied multivariate statistics for the social sciences,* (2nd ed.). Hillsdale, NJ: Lawrence Erlbaum Associates.

Van Dijk, M., De Boer, J., Koot, H., Tibboel, D., Passchier, J., & Duivenvoorden, H. (2000). The reliability and validity of the comfort scale as a postoperative pain instrument in 0–3-year-old infants. *Pain, 84*(2–3), 367–377.

Vullo-Navich, K., Smith, S., Andrews, M., Levine, A., Tischler, J., & Veglis, J. (1998). Comfort and incidence of abnormal serum sodium, BUN, creatinine and osmolality in dehydration of terminal illness. *The American Journal of Hospice & Palliative Care, 15*(2), 77–84.

BIBLIOGRAPHY

Andrews, C., & Chrrzanowski, M. (1990). Maternal position, labor, and comfort. *Applied Nursing Research, 3*(1), 7–13.

Arruda, E., Larson, P., & Meleis, A. (1992). Comfort: Immigrant Hispanic cancer patients' views. *Cancer Nursing, 15*(6), 387–394.

Bottorff, J. L. (1991). The lived experience of being comforted by a nurse. *Phenomenology and Pedagogy, 9*, 237–252.

Bucholtz, J. (1994). Comforting children during radiotherapy. *Oncology Nursing Forum, 21*(6), 987–994.

Cameron, B. (1993). The nature of comfort to hospitalized medical surgical patients. *Journal of Advanced Nursing, 18*, 424–430.

Dowd, T. (2001). Katherine Kolcaba: Comfort theory. In A. Tomey & M. Alligood (Eds.), *Nursing theorists and their works* (5th ed., pp. 430–442). St. Louis, MO: Mosby.

Fox, C., & Kolcaba, K. (1995). Unsafe practice: A lack of strategies for effective decision making. (News, notes, and tips). *Nurse Educator, 20*(5), 3–4.

Gropper, E. (1992). Promoting health by promoting comfort. *Nursing Forum, 27*(2), 5–8.

Hamilton, J. (1989). Comfort and the hospitalized chronically ill. *Gerontological Nursing, 15*(4), 28–33.

Keeling, A., Knight, E., Taylor, V., & Nordt, L. (1994). Post-cardiac catheterization time-in-bed study: Enhancing patient comfort through research. *Applied Nursing Research, 7*(1), 14–17.

Koehn, M. (2000). Alternative and complementary therapies for labor and birth: An application of Kolcaba's theory of holistic comfort. *Holistic Nursing Practice, 15*(1), 66–77.

Kolcaba, K. (1987). Reaching optimum function is realistic goal for elderly (Letter to the Editor). *Journal of Gerontological Nursing, 13*(12), 36.

Kolcaba, K. (1988). A framework for the nursing care of demented patients. *Mainlines, 9*(6), 12–13.

Kolcaba, K. (1998). Comfort. In J. J. Fitzpatrick (Ed.), *The encyclopedia of nursing research*, (pp. 102–104). New York: Springer.

Kolcaba, K. (2001). Holistic care: Is it feasible in today's health care environment? In H. Feldman (Ed.), *Nursing leaders speak out.* (pp. 49–54). New York: Springer.

Kolcaba, K. (2001). Kolcaba's theory of comfort. In D. L.

Robinson & C. P. Kish (Eds.), *Core concepts for advanced nursing practice.* (pp. 418–422). St. Louis, MO: Mosby.

Kolcaba, K. (2003). *Comfort theory and practice: A vision for healthcare and research in the 21st century.* New York: Springer.

Kolcaba, K., & Dowd, T. Kegel exercises: Strengthening the weak pelvic floor muscles that cause urinary incontinence. *American Journal of Nursing, 100*(11), 59.

Pederson, C. (1994). Ways to feel comfortable: Teaching aids to promote children's comfort. *Issues in Comprehensive Pediatric Nursing, 17,* 37–46.

Pineau, C. (1982). The psychological meaning of comfort. *International Review of Applied Psychology, 31,* 271–283.

Schuilling, K., & Sampselle, C. (1999). Comfort in labor and midwifery art. *Image: Journal of Nursing Scholarship, 31*(1), 77–81.

Taylor, B. (1992). Relieving pain through ordinariness in nursing: A phenomenologic account of a comforting nurse–patient encounter. *Advances in Nursing Science, 15*(1), 33–43.

Health-Related Quality of Life

TIMOTHY S. BREDOW AND SANDRA J. PETERSON

DEFINITION OF KEY TERMS

Health-related quality of life	Subset of quality of life representing feelings, attitudes, or the ability to experience satisfaction in an area of life identified as personally important that has been disrupted by disease processes or health-related deficits
Life domains	Basic component of health-related quality of life referring to a specific aspect of life, most commonly physical, psychological, socioeconomic, or psychological/spiritual
Nursing interventions	Not included as a component of health-related quality of life. Involves delivering specific care or treatments targeted for an individual who has deficits in an identified domain of functioning that disrupts or has the potential to disrupt health-related quality of life
Patient-perceived satisfaction	Basic component of health-related quality of life referring to an individual's sense of well-being related to a relevant life domain when a specific nursing intervention has been performed
Quality of life	Sense of well-being reflecting an individual's perception of a level of satisfaction with his/her life over time that is defined as personally significant

INTRODUCTION

Quality of life has been a philosophical and socio-political phenomenon for hundreds, if not thousands of years. In recent years, it has developed into a theory, particularly in response to the growing interest in quality of life as expressed by those involved in health care. Because quality of life is not clearly identified with one theorist, it is difficult to define and describe. This lack of specificity has not diminished its popularity as a theory tested by research. It has been empirically tested in hundreds of studies published both nationally and internationally. Quality of life has been identified as a middle range theory (Meleis, 1997), representing a specific phenomenon, with a limited number of related concepts, that has obvious applications to practice. Quality of life and the related and sometimes interchangeable theory, health-related quality of life (HRQOL), are developing into explanatory theories.

HISTORICAL BACKGROUND

The concept of quality of life, concerned with an individual's personal satisfaction with life, has its roots in classical Greek thought and religious teachings. Aristotle is credited with the initial conceptualization of quality of life, defined as happiness, the good life, or the outcome of a life of virtue (Morgan, 1992). In the New Testament (John 10:10), Jesus stated that he came to give life and give it abundantly (The Lockman Foundation, 1995). The ten stages of enlightenment in Buddhism start out with achieving joy in life (Stryk, 1968).

Quality of life, or in the words of the United States' Declaration of Independence, the pursuit of happiness, was claimed as a right during the founding of the country. Pigou is credited with the introduction of the term in 1920 in his book on economics and welfare (Wood-Dauphinee, 1999). He discussed the need for governmental support for the lower class as a means of not only directly benefiting them financially but also promoting the health of the national economy. Pigou's position and the term "quality of life" that he used to express it did not receive much attention. Politically, use of the concept, quality of life, was limited until it was reintroduced in remarks made by Presidents Johnson and Nixon in speeches on environmental and social issues (Campbell, 1981; Dalkey, Rourke, Lewis, & Snyder, 1972).

Quality of life has its academic roots in the disciplines of psychology and sociology (Spranger, 2001). In the 1970s, these disciplines began to consider the issue of quality of life. For instance, in 1978, the Ninth World Congress of Sociology introduced the concept as a topic of discussion (Szulai & Andrews, 1980). Also in the 1970s, the business world adopted the term "quality of life" to make claims about the ability of a product to enhance a person's life in the milieu of everyday living.

The health care disciplines' recent interest in quality of life can be traced to the work of the World Health Organization (WHO). WHO's more-encompassing definition of health as physical, psychological, and social well-being, and not just the absence of illness or infirmity (World Health Organization, 1948), provided early impetus to the consideration of quality of life as a relevant human experience for health care professionals. In 1978, WHO provided a statement on the application of their definition of health, indicating that individuals have the right "to psychosocial care and adequate quality of life in addition to physiologic care" (King & Hinds, 1998, p. xi). The documents, "Healthy People 2000" and "Healthy People 2010," consistent with the goals identified by WHO, have included not only disease- and disability-related issues, but those concerned with quality of life (Baker, 2000).

Nursing's interest in quality of life is long standing. Florence Nightingale's involvement with the British military provided multiple examples of how nurses can promote the quality of life for individuals. This interest has intensified and become a focus of research in the last 15 to 20 years. In 1991, the Oncology Nursing Society's Research Priority Survey identified quality of life as its highest research priority (Mooney, Ferrell, Nail, Benedict, & Haberman, 1991). Before 1982, there were no references to quality of life in the nursing research literature, but by 1995 the number of citations in the Cumulative Index of Nursing and Allied Health (CINAHL) had grown to more than 400 (Grant & Rivera, 1998).

Health-related quality of life (HRQOL), a specific subcategory of global quality of life sometimes used interchangeably with quality of life, is a more recent concept. Health care trends have contributed to the emergence of HRQOL as an important phenomenon. In the past 15 to 20 years, the concern for patients has become more inclusive, focusing not just on the treatment of disease, but also the restoration and promotion of health (Read, 1993). With increased client longevity, health care professionals are attending to the lifestyle issues that accompany chronic disease and often affect quality of life.

The Food and Drug Administration (FDA) is reflecting this changing emphasis. It can require documentation of not only the safety and efficacy of new products but also their effect on a user's quality of life (Spilker, 1998). In 1985, the guidelines for approval of antineoplastics included documentation of a favorable response in terms of quality of life or survival (Johnson & Temple).

DEFINITION OF THEORY CONCEPTS

Quality of life has emerged as a concept of interest to many disciplines. This multiplicity of discipline-specific perspectives has led to little consensus on a definition. Philosophers consider the nature of existence and what is meant by the "good life." Ethicists are concerned with social utility. Economists pursue cost-effectiveness in producing the greatest good. Physicians focus on health- and illness-specific issues, while nurses approach the issue of quality of life more holistically (Anderson & Burckhardt, 1999).

Taxonomy of Definitions

Farquhar (1995) suggests a taxonomy of quality of life definitions as a means of clarifying the confusion created by the plethora of available conceptualizations. Three major categories are identified: global, component, and focused. Farquhar also notes that some established definitions do not clearly fit into the taxonomy, reflecting more than one category. These definitions are identified as combined and can be designated a fourth category in the taxonomy.

Global definitions (Type I) are considered the most commonly occurring and the most generalized conceptualizations of quality of life. They often refer to satisfaction/dissatisfaction, a cognitive experience, or happiness/unhappiness, an affective realization. Definitions may include both internal and external life factors. The inner factors refer to the individual's thoughts and feelings. The external factors refer to the individual's activities and social milieu. Global definitions are not easily operationalized and, therefore, not as useful for the purposes of research.

Component definitions (Type II) identify the relevant components or domains that constitute quality of life. They often address both objective and subjective dimensions of the concept. General functional ability and socioeconomic status are examples of objective dimensions. Self-esteem and personal determination of life satisfaction are examples of subjective dimensions. Because component definitions are easier to operationalize, they are more useful in research.

Focused definitions (Type III) are the narrowest conceptualization of the phenomenon. They consider only one or a limited number of components of quality of life. Focused definitions may be either explicit or implicit. Definitions that focus on health-related quality of life or a microeconomic quality of life are both considered explicit. Definitions that focus on a limited number of components yet refer to the more general term, quality of life, are considered implicit. Because implicit definitions are imprecise, they are not appropriate for research purposes.

Quality of life has been identified as both a middle range theory (Meleis, 1997) and a meta theory (Ventegodt, Hilden, & Zachau-Christiansen, 1993). Historically referred to as happiness, welfare, life satisfaction, or subjective well-being, the terms "overall quality of life" or "global quality of life" are currently preferred (Dalkey et al., 1972). The subcategory, health-related quality of life, has become of particular interest to nursing and increasingly the focus of nursing research.

DESCRIPTION OF THE THEORY OF HEALTH-RELATED QUALITY OF LIFE

The theory, Health-Related Quality of Life, developed as an entity separate from global quality of life as a means of specifying health-related domains of particular interest to researchers. It is multidimensional (Faden & Leplege, 1992; Staniszewska, 1998), multifaceted (Haase & Braden, 1998), and utilitarian in nature, lending itself to a vast array of clinical applications in a variety of settings (Staniszewska, 1998). Its concepts "tend to cross different nursing fields and reflect a wide variety of nursing situations" (Meleis, 1997, p. 18). HRQOL is also ambiguous and difficult to define. It can be referred to in the literature as quality of life, subjective health status, or functional health status. Some authors prefer the term, subjective health status, considering it a more accurate descriptor of the phenomenon (Staniszewska, 1998).

Model of Health-Related Quality of Life

A model developed by Wilson and Cleary represents the causal relationships between the basic concepts of HRQOL. The model identifies five determinants that exist on a "continuum of increasing biological, social, and psychological complexity" (1995, p. 60). These leveled determinants of HRQOL are referred to as taxonomy and consist of biological factors, symptoms, functioning, general health perceptions, and overall quality of life. They are in turn influenced by characteristics of the individual and environment. Figure 13-1 illustrates these relationships.

The arrows in the figure represent the dominant causal relationships and are not meant to exclude reciprocal connections between either adjacent or nonadjacent components of the model. There is research support for each of the causal relationships identified in the model.

BIOLOGICAL AND PHYSIOLOGICAL VARIABLES

Biological and physiological variables refer to alterations in the function of cells, organs, and organ systems. These factors are assessed through diagnostic examinations. For instance, laboratory values, such as serum hormone tests, measures of physiological functioning, such as exercise electrocardiography; and physical examination results, such as respiratory wheezing, would be used to determine biological and physiological changes that have the potential to impact HRQOL. These data would be available to the nurse but may not have been collected by him or her.

SYMPTOM STATUS

Symptoms are frequently assessed by the nurse. Symptoms are changes in physical and psychological states that the individual determines are abnormal, based on the nature of the altered sensation and the

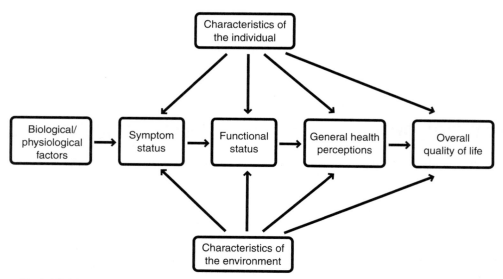

■ **Figure 13.1** HRQOL conceptual model proposed by Wilson and Cleary (1995). Source: *Journal of the American Medical Association, 273,* 59–65. © 1995 by the American Medical Association.

meaning ascribed to it. The development of a symptom is the result of complex relationships between numbers of biological and physiological variables. At times, physiological pathology exists without overt symptoms. Individuals will experience severe hypertension and yet report no symptoms. At other times, acute symptoms will exist without a discernible alteration in the physiologic state. Individuals will complain of severe back pain for which there is no abnormal diagnostic finding. Obviously, much is unknown about the relationships between biological and physiological factors and the onset of symptoms. Factors other than biological and physiological variables will determine an individual's experience of a symptom. For instance, cultural and demographic factors will influence the meaning ascribed to an altered sensation. It is often through the recognition and subjective reporting of a symptom that an individual becomes involved with the health care system and its professionals.

FUNCTIONAL STATUS

"Symptom status is one important determinant of functioning" (Wilson & Cleary, 1995, p. 61). Functional status, the next component in the taxonomy, is defined as the ability to perform specific tasks. In addition to symptoms, individual qualities (e.g., motivation), social factors (e.g., supportive family), and environmental characteristics (e.g., physical layout of home) influence functional status.

Typically, four domains of function are identified: physical, social, role, and psychological (Wilson & Cleary, 1995, p. 61). This list is not comprehensive or exhaustive. For instance, others will identify spiritual as a separate domain. The physical domain includes factors such as strength, sleep, rest, and appetite. The social domain focuses on relationships such as with friends and family, or the neighborhood. The role domain addresses functioning in roles such as student, parent, and worker. The psychological/spiritual domain refers to factors such as happiness, peace of mind, faith in God, and self-sufficiency. "Though not uniformly true, research suggests and the model represents predictive or causal relationships between biological/physiological variables and symptom status and between symptom status and functioning (Wilson & Cleary, 1995, p. 62). Further investigation of the ways in which health or illness conditions affect functioning is needed."

GENERAL HEALTH PERCEPTIONS

The next component in the taxonomy, general health perceptions, represents an integration and subjective expression of all previously discussed components. These general health perceptions are considered the best predictor of the use of the health care system and a strong predictor of mortality, even when clinical factors are controlled (Wilson & Cleary, 1995, p. 62). Because general health perceptions serve as important predictors of health behaviors and outcomes, the factors that contribute to these perceptions warrant extensive study.

OVERALL QUALITY OF LIFE

Overall quality of life refers to an individual's subjective well-being, how happy or satisfied an individual is generally with his or her life. It is considered "a stable synthesis of a wide range of experiences and feelings that people have" (Wilson & Cleary, 1995, p. 62) and can be thought of as a summary measure of quality of life. Because it is related to both HRQOL and a variety of other complex and significant life experiences and circumstances, overall quality of life is not always obviously related to objective life conditions.

INDIVIDUAL AND ENVIRONMENTAL CHARACTERISTICS

Individual and environmental characteristics have an influence on all components of the model but particularly the last two levels: general health perceptions and overall quality of life. They are presented together to represent the multiple linkages between the two. Research has shown that age was positively correlated with a more positive appraisal of physical health, and social isolation, adverse life events, unemployment, dissatisfaction with life circumstances, and lower income were associated with less positive appraisal of self-assessment of health (Sousa, 1999, HRQOL Variable Linkages, para. 8).

Health-Related Quality of Life and Nursing

There are many models of HRQOL (Cowan, Graham, & Cochrane, 1992; Ferrell, Grant, Dean, Funk, & Ly, 1996; Ferrans, 1990; Oleson, 1990; Padilla & Grant, 1998; and Zhan, 1992, as found in King & Hinds, 1998), all of which omit the relationship between specific interventions and the factors that affect HRQOL. Nursing researchers investigating HRQOL often use approaches/interventions from other models and theories, allowing connections to be made between HRQOL and these models or theories. For instance, Stuifbergen, Seraphine, and Roberts (2000) related health-promoting behaviors from Pender's theory with HRQOL as an outcome.

In HRQOL, nursing interventions are related to a specific illness state. They target domains of functioning identified by the patient as being adversely affected by the symptoms of the illness state. Because the domains represent a holistic view of persons, the assessment of functioning and the nursing interventions designed to provide assistance should also reflect that perspective.

The goal of the interventions is to have a positive impact on a patient's perceived satisfaction with HRQOL. This is a central component of HRQOL in that the patient provides a subjective and personal expression of both the level of satisfaction (Staniszewska, 1998) and the degree to which the specific nursing interventions contribute to that level (Robinson, Whyte, & Fidler, 1997). Thus, patient-perceived satisfaction with HRQOL becomes a significant indicator of the success of an intervention. Satisfaction has been defined as a person's sense of well-being related to areas of life that are important to him or her (Ferrans, 1990). "Patient satisfaction is conceptualized as a mediating variable, based on the work of Donabedian (1980), who has consistently regarded patient satisfaction as an outcome. He believes that satisfaction with care represents the patient's judgment of quality of care" (Yang, Simms, & Yin, 1999, p. 3).

APPLICATIONS OF THE THEORY

Health-related quality of life has both general and condition-specific research applications. General HRQOL can be used in the consideration of the general health status of individuals, evaluation of health-policy decisions, and creation of population health profiles. The more common, condition-specific HRQOL is often employed to study the impact of an illness on those experiencing it, or the effectiveness of a specific approach to treat that illness (Staniszeweska, 1998).

Consideration of the general health status of individuals, which includes HRQOL can be used in a number of ways. A survey of general health status of patients could suggest the possibility of an issue of functional status that would be relevant to a specific individual. This information could be further used as a means of focusing attention on areas of concern that typically might not be addressed by health care professionals (Wilkin, Hallam, & Doggett, 1993). Additionally, in clinical practice settings, a routine audit of the health status of patients could provide general information on quality of care.

General population health-status profiles can create a description of the health status at national and international levels and can inform health policy decision-making. Population health profiles would not be limited to mortality or morbidity statistics and would thus be a better indicator of health status, useful in monitoring regional or national health trends (Jenkinson, Wright, & Coulter, 1993). Population health profiles can also be used in cost-effectiveness analysis to make decisions about health care resource allocations.

Condition-specific HRQOL is frequently used to ascertain the impact of a condition from individuals' personal perspectives. It can provide a fuller understanding of the dimensions of life that are being affected by the condition. Interpretation of the significance of the impact can be aided by comparing the responses of those experiencing the condition with the general population. The example in Using Middle Range Theories 13-1 provides a description of a variation of this type of usage.

Determination of the effectiveness of a treatment approach is another common application of condition-specific HRQOL. It can be used to describe treatment outcomes of a single intervention, for instance, in a clinical trial, or to compare the relative efficacy of two or more treatments. The study described in Using Middle Range Theories 13-2 illustrates this type of usage.

INSTRUMENTS USED IN EMPIRICAL TESTING

A variety of instruments have been developed to operationalize HRQOL. A few are general, but many more are condition or illness-specific. These instruments generally employ a Likert scale anchored by a descriptor related to a category of a life domain. Occasionally, a dichotomous, yes/no response is used

13-1 USING MIDDLE RANGE THEORIES

The three main treatment approaches for end-stage renal disease, continuous ambulatory peritoneal dialysis (CAPD), hemodialysis (HD), and transplantation (TP), can affect the health-related quality of life (HRQOL) experienced by the spouses of the treated patients. Researchers in Sweden used a descriptive–comparative study to examine HRQOL of the spouses of patients receiving these three treatments and compared their HRQOL with an age-matched sample from the general population. A group of 55 spouses were recruited from three hospitals in central Sweden. The Swedish Health-Related Quality of Life Survey (SWED-QUAL), consisting of 62 Likert-scale items, measured quality of life. Data were analyzed using descriptive statistics and Pearson's product moment correlations. Student *t*-tests were used to analyze differences between the spouses of the patients being treated with the general population. The researchers found that TP spouses had statistically significant higher values than both CAPD and HD spouses on subscales of satisfaction with physical health, emotional well-being, positive affect, sleep problems, and sexual functioning. In addition, the combined sample of spouses had statistically significant lower values than the general population on the subscales of pain, emotional well-being, positive affect, and sexual functioning.

Lindqvist, R., Carlsson, M., & Sjogen, P. (2000). Coping strategies and health-related quality of life among spouses of continuous ambulatory peritoneal dialysis, haemodialysis, and transplant patients. *Journal of Advanced Nursing, 31*(6), 1398–1408.

13-2 USING MIDDLE RANGE THEORIES

Researchers in the Netherlands compared deterioration of health-related quality of life (HRQOL) in patients suffering from chronic obstructive pulmonary disease (COPD) discharged from a pulmonary rehabilitation center, who received home visits from a specialized respiratory community nurse, with the level of deterioration in HRQOL of patients who were visited by a general community nurse. A pretest–posttest control group study design was used to examine differences. The study's 115 subjects, 40 to 80 years of age, with a confirmed diagnosis of COPD, were assigned to either the experimental or control group, based on their place of residence. Both the specialized and general community nurses discussed relevant topics, provided information and advice, and made referrals as necessary. HRQOL was assessed with the St. George's Respiratory Questionnaire and the "well-being component" of the Medical Psychological Questionnaire for Lung Diseases. Multiple regression analysis revealed that a specialized respiratory community nurse did not contribute to less deterioration in HRQOL than the general community nurse. The researchers did find that HRQOL was improved at the time of discharge from the pulmonary rehabilitation center when compared to baseline levels, suggesting that other intervening factors, such as exercise tolerance and coping strategies, may influence HRQOL

Ketalaars, C. A. J., Huyer, A.-S., Halfens, R. J. G., Scholsser, M. A. G., Mostert, R., & Wouter, E. F. M. (1998). Effects of specialized community nursing care in patients with chronic obstructive pulmonary disease. *Heart & Lung: The Journal of Acute and Critical Care, 27*(2), 109–120.

to represent satisfaction with an aspect of HRQOL. The instruments can be used in prospective, retrospective, cross-sectional, and longitudinal research designs (Baker, 2000). Cross-sectional research designs provide a description of the quality of life at a specific point in time, but do not allow for the consideration of how that might change over time. A retrospective approach uses a description of past quality of life, but relies on recall that may not be reliable. "The use of prospective, population-based, longitudinal designs ...offers a way of overcoming a number of these deficiencies" (Baker, 2000, p. 6). There are two main types of HRQOL assessment tools that can be used in research: health index measures and health profile measures (Staniszeweska, 1998).

The health index measures are of limited usefulness because they result in a single score to represent HRQOL. Along with data on treatment cost and expected life expectancy after a treatment, the HRQOL score can be entered into an equation to determine quality-adjusted life years gained or QUALY (Jenkinson et al., 1993). The statistical utility of a single score for HROL is questionable (Speegelhalter, Gore, & Fitzpatrick, 1992). Health index measures are often used for health care policy decision-making.

The health profile measures provide for a more inclusive and descriptive indication of HRQOL. There are generic versions of health profile instruments (e.g., the SF-36) (Ware & Sherbourne, 1992), and condition-specific instruments such as the Arthritis Impact Measurement Scale (Meenan, Gertman, & Mason, 1980) and the McGill Pain Questionnaire (Melzack, 1975). These measurement tools would most frequently be used to determine the impact of an illness-specific treatment on HRQOL. There are a wide variety of tools available for almost any disease. The Quality of Life Assessment In Medicine (*http://www.qlmed.org/LIST/index.html*) lists at least 800 instruments that are either patient or clinician oriented. Table 13-1 provides examples from this site.

One of the listed instruments is the "The Paediatric Asthma Quality of Life Questionnaire" (See Appendix B for a copy of the instrument) developed by Juniper. It has been designed to measure the problems that children between the ages of 7 and 17 experience as a result of their asthma. The questionnaire has 23 items in three domains: symptoms, activity limitations, and emotional function, in both interviewer and self-administered versions. Items were selected on the basis of their importance to children and are rated on a seven-point scale. At the beginning of the administration of the questionnaire, the child identifies personally important issues from the domains. The test takes about 10 minutes to complete and has been tested for use in several languages. "The Paediatric Asthma Quality of Life Questionnaire" (AQOLQ-P) can be used in nursing research as the following case study illustrates (Research Application 13-1).

SUMMARY

Quality of life is a concept with a long history, which has, in the last 15 to 20 years, become of interest to a number of disciplines. Considered both a meta and middle range theory, its subconcept, health-related quality of life (HRQOL) is of particular interest to health care professionals. Models of the middle range theory, HRQOL, often comprise three components: life domains refer to the areas of life being affected by a specific condition; interventions involve the actions taken to bring about a desired outcome, an improved quality of life; and perceived satisfaction is the patient's subjective appraisal of well-being. Nurses wishing to understand the impact of a condition on their patients or to judge the effectiveness of an illness treatment can make use of this middle range theory and the instruments designed to measure it.

Table 13-1. HEALTH-RELATED QUALITY OF LIFE TOOLS

CATEGORY	ABBREVIATION	EXAMPLES
AIDS	AIDS-SQ	AIDS-Specific Questionnaire
	AIDS HAQ	AIDS Health Assessment Questionnaire
Asthma	AQOLQ(S)	Asthma Quality of Life Questionnaire (standard)
	AQOLQ(P)	Asthma Quality of Life Questionnaire (pediatrics)
Cardiology	CAST-QLI	Cardiac Arrhythmia Suppression Quality of Life Instrument
	RCQ	Rose Cardiovascular Questionnaire
Caregivers	CB	Caregiver Burdens Scale
	CD	Caregiving Demands Scale
	ABCD	Assessment of Basic Care for the Demented Scale
Cognitive function	CAM	Confusion Assessment Method
	CAMDEX	Cambridge Mental Disorders of the Elderly Examination
Coping	COPES-F	Coping Strategies—Family
	CSI	Coping Strategy Indicator
Dementia	DAD	Disability Assessment for Dementia
	DD	Dementia Disability Scale
Dermatology	CDLQI	Children's Dermatology Life Quality Index
Diabetes	DQLCTQ	Diabetes Quality of Life Clinical Trial Questionnaire
Drug addiction	AAS	Addiction Admission Scale
Gastroenterology	GIQLI	Gastrointestinal Quality of Life Index
	GERD-HRQL	Gastroesophageal Reflux Disease—Health-Related Quality of Life
Generic	QLSI	Quality of Life Systemic Inventory
	SF-36	MOS Short Form—36 Items
Geriatrics	GDI	Geriatric Depression Scale
	OAHMQ	Older Adult Health and Mood Questionnaire
Gynecology	HRQOL-E	Health-Related Quality-of-Life Instrument for Symptomatic Patients With Endometriosis
	UIWQ	Urinary Incontinent Women Questionnaire
	MRS	Menopause Rating Scale
Neurology	NCSE	Neurobehavioral Cognitive Status Examination
	MS-QOL	Migraine-Specific Quality of Life Questionnaire
Oncology	OTTAT	Oncology Treatment Toxicity Assessment Tool
	CARES	Cancer Rehabilitation Evaluation System
Ophthalmology	NEI-VFQ	National Eye Institute Visual Function Questionnaire
Oral health	OHQOL	Oral Health-Related Quality of Life
Pain	VAS	Visual Analogue Scale

(Continued)

Table 13-1. HEALTH-RELATED QUALITY OF LIFE TOOLS (*Continued*)

CATEGORY	ABBREVIATION	EXAMPLES
Pediatrics	APPI	Adolescent Parent Perception Inventory
	CAQ	Childhood Asthma Questionnaire
	CHQ	Child Health Questionnaire
	PedsQL	Pediatric Quality of Life Inventory (PedsQL) with Cancer Module
Physical function	DASH	Disabilities of the Arm, Shoulder, and Hand questionnaire
Psychiatry	PANSS	Positive and Negative Syndrome Scale for Schizophrenia
	PDI	Psychological Distress Inventory
Respiratory disease	RIQLQ	Respiratory Illness Quality of Life Questionnaire
Satisfaction	LS	Lifestyle Satisfaction
Self-esteem	SEI	Self-Esteem Inventory
Sexuality	ISF	Index of Sexual Function
	FSAQ	Fallowfield's Sexual Activity Questionnaire
Sleep	SAQLI	Sleep Apnea Quality of Life Index
Social function	SEC	Social Experiences Checklist
Urology/nephrology	UDI	Urogenital Distress Inventory

13-1 RESEARCH APPLICATION

A nurse researcher is interested in determining if the inclusion of a nurse-run education and peer-support group improves the outcomes for elementary school-aged asthmatics. Using a prospective research design, in an asthma clinic, the researcher matches patients by age, nature and severity of symptoms, and treatment regimens. The patients are randomly assigned to either group involvement or no group involvement. Before treatment begins, the nurse researcher administers the AQOLQ-P to a new patient, a 10-year old male. The patient is asked to identify the life domains most affected by the asthma, and he selects "activity limitations" domain, which include riding his bicycle, playing recreational baseball, and playing tag with his friends. The patient also chooses "symptoms" domain, and he identifies getting a good night's sleep and being disturbed at school with coughing. The nurse then completes the administration of the AQOLQ-P.

The patient, through random selection, is placed in the experimental treatment group. The group meets weekly for 3 months. At the end of the 3-month period, the patient returns to the asthma clinic, and the nurse researcher readministers the questionnaire, addressing the same domains that were assessed the first time. Any changes in the ratings will fall along a continuum from positive to negative, with positive indicating that a desired outcome relating to HRQOL was achieved. The individual patient data is grouped with other data, and, through statistical analysis, the researcher can determine if the group treatment made a statistically significant difference in the quality of life outcomes in elementary school-aged children diagnosed with asthma.

ANALYSIS EXERCISE

Using the criteria presented in Chapter 2, critique the theory, Health-Related Quality of Life. Compare your conclusions about the theory with those found in Appendix A. A researcher who has worked with the theory completed the analysis found in the Appendix.

Internal Criticism
1. Clarity
2. Consistency
3. Adequacy

4. Logical development
5. Level of theory development

External Criticism
1. Reality convergence
2. Utility
3. Significance
4. Discrimination
5. Scope of theory
6. Complexity

WEB RESOURCES

1. This site is sponsored by the Sigma Theta Tau Nursing Honor Society Virginia Henderson Library. Type in "quality of life" in the search engine box under library search: *http://www.stti. iupui.edu/library/*
2. The mission statement included on the official Web site of the International Society for the Quality of Life Research reads: "The scientific study of Quality of Life relevant to health and healthcare is the mission of the International Society for Quality of Life Research (ISOQOL). The Society promotes the rigorous investigation of health-related quality of life measurement from conceptualization to application and practice. ISOQOL fosters the worldwide exchange of information through: Scientific Publications, International Conferences, Educational Outreach, and Collaborative Support for HRQOL." They can be reached at: *http://www.isoqol.org/*
3. This site contains various on-line nursing journals with full-text articles on HRQOL: *http://www-sci.lib.uci.edu/HSG/Nursing. html#NN3*
4. This site is sponsored by the International Society of Pharmacoeconomics and Outcomes Research. Type "quality if life" in the search box.

It has an on-line guide to quality of life measurements and outcomes: *http://www.ispor.org/*
5. American Thoracic Society states that "This site was designed for researchers, clinicians, industrial groups, and other interested parties who wish to learn about patient-oriented quality of life (QOL) measures. . .The goal of this Web site is to provide information about quality of life and functional status instruments that have been used in assessing patients with pulmonary disease or critical illness that are useful in the study and management of respiratory disease." This site can be accessed at: *http://www.atsqol.org/*
6. Maintained by the Public Health Foundation, this site is mainly concerned with providing information about the program "Measuring Healthy Days." It can be found at: *http://www. phf.org/measuringhealthydays.htm*
7. The official site of the Centers for Disease Control and Prevention contains basic information and a variety of links to other sites: *http://www.cdc.gov/nccdphp/hrqol/*
8. The Quality of Life Assessment in Medicine Web site provides links to multiple sites, with information about QOL, as well as a list of more than 800 measurement tools: *http://www.qlmed.org/index.html*

REFERENCES

Anderson, K., & Burckhardt, C. S. (1999). Conceptualization and measurement of quality of life as an outcome variable for health care intervention and research. *Journal of Advanced Nursing, 29*(2), 298–306.

Baker, F. (2000, Winter). Assessing the quality of life of cancer survivors. *The Behavioral Measurement Letter* 7, 2–12.

Campbell, A. (1981). *The sense of well being in America.* New York: McGraw Hill.

Dalkey, N. C., Rourke, D. L., Lewis, R., & Snyder, D. (1972). *Studies in the quality of life, delphi and decision making.* Toronto: Lexington Books, D.C. Heath and Company.

Faden, R., & Leplege, A. (1992). Assessing quality of life, moral implications for clinical practice. *Medical Care, 30*(5, Supplement), 166–175.

Farquhar, M. (1995). Definition of quality of life: A taxonomy. *Journal of Advanced Nursing, 22*(3), 502–508.

Ferrans, C. E. (1990). Quality of life: Conceptual issues. Seminars in oncology. *Nursing, 6,* 248–254.

Grant, M. M., & Rivera, L. M. (1998). Evolution of quality of life in oncology and oncology nursing. In C. R. King & P. S. Hinds (Eds.), *Quality of life.* (pp. 3–22). Sudbury, MA: Jones & Bartlett Publishers.

Haase, J. E., & Braden, C. J. (1998). Guidelines for achieving clarity of concepts related to quality of life. In C. R. King & P. S. Hinds (Eds.), *Quality of life.* (pp. 54–73). Sudbury, MA: Jones & Bartlett Publishers.

Jenkinson, C., Wright, L., & Coulter, A. (1993). *Quality of life measurement in health care—A review of measures and population norms for the UK SF-36.* Oxford, UK: University of Oxford.

Johnson, J. R., & Temple, R. (1985). Food and Drug Administration requirements for approval of new anticancer therapies. *Cancer Reports, 69,* 1115–1157.

Ketalaars, C., Huyer, A.-S., Halfens, R. J. G., Schlosser, M. A. G., Mostert, R., & Wouter, E. F. M. (1998). Effects of specialized community nursing care in patients with chronic obstructive pulmonary disease. *Heart & Lung: The Journal of Acute and Critical Care, 27*(2), 109–120.

King, C., & Hinds, P. (1998). *Quality of life.* Sudbury, MA: Jones & Bartlett Publishing.

Lindqvist, R. Carlsson, M., & Sjogen, P. (2000). Coping strategies and health-related quality of life among spouses of continuous ambulatory peritoneal dialysis, haemodialyis, and transplant patients. *Journal of Advanced Nursing, 31*(6), 1398–1408.

The Lockman Foundation (Eds.). (1995). *New American Standard Bible.* Chicago: Moody Press.

Meenan, R. F., Gertman, P. M ., & Mason, J. H. (1980). Measuring health status in arthritis: The arthritis impact measurement scales. *Arthritis and Rheumatism, 23,* 146–152.

Meleis, A. I. (1997). *Theoretical nursing: Development and progress.* (3rd ed.). Philadelphia: Lippincott-Raven.

Melzack, R. (1975). The McGill pain questionnaire: Major properties and scoring methods. *Pain, 1,* 277–299.

Mooney, K. H., Ferrell, B. R., Nail, L. M., Benedict, S. C., & Haberman, M. R. (1991). 1991 Oncology Nursing Society Research Priorities Survey. *Oncology Nursing Forum, 18*(8), 1381–1388.

Morgan, M. L. (1992). *Classics of moral and political theory.* Indianapolis, IN: Hacket.

O'Boyle, C. A. (1994). Quality of life and cardiovascular medication. *The Irish Journal of Psychology, 15*(1), 126–147.

Quality of Life Assessment in Medicine: 800 Instruments Patient and Clinician Oriented. Retrieved October 15, 2001 from *http://www.qlmed.org/LIST/index.html*

Read, J. L. (1993). The new era of quality of life assessment. In S. R. Walker & R. M. Rosser, *Quality of life assessment: Key issues in the 1990s* (pp. 3–10). London: Kluwer Academic Publishers.

Robinson, D., Whyte, L., & Fidler, I. (1997). Quality of life measures in a high security environment. *Nursing Standard, 11*(49), 34–37.

Sousa, K. H. (1999). Description of a health-related quality of life conceptual model. *Outcomes Management for Nursing Practice, 3*(2), 78–82.

Speegelhalter, D. J., Gore, S. M., & Fitzpatrick, R. (1992). Quality of life measures in health care. III: Resource allocation. *British Medical Journal, 305,* 1205–1209.

Spilker, B. (1998). *Quality of life and pharmaco economics in clinical trials.* (2nd ed.). New York: Lippincott -Raven.

Spranger, M. J. (2001). International Society of Quality of Life Newsletter 6(1). Retrieved June 15, 2001 from *www.ISOQOL.org*

Staniszewska, S. (1998). Measuring quality of life in the evaluation of health care. *Nursing Standard* 12(17), 36–39.

Stryk, L. (1968). *World of Budha: A reader.* Garden City, NY: Doubleday.

Stuifbergen, A. K, Seraphine, A., & Roberts, G. (2000). An explanatory model of health promotion and quality of life in chronic disabling conditions. *Nursing Research, 49*(3), 122–129.

Szulai, A., & Andrews, F. M. (Eds.) (1980). *The quality of life.* London: Sage Publications.

Ventegodt, S., Hilden, J., & Zachau-Christiansen, B. (1993). Measuring the quality of life: A methodological framework. Retrieved June 2001 from *www.home2.inet.tele.dk/ felk/mql2.htr.*

Ware, J. E., & Sherbourne, C. D. (1992). The MOS 36-item short form health survey 1: Conceptual framework and item selection. *Medical Care* 30(6), 473–483.

Wilkin, D., Hallam, L., & Doggett, M. (1993). *Measures of*

need and outcome for primary health care. Oxford, UK: Oxford University Press.

Wilson, I. B., & Cleary, P. D. (1995). Linking clinical variables with health-related quality of life. *Journal of the American Medical Association, 273*(1), 59–65.

Wood-Dauphinee, S. (1999). Assessing quality of life in clinical research: From where have we come and where are we going? *Journal of Clinical Epidemiology, 55,* 355–363.

World Health Organization. (1948). Constitution of the World Health Organization. *Chronicle of the World Health Organization, 1*(1/2), 13.

Yang, K., Simms, L. M., & Yin, J. (1999, August 3). Factors influencing nursing-sensitive outcomes in Taiwanese nursing homes. *Journal of Issues in Nursing.* Retrieved June 14, 2001 from *www.nursingworld.org.*

BIBLIOGRAPHY

Andresen, E. M., & Meyers, A. R. (2000). Health-related quality of life outcomes measures. *Archives of Physical Medicine and Rehabilitation, 81*(12, Suppl. 2), 30–45.

Andresen, E. M., Vahle, V. J., & Lollar, D. (2001). Proxy reliability: Health-related quality of life (HRQOL) measures for people with disability. *Quality of Life Research, 10*(7), 609–619.

Bell, C. M., Araki, S. S., & Neumann, P. J. (2001). The association between caregiver burden and caregiver health related quality of life in Alzheimer disease. *Alzheimer Disease & Associated Disorders, 15,* 129–136. Retrieved May 12, 2002 from Ovid database.

Chaboyer, W., & Elliott, D. (2000). Health-related quality of life of ICU survivors: Review of the literature. *Intensive and Critical Care Nursing, 16*(2), 88–97.

Coons, S. J., Rao, S., Keininger, D. L., & Hays, R. D. (2000). A comparative review of generic quality-of-life instruments. *Pharmacoeconomics, 17*(1), 13–35.

Corless, I. B., Nicholas, P. K., & Nokes, K. M. (2001). Issues in cross-cultural quality-of-life research. *Journal of Nursing Scholarship, 33*(1), 15–20.

Cosby, C. F., Holzemer, W. L. Henry, S. B., & Portillo, C. J. (2000). Hematological complications and quality of life in hospitalized AIDS patients. *AIDS, 14*(5), 269–279.

Duggan, C. H., & Dijkers, M. (2001). Quality of life after spinal cord injury: A qualitative study. *Rehabilitation, 46*(1), 3–27.

Galbraith, M. E., Ramirez, J. M., & Pedro, L. W. (2001). Quality of life, health outcomes, and identity for patients with prostate cancer in five different treatment groups. *Oncology Nursing Forum, 28*(3), 551–560.

Hackett, M. L., Duncan, J. R., Anderson, C. S., Broad, J. B., & Bonita, R. P. (2000). Health-related quality of life among long-term survivors of stroke: Results from the Auckland stroke study, 1991–1992. *Stroke, 31*(2), 440–447.

Hollen, P. J. (2000). A clinical profile to predict decision making, risk behaviors, clinical status, and health-related quality of life for cancer-surviving adolescents. Part 1. *Cancer Nursing, 23*(4), 247–257.

Hollen, P. J. (2000). A clinical profile to predict decision making, risk behaviors, clinical status, and health-related quality of life for cancer-surviving adolescents: Part 2. *Cancer Nursing, 23*(5), 337–343.

Lamping, D. L., Constantinovici, N., Roderick, P., Normand, C., Henderson, L., & Harris, S. (2000). Clinical outcomes, quality of life, and costs in the North Thames Dialysis Study of elderly people on dialysis: A prospective cohort study. *Lancet, 356*(9241), 1543–1550.

Nuamah, I. F., Cooley, M. E., Fawcett, J., & McCorkle, R. (1999). Testing a theory for health-related quality of life in cancer patients: A structural equation approach. *Research in Nursing and Health, 22*(3), 231–242.

Pedro, L. W. (2001). Quality of life for long-term survivors of cancer: Influencing variables. *Cancer, 24*(1), 1–11.

Power, M., Bullinger, M., Harper, A., & The World Health Organization Quality of Life Group. (1999). The World Health Organization WHOQOL-100: Tests of the universality of quality of life in 15 different cultural groups worldwide. *Health, 18*(5), 495–505.

Raak, R., Wikblad, K., Raak, A. Sr, Carlsson, M., & Wahren, L. K. (2002). Catastrophizing and health-related quality of life: A 6-year follow-up of patients with chronic low back pain. *Rehabilitation Nursing, 27*(3), 110–116.

Sousa, K. H., Holzemer, W. L., Henry, S. B., & Slaughter, R. (1999). Dimensions of health-related quality of life in persons living with HIV disease. *Journal of Advanced Nursing, 29*(1), 178–187.

Westlake, C., Dracup, K., Creaser, J., Livingston, N., Heywood, J. T., Huiskes, B. L., Fonarow, G., & Hamilton, M. (2002). Correlates of health-related quality of life in patients with heart failure. *Heart and Lung, 31*(2), 85–93.

Williams, S., Sehgal, M., Falter, K., Dennis, R., Jones, D., Boudreaux, J., Homa, D., Raskin-Hood, C., Brown, C., Griffith, M., & Redd, S. (2000). Effect of asthma on the quality of life among children and their caregivers in the Atlanta Empowerment Zone. *Journal of Urban Health, 77*(2), 268–279.

Health Promotion

MARJORIE COOK MCCULLAGH

DEFINITION OF KEY TERMS

Activity-related affect	Subjective feelings associated with the health-promoting behavior
Commitment to a plan of action	Commitment to carry out a health-promoting behavior. The plan should be specific to time and place, and specify whether it will be with identified persons or alone.
Health-promoting behavior	Behaviors or actions that people carry out with the intention of improving their health
Immediate competing demands	Distracting ideas about other things that must be done (e.g., childcare) immediately before the person's intention to carry out a health-promoting behavior
Immediate competing preferences	Distracting ideas about other attractive activities to do (e.g., shopping) immediately before engaging in a health-promoting behavior.
Interpersonal influences	Beliefs concerning the behaviors, beliefs, or attitudes of others regarding a health-promoting behavior. Sources of influence include social norms, social support, and modeling.
Perceived barriers to action	Beliefs about the unavailablity, inconvenience, expense, difficulty, or time-consuming nature of a health-promoting behavior
Perceived benefits of action	Beliefs about the positive or reinforcing consequences of a health-promoting behavior
Perceived self-efficacy	A person's judgment of his or her own abilities to accomplish a health-promoting behavior
Personal factors: biological, psychological, sociocultural	Factors about the person that influence health-promoting behavior. Examples of biological factors: age, BMI, aerobic capacity. Examples of psychological factors: self-esteem, self-motivation, perceived health status. Examples of sociocultural factors: race,

	ethnicity, acculturation, education, socioeconomic status. The variables may be specific to each health-promoting activity (i.e., factors influencing healthy dietary behaviors may not be the same as those affecting exercise behavior).
Prior related behavior	Experience with the health-promoting behavior
Situational influences	Beliefs about the situation or context of the health-promoting behavior. These beliefs may include perceptions of the available options, demand characteristics, and aesthetic features of the environment in which a given behavior is proposed to take place.

INTRODUCTION

Nurses, as well as many other health professionals, are interested in learning more about helping their patients, families, and communities to improve their lives. In seeking a way to bring greater longevity and a higher quality of life, some nurses are attracted to interventions that enhance health and quality of living. The Health Promotion Model has achieved popularity among nurses as a model that serves this purpose.

Health promotion has many benefits. The benefits of living a healthier lifestyle go beyond the prevention of disease to include greater vigor and a subjective feeling of wellness. While these benefits can be enjoyed by the individual, society as a whole profits from health promotion, when people create personal and family lifestyles that are consistent with economic prosperity and interpersonal harmony. Health promotion can decrease social problems, such as violence, suicide, and sexually transmitted diseases. Furthermore, health promotion has the potential to significantly decrease health care costs in the years ahead.

Health promotion is a concept well suited to the needs and interests of nurses and their clients. Nurses commonly work in schools, churches, homes, workplaces, and health care agencies, settings ideal for the promotion of health. Nurses are skilled in many areas necessary for health promotion, such as education, counseling, and advocacy. For example, a parish nurse may offer classes to congregational members on a variety of health-related topics, such as parenting and caring for aging family members. A school nurse may facilitate self-help group meetings for bereaved children. An occupational health nurse may advocate for inclusion of mental health services in employee health-benefit packages. In addition, clients are likely to be receptive to nursing interventions to promote health, because they trust nurses and are accustomed to seeking assistance from these professionals in dealing with their health care needs.

HISTORICAL BACKGROUND

During the past century, the major cause of health problems has shifted from infectious disease to chronic illness. Many chronic illnesses are closely related to lifestyle factors, such as diet, exercise, and stress management. To improve the health of a population experiencing high rates of chronic illness, it is apparent that changes in lifestyle factors are required.

Nola Pender first published her Health Promotion Model (HPM) in *Health Promotion in Nursing Practice* in 1982. It was subsequently revised (Pender, 1996) and published recently in the fourth edition (Pender, Murdaugh, & Parsons, 2002). The latest edition incorporates additional concepts and relationships. These additions to the model, based on recent research and theoretical considerations, were made to increase its explanatory power and its potential for use in structuring health-promoting nursing interventions.

DEFINITION OF THEORY CONCEPTS

Nurses are accustomed to assessing their patients for evidence of disease or dysfunction. However, the assessment process commonly reflects a focus on illness rather than health. This approach is limiting in several ways. First, it risks reducing the patient to a sum of his or her parts (e.g., respiratory, neurological, cardiovascular). Second, it does not determine the meaning the client attaches to health and illness. This approach to health is a negative one in that it views health as an absence of disease. Some consider health and illness to be opposite concepts. This way of thinking suggests that persons with disabilities, chronic illness, and those who are near death cannot achieve health. However, many nurses experienced in working with these clients may oppose this view. Negative approaches to health as the absence of illness are inadequate for health professionals when they are increasingly concerned with quality of life and healthy longevity.

Pender's (1990) definition of health is positive, comprehensive, unifying, and humanistic. She believes that health includes a disease component, but does not make disease its principal element. Her definition of health encompasses the whole person and his or her lifestyle, and includes strengths, resiliencies, resources, potentials, and capabilities. Pender (2002, p. 22) defines health as the actualization of inherent and acquired human potential through goal-directed behavior, competent self-care, and satisfying relationships with others, while adjustments are made as needed to maintain structural integrity and harmony with relevant environments.

A major strength of Pender's definition of health is that it offers an expanded view of health. This expanded view provides for greatly increased opportunities to improve client health because it is not limited to absence of disease, or even limitations in functioning or adaptation. For example, Pender's positive view of health permits the development of nursing interventions that are not limited to decreasing risks for disease, but are also aimed at strengthening resources, potentials, and capabilities. This creates broader opportunities for nurses to assist individuals, families, and communities to achieve improved health, enhanced functional ability, and better quality of life.

Health Promotion

Health professionals have long recognized the benefits of early detection and treatment of illness, or secondary prevention. However, recently there has been increased appreciation for the role of primary prevention and health promotion in improving health and quality of life. Primary prevention involves activities aimed at the prevention of health problems before they occur and the avoidance of disease. An example of primary prevention is the administration of tetanus immunization to prevent tetanus infection. Health promotion is intended to increase the level of well-being and self-actualization of an individual or group. Examples of health promotion activities include physical activity and healthy nutrition.

While health promotion and primary prevention are distinct theoretical concepts, in practice they often overlap. Many activities directed toward health promotion will also have preventive effects. Indeed, many adults engage in healthy behaviors with the intent of increasing wellness and avoiding illness. For example, an adult may adopt a low-fat diet with dual purposes in mind. One intention may be to lower blood cholesterol and therefore prevent future cardiovascular problems (primary prevention, also referred to by Pender as health protection). An accompanying intention may be to gain the benefits of weight loss, such as feeling more energetic (health promotion). Other examples of health behaviors that may have both health promotion and preventive benefits include physical activity, adequate rest, and management of stress.

Health promotion is activity directed toward actualization of human potential through goal-directed behavior, competent self-care, and satisfying relationships with others, while adjustments are made as needed to maintain structural integrity and harmony with relevant environments (Pender, Murdaugh, & Parsons, 2002, p. 22). The concept of health promotion is based on Pender's expanded definition of health that focuses on the whole person and promotes the positive aspects of health. This definition applies to all persons, including persons who are well and those who are experiencing an illness or disability.

Pender advocates the use of health promotion at a variety of levels and settings. Although health promotion is most commonly directed toward the individual, she suggests that interventions directed toward the family and community are most likely to be successful in creating a healthy society. Furthermore, Pender discusses health promotion in a variety of settings, including schools, workplaces, homes, and nurse-managed community health centers. In a broad sense, health promotion involves education, food production, housing, employment, and health care. It is multidimensional, encompassing individual, family, community, environmental, and societal health.

DESCRIPTION OF THE THEORY OF HEALTH PROMOTION

Pender's model is based on theories of human behavior. There is increased recognition of the role of behavior in primary prevention and health promotion, and health professionals are giving more attention to helping clients adopt healthy behaviors. Motivation for healthy behavior may be based on a desire to prevent illness (primary prevention) or to achieve a higher level of well-being and self-actualization (health promotion). The Pender HPM is based primarily on three theories of health behavior: the theory of reasoned action, the theory of planned behvior, and social-cognitive theory. The first, the theory of reasoned action, is based on work by Ajzen and Fishbein (Montano, Kasprzyk, and Taplin, 1997). The theory explains that the major determinant of behavior is the person's intent for that behavior. The theory further explains that a person is more likely to intend to do a behavior when he or she believes that the outcomes of that behavior are desirable. A person is also more likely to engage in a behavior when the person believes that other people think that he or she should do the behavior. In an extension of the theory of reasoned action, the theory of planned behavior suggests that a person is more likely to do a behavior when she believes that she has control over the situation.

The third parent theory is Bandura's (1986) social-cognitive theory. A major tenet of social-cognitive theory is self-efficacy. Self-efficacy is the confidence a person has in his or her ability to successfully carry out an action. Bandura's theory proposes that the greater a person's self-efficacy for a behavior, the more likely that the person will engage in it, even when faced with obstacles. The concept of self-efficacy is one of the behavior-specific cognitions of Pender's model. Pender's belief is that when a person has high-perceived competence or self-efficacy in a certain behavior, it results in a greater likelihood that the person will commit to action and actually perform the behavior.

Some have observed that the HPM resembles the Health Belief Model (HBM). While it is true that the HPM shares some concepts with the HBM, the HPM differs from the HBM in at least one important way. The HPM is a competence- or approach-oriented model that focuses on attainment of high-level wellness and self-actualization. This is contrasted with the HBM, which was intended for use in explaining patients' use of medical diagnosis and treatment of disease, such as tuberculosis. Further, the HBM incorporates fear or threat of disease as a motivation for action. While this perspective may be valid for diseases that have shorter prodromal periods, the HPM does not consider fear or threat as a powerful motivation for distant threats to health.

The HPM has undergone a modification since its initial introduction in 1982. The original model has been examined in a variety of research studies, using model-based hypotheses to test the validity of relationships proposed by the model. These studies of the model have taken place in a variety of settings, health behaviors, and populations. The results of these studies have been mixed. Some studies have demonstrated that the model has been very useful in explaining or predicting health-promoting behavior in a group of research participants. For example, in a study by Kerr (1994), HPM concepts explained 55% of the variance in use of hearing protection among Mexican-American industrial workers. Results of studies in which a large proportion of variance in behavior is explained, such as that by Kerr, provide support for the model.

Some study results have been less successful in explaining client behavior. For example, in a study of preadolescents and adolescents, Garcia et al. (1995) were able to explain only 19% of the variance in exercise behavior. Garcia suggested the need for the addition of concepts to the model to increase its predictive power. Pender (1996) analyzed the empirical support provided by each of the studies based on the model. This analysis resulted in the retention of selected model concepts and the deletion of others. In addition, three new concepts and associated relationships have been added to the model. The newly added concepts include previous related behavior, immediate competing demands and preferences, and commitment to a plan of action.

The revised model (Pender, 1996; Pender et al., 2002) consists of individual characteristics and experiences, behavior-specific cognitions and affect, and other factors leading to the behavioral outcome. Pender identifies the behavior-specific cognitions and affect as the major motivational mechanisms for health-promoting behavior. These include perceived benefits of action, perceived barriers to action, perceived self-efficacy, activity-related affect, interpersonal influences, and situational influences. Individual characteristics and experiences included in the model are previous related behavior and personal factors. The additional concepts of the model are immediate competing demands and preferences, commitment to a plan of action, and health-promoting behavior. These concepts are briefly described in Definition of Key Concepts, at the beginning of the chapter. Relationships of the concepts are described in the model's theoretical propositions (Box 14-1). The schematic representation of the model (Fig. 14-1) shows the relationship of model concepts to the behavioral outcome—health-promoting behavior.

The model includes multiple concepts and relationships. However, some concepts and relationships may be more salient than others to a given health behavior. The model does not provide assistance in selecting which concepts and relationships are appropriate for specific behaviors. Therefore, the researcher who seeks to use the model should select concepts and relationships based on previous research, theoretical foundations, clinical experience, or practical limitations regarding a specific behavior. Indeed, extant research using the HPM shows the selectivity of researchers in determining which model concepts to include in their study designs.

BOX 14.1   Theoretical Propositions of the Health-Promotion Model

- Previous related behavior and inherited and acquired characteristics influence beliefs, affect, and enactment of health-promoting behavior.
- Persons commit to engaging in behaviors from which they anticipate deriving personally valued benefits.
- Perceived barriers can constrain commitment to action, a mediator of behavior, as well as actual behavior.
- Perceived competence or self-efficacy to execute a given behavior increases the likelihood of commitment to action and actual performance of the behavior.
- Greater perceived self-efficacy results in fewer perceived barriers to a specific health behavior.
- Positive affect toward a behavior results in greater perceived self-efficacy, which can, in turn, result in increased positive affect.
- When positive emotions or affect are associated with a behavior, the probability of commitment and action are increased.
- Persons are more likely to commit to and engage in health-promoting behaviors when significant others model the behavior, expect the behavior to occur, and provide assistance and support to enable the behavior.

- Families, peers, and health care providers are important sources of interpersonal influence that can increase or decrease commitment to and engagement in health-promoting behavior.
- Situational influences in the external environment can increase or decrease commitment to or participation in health-promoting behavior.
- The greater the commitment to a specific plan of action, the more likely health-promoting behaviors are to be maintained over time.
- Commitment to a plan of action is less likely to result in the desired behavior when competing demands over which persons have little control require immediate attention.
- Commitment to a plan of action is less likely to result in the desired behavior when other actions are more attractive, and thus preferred over the target behavior.
- Persons can modify cognitions, affect, and the interpersonal and physical environments to create incentives for health actions.

Source: Pender, N., Murdaugh, C., & Parsons, M. (2002). *Health promotion in nursing practice* (4th ed.). Reprinted by permission of Pearson Education, Inc., Upper Saddle River, NJ.

APPLICATION OF THE THEORY

The HPM offers a conceptual framework for the provision of effective nursing care directed at improved health and functional ability. First, the model provides a method for the assessment of client health-promoting behaviors. The model directs nurses to systematically assess clients for their perceived self-efficacy, perceived barriers, perceived benefits, interpersonal influences, and situational influences that are relevant to the selected health behavior.

Second, the model identifies several additional client characteristics as targets for assessment. These client characteristics include previous behavior, demographic characteristics, and perceived health sta-

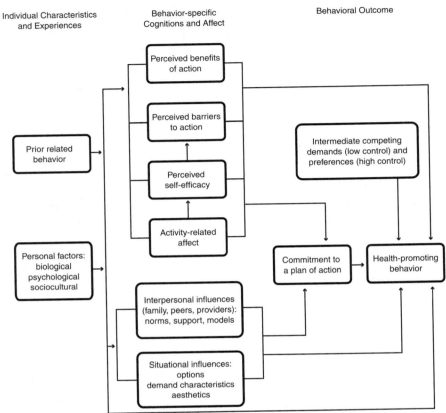

■ **Figure 14-1.** Health promotion model. Source: Pender, N., Murdaugh, C., & Parsons, M. (2002). *Health promotion in nursing practice* (4th ed.). © Reprinted by permission of Pearson Education, Inc., Upper Saddle River, NJ.

tus. While these characteristics are not amenable to alteration, they offer a basis for the tailoring of nursing interventions, discussed below.

Third, the model suggests that nursing interventions can be designed to alter clients' perceptions in these areas. Success in these interventions is expected to result in more frequent health-promoting behaviors and resultant improved wellness.

Although the model identifies foci for nursing interventions, it does not explicitly describe how nurses can effect changes in client perceptions. While these nursing interventions directed at changing client perceptions are proposed by the HPM, few studies testing the effectiveness of these proposed interventions have been completed.

Pender prescribes use of the nursing process as the method of producing behavior change. She emphasizes nursing assessment of health, health beliefs, and health behavior, using established frameworks such as North American Nursing Diagnosis Association (NANDA) and Gordon's functional health patterns. In addition, she recommends use of model-based assessments such as the Health-Promoting Lifestyles Profile II (HPLP-II). Pender emphasizes use of the nursing process in empowering self care across the life span. She outlines a multistep process for health planning that includes reinforcing client strengths, developing a plan based on client preferences and Prochaska's (1994) stages of change, addressing facilitators and barriers, and committing to goals.

Areas of intervention for health promotion include exercise, nutrition, stress management, and social support. Pender et al. (2002) review several interventions in each of these areas, many of which are research-based, but not model-based. These are directed toward increasing the client's capacity for a vigorous and productive life.

Use of the Health Promotion Model in Tailoring Nursing Interventions

Model variables, such as client characteristics, cognitions, and affect may be used to tailor nursing interventions to clients. Tailoring of interventions involves shaping of health messages based on characteristics unique to that person. Tailoring interventions has been found to increase intervention effectiveness (Strecher et al., 1994). This innovative intervention strategy offers exciting opportunities for planning health-promotion interventions that are designed to meet the unique needs of each individual client. Once the nurse assesses the client on each of the relevant factors of the model, this information can be used to custom-design a health promotion program for that individual client. Recent applications of the HPM have used computers to quickly and accurately assess the health of the client on model-based variables. With the help of computer technology, the nurse has used this information to design a health promotion intervention that is unique to the needs of this individual (Lusk, Kerr, Ronis, & Eakin, 1999). This computer-assisted approach offers nurses the opportunity to provide interventions that are more appropriate to the individual, and may, as a result, greatly enhance intervention effectiveness.

Selecting the Health Promotion Model

Nurses are faced with selecting from a variety of models for use in clinical practice and research. This selection may be based on a variety of factors, including philosophy, research, clarity, and utility.

The HPM is appealing to many nurses because it offers a view of health consistent with their motivation for pursing the profession of nursing. Its holistic and humanistic view is congruent with many nurses' own personal philosophy of health and nursing. The model reflects a belief that persons are capable of introspection and personal change. In turn, the model proposes that health care is more than treatment and prevention of disease, but also involves the creation of conditions in which clients can express their unique human potential. The nurse is presented as an agent for creating behavioral and environmental changes.

The HPM has been used successfully in several research studies, as discussed earlier in this chapter. While some models have been tested more extensively, the HPM does have a body of extant literature that provides support for its use. A more thorough discussion of studies using the HPM is presented in Pender's 4th edition (Pender et al., 2002).

Most nurses will find that the HPM is straightforward and easy to understand. It uses terms that are readily understood, and its propositional statements are clearly presented. The phenomena addressed by the model are familiar to nurses, and most nurses will require minimal learning of new terms and concepts to use and understand the model, which is clearly presented in graphic form.

The HPM has been used in a variety of settings, including schools, workplaces, ambulatory treatment facilities, rehabilitation centers, and a prison. It has been used with a wide variety of health behaviors, including exercise, nutrition, and hearing protection use. See Using Middle Range Theories 14-1 for a study based on the HPM to promote use of hearing protection devices. The studies have involved clients diverse in gender and age. The model has a limited history of application in culturally

---

14-1 USING MIDDLE RANGE THEORIES

Workers who work in high-noise environments are at risk for development of noise-induced hearing loss. Although hearing loss can be prevented with the consistent use of hearing-protection devices, use of these devices among a group of construction workers ranged from 18% to 41%. These usage rates are too low for effective hearing protection. The Health Promotion Model (HPM) was originally intended for application with health-promoting behaviors such as exercise, nutrition, and stress management. However, its application has been extended to examine a health-protective behavior (hearing protector use). In an intervention effectiveness study, Lusk, Hong, Ronis, Kerr, Eakin, and Early (1997) examined an HPM-based intervention to increase workers' use of hearing protection.

The HPM served as a basis for assessing this group of construction workers' use of hearing protection. The results of this model-based assessment were used to generate a training program that was responsive to the attitudes and beliefs of the workers. Construction workers were recruited for the training program through their trade association, while plumber/pipe fitter trainers were recruited at their national conference. Because the researchers suspected an effect of pretesting on participants, a Solomon four-group design was employed. This design offers the advantage of examining for effects of the intervention among subjects who have and have not been pretested.

The intervention consisted of a video encouraging use of hearing protection devices by building worker self-efficacy for use of hearing protection and overcoming common barriers to hearing protector use. The video was supplemented with guided practice, handouts, and sample hearing protection devices. Teaching was accomplished with the use of specially prepared trainers.

ANOVA analysis showed a significant main effect of the intervention as well as no effect of pretesting. Among pretested workers, the analysis showed a statistically significant increase in use of hearing protection (53%), compared to workers' baseline level of use (44%). In addition, workers who received the intervention reported rates of use of hearing protection (52%) that were higher than the comparison groups (46%). Although the intervention was successful in improving use of hearing protection devices, workers' use of these devices remained lower than can be considered effective. The study authors call for future studies to develop interventions that are more effective in encouraging construction workers' use of hearing protection devices.

Lusk, S., Hong, O., Ronis, D., Kerr, M., Eakin, B., & Early, M. (1997). Test of the effectiveness of an intervention to increase use of hearing protection devices in construction workers. *Research in Nursing and Health; 20*(3), 183–194.

diverse groups. However, Korean, Taiwanese, Thai, and Japanese individuals have participated in previous studies. It is noteworthy that persons included as study participants have been either well or experiencing chronic illness, such as HIV infection.

The HPM has been used by nurses working in a variety of community-based settings, such as occupational health and public health. The model is well suited to clients whose health status is stable and whose basic needs are met. See Using Middle Range Theories 14-2. Although Pender's definition of health is broad and encompasses persons who are experiencing illness, application of the HPM is untested in acute care settings, and with clients whose health concerns are urgent or living conditions are unstable.

INSTRUMENTS USED IN EMPIRICAL TESTING

Instruments have been developed to measure a variety of concepts related to the Health Promotion Model. Primary of these is the Health-Promoting Lifestyles Profile II (HPLP-II) (Susan Walker, personal communication, June 24, 2002). Due to the broad nature of the model, many instruments have

14-2 USING MIDDLE RANGE THEORIES

Although exercise has been shown to have positive effects on health, only a small percentage of the population engages in exercise at a level effective enough to produce these health benefits. A precipitous drop in the level of physical activity among adolescents contributes to a sedentary adult population. Garcia et al. (1995) studied the exercise behavior and related beliefs of a group of male and female preadolescents and adolescents.

Two cohorts of children, 5th/6th grade and 8th grade, were recruited to participate in the study. Participants completed surveys measuring their self-esteem, perceived health status, exercise self-efficacy, benefits of exercise, barriers to exercise, extent of previous exercise, exercise models, exercise norms, social support for exercise, and access to places for exercise. In addition, students completed exercise logs each day for 5 days. Results of perceived barriers were subtracted from results of perceived benefits to produce a benefits–barriers differential.

The results showed that gender had a significant effect on exercise behavior and beliefs of preadolescents and adolescents. Females reported less exercise, lower self-esteem, poorer health status, and less previous exercise. The results also showed an interaction effect between gender and developmental stage on the benefits–barriers differential. That is, adolescent girls were less likely to believe that the benefits of exercise were greater than the barriers, when compared to males.

When exercise scores were regressed on all the model factors, 19% of the variance in exercise behavior was explained. Three factors (gender, benefits–barriers differential, and access to facilities) reached significance. An exploratory path analysis suggested that beliefs about benefits and barriers mediate effects of developmental stage, perceived health status, exercise self-efficacy, social support for exercise, and exercise norms on exercise behavior.

Garcia, A., Broda, M., Frenn, M., Coviak, C., Pender, N., & Ronis, D. (1995). Gender and developmental differences in exercise beliefs among youth and prediction of their exercise behavior. *Journal of School Health, 65*(6), 213–219.

been developed to measure behavior-specific attitudes and beliefs. A sample of these is described in Table 14-1. Examples of measures of all model variables can be found on the following Web site: *http://www.nursing.umich.edu/faculty/pender_nola.html*. Research Application 14-1 provides an example of using selected physical assessments as measures of a fitness program.

Table 14-1. HEALTH PROMOTION MODEL INSTRUMENTS

INSTRUMENT	FIRST AUTHOR (DATE)	DESCRIPTION
Health-Promoting Lifestyles Profile II (HPLP-II)	Susan Walker (personal communication, June 24, 2002)	52-item questionnaire in a 4-point response format measures the frequency of health-promoting behaviors in six domains (health responsibility, physical activity, nutrition, spiritual growth, interpersonal relations, and stress management).
HPLP—Spanish Version	Walker, Kerr, Pender, & Sechrist, 1990	This instrument provides a Spanish language version of the HPLP.
HPLP—Japanese Version	Wei et al., 2000	This instrument provides a Japanese language version of the HPLP.
Exercise Benefits/Barriers Scale (EBBS)	Sechrist, Walker, & Pender, 1987	This Likert scale measures the person's perceived benefits to undertaking preventive behaviors that reduce risk factors in CAD.
Perceived Self-Efficacy of Hearing Protector Use Scale	Lusk, 1997	This 10-item scale asks respondents to rate the extent to which they have confidence in their ability to use hearing protection. An example of an item from this scale is, "I am sure I can use my hearing protection so it works effectively."
Perception of Accessibility and Availability of Hearing Protectors Scale	Lusk, 1997	This 9-item scale asks respondents to report on this dimension of situational factors influencing health behavior. A sample item from this scale is, "Ear plugs are available to pick up at my job sites."
Interpersonal Influences on Hearing Protector Use Scale	Lusk, 1997	This scale includes three subscales measuring dimensions of these variables: interpersonal norms, interpersonal modeling, and interpersonal support. The Interpersonal Norms Subscale includes 4 items that query respondents about their beliefs as to how much others (family members, friends, supervisor, and coworkers) think they should wear hearing protection. The Interpersonal Support Subscale measures encouragement or praise from family, friends, coworkers, and supervisors about the respondent's use of hearing protection. The Interpersonal Modeling Subscale measures how much they believe others use hearing protection when exposed to noise.

14-1 RESEARCH APPLICATION

An occupational health nurse was interested in improving the health status of employees through implementation of a fitness program. A baseline assessment of employee health was offered to a random sample of 397 employees. The Health Promotion Model-based assessment consisted of a survey of health behaviors, personal factors, perceived barriers to exercise, perceived benefits of exercise, self-efficacy, situational influences, and interpersonal influences. The survey was supplemented with selected physical measurements, including height, weight, BMI, blood pressure, and serum cholesterol. Employee health care claims were also monitored. A review of a summary of employee survey results revealed that the major barrier to fitness for this group included a perception that fitness programs were too time consuming. One situational influence that many employees shared was the lack of year-round access to exercise facilities.

Based on survey responses, the occupational health nurse planned a multifocal fitness promotion program that featured policy development and health education. The educational interventions included work site classes, paycheck inserts, and an employee health newsletter. These educational interventions included suggestions for incorporating physical activity into routine activities, such as walking and climbing stairs. The nurse was also successful in obtaining a group discount for employees at a local health club.

After a 6-month period, the survey and physical measures were readministered to employees and results were compared. Moderate gains in employee perception of barriers to exercise and situational influences on exercise were achieved. Employee participation in exercise was found to increase from an average of 48 to 65 minutes per week. In addition, average serum cholesterol levels were found to drop from 231 to 218 mg/dL, and a 22% difference in health care claims was observed between participants and nonparticipants.

The nurse plans to continue the program, with the goal of improving employee self-efficacy for exercise, while continuing to monitor for effects on exercise behavior and health outcomes.

SUMMARY

Pender has proposed a model of health promotion to guide nurses in helping clients achieve improved health, enhanced functional ability, and better quality of life. The need for behavioral and environmental changes to effect improvements in a society where lifestyle factors account for a large proportion of health problems provides justification for the model. The model is based on established theories of human behavior, including the theory of reasoned action, the theory of planned behavior, and social-cognitive theory. The Health Promotion Model claims that a variety of client characteristics and cognitive-affective factors combine with competing demands and preferences, as well as commitment to a plan of action to explain the likelihood of health-promoting behavior. The model has been tested in several clinical studies, using a variety of settings, health behaviors, and client characteristics. It presents exciting possibilities for the creation of interventions that are tailored to the unique characteristics and needs of individual clients.

The model was revised in 1996 following review and analysis of the results of model testing and the intervention-effectiveness research based on the model. While the authors expect the revised model to have greater explanatory and predictive power, this is as yet untested by multiple scientific studies. The model authors acknowledge the need for measures of model concepts that fit the target population and the design of robust interventions that can change model beliefs and, subsequently, health outcomes. Interventions that address not only individuals but families and communities in creating multilevel interventions employing the HPM in combination with community action models are most likely to achieve success.

ANALYSIS EXERCISE

Using the criteria presented in Chapter 2, critique the Health Promotion Model. When you are finished, you can compare your ideas about the model with those of a researcher who has worked with the model (Appendix A).

Internal Criticism

1. Clarity
2. Consistency

3. Adequacy
4. Logical development
5. Level of theory development

External Criticism

1. Reality convergence
2. Utility
3. Significance
4. Discrimination

WEB RESOURCES

1. The Canadian Public Health Association, together with Health and Welfare Canada, and WHO, sponsors a page that describes a charter for action to achieve Health for All by the year 2000 and beyond: *http://www.who.int/hpr/archive/docs/ottawa.html*
2. This link provides information about WHO's Department of Noncommunicable Diseases and Health Promotion (NCD), and its global conferences on health promotion. The goal of this agency is to reduce the incidence of NCDs and promote positive health and well-being, with particular focus on developing countries: *http://www.who.int/hpr/archive/oldhpr/aboutus.html*
3. Healthy People 2010 is the prevention agenda for the nation. It is a statement of U. S. health objec-

tives designed to identify the most significant preventable threats to health and establish national goals to reduce these threats: *http://www.health.gov/healthypeople/*
4. The Combined Health Promotion Database is a service of the National Center for Chronic Disease Prevention and Health Promotion (part of the Centers for Disease Control and Prevention). The stated goal of this agency is to collect and provide health promotion/ health education information emphasizing methodology and the application of effective health promotion and education programs and risk reduction interventions: *http://chid.nih. gov/subfile/contribs/he.html*
5. The National Council on Aging sponsors research and demonstration projects to promote vital aging. The Institute accomplishes its mission through advocating for and empowering

older adults to achieve health and well-being through a multidisciplinary approach: *http://www.ncoa.org/index.cfm*

6. Many universities have schools of public health, nursing, medicine, and related fields, offering a variety of resources (e.g., research, teaching, service programs) related to health promotion. An example of one of these is the Center for Health Promotion and Disease Prevention at the University of North Carolina at Chapel Hill (HPDP): *http://www.hpdp.unc.edu/ hpdp/index.cfm?fuseaction=about.home*

7. The AHRQ's mission includes both "translating research findings into better patient care and providing policy makers and other health care leaders with information needed to make critical health care decisions." This site includes information about improving health care and prevention research: *http://www.ahcpr. gov/news/focus/index.html*

8. The American Public Health Association (APHA) is a professional association of researchers, health service providers, administrators, teachers, and other health workers. This site includes a rich resource of selected internet resources for health education and health promotion: *http://www.apha.org/public_health/ hphe.htm*

9. Many state health departments sponsor health promotion programs for their residents, and include related information on their home pages. One example is the Minnesota Department of Health:*http://www.health.state.mn.us/ index.html*

10. Dr. Pender maintains a web site of FAQs about the HPM: *http://www.nursing.umich.edu/ faculty/pender_nola.html*

REFERENCES

Bandura, A. (1997) *Self-efficacy: The exercise of control.* New York: W.H. Freeman.

Garcia, A., Broda, M., Frenn, M., Coviak, C., Pender, N., & Ronis, D. (1995). Gender and developmental differences in exercise beliefs among youth and prediction of their exercise behavior. *Journal of School Health, 65*(6), 213-219.

Kerr, M. (1994). Factors related to Mexican-American workers' use of hearing protection, #9501083. Ann Arbor, MI: Dissertation Abstracts International.

Strecher, V. J., Kreuter, M., Den-Boer, D. J., Kobrin, S., Hospers, H. J., & Skinner, C. S. (1994). The effects of computer-tailored smoking cessation messages in family practice settings. *Journal of Family Practice, 39*(3), 262–270.

Lusk, S., Hong, O., Ronis, D., Kerr, M., Eakin, B., & Early, M. (1997). Test of the effectiveness of an intervention to increase use of hearing protection devices in construction workers. *Research in Nursing and Health, 20*(3), 183–194.

Lusk, S., Kerr, M., Ronis, D., & Eakin, B. (1999). Applying the health promotion model to development of a worksite intervention. *American Journal of Health Promotion, 13*(4), 219–226.

Montano, D., Kasprzyk, D., & Taplin, S. (1997). The theory of reasoned action and the theory of planned behavior. In K. Glanz, I.M. Lewis, & B.K. Rimer (Eds.), Health behavior and health education: Theory, research, and practice (2nd ed,) San Francisco: Jossey-Bass.

Pender, N., Murdaugh, C., & Parsons, M. (2002). *Health promotion in nursing practice* (4th ed.). Upper Saddle River, NJ: Prentice Hall.

Pender, N. (1996). *Health promotion in nursing practice* (3rd ed.). Stamford, CT: Appleton & Lange.

Pender, N. (1990). Expressing health through lifestyle patterns. *Nursing Science Quarterly, 3*(3) 115–122.

Sechrist, K., Walker, W., & Pender, N. (1987). Development and psychometric evaluation of the exercise benefits/barriers scale. *Nursing in Research and Health, 10*(6), 357–365.

Walker, S., Sechrist, K., & Pender, N.(1997). The Health-Promoting Lifestyle profile: Development and psychometric characteristics. *Nursing Research, 39*(5), 268–273.

Walker, S., Kerr, M., Pender, N., & Sechrist, K. (1990). A Spanish language version of the health-promoting lifestyle profile. *Nursing Research, 39*(5), 268–273.

Wei, C. N., Yonemitsu, H., Harada, K., Miyakita, T., Omori, S., Miyabayashi, T., & Ueda, A. A. (2000). Japanese language version of the health-promoting lifestyle profile. *Nippon-Eiseigaku-Zasshi, 54*(4), 597–606.

Deliberative Nursing Process

MERTIE L. POTTER

DEFINITION OF KEY TERMS

Automatic nursing process Actions (visible behaviors) the nurse takes based on reasons other than the patient's immediate needs

Deliberative nursing process Means by which the professional nurse purposefully explores with the patient the nurse's perceptions (stimulation of any one of the five senses), thoughts, and/or feelings related to the patient's immediate need for help

Dynamic nurse–patient relationship Interactive contact/connection between nurse and patient, when the nurse begins to explore the meaning behind the patient's verbal and nonverbal behaviors

Immediate need for help Requirement of the patient in a specific situation. Help for the need relieves or diminishes the patient's immediate distress or improves the patient's immediate sense of adequacy or well-being.

Nursing situation Circumstance that involves a patient's behavior, the nurse's reaction (perceptions, thoughts, and feelings combined together), and the nurse's action (activity the nurse completes with or for the patient)

Patient distress Feeling experienced by a patient when the patient cannot meet certain needs and is not helped in meeting such needs

Patient outcomes/product Improved verbal and nonverbal patient behaviors that can result from the nurse's deliberative and effective action(s) with the patient

Validation Ongoing process of exploring and determining with a patient if the nursing reaction was accurate and if the nursing action was helpful

INTRODUCTION

The birthing of Deliberative Nursing Process by Ida J. Orlando culminated in 1961, after a number of years laboring to define both the function and product of professional nursing (Orlando, 1961). The theory began to take shape through Orlando's experiences within nursing practice and nurse education. Orlando reviewed more than 2000 anecdotal recordings written by faculty, students, and nurses related to their interactions with patients and began to see patterns of effective and ineffective nursing process in various nurse–patient situations (Pelletier, 1976). Emerging from these early experiences, Deliberative Nursing Process since has matured into a significant, enduring, and practical nursing theory.

As a middle range theory, Deliberative Nursing Process has a limited number of variables and is limited in scope (McEwan, 2002; Walker & Avant, 1995). However, it is specific and adequate enough to apply and test in research and practice. Although categorized as a grand theory by some (Walker & Avant, 1995; Wills, 2002), Deliberative Nursing Process demonstrates the following middle range theory characteristics: comprehensive yet focused, generalizable, restricted in its concepts, clear in its propositions, and conducive to testable hypotheses (McEwan, 2002).

An unusual paradox within Deliberative Nursing Process is its proclivity toward both simplicity and complexity as a theory. This paradox partially explains the attractiveness of using this theory. Generally, it is straightforward in its presentation, while being multifaceted in its applications. For example, developing a nurse–patient relationship that is dynamic and unique is not complicated. However, the dynamics of the nurse–patient relationship itself may be very complex (Orlando, 1961).

A unique feature related to development of this theory is the inductive manner in which Orlando defined effective nursing (Schmieding, 2002). Orlando determined effective nursing and ineffective nursing from her observations of "good" and "bad" nursing practice (Orlando, 1961, 1972; Pelletier, 1976; Schmieding, 1993a). From her observations of specific phenomena (nurse–patient interactions), Orlando identified relationships with other phenomena to develop propositions that led to the development of larger concepts and, ultimately, the theory (Johnson & Webber, 2001).

Orlando desired that nurses become educated to assist patients to express what help they actually need (Pelletier, 1967). Another distinctive feature of Deliberative Nursing Process is that patient input is critical. It is the nurse's professional responsibility to involve the patient in the process of identifying and meeting the patient's immediate needs for help (Orlando, 1961, 1972, 1990).

HISTORICAL BACKGROUND

The need for nurses to have a distinct body of knowledge to direct and enhance nursing practice and the movement of nursing towards becoming a profession were beginning to take place at the turn of the 20th century (Alligood, 2002). Orlando's Deliberative Nursing Process evolved during an era when nurses were attempting to distinguish nursing from other disciplines, and when psychiatric-mental health nurses were determining their place among nurses of other specialties. Deliberative Nursing Process came into being as Orlando realized that nursing needed to address three areas:

"nurse–patient relationships, the nurse's professional role and identity, and the development of knowledge which is distinctly nursing" (Orlando, 1961, p. viii).

Orlando first published work related to this theory after she examined what made nursing interventions effective or ineffective. She asserted early on that effective nursing was "good nursing," and ineffective nursing was "bad nursing" (Orlando, 1976; Schmieding, 1993a). Although this terminology might not be acceptable during today's trend of political correctness and relativity, Orlando was bold in her assertion that nursing was either "good" or "bad." She also stressed that nursing needed to define exactly what "nursing" was, and contended that nursing could not be a profession unless it was able to distinguish what nurses did that was unique (Orlando, 1961).

Orlando was asked to determine what mental health principles were needed in a nursing curriculum. However, she became acutely aware during the project that professional nursing did not have a clear function or product. Nursing was at a crossroads. Orlando understood that nurses were unclear in their attempts to define what nursing was (Orlando, 1961). For someone concerned with meeting patients' immediate needs, here was an immediate need for nurses—to define and to distinguish nursing's function and product. She recognized that the patient and the patient's needs were getting lost in nurses' assumptions of what those needs were. During a project funded by the National Institute of Mental Health, Orlando began to examine nurses' interactions with patients.

Resolute in her mission, Orlando set forth in her later work to assist nurses further in defining what nursing is and what it should entail to distinguish it from other disciplines. Key goals became the following: to define the distinct professional function of nurses; to encourage nurses to assume authority to carry out that function; and to educate nurses to use process discipline (deliberative nursing process) to assure that the product of nursing function involves the patient and others who impact the patient's care (Orlando, 1972). She developed a user-friendly theory that was readily understandable and broadly applicable.

Orlando held that "to nurse" and "nursing" were very different from "to doctor" and "doctoring" (Orlando, 1961, 1972; Orlando & Dugan, 1989). She asserted that doctors' orders are designed for patients, not nurses, and that nurses keep themselves on a dependent path when they focus on following doctors' orders rather than assisting patients to meet their needs for help, which may include the patient's needing to comply with doctors' orders (Orlando, 1987). Orlando contended that licensure authorizes nurses to fulfill a professional role, but authority is only implicit until the nurse engages in a process with the patient to meet the function of nursing, namely, to help the patient meet immediate needs for help that the patient is unable to meet on his or her own (Orlando, 1972).

Orlando suggested that the concept of "nursing" derives its meaning from the nursing of infants and the need to have someone nurture and assist infants in obtaining what they need from the environment to survive. She postulated that, at times, individuals might need assistance from others to obtain what is needed from the environment to meet their needs when they are unable to nurse themselves (Orlando, 1961, p. 4; Orlando & Dugan, 1989). Orlando (1972, 1987) distinguished the difference between lay and professional nursing by stating that a professional nurse is needed when a lay person cannot assure that the patient's distress will be identified or relieved.

In some of her works, she questioned whether or not expanded roles of nursing should be considered in the realm of nursing or in the realm of doctoring at a lower cost (Orlando & Dugan, 1989). She used straightforward and uncomplicated language. She contemplated and encouraged nurses to discern what the words "to nurse" meant and referred to a dictionary to emphasize her point of what nursing should entail. She accepted Funk & Wagnall's definition of "to nurse" to mean: "to encourage, to look after; to nourish, protect, and nurture; to give curative care to an ailment" (Orlando, 1987, p. 408).

Notably, Orlando was ahead of her time in her concern for and measurement of outcome variables. She promoted progressive ideas, such as defining professional nursing, employing critical thinking within the nursing process, involving the patient in the nursing process, and measuring patient outcomes. Orlando was aware that ineffective nursing activities impacted areas, such as nursing care costs, patient progress, material costs, and medication costs. She was concerned that nursing was acquiring too many nonprofessional tasks that would take the nurse away from helping the patient (Orlando, 1961). Always seeking patient involvement in the provision of nursing care, Orlando looked for a "helpful outcome" as validated with the patient to include "change in the behavior of the object indicating either relief from distress or that a solution to a living or work problem had been found" (Orlando, 1972, p. 61). She addressed work problems involving staff members, as well as patient problems in her 1972 reported studies.

Work on Deliberative Nursing Process theory has spanned more than a half century. Orlando's initial development on this theory began in the early 1950s, and work on the theory's development continues. Her early works referred to the "deliberative nursing process." Orlando began using the term "nursing process discipline" in 1972 because she asserted that nursing process was a discipline that could be learned (Orlando, 1972, p. 2). The term "deliberative nursing process" will be used throughout this chapter for consistency.

It is obvious in both her published and unpublished writings that Orlando is not only an intensely passionate individual about nursing but also a determined advocate for nursing (Orlando, 1961, 1972, 1976, 1983, 1987). Several basic tenets come through strongly in her work, primarily: (a) the function of nursing is to meet the patient's immediate need for help when the patient is unable to do so without the nurse's help; and (b) that the product of nursing is to relieve the patient's distress caused by the immediate need for help and to be able to observe improvement either verbally or nonverbally (Orlando, 1961, 1972). Furthermore, Orlando's theory promotes the uniqueness of nurses and maintains that patients must be involved in the identification and determination of their immediate needs for help (Orlando, 1961). Orlando was not hesitant to express her grave concern with the definition of nursing promoted in the American Nurses Association Social Policy Statement of 1980—she found "no operational meaning" in it and no differentiation between professional and lay nursing (Orlando, 1983, p.2). Her passion for nursing continues to be evident, and her assertion that the profession still needs to define nursing persists (I. J. Orlando, personal communication, June 24, 2002).

DEFINITION OF THEORY CONCEPTS

Deliberative Nursing Process

Deliberative Nursing Process remains relevant and significant as a nursing theory due to its patient-focused approach, nurse exploration of nurse perceptions, thoughts, and feelings with patients, and effective outcomes that result from its use. Orlando (1961) proposes a practical approach, with a broad application within nursing education, practice, and research. She focuses on the nurse's unique and deliberative response to the patient who has expressed an immediate need for help. This

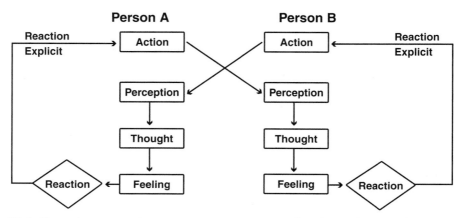

■ **Figure 15-1.** The action process in a person-to-person contact functioning by open disclosure. The perceptions, thoughts, and feelings of each individual through the observable action. Used with permission from Orlando, I. J. (1972). *The discipline and teaching of nursing process (An evaluative study)* (p. 26). New York: G. P. Putnam's Sons.

is accomplished by the nurse's exploration and validation of the nurse's perceptions, thoughts, and feelings about the patient's behavior with the patient. Furthermore, it is the nurse's responsibility in deliberative nursing to see to it that the patient's need for immediate help is met either by the nurse's own activity or by eliciting the help of others (Orlando, 1961).

Orlando acknowledges and affirms the nurse's distinctive interpretation and validation of observations made. Furthermore, she stresses the independent function performed during a deliberative nursing interaction. Orlando recognizes that nurses' continually sharing their unique perceptions, thoughts, and feelings (i.e., their immediate reaction) about patients' unique behaviors within a deliberative process with patients is what makes nurse–patient relationships dynamic (Orlando, 1961, 1972).

Orlando asserts that good nursing initially involves a nurse's determining with the patient a number of elements: (a) What does the patient think is occurring?; (b) What does the patient define as the immediate distress?; (c) Is the patient's distress related to an immediate need for help?; and (d) Is the nurse's help needed for the patient to obtain relief? Orlando also observed that nurse–patient interactions involving Deliberative Nursing Process resulted in positive outcomes, namely both verbal and nonverbal positive changes within the patient (Pelletier, 1976).

Deliberative Nursing Process was renamed Nursing Process Discipline by Orlando (1972). She also refers to Deliberative Nursing Process as Effective Nursing (Orlando, 1961, 1972), or good nursing (Orlando, 1976). She analyzed nurse–patient interactions and determined that effective interactions involved open disclosure of the nurse of perceptions, thoughts, and feelings and validation of the same with the patient. After implementing a nursing action, the nurse validates with the patient if the nursing action met the patient's immediate need for help (Orlando, 1961) (Figure 15-1).

Orlando also noted that ineffective interactions often involved a more secretive style. Both patient and nurse were not aware of each other's perceptions, thoughts, and feelings in such interactions (Figure 15-2).

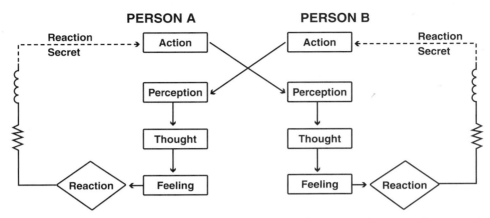

■ Figure 15-2. The action process in a person-to-person contact functioning in secret. The perceptions, thoughts, and feelings of each individual are not directly available to the perception of the other individual through the observable action. Used with permission from Orlando, I. J. (1972). *The discipline and teaching of nursing process (An evaluative study)* (p. 26). New York: G. P. Putnam's Sons.

Orlando (1972, p. 28) developed a Nursing Process Record to assist in learning deliberative nursing process (process discipline) and to be better able to discern nursing process done in secret or using open disclosure (Figure 15-3). Orlando referred to the nurse's perceptions, thoughts, and feelings as part of the nurse's reaction, and whatever the nurse said and/or did to, with, or for the patient as the nurse's action (Orlando, 1972, p. 56) (see Figure 15-3).

Automatic Nursing Process

Automatic nursing process refers to any actions or interventions a nurse takes to help a patient that may not be related to the process of helping the patient. Automatic nursing process may be impacted by other influences, such as nursing care costs, patient progress, or additional expenses. Automatic nursing process also is referred to as Nursing Process Without Discipline (Orlando, 1972), Ineffective Nursing, (Orlando, 1961, 1972) and bad nursing (Orlando, 1976).

Orlando asserted that automatic nursing process activities were ineffective when they: (a) involved nursing action without determining the meaning of the patient's behavior to the patient or the need that caused the behavior; (b) did not assist the patient to inform the nurse how the activity influenced the patient; (c) did not connect the nursing activity to the patient's need; (d) were implemented because of the nurse's inability to explore the nurse's reaction to the patient's behavior; or (e) did not indicate that the nurse was attuned to how the nursing activity influenced the patient (Orlando, 1961, p. 65). Such activities are not necessarily wrong or negative, but they do not determine if the activity is perceived as helpful in relieving the patient's immediate needs. Furthermore, automatic nursing activities indicated to Orlando that nursing care had been given without a disciplined or deliberative professional process (Orlando, 1976).

An example of the difference between use of an automatic nursing process, which involves nurses' assumptions, and a deliberative nursing process, which involves nurses' exploration of the patients' immediate needs for help, is demonstrated in a study by Bochnak, Rhymes, and Leonard (1962).

Nursing Process Record

Perception of or About the Patient	Thought and/or Feeling About the Perception	Said and/or Did To, With, or For the Patient.
PROCESS A Mr. G walking back and forth; face red	Looks angry; something must have happened. I'm afraid to ask because he might hit me.	"Good morning, Mr. G."
PROCESS B Mr. G walking back and forth; face red	Looks angry; something must have happened. I'm afraid to ask because he might hit me.	"I'm afraid you will hit me if I ask a question. Should I be afraid?"

■ **Figure 15-3.** Process A illustrates the nursing process functioning in secrecy. Process B illustrates the nursing process functioning by open disclosure. Used with permission from Orlando, I. J. (1972). *The discipline and teaching of nursing process (An evaluative study)* (p. 28). New York: G. P. Putnam's Sons.

When two different types of nursing activities to address patients' complaints of pain were examined, statistically significant results occurred at the .05 level. In the control group, it was assumed that any complaint of pain indicated a need for pain-relieving medication, and when patients complained of pain, they were given pain-relieving medication. Relief was variable and slow. However, in the experimental group, nurses who used a deliberative approach to determine more accurately what the patients' complaints of pain were about did not automatically administer pain-relieving medication. Their explorations with the patients led to various interventions that provided more extensive relief and quicker relief for the patients (Bochnak, Rhymes, & Leonard, 1962).

Dynamic Nurse–Patient Relationship

According to a recent study, patients are most concerned with personal care issues related to five essential themes: having their needs met, being treated pleasantly, being cared for, having competent nurses, and having care provided promptly (Bolden & Larrabee, 2001). These areas relate to meeting patients' immediate needs for help, which are foundational in Orlando's Theory of Deliberative Nursing Process. Orlando based her ideas about a dynamic nurse–patient relationship on principles from other theories, such as behavioral theory, which postulates that humans are living and behaving organisms who interact continually with one another and within the environment (Orlando, 1961).

Defining the function and product of nursing is explicit in Orlando's definition of the dynamic nurse–patient relationship. Orlando fervently strove to have nurses define the unique function and product of nursing. She defined nursing function as helping the patient and defined nursing product as the improvement or helpful result in the patient's behavior, observable both verbally and nonverbally (Orlando, 1961, 1972, 1983).

Immediate Need for Help

Immediate need for help refers to the patient's inability to fulfill a need for help; the patient may or may not need assistance identifying and/or communicating what the actual need for help is (Orlando, 1961). The observed behavior of the patient is assumed until the meaning behind the behavior is explored (Orlando, 1961, p. 23). Behaviors observed by the nurse may be nonverbal or verbal. Nonverbal behaviors include motor activity, physiological manifestations, and vocalizations. Verbal behaviors take into account complaints, requests, questions, refusals, demands, comments, and statements (Orlando, 1961, pp. 36–37). Immediate needs for help also are referred to simply as "need" in earlier writings (1961).

Therefore, an immediate need for help is any condition in which patients need to have immediate distress relieved or diminished, or their sense of sufficiency or welfare improved (Orlando, 1961, p. 5). Immediate need for help definitely implies that the patient cannot meet the need without professional help.

Patient Distress

Patient distress occurs when a patient's immediate needs are unmet. It is a sense of discomfort that arises when a patient is unable to communicate his or her needs adequately or clearly. Orlando cited physical challenges, unfavorable reactions to the environment, and unfavorable occurrences as examples of circumstances that keep the patient from being able to meet immediate needs (Orlando, 1961, p. 11).

Patient distress is what the patient perceives to be stressful. Orlando holds that behavior has meaning, and that nurses cannot assume what the behavior means without exploring with the patient what the behavior and accompanying distress mean to the patient.

Nursing Situation

According to Orlando (1961, p. 36), a nursing situation encompasses three elements and is dependent upon the nurse's use of them: (1) the patient's behavior; (2) the nurse's reaction; and (3) the nurse's actions intended for the patient's benefit. The interaction of these three elements comprises nursing process.

Validation

Validation is an ongoing nursing action within the Deliberative Nursing Process. It involves checking with the patient if the nurse's perceptions, thoughts, and/or feelings were accurate in relation to the patient's behavior, and if the nurse's interventions were "correct, helpful, or appropriate" (Orlando, 1961, p. 56). In addition, Orlando sees the nurse as primarily responsible for initiating the process of exploration and discovery in relation to how the patient is responding to any nursing action (Orlando, 1961).

Patient Outcomes/Product

The end result of a nursing action is to "bring about improvement" (Orlando, 1961, p. 6). That improvement should be observable both verbally and nonverbally in the patient's behavior (Orlando, 1972, p. 21). Patient outcomes also should be both "predictable and helpful," and may include such outcomes as "avoidance, relief or diminution of helplessness suffered or anticipated by the individual in an immediate experience" (Orlando, 1972, p. 9). The nurse's activity may result in help, no help, or be unknown (Orlando, 1961, p. 67). If the outcome does not transpire as predicted, then the nurse must continue to explore what else may be needed to meet the patient's immediate need for help.

DESCRIPTION OF THE THEORY OF DELIBERATIVE NURSING PROCESS

Simple Yet Complex Theory

Deliberative Nursing Process is a theory that is readily understood, has a specific focus (i.e., meeting patients' immediate needs for help), addresses patient problems and probable outcomes (felt distress and lowered distress, respectively), and is explicit to nursing. Its concepts and their relationships are testable and they answer questions about nursing, which are indicators of a middle range nursing theory (Marriner-Tomey, 1998). Orlando's work helped refocus nurses on patients rather than on tasks and on an active, rather than passive, role of patients in their own care.

Complexity refers to the "richness" of a theory to elucidate more variables and their interrelationships (Stevens-Barnum, 1990, p. 97). Part of the theory's complexity involves learning how to use it. Becoming proficient in the use of Deliberative Nursing Process necessitates time, practice, and self-reflection, often in the form of a supervisory experience. Use of Nurse Process Recordings (see Figure 15-3) helps the nurse distinguish between perceptions, thoughts, and feelings—no small task in itself. Learning Deliberative Nursing Process often involves a close supervisory experience in which the learner reconstructs and examines interactions. The process of becoming comfortable in owning one's perceptions, thoughts, and feelings and sharing them with patients is at times difficult and complex.

Function of Nursing

Orlando observed patients in distress and asserted that it was professional nursing's role to determine and meet their immediate needs for help by exploring with the patient the nurse's unique thoughts and feelings resulting from perceptions related to the observed patient behaviors (Orlando, 1961, 1972, 1990). When the nurse shares perceptions, thoughts, and/or feelings, it is considered to involve open disclosure; by not sharing, the patient is unaware of the nurse's reaction (Orlando, 1972, p. 26). Nurses must not make assumptions, but must explore their perceptions, thoughts, and feelings about the patient's behavior with patients. Orlando's (1961) incorporation of nurses' exploration of their thoughts with patients as part of a deliberative process indicates how critical thinking is an essential part of the deliberative nursing process (Schmieding, 2002).

Major Components and Their Relationships

Nursing is independent, has its own unique professional function, and has its own distinct product (Pelletier, 1976, p. 17). The dynamic nurse–patient relationship involves reciprocity between the nurse and patient; each is influenced by what the other does and says (Marriner Tomey, 1998). It is dependent upon a nurse-initiated exploration of perceptions, thoughts, and feelings about the patient's behavior, and validation that the nurse's perceptions, thoughts, and feelings are accurate.

The nurse initiates the deliberative process to determine the immediate need for help by helping the patient identify and express the meaning of his or her behavior (Orlando, 1961). Further, the nurse helps the patient explore distress related to the immediate need for help to determine the help needed (p. 29). Within the *dynamic nurse–patient* relationship, the nurse observes a patient whom the nurse thinks is in *distress*. This dynamic relationship is dependent upon "what the nurse and patient start with, to the length of their contact and to what they are able to accomplish" (Orlando, 1961, p. 91).

As Schmieding points out, nurses using Deliberative Nursing Process realize "that the patient is the source of the nurse's power" (Schmieding, 2002, p. 327). The nurse uses reflection as part of a critical thinking process to help ascertain the meaning of the patient's behavior according to the patient, and to determine how the behavior relates to the nurse's assumption that an immediate need exists, which is leading to distress for the patient. Nurses obtain information either directly from the patient or indirectly from other sources, such as family, friends, nursing staff, etc. Orlando considers nurses have access to a tremendous amount of information about the patient (Orlando, 1961).

The nurse using a *deliberative process* will check what the meaning of the information is with the patient. In an *automatic process,* the nurse assumes what the information means. Most likely, the outcomes would be significantly different, depending upon which process the nurse uses. Using the deliberative process, the patient partners with the nurse to identify the need, and a successful outcome is more likely. When an automatic process is used, the patient is not included in the assessment or decision-making processes, making a successful outcome less likely (Orlando, 1961, 1972).

Deliberative Nursing Process is a learned and practiced process (Orlando, 1972). The nurse *validates* with the patient that the patient has an *immediate need for help*, and that the immediate need for help cannot be met without a professional nurse's help. The nurse intervenes, after exploring with the patient what meaning the patient ascribes to behaviors related to the situation that resulted in an immediate need for help. The *nursing situation* involves: (a) the patient's behavior, (b) the nurse's reaction, and (c) the nurse's activity or actions to assist the patient. Nursing process is the interaction of the three elements contained within a nursing situation (Orlando, 1961, p. 36).

The nurse validates that the immediate need for help has been met by asking the patient and evaluating if the anticipated *product or patient outcome* of the nursing action, namely improvement and relief of distress, have occurred. If the nursing action has resulted in the patient's relief, the nursing action has been effective in achieving the desired and predicted patient outcome or product. As mentioned, Orlando used Nursing Process Recordings to study nursing process and to educate nurses in Deliberative Nursing Process.

Assumptions and propositions will be described, based upon Johnson & Webber's (2001) definitions. *Assumptions* are assumed truths that are associated with the relationships (p. 15). Patients becoming distressed when they cannot meet their own needs is an example of an assumption within Deliberative Nursing Process (Orlando, 1961). A more complete listing of assumptions implied within Orlando's Deliberative Nursing Process Theory can be found in Table 15-1.

Propositions direct the relationship between concepts and provide a description of the relationship between concepts (Johnson & Webber, 2001, p. 15). An example that Orlando cited was that "the professional function of nursing is distinct and of central importance to patients in any treatment setting" (Pelletier, 1967, p. 30). Implied propositions within Orlando's Deliberative Nursing Process Theory are listed in Table 15-1.

Table 15-1. ASSUMPTIONS AND PROPOSITIONS WITHIN ORLANDO'S (1961) DELIBERATIVE NURSING PROCESS

ASSUMPTIONS	PROPOSITIONS
1. Patients require the expertise of professional nurses to meet certain immediate needs for help.	1. Nurses can determine patients' immediate needs for help by using a deliberative nursing process to ascertain with the patient what the immediate need is.
2. Patients experience distress when they cannot meet their own needs.	2. Nurses can help alleviate patients' distress most effectively when implementing actions based upon a deliberative nursing process because the actions will be designed to meet the need causing distress.
3. Nursing can be evaluated as either good or bad.	3. Good nursing involves open disclosure of and validation with the patient of the nurse's perceptions, thoughts, and/or feelings related to the patient's behavior, and validation with the patient that the nursing action taken met the patient's immediate need for help.
4. It is the responsibility of professional nurses to meet patients' immediate needs for help or to assure that those needs are met by someone else.	4. Professional nurses using a deliberative nursing process function differently than lay nurses because they are trained in a process whereby they validate with patients: (a) what the patients' needs are, and (b) if the needs have been met effectively by the nursing actions implemented.
5. Each nursing situation with a patient is unique and dynamic.	5. Patients' individualized needs and nurses' distinctive styles create individually unique nursing situations, and each nursing situation is dynamic because it involves ongoing deliberation by the nurse.
6. The desired outcome of good nursing is that the patient reports or demonstrates: (a) relief from distress, (b) experience of less distress, or (c) improvement in "adequacy or well-being" (p. 5).	6. The nurse can determine with the patient if nursing actions based on the deliberative nursing process alleviated or decreased the distress or helped the patient gain a sense of improved "adequacy or well-being" (p. 5).

APPLICATIONS OF THE THEORY

Example of Use of Deliberative Nursing Process in a Group Context

The author supervises nurses in 12-week group leadership training experiences. Nurses receive contact hours for co-leading a weekly group session, completing written assignments and readings, and participating actively in supervision throughout the group experience. Each group focuses upon meeting patients' immediate needs for help, validating that the nurse co-leaders understand that what the group members are stating is their immediate need for help, and sharing with the patients the nurse co-leaders' perceptions, thoughts, and/or feelings in response to what behaviors (verbal or nonverbal) that the group members present within the group. Group members often comment when leaving, if not during the group sessions, how helpful they feel the group was. Frequently, members will comment that they feel better. Check-ins and checkouts are extremely helpful in addressing patient immediate needs for help and decreasing patient distress.

Nurses are educated to use a deliberative nursing process within a nursing situation (involving the patient's behavior, the nurse's reaction, and the nurse's action) to identify with the patient what the meaning of the patient's behavior is, so that the patient's immediate need for help can be met and distress can be relieved. Involvement of the patient in discerning the meaning of his or her behavior promotes a dynamic nurse–patient relationship. Validation with the patient that the need has been correctly identified and met results in positive patient outcomes.

Example of Use of Deliberative Nursing Process with Potential Nursing Students

Nursing Camp 2002 was a 2-week camp for 8th-grade students that ran during the summer at Saint Anselm College in Manchester, New Hampshire. Nursing Camp 2002 was a partnership between the Manchester School-to-Careers Partnership, Saint Anselm College, Elliot Hospital, Hanover Hill Healthcare, New Hampshire Hospital, and Visiting Nurses Association Childcare Center. Sylvia Durette, camp director, and this writer introduced the 27 students to Orlando's Deliberative Nursing Process as part of their overview of the nursing profession. Students also participated in an interactive experience related to Deliberative Nursing Process.

Research Applications

Deliberative Nursing Process has been categorized as a nursing process theory (Orlando, 1990), a prescriptive theory (Wooldridge, Skipper, & Leonard, 1968), and a reflective practice theory (Schmieding, 2002). The inductive, research-based approach Orlando used to develop Deliberative Nursing Process as a theory was unique. Meleis (1997, p. 348) points out that Orlando used field methodology before it became widely accepted in research use.

Orlando's theory has been widely used as a framework for numerous studies in a variety of settings. Areas studied encompass nursing theory, practice, education, and administration. Both qualitative and quantitative approaches have been employed.

Deliberative Nursing Process has been applied in theory analysis (Alligood & Choi, 1998; Andrews, 1989; Walker & Avant, 1995). A number of patient outcomes have been studied using Deliberative Nursing Process including, but not limited to, pain (Barron, 1966; Bochnak, 1963; Bochnak, Rhymes, & Leonard, 1962); postoperative recovery (Eisler, Wolfer, & Diers, 1972); blood pressure and pulse rates (Mertz, 1963); vomiting (Dumas & Leonard, 1963); and levels of distress (Potter & Bockenhauer, 2000). Additional areas explored using Deliberative Nursing Process include spousal grieving (Dracup & Breu, 1978); breastfeeding (Clausen, 1983); and cancer (Reid-Ponte, 1988). Nursing education (Haggerty, 1987; Orlando, 1972) and nursing administration (Schmieding, 1984, 1992) also have been examined using the Deliberative Nursing Process. For additional studies using Deliberative Nursing Process, refer to the Bibliography.

Potter, Dawson, and Vitale-Nolen (2002) have designed a study to determine if implementation of Safety Agreements makes a difference in the rate of patient self-harm incidents and in nurses' feeling more comfortable interacting with patients at risk for self-harm. A Safety Agreement was designed to assist nurses in incorporating Deliberative Nursing Process when interacting with patients at risk for self-harm (see Research Application 15-1 on page 317).

 15-1 USING MIDDLE RANGE THEORIES

A quasi-experimental pilot study was undertaken in a large, university-affiliated state psychiatric facility to determine if implementation of Orlando's nursing theory-based practice (Deliberative Nursing Practice) made a difference in patient outcomes when compared with patient outcomes resulting from interventions using nonspecified nursing practice. Two inpatient units were selected that matched most closely in staffing patterns, patient census, and acuity levels. Ten registered nurses (RNs) participated—six in the experimental group and four in the control group. The experimental and control groups of RNs had no significant differences in their demographic composition. Thirty patients were involved in the study—19 in the experimental group and 11 in the control group. Patient experimental and control groups were statistically similar. The RNs were educated in use of the Bockenhauer-Potter Scale of Immediate Distress (BPSID), a 5-point Likert-scaled instrument that quantifies the level of patient-demonstrated distress. The BPSID was developed to control for subjectivity when assessing patients' levels of distress. The two investigators, a consultant in Orlando's theory, and three hospital RN nurse specialists reviewed and enhanced reference points on the scale. Video-taped simulated interactions helped nurses to learn how to use the BPSID, thus increasing inter-rater reliability. RNs in the experimental group received instruction in Deliberative Nursing Process. Data collection took place over a 12-week time frame. Distress levels of patients were measured before and after RN interventions. A greater reduction ($p = .04$) in patients' levels of distress occurred in the group in which RNs used the Deliberative Nursing Process. Interestingly, RNs who used the Deliberative Nursing Process reported that having a "road map" helped them feel more effective in their nursing interventions. Further research is suggested to control for the possible "halo effect" of additional attention provided to the experimental group of RNs via weekly support and education and to obtain verbal feedback from patients who experience nursing interventions that incorporate Deliberative Nursing Process.

Potter, M. L., & Bockenhauer, B. J. (2000). Implementing Orlando's nursing theory: A pilot study. *Journal of Psychosocial Nursing and Mental Health Services, 38*, 14–21.

Bezanson (2002) proposed a theoretical application of Deliberative Nursing Process for an outpatient surgery center of an acute care, community-based hospital. Bezanson asserts implementation of Deliberative Nursing Process could provide opportunities to improve nursing practice, increase patient satisfaction, and enhance staff satisfaction with their nurse–patient interactions. Bezanson suggests that mechanisms of evaluation might include patient-focused satisfaction surveys, staff self-reports of satisfaction in practice, and improved patient outcomes.

Deliberative Nursing Process can be used as a framework to design research in various settings and to examine specific patient outcomes. The study illustrated in Using Middle Range Theories 15-1 demonstrates patient outcomes related to reduction in levels of distress when Deliberative Nursing Process was implemented in an acute care psychiatric hospital setting.

Olson and Hanchett (1997) carried out a study examining Orlando's assertion that relationships exist between nurse-expressed empathy and several patient outcomes. They used a descriptive, correlational format, described in Using Middle Range Theories 15-2.

INSTRUMENTS USED IN EMPIRICAL TESTING

There are no set means or tools to measure Deliberative Nursing Process. This is indicative of the nature of the theory because Orlando emphasized that Deliberative Nursing Process involves a nurs-

---

 15-2 USING MIDDLE RANGE THEORIES

Relationships between nurse-expressed empathy and two patient outcomes (patient-perceived empathy and patient distress) were explored in a descriptive, correlational study. The hypotheses were: (1) a negative relationship will exist between measures of nurse-expressed empathy and measures of patient distress; (2) a positive relationship will exist between measures of nurse-expressed empathy and patient-perceived empathy, and (3) a negative relationship will exist between patient-perceived empathy and measures of patient distress.

One hundred and forty subjects comprised the sample. Seventy staff registered nurses (RNs) were selected from a pool of 50% of all eligible nurses who were invited. Seventy patients for whom the nurses cared during a day shift were randomly selected to participate.

Nurse participants completed the Staff-Patient Interaction Response Scale (SPIRS) and the Behavioral Test of Interpersonal Skills (BTIS). Both measure nurse-expressed empathy. Patient participants completed the Empathy Subscale of the Barrett-Lennard Relationship Inventory (BLRI) to determine patient-perceived empathy measures; their patient distress scores were measured using the Profile of Mood States (POMS) and the Multiple Affect Adjective Check List (MAACL).

Testing of hypothesis was as follows: (1) hypothesis one and three were tested together by means of one canonical correlation and (2) hypothesis three was tested by means of multiple regression analysis. All three hypotheses received statistically signiicant support with the BTIS measurement. A fuller description of methodology and findings are recorded in a report by Olson (1995). This study supported Orlando's (1961, 1972) assertion that realtionships exist between accurate perceptions of patients' needs (nurse-expressed empathy and patient-expressed empathy) and patient distress.

Olson, J., & Hanchett, E. (1997). Nurse-expressed empathy, patient outcomes, and development of a middle-range theory. *Image: Journal of Nursing Scholarship, 29,* 71–76.

ing situation in which the uniqueness of the nurse is brought to the experience to meet the immediate needs for help, as expressed by the patient, explored by the nurse and patient, and validated by the nurse with the patient. Each circumstance or nursing situation will be unique and different, because each nurse perceives, feels, and thinks differently than any other nurse entering the same nursing situation.

Different tools have been developed and/or used to measure different aspects of Deliberative Nursing Process. These tools facilitate examination of such factors as patient outcomes, nursing process, nurse empathy, and patient-perceived empathy. The instruments have been developed and/or used to test Deliberative Nursing Process qualitatively and quantitatively. Instruments used in different studies explore different aspects of the Deliberative Nursing Process, such as theory description and analysis, use in research, use in clinical practice, and use in administrative practice.

Much of the testing done with Deliberative Nursing Process involves questionnaires and surveys. Examples of tools that have been used for studies involving Orlando's Deliberative Nursing Process are listed in Table 15-2.

Table 15-2. DELIBERATIVE NURSING PROCESS TOOLS

CATEGORY	ABBREVIATION	EXAMPLE
Anxiety		State Anxiety Inventory (Spielberger, Gorsuch, & Lushene, 1970).
Attitude change		Spouse Questionnaire (from Silva, 1979) Spouses' Perception Scale (Silva, 1979)
Emotional state	WI	Welfare Inventory (Eisler, Wolfer, & Diers, 1972)
Nurse-expressed empathy	BTIS SPIRS	Behavioral Test of Interpersonal Skills (Gerrard & Bussell, 1980) Staff-Patient Interaction Response Scale (Gallop, 1989)
Patient-perceived empathy	BLRI	Barrett-Lennard Relationship Inventory (Barrett-Lennard, 1962)
Patient distress	POMS MAACL BPSID	Profile of Mood States (McNair, Lorr, & Droppleman, 1981) Multiple Affect Adjective Check List (Zuckerman & Lubin, 1965) Bockenhauer/Potter Scale of Immediate Distress (Bockenhauer & Potter, 2000)
Patient's self-harm incidents	SA	Safety Agreement (Potter, Dawson, & Vitale-Nolen, 2002, research in process)
Nurse-perceived comfort with use of safety agreements		Registered Nurses Evaluation Survey (Potter, Dawson, & Vitale-Nolen, 2002, research in process)
Therapeutic effectiveness	EPPS SII	Edwards Personal Preference Schedule (Edwards, 1959) Social Interaction Inventory (Methven & Schlotfeldt, 1962)
Postoperative physical recovery	RI	Recovery Inventory (Eisler, Wolfer, & Diers, 1972)
Social approval	SD Scale	Social Desirability Scale (Crowne & Marlowe, 1964)

One instrument used in the study of Deliberative Nursing Process is the Safety Agreement. The Safety Agreement is an instrument developed by nurses at New Hampshire Hospital (NHH) and is designed to measure patients' risk for self-harm and willingness and ability to agree to remain safe (see Table 15-2). Most of the agreement is designed in Likert-style format. A question related to a patient's perceived ability to remain safe requires a "yes" or "no" response. In addition, a question that seeks to determine how the patient and registered nurse (RN) might work together to manage the current risk for self-harm elicits a response from a number of given choices with an "other" option included. The intent of the Safety Agreement is to assist the RN in a deliberative process of determining with the patient the patient's risk for self-harm.

A Safety Agreement is to be implemented nonrandomly, with all patients admitted or considered at risk for self-harm. Patients will be asked to self-rate the following areas with the RN: (1) their current harm level, (2) the likelihood of their acting on their thoughts of self-harm, (3) their thoughts about managing the risk with the RN, (4) their willingness to enter an agreement for safety with the RN, and (5) their thoughts about how long they think they can remain safe.

RNs will be given the Registered Nurses Evaluation Survey, which also is in Likert-type format except for one question. RNs will be asked to evaluate: (1) the number of times they used the Safety Agreement in a 3-month period, (2) if the Safety Agreement assisted them in feeling more comfortable while helping patients at risk for self-harm, (3) if they thought self-harming incidents decreased since implementation of Safety Agreements, and (4) if they have any other comments to share related to use of Safety Agreements. Research Application 15-1 describes research planned for implementation of Safety Agreements at NHH.

15-1 RESEARCH APPLICATION

Nurses at New Hampshire Hospital (NHH), a university-affiliated, state psychiatric facility, are interested in determining if implementation of Safety Agreements effects patient outcomes and nursing comfort levels when working with patients at risk for self-harm (Potter, Dawson, & Vitale-Nolen, 2002). Registered nurses (RNs) serving on a Continuous Quality Improvement (CQI) committee had examined the use of safety contracts by nurses at the facility and developed a Safety Agreement tool that they thought would facilitate incorporating Orlando's Deliberative Nursing Process when assessing patients at risk for self-harm.

Validity of safety contracts in general has not been tested. Confusion and controversy exist in relation to the definition and use of safety contracts with patients who are suicidal (Potter & Dawson, 2001). It is suspected that this confusion and controversy lead to a discomfort and lack of direction when nurses "contract" with patients for safety.

It has been demonstrated by nurses at NHH that Deliberative Nursing Process can make a difference in patient outcomes (Potter & Bockenhauer, 2000). Hence, these investigators postulate that a more standardized process, using Orlando's Deliberative Nursing Process to enhance communication, might promote patients' agreeing to be safe and, in turn, decrease the

(Continued)

(Continued) **15-1 RESEARCH APPLICATION**

rate of self-harm incidents and increase RNs' comfort levels when working with patients at risk for self-harm.

Safety agreements will be implemented as the standard of care on all units in Acute Psychiatric Services (APS) for 3 months. Incidents of self-harm will be collected via the organizational-wide data collection system pre- and postimplementation. Instruction for RNs in use of safety agreements will occur the month before implementation of Safety Agreements. RNs already use Deliberative Nursing Process as a framework for nursing care. The RNs will be invited to complete a survey on use of Safety Agreements at the end of the 3-month period. There are two convenience sample databases: (1) anonymous lists of self-harm incidents (only chart numbers used, not patient names), and (2) all RNs performing direct patient care (approximately 60 RNs) in APS.

The investigators plan to examine data pre- and postimplementation of safety agreements. *t*-tests will be used to detect differences in pre- and postintervention outcomes. Stat Pac Gold computer software will be used to analyze data for statistical differences. Trend analysis will be done to examine trends in specific years. Data from RNs' evaluations of Safety Agreements will be collated and summarized.

SUMMARY

Gowan and Morris (1964) speculated that the nursing shortage of that era and the increased expectations upon nurses led to nurses' spending more time designing care than providing care. Results from their study indicated that patients experienced undue delays in receiving care and withheld requests that involved their well-being due to patient perceptions that the nurses were too busy, would disapprove, would not like to be interrupted, or would think the request was not helpful to the patient. Might this same scenario be repeating itself today?

In 1990, the National League for Nursing honored Orlando by reprinting *The Dynamic Nurse–Patient Relationship*. Orlando noted in the Preface to that edition that interest in the United States using her theory had waned (Orlando, 1990, p. viii). Interest and use of the theory may have subsided temporarily, but it never ceased. As noted by Orlando herself, her work has been published in five foreign countries, and there have been numerous publications in recent years related to Deliberative Nursing Process (Potter & Bockenhauer, 2000; Potter & Dawson, 2001; Potter & Tinker, 2000; Schmieding, 1993b, 1999, 2002; Rosenthal, 1996). Many changes have occurred in nursing. However, the essence of nursing, described so simply yet eloquently by Orlando, has not changed—namely that the nurse–patient relationship involves a dynamic and unique process that evolves between nurse and patient when approached deliberatively and validated with the patient on an ongoing basis.

Deliberative Nursing Process is a nursing theory for all times. Use of Deliberative Nursing Process helps nurses maintain a patient-centered approach when providing nursing care amidst additional and varied expectations of the nurse. Orlando has kept the message of Deliberative Nursing Process clear throughout the years: "It is the nurse's direct responsibility to see to it that the patient's needs for help are met, either directly by her own activity or indirectly by calling in the help of others" (Orlando, 1961, p. 29). Adopting such a clear function promotes effective and efficient nursing practice as has been demonstrated through empirical studies on Deliberative Nursing Process for more than 40 years.

ANALYSIS EXERCISE

Using the criteria presented in Chapter 2, critique the theory, Deliberative Nursing Process. Compare your conclusions about the theory with those found in Appendix A. A nurse scholar who has worked with the theory completed the analysis found in the Appendix.

Internal Criticism
1. Clarity
2. Consistency
3. Adequacy
4. Logical development
5. Level of theory development

External Criticism
1. Reality convergence
2. Utility
3. Significance
4. Discrimination
5. Scope of theory
6. Complexity

WEB RESOURCES

1. The Ida J. Orlando Web site gives a brief biography and summary of her theory. There are also many links to additional publications and research studies. This site is sponsored by the University of Rhode Island College of Nursing: *http://www.uri.edu/nursing/schmieding/orlando/index.html*

Much appreciation is expressed to: Mimi Dye, MSN, ARNP, who completed the critique on Deliberative Nursing Process in the Appendix A and studied Deliberative Nursing Process as a student with the theorist, Ida J. Orlando, MS, RN; Joy L. Potter, who served as research assistant in the development of this chapter; and Dorothy Y. Kameoka, MLS, MSW, RN, who provided valuable assistance in seeking out materials for this chapter.

REFERENCES

Alligood, M. R. (2002). The nature of knowledge needed for nursing practice. In M. R. Alligood & A. Marriner-Tomey, *Nursing theory—Utilization & application* (2nd ed., pp. 3–14). St. Louis: Mosby, Inc.

Alligood, M. R., & Choi, E. C. (1998). Evolution of nursing theory development. In A. Marriner-Tomey & M. R. Alligood (Eds.), *Nursing theorists and their work* (4th ed.) (pp. 55–66). St Louis: Mosby.

Andrews, C. M. (1989). Ida Orlando's model of nursing practice. In J. J. Fitzpatrick & A. L. Whall (Eds.), *Conceptual models of nursing: Analysis & application* (2nd ed.) (pp. 69–87). Norwalk, CT: Appleton & Lange.

Barron, M. A. (1966). The effects varied nursing approaches have on patients' complaints of pain. *Nursing Research, 15,* 90–91.

Bezanson, A. (2002). Theoretical application of Orlando's Theory of Deliberate Nursing Process in an outpatient surgery center. Unpublished manuscript.

Bochnak, M. A. (1963). The effect of an automatic and deliberative process of nursing activity on the relief of patients' pain: A clinical experiment. *Nursing Research, 12*, 191–192.

Bochnak, M. A., Rhymes, J. P., & Leonard, R. C. (1962). The comparison of two types of nursing activity on the relief of pain. In *Innovations in nurse–patient relationships: Automatic or reasoned nurse action* (Clinical Paper No. 6). New York: American Nurses Association.

Bolden, L. V., & Larrabee, J. H. (2001). Defining patient-perceived quality of nursing care. *Journal of Nursing Care Quality, 16*, 34–60.

Clausen [Cameron], J. C. (1983). Clinical nursing research on the science and art of breastfeeding using a deliberative nursing care approach. *Western Journal of Nursing Research, 5*, 29.

Dracup, K. A., & Breu, C. S. (1978). Using nursing research findings to meet the needs of grieving spouses. *Nursing Research. 27*, 212–216.

Dumas, R. G., & Leonard, R. C. (1963). The effect of nursing on the incidence of postoperative vomiting. *Nursing Research, 12*, 12–15.

Eisler, J., Wolfer, J. A., & Diers, D. (1972). Relationship between need for social approval and postoperative recovery and welfare. *Nursing Research, 21*, 520–525.

Gowan, N. I., & Morris, M. (1964). Nurses' responses to expressed patient needs. *Nursing Research, 13*, 68–71.

Haggerty, L. A. (1987). An analysis of senior nursing students' immediate responses to distressed patients. *Journal of Advanced Nursing, 12*, 451–461.

Johnson, B. M., & Webber, P. B. (2001). *Theory and reasoning in nursing.* New York: Lippincott Williams & Wilkins.

Marriner-Tomey, A. (1998). Introduction to analysis of nursing theories. In A. Marriner-Tomey & M. R. Alligood, (Eds.), *Nursing theorists and their work* (4th ed., pp. 3–15). St. Louis: Mosby.

McEwan, M. (2002). Middle-range nursing theories. In M. McEwan & E.. M. Wills, (Eds.), *Theoretical Basis for Nursing,* (pp. 202–225). Philadelphia: Lippincott Williams & Wilkins.

Meleis, A. I. (1997). *Theoretical nursing: Development & progress* (3rd ed., pp. 343–353). Philadelphia: Lippincott-Raven.

Mertz, H. (1963). A study of the process of the nurse's activity as it affects the blood pressure readings and pulse rate of patients admitted to the emergency room. *Nursing Research, 12*, 197–198.

Orlando, I. J. (1961). *The dynamic nurse–patient relationship.* New York: G. P. Putnam's Sons.

Orlando, I. J. (1972). *The discipline and teaching of nursing process (an evaluative study).* New York: G. P. Putnam's Sons.

Orlando, I. J. (1976, August). *The fundamental issue in professional nursing.* Paper presented at the University of Tulsa College of Nursing, Tulsa, OK.

Orlando [Pelletier], I. J. (1983, October). *Comments on ANA's social policy statement of 1980.* Paper presented at Southeastern Massachusetts University, College of Nursing, Honor Society, South Dartmouth, MA.

Orlando, I. J. (1987). Nursing in the 21st century: Alternate paths. *Journal of Advanced Nursing, 12*, 405–412.

Orlando, I. J. (1990, reissue). *The dynamic nurse–patient relationship.* New York: National League for Nursing.

Orlando, I. J., & Dugan, A. B. (1989). Independent and dependent paths: The fundamental issue for the nursing profession. *Nursing and Health Care, 10*, 77–80.

Pelletier, I. O. (1967). The patient's predicament and nursing function. *Psychiatric Opinion, 4*, 25–30.

Pelletier, I. O. (1976). The fundamental issue in professional nursing. Unpublished manuscript, pp. 1–22.

Potter, M. L., & Bockenhauer, B. J. (2000). Implementing Orlando's Nursing Theory: A pilot study. *Journal of Psychosocial Nursing and Mental Health Services, 38*, 14–21.

Potter, M. L., & Dawson, A. M. "From safety contract to safety agreement." (2001). *Journal of Psychosocial Nursing and Mental Health Services 39*, 38–45.

Potter, M. L., Dawson, A. M., & Vitale-Nolen, R. A. (2002). Implementation of safety agreements in an acute psychiatric facility. Study in progress.

Potter, M. L., & Tinker, S. W. (2000). "Put power in nurses' hands: Orlando's Nursing Theory supports nurses—simply." *Nursing Management, 31*, 40–41.

Reid-Ponte, P. (1988). The relationship among empathy and the use of Orlando's deliberative process by the primary nurse and the distress of the adult cancer patient. Doctoral dissertation, Boston University, Boston.

Rosenthal, B. C. (1996). An interactionist's approach to perioperative nursing. *Association of Operating Room Nurses Journal, 64*, 254–260.

Schmieding, N. J. (1984). Putting Orlando's theory into practice. *American Journal of Nursing, 84*, 759–761.

Schmieding, N. J. (1992). Relationship between head nurse responses to staff nurses and staff nurse response to patients. *Western Journal of Nursing Research, 13*, 746–760.

Schmieding, N. J. (1993a). *Ida Jean Orlando: A nursing process theory.* London: Sage Publications, Inc.

Schmieding, N. J., (1993b). Successful superior-subordinate relationships require mutual management. *Health Care Supervisor,* 11, 52–63.

Schmieding, N. J. (1999). Reflective inquiry framework for nurse administrators. *Journal of Advanced Nursing, 30*, 631–639.

Schmieding, N. J. (2002). Orlando's nursing process theory. In M. R. Alligood & A. Marriner-Tomey, (Eds.),

Nursing theory utilization & application (2nd ed.) (pp. 315–337). St Louis: Mosby.

Stevens-Barnum, B. J. (1990). *Nursing theory: Analysis, application, evaluation*. Glenview, IL: Scott, Foresman, Little, & Brown.

Walker, L. O., & Avant, K. C. (1995). *Strategies for theory construction in nursing*. (3rd ed.). Norwalk, CT: Appleton & Lange.

Wills, E. M. (2002). Overview of grand nursing theories. In M. McEwan & E. M. Wills (Eds.), *Theoretical basis for nursing*, (pp. 111–124). Philadelphia: Lippincott Wilkins & Williams.

Wooldridge, P. J., Skipper, J. K., Jr., & Leonard, R. C. (1968). *Behavioral science, social practice, and the nursing profession*. Cleveland, OH: Case Western Reserve University.

BIBLIOGRAPHY

Cameron, J. (1963). An exploratory study of the verbal responses of the nurse–patient interactions. *Nursing Research, 12*, 192.

Chapman, J. S. (1969). Effects of different nursing approaches upon psychological and physiological responses of patients. Unpublished doctoral dissertation. Case Western Reserve University, Frances Payne Bolton School of Nursing, Cleveland, Ohio.

Clausen [Cameron], J. C. (1983). Clinical nursing research on the science and art of breastfeeding using a deliberative nursing care approach. *Western Journal of Nursing Research, 5*, 29.

Dumas, R.G., & Johnson [Anderson], B. A. (1972). Research in nursing practice: A review of five clinical experiments. *International Journal of Nursing Studies, 9*, 137–149.

Dumas, R.G., & Leonard, R.C. (1963). The effect of nursing on the incidence of postoperative vomiting. *Nursing Research, 12*, 12–15.

Dye, M. C. (1963a). Clarifying patients' communication. *The American Journal of Nursing, 63*, 56–59.

Dye, M. C. (1963b). A descriptive study of conditions conducive to an effective process of nursing activity. *Nursing Research, 12*, 194.

Elms, R. R., & Leonard, R. C. (1966). Effects of nursing approaches during admission. *Nursing Research, 15*, 39–48.

Farrell, G. A., (1991). How accurately do nurses perceive patients' needs? A comparison of general and psychiatric settings. *Journal of Advanced Nursing, 16*, 1062–1070.

Faulkner, S. A. (1963). A descriptive study of needs communicated to the nurse by some mothers on a postpartum service. *Nursing Research, 4*, 260.

Forchuck, C. (1991). A comparison of the works of Peplau and Orlando. *Archives of Psychiatric Nursing, 5*, 38–45.

Gillis, Sister L. (1976). Sleeplessness: Can you help? *The Canadian Nurse, 72*, 32–34.

Hampe, S. O. (1975). Needs of grieving spouses in a hospital setting. *Nursing Research, 24*, 113.

Kokuyama, T., & Schmieding, N. J. (1995). Responses staff nurses prefer compared with their perception of head nurse responses. *Japanese Journal of Nursing Administration, 5*, 33–38.

Laurent, C. L. (1999). A nursing theory for nursing leadership. *Journal of Nursing Management, 8*, 83–87.

Mahaffy, P. P. (1965). The effects of hospitalization on children admitted for tonsillectomy and adenoidectomy. *Nursing Research, 14*, 12–19.

Nelson, B. (1978). A practical application of nursing theory. *Nursing Clinics of North America, 13*, 157–169.

Olson, J. K. (1995). Relationships between nurse expressed empathy, patient perceived empathy, and patient distress. *Image: Journal of Nursing Scholarship, 27*, 323–328.

Olson, J., & Hanchett, E. (1997). Nurse-expressed empathy, patient outcomes, and development of a middle-range theory. *Image: Journal of Nursing Scholarship, 29*, 71–76.

Peitchinis, J. A. (1972). Therapeutic effectiveness of counseling by nursing personnel. *Nursing Research, 21*, 138–148.

Pride, L. F. (1968). An adrenal stress index as a criterion measure of nursing. *Nursing Research, 17*, 292–303.

Schmieding, N. J. (1987). Problematic situations in nursing: Analysis of Orlando's theory based on Dewey's theory of inquiry. *Journal of Advanced Nursing, 12*, 431–440.

Schmieding, N. J. (1987a). Analyzing managerial responses in face-to-face contacts. *Journal of Advanced Nursing, 12*, 357–365.

Schmieding, N. J. (1987b). Face-to-face contacts: Exploring their meaning. *Nursing Management, 12*, 82–86.

Schmieding, N. J. (1988). Action process of nurse administrators to problematic situations based on Orlando's theory. *Journal of Advanced Nursing, 13*, 99–107.

Schmieding, N. J. (1990a). A model for assessing nurse administrator's actions. *Western Journal of Nursing Research, 12*, 293–306.

Schmieding, N. J. (1990b). Do head nurses include staff nurses in problem solving? *Nursing Management, 21*, 58–60.

Silva, M. C. (1979). Effects of orientation information on

spouses' anxieties and attitudes toward hospitalization and surgery. *Research in Nursing and Health, 2,* 127–136.

Tarasuk [Bochnak], M. B., Rhymes, J., & Leonard, R. C. (1965). An experimental test of the importance of communication skills for effective nursing. In J. K. Skipper, Jr. & R. C. Leonard (Eds.), *Social interaction and patient care* (pp. 110–120). Philadelphia: J. B. Lippincott.

Tryon, P. A. (1966). Use of comfort measures as support during labor. *Nursing Research, 15,* 109–118.

Tryon, P. A., & Leonard, R. C. (1964). The effect of patients' participation on the outcome of a nursing procedure. *Nursing Forum, 3,* 79–89.

Williamson, Y. M. (1978). Methodologic dilemmas in tapping the concept of patient needs. *Nursing Research, 27,* 172–177.

Planned Change

EILEEN PAT GERACI

INTRODUCTION

In rapidly changing health care environments, professional nurses are expected to identify opportunities and implement well-coordinated strategies for planned change on several levels:

- Within the health care system, as nurses help to plan and organize strategies for the delivery of comprehensive services to individuals, families, and communities
- At the organizational level, such as implementing quality improvement programs
- By assisting individual clients to develop and maintain healthy behaviors.

Nursing researchers have examined and applied several theories of change to problems in education, practice, and management. This chapter will discuss Lewin's *Force Field Analysis* (1947, 1951), Lippitt's Seven Stages of Planned Change from *The Dynamics of Planned Change* (Lippitt, Watson, & Westley, 1958), Rogers' *Diffusion Theory* (1983), and The Transtheoretical Model (TTM) *Stages of Change* (Prochaska, DiClemente, & Norcross, 1992; Prochaska & Prochaska, 1999) and their research applications.

Death and taxes have long been on the short list of those things considered to be the only "sure things" in life. However, reflection on the last decade in health care reveals change as another absolute certainty. Change has been described as inevitable, continuous, compelling, inescapable, painful, and powerful (Workman & Kenney, 1988). Change affects people, both positively and negatively, in their behavior, their relationships, and in how and where they work. Equilibrium and stability are more comfortable and considerably easier to deal with than the ambiguity and conflict that are inherent in change. Change means giving up control within one's zone of comfort and moving into unfamiliar and uncertain territory and, therefore, can create stress and doubt within those who are affected by the change (Grohar-Murray & DiCroce, 2003). Yet change also can impel growth and progress as nurses move into an exciting and challenging future in health care; failure to participate in change results in stagnation and immobility. Initiating and managing change in increasingly complex environments are critical skills for the professional nurse, requiring knowledge of the change process, creativity and flexibility in applying an appropriate theory of change, and commitment to see a proposed change project through to successful completion, including measurement of the outcomes of the change process. This chapter will present a brief overview of the most widely used theories, with a discussion of how nursing scholars have used these theories to support their work in several different areas, including planned changes within individuals, groups, organizations, and communities.

Shifting economic, social, and technological trends in the United States are transforming the entire health care delivery system. Efforts to curb escalating health care costs and to improve quality, efficiency, and access to health care services are among the current driving forces of change in the health care delivery system. Other external influences that have affected nursing and health care delivery also include an exponential growth in information systems, restructure of health care organizations in response to changes in funding and reimbursement, and changes in demographics as the "Baby Boomers" age. Among the internal influences affecting nursing are changing patterns of who, where, and how we practice. An aging nursing workforce (Moses, 1997), fewer students entering into nursing programs (Tanner, 2001), a shift of outpatient care from hospitals to community-based settings, and dissatisfaction of experienced nurses because of workload/staffing shortages have all contributed to massive changes in the practice of nursing (Peterson, 2001). The frequency and rapidity of the pace of change creates tension and stress in the individual, the workplace, and in the larger social system. In an attempt to understand, manage, and direct change, nursing scholars have used a variety of theories, largely borrowed from other disciplines, to clarify and describe the processes necessary to effect successful planned change within nursing.

HISTORICAL BACKGROUND

Throughout history, chance, natural evolution, luck, and divine intervention have all served as possible explanations for the moving forces behind change, yet most historians and social scientists would now agree that the current focus of study regarding planned change is man's ability to create and to manage change. Through creative effort, application of superior intellect and scientific reasoning, along with a willingness to take risks and to persevere in the face of adversity, man has attempted to control the scope, the pace, and the progression of change (LaPiere, 1965).

The study of planned change in the United States began in the early 1900s with a controversy over a broad ideological question: Should man attempt to mold his own individual and collective future through purposeful forethought and deliberate, calculated effort, or should he trust the evolution of time and nature to determine the course of his future? Historians, politicians, and economists looked to the past for answers, while behavioral scientists, a newly emerging group of intellectuals, sought to actively engage in social change through intentional, planned, and often, collaborative efforts (LaPiere, 1965). Thinking shifted from whether change should occur, to how and who should direct and manage the changes in society as we moved from an industrial age to an information and technology era. With this shift came the need for a different type of worker, equipped with the knowledge and skills necessary to actively support people through change. New helping professionals such as professional nurses, social workers, counselors, and managers were deliberately introduced to assist clients in managing, directing, and controlling the effects of change (LaPiere, 1965).

Building on his earlier work on force field analysis, Lewin (1947, 1951) introduced the concept of planned change as a logical process that proceeded through three phases: unfreezing, moving, and refreezing. Lewin also further suggested that there are forces within and outside of a situation that will either facilitate or impede the change process, and that must be carefully considered when initiating a change project. Much of Lewin's original work was built on analyzing what happens within organizations when change is introduced. Lippitt, Watson, and Westley (1958), colleagues of Lewin's, later refined his work by proposing four additional phases that included obtaining the help of a change agent, an individual with the skills necessary to implement and facilitate change, such as problem solving and interpersonal skills. Rogers' (1983) Innovation-Diffusion Theory, while not specifically a theory of planned change (Hagerman & Tiffany, 1994), took into account the nature of the proposed change, the environment in which it would occur, and the skills of the individuals involved in implementing the innovation. Rogers (1983) suggested that one must progress through five phases before the change is adopted, and he described the characteristics that are associated with successful planned change projects. The Transtheoretical Model of Change (TTM) grew out of research by Prochaska, DiClemente, Norcross, and others (1983, 1992, 1999) in psychology and sociology. This model focuses on the stages, processes, and levels of change through which individuals progress when changing behaviors.

Nurse researchers have largely adapted theories borrowed from other disciplines to study problems effecting nurses, nursing practice, and health behaviors. While few original theories of planned change have been generated from nursing studies, Lutjens and Tiffany (1994) developed a criterion-referenced instrument to determine the content validity or "goodness of fit" of theories of planned change for use in nursing situations. Their instrument, which was designed to quantify the suitability of the borrowed theories to nursing situations, identified seven criteria for evaluating a planned change theory: significance, agreement with nursing's worldview, clarity and consistency, economy, generality, practicality, and testability (Lutjens and Tiffany, 1994, p. 55). Several theories of planned change were evaluated using the Planned Change Evaluation Scale (Lutjens and Tiffany, 1994), including Bennis, Benne, and Chin (1985), Bhola (1965), Lewin (1947, 1951) and Rogers (1983). Of these four, Bhola's theory was rated the highest for its applicability to nursing situations. However, other than initial inter-rater reliability, no other reliability information on the instrument was available.

DEFINITION OF THEORY CONCEPTS

Change occurs on a continuum ranging from random, unplanned or unintentional change, to structured or planned change. The focus of this chapter is on planned change as it applies to the individual, the organization, or the health care system.

Strategies used by the change agent to implement the planned change process can include both proactive methods, as well as assertive and coercive methods, depending on the circumstances surrounding the proposed change. Proactive steps include encouraging early and consistent participation in planning for the change, and clear communication about the steps of the process. These proactive steps assist individuals who will be a part of the change and those who will be affected by the change to learn about the process and become part of it. When encountering resistance, encouraging open discussion and negotiation can lead to improved cooperation throughout the process. Coercion, co-optation, and manipulation are also strategies for change that involve the use of power to force the change rather than through cooperative efforts (Yoder-Wise, 1997, 2003). The most effective change projects combine a number of strategies simultaneously.

Planned Change

Planned change is a deliberate, controlled, and conscious effort to alter the status quo (Bennis et al., 1985, p. 4). Huber (1996, 2003) suggests that the goal of nursing in managing planned change is to maintain control over our professional practice through careful planning and control of the events occurring during the change process and throughout evaluation of the change. According to Bennis, Benne, and Chinn (1985), successful change requires several key elements: recognition of a need, a choice of a direction for the change, people who are willing to make and follow decisions, and time for re-education of those who will be most affected by the change.

The Change Agent

Successful change requires a leader and a visionary who is able to imagine the future and is willing to make and implement difficult decisions about how to get there. Accepting and embracing change implies risk-taking and willingness to leave the "comfort zone" to achieve a new reality. According to Lippitt, Watson, and Westley (1958), planned change requires a change agent, an individual who has expertise in the theory and practice of planned change and who has the capacity to lead others through the change process. The change agent can be a member of the organization undergoing the change or may come from outside the organizations, depending on the problem and the resources available to implement the change project.

Noone (1987) described the role of the clinical nurse specialist as a change agent involved in improving nursing practice through problem solving and deliberate planning for change. While most authors (Huber, 1996, 2000; Marquis & Huston, 2000; Olson, 1979; Welch, 1979) agree that professional nurses are ideal candidates to act as change agents, there are no studies that critically examine this assumption. A review of the literature reveals no nursing research that investigates the best ways to develop nurses as change agents or which combination of skills in the nurse/change agent leads to successful adoption of a planned change. However, several descriptive studies report that nurses have successfully acted as leaders and change agents in completing planned change projects (Dean, 1979; Geraci, 1997).

SKILLS OF THE SUCCESSFUL CHANGE AGENT

According to Olson (1979) and Huber (1996, 2000), the successful change agent, or change facilitator, possesses expertise in three critical skills: problem solving, decision-making, and interpersonal communication skills to lead others through the often-painful process of leaving the old system and embracing the new (Box 16-1).

> ### BOX 16-1   Formula for Planned Change
>
> Planned change = problem-solving skills + decision-making skills + interpersonal competence ÷ change agent
>
> $$PC = \frac{PS + DM + IC}{Change\ agent}$$

Problem Solving. The change agent's ability to apply problem-solving skills is key to managing the change process because the two processes are closely linked (Huber, 1996, 2000). The steps of the problem-solving process are to:

- Gather all available information about the problem and the environment in which it is occurring accurately and concisely define the problem
- Develop a range of alternative responses, considering the consequences of each alternative
- Decide on the best option given all the information that is available
- Implement the change
- Evaluate the solution and its effects on the organization (Huber, 1996, 2000).

Decision-Making. In addition to the ability to apply the problem-solving steps, the change agent must also demonstrate a willingness and capacity to make logical decisions based on factual information. Knowing the desired outcome of the decision and identifying the criteria to be used to measure the outcomes are also part of the decision-making process (Huber, 2000).

Interpersonal Skills. Interpersonal skills of the change agent include the ability to motivate others and an ability to articulate the need for a change to all constituents of the change project without alienating anyone. Encouraging open communication and active participation in the process is invaluable to the success of the project, as well as to future projects. The change agent who is able to maintain contact with what is valued from the old system while empowering others to participate in the process can make a critical difference to whether the change is adopted or rejected (Huber, 1996, 2000).

Responses to Change

Responses to change by individuals and groups are widely variable and often inconsistent (Yoder-Wise, 1997, 2003). Depending on the nature, pace, and scope of the change, responses can range from enthusiastic acceptance of the change, to little or no perceptible reaction, or outright rejection. No two groups, individuals, or even the same individual, are likely to respond in the same manner to each change. Individual response to change is largely dependent on the degree to which the individual is cognitively and emotionally involved in the change. Change is often stressful and, therefore, evokes strong emotional, psychological, and even physical responses, similar to the emotional responses seen with the process of death and dying as the individual or group lets go of the status quo (Olson, 1979). While not an empirically tested theory, Perlman and Takacs (1990) describe 10 stages of emotional responses to change that are based on Kuebler-Ross's (1969) stages of death and dying:

1. Equilibrium: A sense of balance and comfort with personal and professional goals in sync
2. Denial: Defense mechanisms arise, and emotional energy is spent on denying the reality of the change
3. Anger: Active resistance to the change expressed through anger and frustration with the change
4. Bargaining: The individual uses more emotional energy in his or her attempts to compromise or bargain to eliminate or postpone the change
5. Chaos: Energy is diffused, with a loss of direction, and thoughts and emotions scattered
6. Depression: Energy has been spent leaving an emotional emptiness and a lack of will to go on
7. Resignation: With no energy or enthusiasm remaining, the individual resigns himself or herself to the change
8. Openness: Renewed energy to explore new options
9. Readiness: Willingness to "let go" of the old and a willingness to adopt changes
10. Re-emergence: Renewed energy allows the individual to become more proactive and comfortable with the change as they fully re-engage into the new environment or behavior.

In addition to emotional reactions to change, resistance is also an expected response of those undergoing change. Problems usually arise as individuals struggle with conflicting values and ideas of what needs to be changed, the scope and pace of the change, and how the change should be managed. Opposition to change is often based on a threat to the security of the individual, as change disrupts their normal patterns of behavior (Swansburg & Swansburg, 2002). Fear of what the change will mean to one's ability to maintain status, power, and control in his or her job or personal relationships are some of the underlying reasons for resistance to change (Huber, 1996, 2000).

Nursing studies that use planned change as the theoretical framework have led to greater insight into responses to change. Lepola and Blom-Lange (1999) investigated staff response to change through analysis of self-reflective essays that described the individual's orientation of action toward the planned change. The authors concluded that staff reaction and participation in the change project varied from enthusiasm, hesitation, to withdrawal. In another study, conducted by Schoolfield and Orduna (1994), a case-study approach was used to describe the responses of staff nurses to organizational change. After recognizing that Lewin's concept of change failed to take into account the emotional aspects of change on individuals and groups, the authors modified Lewin's concept of change to include Perlman and Takacs' (1990) *Ten Stages of Change* to better explain and describe the emotional context of change.

DESCRIPTION OF THE THEORIES OF PLANNED CHANGE

Lewin's Theory of Change

The most frequently cited theory of planned change used in nursing studies is the classical change theory of Kurt Lewin (1947, 1951, 1958), who identified three simple and basic stages of planned change: unfreezing, moving, and refreezing (Box 16-2).

The first stage of *unfreezing* is largely "a thawing out stage," which occurs with the client's awareness of a problem, along with an openness and willingness to disturb the status quo. Lewin (1951) suggests that this awareness of the need for change may develop from several different sources, such as when events occur that either confirm (or disconfirm) one's unmet expectations about an event, when

---

BOX 16-2   Lewin's Theory of Change

- Unfreezing
- Moving
- Refreezing

---

one becomes uncomfortable or anxious about actions that were taken (or no action at all occurs), or when former barriers have been removed in a situation that now allows for changes to be implemented. After recognizing and acknowledging that a problem exists, the individual thoroughly investigates the factors affecting the situation and determines the willingness and commitment of the group members to adopt change and looks at alternative solutions to the problem. Careful analysis of the environment in which the change will occur and all of the factors that may facilitate or hinder resolution of the problem are of vital importance. Lewin refers to the elements that push the situation toward change as *driving forces*, and those forces that inhibit or restrict change, as *restraining forces*. Lewin also suggests that analysis of these forces should be conducted and their relative strength estimated, so that a plan can be developed that either modifies or eliminates the opposition, thereby enhancing the chances of implementing a successful change.

The second stage of *moving* is the "acting and implementation stage," which occurs when the data that have been collected about the situation are analyzed and new responses are developed. Detailed plans, along with a timetable for the project, and appropriate strategies to support the driving forces and reduce or eliminate the restraining forces, are initiated and implemented, with the expectation that the proposed changes will improve the situation.

The last stage of *refreezing* is the stage of "a return to stability," where the new changes are adopted and integrated into a new system, which then eventually becomes the status quo.

Lippitt's Theory of Change

Using Lewin's work as a framework, Lippitt (1973) proposed a model that emphasized problem-solving skills as well as the interpersonal aspects of the change process. Lippitt's model includes seven phases of planned change (Box 16-3).

According to Lippitt and colleagues (1958), the first stage in planned change is the accurate *diagnosis of the problem*. This stage begins with awareness that "something just isn't working as it should be." Problem awareness may be in the form of recognition of internal or external forces that are affecting the organization; however, the system has not yet adjusted to those forces and disequilibria exists. According to Lippitt, to accurately diagnose the exact nature and extent of the problem, complete data collection from all available resources is critical. Identifying and involving key people, such as those who will be directly affected by the change, as well as the decision makers, is vital to the success of the proposed change project. Group discussions with representatives of each department to thoroughly examine the problem and to identify strengths and weaknesses in the current system allows time for individuals to share how the problem affects their work and affords an early opportunity to "buy into" a plan to solve the problem as a group. Because members of the group will most likely define the problem primarily using their own frames of reference, without necessarily seeing the whole

---

BOX 16-3 Lippitt's Stages of Change

UNFREEZING

1. Diagnosing the problem
2. Assessing the motivation and capacity for change
3. Assessing the change agent's motivation and resources

MOVING

4. Selecting progressive change objectives
5. Choosing the appropriate role for the change agent

REFREEZING

6. Maintaining the change once it has been started
7. Ending the helping relationship

Welch, L. B. (1979). Planned change in nursing: the theory. *Nursing Clinics of North America, 14*(2), 307–321.

---

picture, it is likely that this first stage will be a continuing process of defining and redefining the problem as more information becomes available (Geraci, 1997).

The second stage of Lippitt's model involves *accurately assessing the system and the personnel who will be involved in the change along with their motivation and capacity to implement a change.* Included at this point are a thorough appraisal of the organizational structure, the formal and informal power base, and a thorough and accurate assessment of the motivation and resources available for initiating a change. Development of a plan for change begins to take shape as critical factors that can potentially restrict or enhance the project are examined.

Lippitt's third stage involves first *identifying a qualified and credible change agent* to guide the organization and its personnel through the proposed project. Depending on the type of identified problem, the resources available to support the project, and the specificity of the skills needed to implement the change, the person or persons needed to lead the project must be identified. The change agent can come either from within the organization itself or from outside the organization, or may actually be several people designated to act as change agents at various stages of the process. Tasks of this stage include matching the leadership style of the change agent with the organization, assessing the change agent's motivation for initiating the change, and evaluating the change agent's ability to access resources quickly and efficiently.

The fourth stage of planned change involves *specifying objectives of the change*, which includes mapping out exactly how to get the organization where it is headed, and estimating the length of time the project will take. Gathering data from the literature or from other resources that describe organizations that have implemented similar changes is very useful when planning the change process. Having a pilot or trial period for the project may be helpful to allow for periodic evaluation of the plan prior to full implementation.

Choosing the exact role of the change agent during the change process is critical to the success of the plan and is the fifth stage in Lippitt's model. Failure to clearly describe the role of the change agent and his/her power in the decision-making process usually leads to complications in communication between the parties, which can subsequently and often lead to breakdown of the process.

Stage six includes *diffusing the change beyond the pilot project to the larger organization and maintaining the change once it has been initiated.* The key to success at this stage is keeping the lines of communication open between the parties, as well as maintaining flexibility and creativity in solving problems as they arise.

Stage seven involves *withdrawing the change agent from the process as the organization reintegrates and assimilates the new changes into the system.* Ideally, individuals who are motivated and committed to the change have been identified during the implementation of the project and have been groomed to take over from the original change agent.

Rogers' Theory of Diffusion and Innovation

Rogers' Diffusion Theory differs from Lewin's and Lippitt's theories in that Rogers' model looks at the progressive stages used in the process of adopting change. Rogers considers both the background of the individual and the environment for change as variables in his model. He described five phases necessary in the adoption of change (Box 16-4).

Rogers' (1983) also described several characteristics that are associated with the successful implementation of a planned change project. He suggests that outcomes can be improved for adoption of the change when planning includes consideration of the following factors:

- Relative advantage: Are the changes perceived to be improvements over the current system?
- Compatibility: Are the existing values, norms, and corporate culture compatible with the suggested change?
- Complexity: Is the change too complex for people to comprehend, thus rendering it less likely to be adopted?

BOX 16-4   Rogers' Stages of Change

UNFREEZING

1. Awareness
2. Interest

MOVING

3. Evaluation
4. Trial

REFREEZING

5. Adoption

- Divisibility: Can portions of the change be divided or delegated in small increments before adopting the entire change?
- Communicability: Can the intended changes be clearly articulated to others both inside and outside the organization?

Rogers' (1983) later contributions regarded his theory of adoption and diffusion of change in which he suggests that people adopt change in their own unique ways and at their own pace. He describes the behavioral patterns commonly seen as the individuals respond to change as: *innovators, early adopters, early majority, late majority, laggards and rejecters.* One could describe the various stages of acceptance by using running a marathon as a metaphor for the change process. Innovators "lead the pack" in the race, enthusiastically embracing change, perhaps even deliberately seeking it out, despite the potential to cause upheaval in the organization. Early adopters are open to change and new ideas and are often among the first in the race in their willingness to be "ahead of the pack" as the first to try a new innovation. Those in the early majority are not usually among the very first to try the new innovation, but are solidly in the middle of the crowd of runners—they aren't in the "front of the pack" but they're not last either. The late majority follows the pack in front of them and brings up the rear; they only go when and where everyone else has already gone. Laggards, the last to adopt change, are the stragglers at the end of the pack, who wait until the last minute to get into the race, kicking and fighting the whole time. Rejecters don't even show up for the race; they openly oppose it and refuse to participate, often encouraging others to do the same.

The Transtheoretical Model of Change

The Transtheoretical Model of Change (TTM) differs from previous models in that though it includes multiple sequential stages, it focuses on individual change (Petrocelli, 2002). The TTM model emphasizes the personal dimensions of change as opposed to managerial or institutional changes. Based on the work of psychologists DiClemente and Prochaska (1998), this model recognizes the importance of an individual's readiness and intention to alter behavior as a critical ingredient to implementing change.

STAGES OF CHANGE

DiClemente and Prochaska (1998) describe five stages of change used by an individual when implementing a successful behavioral change (Box 16-5).

People are said to be in the first stage, *precontemplation*, when they refuse to acknowledge that a problem exists and are resistant to any change in behavior for at least the next six months. Individuals enter the *contemplation* stage when they are considering a change in behavior but have not already enacted any changes. Individuals are often weighing the pros and cons of change, collecting information about the change, and deciding on whether to actually implement a plan for the behavioral change within the next 6 months.

After individuals have weighed the options, both positive and negative, for initiating a change, they often recognize that a new behavior is required. They often state that they are highly motivated to initiate a change within 1 month. At this point, the individuals would then enter the *preparation* phase, wherein they move from thinking about a change to actually embarking on a plan to make the change.

The *action* stage is where people actually begin the work of changing their behavior. The final stage is *maintenance*, which typically occurs 3 to 6 months after the initial change in behavior. This stage fo-

> **BOX 16-5   Stages in the Transtheoretical Model of Change**
>
> 1. Precontemplation
> 2. Contemplation
> 3. Preparation
> 4. Action
> 5. Maintenance

cuses on lifestyle modifications that support the new behavior and which aid in resisting relapse into former negative behaviors.

PROCESSES OF CHANGE

According to DiClemente and Prochaska, (1998), 10 processes of change help to facilitate movement through the actual stages of change. The first five of the processes, which include consciousness raising, dramatic relief, environmental reevaluation, social liberation, and self-reevaluation, are internal processes that deal primarily with the individual's beliefs, values, and emotions. In these phases, the individual becomes aware of the behavior that requires changing and seeks out new information about how and what the change will entail. In reevaluating his environment for the means and methods for implementing the change, he is becoming increasingly aware of the impact of his behavior and, thus, sees himself in a new light.

In contrast to the first five processes, the second five deal largely with an individual's behavior in surrounding himself with positive forces in which to enhance and support the change and to assist in maintaining the change permanently. These processes are counter conditioning, helping relationships, reinforcement management, stimulus control, and self-liberation.

APPLICATIONS OF THE THEORIES

What is usually found in the literature when planned change theories are mentioned, are descriptions or case studies of a change process. There are studies of factors that lead to successful implementation of change and evaluation of the outcomes of a change process, but these are few in number. The paucity of studies can be attributed in part to the few valid instruments to measure planned change as either an independent or dependent variable.

Lewin's Theory

According to Loudermelt and Doornbos (1997) in their review of the nursing literature on planned change theories, among the most frequently cited theories by nurse researchers is Lewin's concept of planned change, largely due to its simplicity, broad applicability, and generalizability. However, a review of the nursing studies that cite Lewin reveals that most are descriptive case studies that apply planned change theory to explain what happened during a single change event. Few nursing studies report the use of a valid instrument to measure the planned change as either an independent or dependent variable; several studies used Lewin's concepts as the theoretical framework to support their descriptive study.

Two nursing studies that used Lewin's concept of planned change as their theoretical framework investigated the factors leading to successful implementation of computer-assisted instruction (CAI) in nursing programs. Brose (1981), recognizing the importance of decision-making in implementing any change, measured six factors that were either positive or restraining forces in the decision to use CAI by nursing administrators in one baccalaureate nursing program. She developed a schema to assist administrators with their decision and concluded that the schema was useful in planning and implementing the decision to implement CAI. Perciful (1992) also cited Lewin as the theoretical framework in her investigation of the relationship between planned change and successful implementation of CAI in nursing programs. Data were collected on the predictor variable, planned change, using an author-developed instrument, the Planning and Implementing Phases for CAI (PIP-CAI), which had a reported reliability coefficient alpha of .91 (Perciful, 1990). Perciful (1992) concluded that successful implementation of CAI was best predicted by the degree of planning used to implement the CAI and, thus, supported the validity of Lewin's concept of planned change.

Lippitt's Theory of Planned Change

Geraci (1997), using Lippitt's model of planned change in her study, reported on nurses' responses to working with laptop computers in home-care settings. She concluded that successful change was facilitated through proactive planning and careful appraisal of the driving and restraining forces that both impede and facilitate individuals and organizations undergoing planned change. Further research to determine the best ways to support staff through the transition from the old to the new system, is recommended.

Roger's Theory of Diffusion and Innovation

Hagerman and Tiffany (1994) contend that Rogers' diffusion theory has a low level of significance for nursing as a change theory. The authors suggest that this is primarily due to the fact that it focuses on technological concerns and is, therefore, illogical to use in nursing situations. However, the authors acknowledge that this theory has been useful in tracking adoption of innovations within nursing systems (Hagerman & Tiffany, 1994). Hilz (2000), in her investigation of the informatics nurse specialist as a change agent, concluded that Rogers' Innovation-Diffusion model facilitates nurses' adoption of technology in clinical practice settings but suggested that further investigations be conducted to determine the specific factors that lead to adoption of technology.

Vojir, Howell, Foster, Hester, and Miller (1999) investigated the integration of a planned innovation into nursing practice using Rogers' Innovation-Diffusion model as the theoretical framework. Qualitative data were collected to determine the meaning nurses assigned to the adoption. The authors concluded that Rogers' model was useful in evaluating a practice change in the practice setting.

The Transtheoretical Model of Change (TTM)

Nursing researchers have applied this model to descriptive studies linking theory to nursing practice in a smoking-cessation program (Miller, 1999), and use of motivational interviewing techniques by public health nurses to facilitate change and promote healthy behaviors (Shinitzky & Kub, 2001). Hulton (2001) examined adolescent sexual decision-making using TTM. Hulton's (2001) study supported the applicability of the TTM to the behavior of sexual abstinence in adolescents (Using Middle Range Theories 16-1).

Jue and Cunningham (1998) examined exercise behaviors in postcoronary-bypass graft surgery patients. Findings from that study supported the stages of change theory but also recommend additional study of relapse prevention.

Research Application 16-1 provides an additional example of the use of a planned change theory in research.

16-1 USING MIDDLE RANGE THEORIES

The increased incidence of unplanned pregnancies and sexually transmitted disease (STD) in the United States is well documented. Though there has been a growing interest in promoting sexual abstinence in adolescents as the primary method of preventing pregnancy and STDs, few of the efforts to promote abstinence have been evaluated. Using the Transtheoretical Model of Change (TTM) as a foundation, the following hypothesis was tested: "significant differences would be found in the variable of decisional balance among adolescents in the precontemplation, contemplation, preparation, action, and maintenance stages of sexual abstinence among both virgins and nonvirgins" (Hulton, 2001, p. 97).

Subjects consisted of 694 7th-graders from a school system in central Virginia. They were selected through a purposive cluster sampling procedure and had participated in the program "Models of the Heart," funded by the Virginia Abstinence Initiative. Subjects from four middle schools were assigned to program groups (three schools) or comparison group (one school).

During a regular class period, trained staff administered two questionnaires to the subjects, a demographic tool, the Adolescent Stages of Change Scale for Sexual Abstinence (ASCSSA), and the Adolescent Decisional Balance Scale for Sexual Abstinence (ADBSSA). The demographic tool included scales for gender, age, birth date, school grade completed, race/ethnicity, and family structure. A coding system was used to provide for confidentiality. The ASCSSA, developed for this study, had a content validity index of .82 and consisted of subscales for virgins and nonvirgins, using one-sentence descriptors. The ADBSSA comprised 17 statements, rated on a 5-point Likert scale and divided into three factors representing perceptions of abstinence: Cons, Pros/External, and Pros/Internal. The Coefficient alpha for the factors ranged from .80 to .88.

One-way analysis of variance with follow-up *t*-tests was used to examine the differences among the stages of change of virgins and nonvirgins and the Pros and Cons factors. The hypothesis was supported only for subjects who were virgins. These subjects evaluated the Pros of sexual abstinence progressively more important as they moved to the action stage for abstinence behavior. For subjects who were nonvirgins, there were no statistically significant differences between the Stages of Change and Decisional Balance constructs.

Hulton, L. J. (2001). The application of the Transtheoretical Model of Change to adolescent sexual decision-making. *Issues in Comprehensive Pediatric Nursing, 24,* 95–115.

16-1 RESEARCH APPLICATION

For the implementation of a system-wide change to computer-based medical records, a researcher wanted to investigate the impact of a unit-selected project manager/change agent rather than an administration-selected project manager/change agent. The importance of the change agent is noted in Lippitt's model of change. A study was designed to answer the question: What is the impact of the project-manager selection process on length of time to complete the project, and also on resistance to change during the implementation of the system throughout two related hospitals in a larger medical system?

The hospitals are both located in suburbs of a metropolitan area and both have comparable capacities of 250 to 300 patients. The decision by the administrations of the hospitals to implement the change to computer-based medical records had been communicated to staff 3 months before the onset of the study. For this study, 12 units from the two hospitals were matched according to primary medical services provided. For the paired units, random assignment was made to either a project manager selected by administration from the clinical education department, or to a project manager selected by the unit personnel from its staff. All project managers needed to be full-time registered nurses. All project managers engaged in a basic 4-hour program on project management and specific training on the computer-based medical record, consisting of 2-hour classes, twice a week for 4 weeks. At the conclusion of the training, the project managers were informed that the implementation of the change had to be completed within 3 months, but that it would be an advantage to complete the project in a shorter time frame. An expert on clinical information systems was available to all project managers throughout the study.

Data on resistance to change would be collected through interviews. At the end of the training period and the onset of the actual implementation process, the researcher interviewed two nurses from each of the involved units. Nurse managers identified the nurses to be interviewed, one believed to be predisposed to the change and one believed to be resistant to it. The nurses needed to be employed at least half-time. The nurses were permitted to refuse to participate in the interviews without penalty. If they chose to be interviewed and were involved throughout the study, they were given 4 hours of paid vacation. The audio-taped interviews focused on their thoughts and feelings about the innovation. Interviews were conducted every other week until the computer-based medical record was fully implemented on their units. Data on the length of time of project completion were determined by the project manager's report that computer-based medical records were fully implemented on the unit.

Data analysis included both qualitative and quantitative processes. To aid in the analysis of the qualitative data, the transcribed texts of the interviews were entered into a computer program, HyperQual. The researcher analyzed the data for themes within the stages of change suggested by Lippitt's model, particularly: selecting progressive change objectives, choosing the appropriate role for the change agent, maintaining the change once it has been started, and ending the helping relationship. Though the number of pairs makes the use of inferential statistics problematic, quantitative data will be analyzed using a basic *t*-test.

SUMMARY

During the last several decades, change theory has been widely applied in nursing as well as in other disciplines, as a means of describing and explaining the exponential rate of change occurring within the health care system. Several models of change, each with its own strengths and weaknesses, ranging from simple theories to complex models have been applied in nursing research studies. However, few of the theories used by nurse scholars have been generated by nurses. Rather, the theories are largely borrowed from other disciplines and applied to explain or describe an incident or change event occurring in the nurse's immediate environment. This use of convenience samples and local situations may not serve nursing's overall purpose, by failing to generate unique nursing theories of planned change and change management (Tiffany & Lutjens, 1998).

Some areas for further investigation of planned change could be: studying the essential attributes of the nurse as change agent, describing the variables that encourage/discourage successful change in nursing situations, or describing the "best practices" for implementing change in individuals, organizations, and systems.

Nurses can develop and use planned change as a middle range theory, as they study the best ways to implement and manage change, as well as to measure the effects of change on individuals, groups, and institutions. Nurse-developed planned change theories will foster nursing's efforts to develop research-based nursing practice and, ultimately, improve the quality of nursing services provided to the public.

ANALYSIS EXERCISE

This chapter provides several constructs with which to view the phenomenon of planned change. Using the criteria presented in Chapter 2, critique the body of knowledge presented in this chapter. You will be using each criterion in a manner different from its use when applied to one specific theory. Specific questions related to the use of each criterion in this new context follow. Compare your conclusions about the constructs across theories with those found in Appendix A. A nurse scholar who has worked with this phenomenon completed the analysis found in the Appendix.

Internal Criticism

1. Clarity (Do we have theories of planned change that are clear?)
2. Consistency (Is there consistency in approach, i.e., terms, interpretations, principles, and methods across theories?)

3. Adequacy (How adequate is the body of theories in accounting for planned change?)
4. Level of theory development (At what level of development are the planned change theories?)

External Criticism

1. Reality convergence (Do these theories reflect "real world" nursing experiences of planned change?)
2. Utility (How useful are present theories when applied in practice and research?)
3. Significance (Do the theories reflect issues essential to nursing?)
4. Discrimination (Do the theories help distinguish planned change from other social processes?)
5. Scope of theory (What seems to be scope of the theories?)
6. Complexity (As a group, how would you judge the complexity of planned change theories?)

WEB RESOURCES

1. This site provides brief summaries of the work of several change theorists: Ely's factors that explain successful change implementation, Fullan's change forces, Havelock and Zlotolow's C.R.E.A.T.E.R. Model, and Rogers' Diffusion of Innovations Theory:
   http://ide.ed.psu.edu/itsc/janice/port/difadop.htm

2. This site describes theory of Diffusion of Innovations by providing a list of characteristics of an innovation, categories of adopters, roles in the innovation process, and functions of change agents. Also provides a link to resource page that included additional references:
   http://www.anu.edu.au/people/Roger.Clarke/SOS/InnDiff.html

REFERENCES

Barr B. (2002). Managing change during an information systems transition. *Journal of Operating Room Nursing (AORN), 75* (6), 1085–1088.

Bennis, W. G., Benne, K. D., & Chin, R. (1985). *The planning of change* (4th ed.). New York: Holt, Rinehart and Winston.

Bhola, H. S. (1994). The CLER model: Thinking through change. *Nursing Management, 25*(5), 59–63.

Brose, C. (1981). The design and application of a decision-making scheme concerning implementation of computer-assisted instruction in baccalaureate schools of nursing. *Dissertation Abstracts International, 42,* 2778B.

Dean, L. (1979). The change from functional to primary nursing. *Nursing Clinics of North America, 14*(2), 407–423.

DiClemente, C., & Prochaska, J. (1998). Toward a comprehensive transtheoretical model of change. In W. R. Miller & N. Healther (Eds.), *Treating addictive behaviors* (pp. 3–24). New York: Plenum Press.

Geraci, E. P. (1997). Computers in home care: Application of change theory. *Computers in Nursing, 15* (4), 199–203.

Grohar-Murray, M. E., & Di Groce, H.R. (2003). *Leadership and Management in Nursing* (3rd ed.). Upper Saddle River, NJ: Prentice Hall.

Hagerman, Z., & Tiffany, C. (1994). Evaluation of two planned change theories. *Nursing Management, 25*(4), 57–62.

Hein, E. C., & Nicholson, M. J. (1996). *Contemporary leadership behavior* (4th ed.). Philadelphia: J. B. Lippincott Co.

Hilz, L. (2000). The informatics nurse specialist as change agent: Application of innovation-diffusion theory. *Computers in Nursing, 18*(6), 272–281.

Huber, D. (1996). *Leadership and nursing care management.* Philadelphia: W. B. Saunders.

Huber, D. (2000). *Leadership and nursing care management.* (2nd ed.) Philadelphia: W. B. Saunders.

Hulton, L. (2000). The application of the Transtheoretical Model of change to adolescent sexual-decision making. *Issues in Comprehensive Pediatric Nursing, 24,* 95–115.

Jue, N., & Cunningham, S. (1998). Stages of exercise behavior change at two time periods following coronary bypass graft surgery. *Progress in Cardiovascular Nursing, 13*(1), 23–33.

Kuebler-Ross, E. (1969). *On death and dying.* New York: Macmillan Publishing.

LaPiere, R. T. (1965). *Social change.* New York: McGraw-Hill.

Lepola, I., & Blom-Lange, M. (1999). Participation in change: Self-reflection of staff in a psychiatric admission unit. *Nursing and Health Sciences, 1,* 171–177.

Lewin, K. (1947). Frontiers in group dynamics: Concept, method, and reality in social science; social equilibria and social change. *Human Relations, 1*(1), 5–41.

Lewin, K. (1951). *Field theory in social science: Selected theoretical papers.* New York: Harper and Row.

Lewin, K. (1958). *Group decision and social change.* In E. Macoby (Ed.), *Readings in social psychology* (3rd ed., pp. 197–211). New York: Holt, Rinehart and Winston.

Lippitt, G. L. (1973). *Visualizing change: Model building and the change process.* La Jolla, CA: University Associates, Inc.

Lippitt, G. L., Watson, J., & Westley, B. (1958). *The dynamics of planned change.* New York: Harcourt, Brace and Company.

Loudermelt, L., & Doornbos, D. (1992). Change theories in recent nursing literature.Retrieved September 28, 2002, from *http://www.stti.inpui.edu/rnr/search/hts/fullview.hts?sid=523*

Lutjens, L., & Tiffany, C. (1994). Evaluating planned change theories. *Nursing Management, 25*(3), 54–57.

Marquis, B. M., & Huston, C. J. (2000). *Leadership roles and management functions in nursing: theory and application* (3rd ed.) Philadelphia: Lippincott Williams & Wilkins.

Miller, C. E. (1999). Stages of change theory and the nicotine-dependent client: Direction for decision making in nursing practice. *Clinical Nurse Specialist, 13*(1), 18–22.

Moses, E. (1997). *The registered nurse population: Findings from the national sample survey of registered nurses 1996.* Rockville, MD: Health Resources and Services Administration, U.S. Department of Health and Human Services.

Noone, J. (1987). Planned change: Putting theory into practice...utilizing Lippitt's theory. *Clinical Nurse Specialist, 1*(1): 25–9.

Olson, E. (1979). Strategies and techniques for the nurse change agent. *Nursing Clinics of North America, 14*(2), 323–336.

Perciful, E. (1990). The relationship between planned change and successful implementation of computer-assisted instruction (CAI) within higher education in nursing as perceived by faculty. *Dissertation Abstracts International, 52*(05), 2504B.

Perciful, E. (1992). The relationship between planned change and successful implementation of computer-assisted instruction. *Computers in Nursing, 10*(2), 85–90.

Perlman, D., & Takacs, G. (1990). The ten stages of change. *Nursing Management, 21* (4), 33–38.

Peterson, C. A. (2001). Nursing shortage: Not a simple problem—no easy answers. *Online Journal of Issues in Nursing, 6*(1), manuscript 1. Retrieved June 26, 2002 from *http://www.nursingworld.org/ojin/topic14/tpc14_1.htm.*

Petrocelli, J. V. (2002, Winter). Processes and stages of change: Counseling with the transtheoretical model of change. *Journal of Counseling and Development, 80*, 22–30.

Prochaska, J., & DiClemente, C. (1983). Stages and processes of self-change of smoking: Toward an integrative model of change. *Journal of Consulting and Clinical Psychology, 51*(3), 390–395.

Prochaska, J., DiClemente, C., & Norcross, J. (1992). In search of how people change: Applications to addictive behaviors. *American Psychologist, 47*(9), 1102–1114.

Prochaska, J. O., & Prochaska, J. M. (1999). Why don't continents move? Why don't people change? *Journal of Psychotherapy Integration, 9*(1), 83–102.

Rogers, E. M. (1983). *Diffusion of innovations* (3rd ed.). New York: The Free Press.

Schoolfield, M., & Orduna, A. (1994). Understanding staff nurses responses to change: Utilization of a grief-change framework to facilitate innovation. *Clinical Nurse Specialist, 8*, 57–62.

Shinitzky, H. E., & Kub, J. (2001). The art of motivating behavior change: The use of motivational interviewing to promote health. *Public Health Nursing, 18*(1), 178–185.

Swansburg, R. C., & Swansburg, R. J. (2002). *Introduction to management and leadership for nurse managers* (3rd ed.). Sudbury, MA: Jones and Bartlett.

Tanner, C. (2001). Resolving the nursing shortage: Replacement plus one! *Journal of Nursing Education, 40*(3), 99.

Tiffany, C. R., & Lutjens, L. R. (1998). *Planned change theories for nursing: Review, analysis, and implications.* Thousand Oaks,CA: Sage.

Vojir, C., Howell, R., Foster, N., & Miller, K. (1999). Evaluating a planned practice change using Rogers' innovation-decision model. Retrieved on September 28, 2002, from *http://www.stti.iupui.edu/nrn/search/hts/fullview/ hts?sid=963.*

Welch, L. B. (1979). Planned change in nursing: the theory. *Nursing Clinics of North America, 14*(2), 307–321.

Workman, R., & Kenney, M. (1988). The change experience.

In S. Pinkerton & P. Schroeder (Eds.), *Commitment to excellence: Developing a professional nursing staff.* (pp. 17–25). Rockville, MD: Aspen.

Yoder-Wise, P. (1997). *Leading and managing in nursing.* (2nd ed.). St. Louis, MO: Mosby.

Yoder-Wise, P. (2003). *Leading and managing in nursing.* (3rd ed.). St. Louis, MO: Mosby.

BIBLIOGRAPHY

Archer, S. E., Kelly, C. D., & Bisch, S. A. (1984). *Implementing change in communities: A collaborative process.* St. Louis: Mosby.

Asprec, E. (1975). The process of change. *Supervisor Nurse, 6*, 15–24.

Bhola, H.S. (1977). Configurations of change: The framework for a research review. *Resources in Education, 12*(1). [ERIC Document No ED. 127–702].

Bhola, H. S. (1994). The CLER Model: Thinking through the change. *Nursing Management, 25*(5), 59–63.

Bozak, M. G. (2003). Using Lewin's Force Field Analysis in implementing a nursing information system. *CIN: Computers, Informatics, Nursing, 21*(2), 80–85.

Bushy, A. (1992). Managing change: Strategies for continuing education. *Journal of Continuing Education in Nursing, 23*, 197–200.

Conger, M. M. (1992). Application of change theory to a clinical problem. *Nursing Management, 23*(10), 89, 90.

Coyle, L. A., & Sokop, A. G. (1990). Innovation adoption behavior among nurses. *Nursing Research, 39*, 176–180.

Curtis, E., & White, P. (2002). Resistance to change: Causes and solutions. *Nursing Management, 8*(10), 15–20.

Dufault, M. A., Bielecki, C., Collins, E., & Willey, C. (1995). Changing nurses' pain assessment practice: A collaborative research utilization approach. *Journal of Advanced Nursing, 21*, 634–645.

Gender, A. (1996). Planned change. In C. E. Loveridge & S. H. Cummings (Eds.), *Nursing management in the new paradigm* (pp. 379–408). Gaithersburg, MD: Aspen.

Haynes, S. (1992). Let the change come from within: The process of change in nursing. *Professional Nurse, 10*, 635–638.

Manix, K. D. (2000). Educating to manage the accelerated change environment effectively: Part 1. *Journal for Nurses in Staff Development, 16*(6), 282–288.

McCaugherty, D. (1991). The theory-practice gap in nursing education: Its causes and possible solutions. Findings from an action research study. *Journal of Advanced Nursing, 16*(9), 2055–2061.

McDonald, H. (2001). Changing practice: Modified clean technique for intermittent catheterization. *Spinal Cord Injury Nursing, 18*(1), 30–33.

Pearcey, P., & Draper, P. (1996). Using the diffusion of innovation model to influence practice: A case study. *Journal of Advanced Nursing, 23*, 714–721.

Riddle, C.R. (1994). Development of an adolescent inpatient sexual abuse group: Application of Lewin's model of change. *Journal of Children and Adolescent Psychiatric Nursing, 7*(1), 17–24.

Saarmann, L., Daughtery, J., & Riegel, B. (2000). Patient teaching to promote behavioral change. *Nursing Outlook, 48*, 281–287.

Schwartz, K., & Tiffany, C. R. (1994). Evaluating Bhola's Configurations Theory of Planned Change. *Nursing Management, 25*(6), 56–61.

Stulginsky, M. (1993). Nurses' home care experience. *Nursing and Health Care, 14*, 402–407.

Swan, J., & Mac Vicar, B. (1992). The rough guide to change. *Nursing Times, 88*(13), 48–49.

Taft, S. H., & Stearns, J. E. (1991). Organizational change toward a nursing agenda: A framework from the Strengthening Hospital Nursing Program. *Journal of Nursing Administration, 21*(2), 12–21.

Tiffany, C. R., Cheatham, A. B., Doornbos, D., Loudermelt, L., & Momadi, G. G. (1994). Planned change theory: Survey of nursing periodical literature. *Nursing Management, 25*(7), 54–59.

Walter, G. A., & Marks, S. E. (1981). *Experiential learning and change.* New York: John Wiley & Sons.

Williams, N., McDonough, J., & Boettcher, J. (1990). Nurse faculty practice: From theory to reality. *Journal of Professional Nursing, 6*(1), 11–20.

Resilience

JOAN E. HAASE

DEFINITION OF KEY TERMS

Boundaries of resilience
The contextual influences, dimensions and assumptions that are considered in determining the attributes of resilience

Meaning-based models
Explanatory models focused on the patterns and experiences of illness from a subjective and holistic perspective

Person-focused research to resilience
Research to identify the patterns of variables that naturally occur, then examining what might contribute to these outcomes; or using cut-off scores on selected variables to categorize adversity sub-groups, then examining outcomes in these groups.

Positive health research
Efforts to gain understanding of ways individuals sustain or regain optimal health

Protective factors
The individual, family, social or other contextual factors that enhance resilience processes and outcomes

Quality of life
A sense of well-being

Resilience
General definition: Positive adjustment in the face of adversity

Context-derived definition: The process of identifying or developing resources and strengths to flexibly manage stressors to gain a positive outcome, a sense of confidence/mastery, self-transcendence, and self-esteem

Risk factors
The individual, family, social, or other contextual factors that impede development of resilience processes and outcomes

Strengths-based research
Research that focuses on individual, family, or community "promise" rather than on risk.

Triangulation
Use of quantitative or qualitative research approaches either sequentially or simultaneously to refine, evaluate, and/or extend theory

DEFINITION OF KEY TERMS

Variable-focused approaches to resilience	Use of multivariate statistics to test for linkages among measures of adversity, outcomes, and environmental or individual qualities that may protect from or compensate for negative consequences.

INTRODUCTION

Researchers and practitioners have long sought answers to questions about psychosocial adjustment to illness, especially chronic conditions. While much research is guided by pathology and deficit-based models that examine risk, adjustment problems, and developmental delays (Hymovich & Roehnert, 1989), salutogenic and strengths-based models are gaining recognition as useful perspectives in nursing and other health care disciplines (Antonovsky, 1979; Hymovich & Roehnert, 1989; Singer, 2001; Woodgate, 1999). Theories such as resilience (Rutter, 1979, 1987), hardiness (Kobasa, 1982), self efficacy, and learned resourcefulness (Bandura, 1977; Rosenbaum, 1983) were developed to explain positive adjustment to illness, based on the belief that such theories may yield information about effective interventions (Forsyth, Delaney, & Gresham, 1984; Garmezy, 1991; Kadner, 1989; Sinnema, 1991). Resilience was recently identified by the Committee on Future Direction for Behavioral and Social Sciences as a research priority for the National Institutes of Health (Singer, 2001). The committee highlighted the significance of behavioral and psychosocial processes in disease etiology, well-being, and health promotion. Additionally, the committee recommended increased study of the protective factors that are correlates of resilience, such as optimism, meaning and purpose, social and emotional support, and related neurobiological mechanisms, that promote recovery and increased survival rates (Singer, 2001). Nurses also recognize the importance of positive health concepts and are increasingly seeing an understanding of resilience as potentially useful to: (1) guide development of interventions to enhance positive outcomes; (2) improve outcomes for at-risk populations; (3) prevent poor outcomes; and (4) influence public policy related to individuals, families, and communities.

Resilience is broadly defined as a phenomenon of positive adjustment in the face of adversity. Historically, resilience was most frequently studied in children and adolescents and was characterized by attributes usually identified as positive. Examples of such positive attributes found in research include competence (Garmezy, Masten, & Tellegen, 1984; Rutter, 1979); self-esteem (Garmezy, 1981); continual growth and 'elasticity' in relation to change (Block, 1980); superior coping (Garmezy, 1991; Murphy & Moriarty, 1976); advanced self-help, communication and problem-solving skills (Garmezy, 1981; Hauser, Vieyra, Jacobson, & Wertlieb, 1985); tendency to perceive experiences constructively (Werner & Smith, 1982); and ability to use spirituality to maintain a positive vision of a meaningful life (Rutter, 1979; Wells & Schwebel, 1987).

HISTORICAL BACKGROUND

Since the 1970s, shifting perspectives on resilience inquiry have occurred. Two authors' descriptions of these shifting perspectives are especially informative. Richardson (2002) describes resilience research as occurring in three waves:

1. Efforts to describe personal qualities that predict success
2. Resilience as a process
3. Resilience as a motivational life force to be fostered in all individuals.

Similarly, Masten (2001) portrays a gradual change in perspectives of resilience, from a view of resilience as an extraordinary occurrence, to the current evidence-based perspective that resilience is a commonly occurring phenomenon that is essentially a basic function of adaptational systems.

Positive adaptation research began with studies on the premorbid competence of patients with schizophrenia (Garmezy, 1974; Masten, Best, & Garmezy, 1990). Those studies were precursors to the seminal theoretical and empirical groundwork on resilience done with children of mothers with schizophrenia. The major characteristic of these children was the fact that they thrived despite their high-risk status. After describing children who thrived despite adversity, subsequent studies were directed to understanding individual differences in response to adversity. This effort to understand individual differences was gradually expanded to other contexts, such as childhood exposure to adverse conditions of socioeconomic adversity (Rutter, 1979), abuse (Henry, 2001), urban poverty and community violence (Luthar, Cicchetti, & Becker, 2000b), and chronic illness (Wells & Schwebel, 1987). In the early 1990s, researchers began to identify external factors that contributed to development of resilience. Three general classes of protective factors—individual, family, and social—are now generally recognized as influencing resilience development (Rutter, 1987). Currently, in addition to continuing to identify protective factors, researchers are seeking to understand how the protective factors influence resilience outcomes (Luthar et al., 2000b).

DEFINITION OF THEORY CONCEPTS

There is widespread agreement that resilience is a complex, multidimensional construct. Largely because of the complexity of the construct, there is a lack of consensus about terminology, characteristics, or boundaries of resilience. This section examines the various perspectives in these three areas from both the general and the nursing literature.

General Literature

TERMINOLOGY AND ATTRIBUTES OF RESILIENCE

To adequately define a construct, terminology needs to be consistent. In the case of resilience, even the labels for the phenomenon have been inconsistently used. Labels variously applied to the phenomenon have included resilience, resiliency, and ego-resilience. Researchers currently recommend the term "resilience," rather than "resiliency," to describe positive adjustment in face of adversity (Luthar et al., 2000b; Masten, 1994). "Resiliency" is not recommended, because it implies a personality trait that is difficult to alter, much like hardiness. The term "ego-resilience" characterizes resilience as a distinct personality trait. Hence, ego-resilience decreases the options for intervention and increases the danger of labeling individuals as innately "inadequate."

There are two generally recognized essential attributes of resilience present in most definitions. These are the presence of (1) "good" or positive outcomes that occur in spite of (2) adverse conditions (Masten, 2001).

Good Outcomes. "Good" or positive outcomes are not consistently theoretically or operationally defined in the literature. Debate centers on what constitutes "good" outcomes and who decides. Additional questions include whether external criteria (e.g., academic achievement) or intrapersonal characteristics (e.g., sense of well-being, self-esteem), or a combination of both are defining characteristics of positive outcomes (Masten, 2001).

Paradigmatic approaches also contribute to differences in ways positive outcomes are defined. A pathology-based worldview often defines positive outcomes as the absence of psychopathology or low levels of symptoms or impairments (Masten & Coatsworth, 1998). Developmental and life-span perspectives usually define positive outcomes as those that meet or exceed expectations. More recently, a subtle shift in worldviews has occurred that emphasizes dynamic ecosystems influenced by complex, ever-changing, and interacting forces (Richardson, 2002; Waller, 2001) and the notion that resilience is possibly a common human characteristic—"ordinary magic" (Masten, 2001).

Adverse Conditions. The theoretical and operational definitions of "adverse conditions" are also inconsistent in the literature. Frequently, definitions infer threats or risk factors that occur in contexts such as war, illness, community deficits, or family adversity. Beyond the requirement that such factors negatively affect resilience outcomes, there is not agreement on how such risks should be operationalized. Options include either: (1) current or past occurrence: (2) predictors of poor outcomes or status (moderating) variables such as low socioeconomic status; and, (3) single exposure variables or cumulative combinations of factors. Adding to the inconsistency of defining characteristics, risk factors can be continuous bipolar variables classified as either less or more aversive (e.g., mild to severe symptoms) or as negative to positive assets (e.g., low to high economic status, negative to positive coping) (Masten, 2001). In general, much research indicates that risk factors, however operationalized, often co-occur (Masten, 2001).

BOUNDARIES OF RESILIENCE

Boundaries of resilience are the contextual influences (conditions under which resilience exists/varies/disappears), dimensions (e.g., objective/subjective, physiological/psychological) and underlying assumptions (e.g., growth vs. stability and state vs. trait) that are considered in determining the attributes of resilience. Boundaries of resilience that need further research and clarification include state/trait/process, psychological/physiological, individual/aggregate, and objective/subjective perspective.

Trait/State/Process. Although the definition of resilience as the presence of "good" outcomes that occur in the presence of adverse conditions implies a process, there is no consensus on the issue of resilience as trait, state, or process. Again, the confusion is exacerbated by inconsistent terminology and the inability to draw conclusions of causality (Jacelon, 1997; Pettit, 2000). As indicated above, the term "ego-resiliency," for example, is frequently used interchangeably with resilience, but the former refers to a set of personal characteristics (traits) that may or may not be specifically linked to adversity (Luthar et al., 2000b). In addition, terms such as "resilient children" cause confusion. Although this term implies that resilience is a trait, it is used most often in conjunction with the two co-existing conditions of adversity and positive adaptation, and adaptation is usually conceptualized as a process. Even the terms 'outcome' and 'process' contribute to the confusion, when researchers do not clearly identify a model of resilience that stipulates how the underlying mechanisms in a resilience process may result in specific resilience outcomes. Luthar and Cicchetti (2000) encourage researchers to clearly specify the context to which resilience outcomes apply and to clearly delineate the outcomes by using terms such as "emotional resilience," "behavioral resilience," or "educational resilience." It would also be helpful, through staged-model specification, to distinguish proximal resilience outcomes such as self-transcendence and confidence/mastery, from more distal outcomes, such as quality of life, which result from the resilience process and resilience outcomes.

Psychological/ Physiological. Psychological concepts associated with resilience have been more widely studied than physiological concepts. Concepts such as self-esteem, self-perception, personality, temperament, intellect, coping, problem-solving skills are just a few of the psychological concepts that have been studied in relation to resilience. What is not clear is whether these identified psychological variables influence the process and outcomes associated with resilience, or whether they are components of resilience (Jacelon, 1997).

Fewer studies have examined physiological dimensions of resilience. Singer and Ryff (2001) identify several positive physiological mechanisms, including those that involve the hypothalamic-pituitary-adrenal (HPA) axis and the autonomic nervous system, which may be linked to positive health and resilience. They further argue for integrative levels of analysis that include the physiological, behavioral, environmental, and psychosocial systems to better understand how each contributes individually and interactively to resilience.

Individual/Aggregate. Resilience is most often studied in individuals, but to avoid confusion in yet another boundary, it is important for researchers to clarify the level of analysis. At an individual level, family factors have been identified that influence resilience. For example, Hauser, Vieyra, Jacobson, and Wertlieb (1989) identified both direct and indirect effects of family factors on individual resilience. Family direct effects included household composition and family structure, as well as family atmosphere factors such as patterns of communication, adaptability, and flexibility. Family factors apparently also have an indirect effect on individual and social protective factors, since child personality factors (temperament, attitudes, self-esteem, etc.) and social milieu process are often shaped by family processes.

There are growing bodies of literature focused on additional levels of analysis—resilient families (Hawley & DeHaan, 1996; Patterson, 2002) and resilient communities (Bosworth & Earthman, 2002). At these levels, studies most frequently take a systems approach. The family research on resilience is primarily built on family systems theory, and much of the work was done from a family-stress and coping framework. Resilience is equated with family adaptation; that is, the balancing of family demands and capabilities through interaction with family meanings (McCubbin, Balling, Possin, Frierdich, & Bryne, 2002; Patterson, 1995, 2002). Further work on resilience at the family and community level may provide strong significance for public policy decisions.

Objective/Subjective. In a qualitative study of homeless adolescents, Hunter and Chandler (1999) found adolescents who considered themselves resilient. According to the adolescents, being resilient was "surviving." The characteristics self-attributed by the adolescents as being resilient were quite different than the characteristics of resilience found in the literature. Hunter and Chandler's research indicated that resilience in homeless adolescents may be a "process of defense using such tactics as insulation, isolation, disconnecting, denial, and aggression or as a process of survival using such responses as violence" (p. 246). These findings indicate that self-attributed resilience in homeless adolescents seems to lack a positive or good outcome, a key characteristic of resilience in the literature. These findings were further supported in a subsequent study by Hunter (2001) that examined cross-cultural perspectives of resilience in adolescents from New England and Ghana. All the adolescents viewed themselves as resilient, regardless of age, gender, culture, or socioeconomic status. Yet, depending on the presence or absence of consistent, loving, caring, mentoring adults, there were qualitative differences in how the adolescents overcame adversities. Hunter classified these as two different "forms of resilience," self-protective survival resilience or connected resilience.

Hunter and Chandler's findings imply that if the objective and subjective dimensions of resilience are not carefully delineated, much of what determines the process and outcomes of resilience will be difficult to ascertain. For example, the cognitive appraisal of the adversity, the actions that are taken to deal with the adversity, and subsequent evaluation of how one is dealing with the adversity can all influence how resilience as a process proceeds (Fine, 1991). Further, if the objective and subjective appraisal, actions, and evaluation differ, evaluation of outcomes and development of interventions will be more complex.

One potentially helpful way to delineate the objective/subjective dimensions of resilience is to consider whether resilience may be interpersonally assigned to an individual, much like courage is interpersonally assigned (Haase, 1987). Research indicates that individuals usually do not attribute courage to themselves, unless someone else initially indicates that their behavior could be interpreted as courageous (Haase, 1987). Likewise, it is possible that persons who have resilience require time to reflect on the meaning of their actions. That is, resilience may occur through a process that includes deriving meaning from the experience through interaction with others (Haase, Heiney, Ruccione, & Stutzer, 1999). After interviews were conducted, Hunter and Chandler's findings support this perspective in that the adolescents' resilience scores increased from baseline measures (Hunter, 2001). A second consideration regarding the subjective perspective is the social desirability of being labeled "resilient." It is possible that a label of being resilient parallels a label such as "honest," in that, when asked, one would not readily deny having such a characteristic.

Resilience Perspectives in Nursing

Not surprisingly, information in Table 17-1 indicates there is no greater consensus on definitions, characteristics, or boundaries of resilience in the nursing literature than there is in the literature from other disciplines. The nursing literature on resilience parallels that of the general literature. Although nurses historically have focused more extensively on individual and family strengths than many disciplines, systematic study of resilience by nurses only began in the mid to late 1980s. A major contribution to understanding resilience from the nursing literature is the focus on resilience in the context of health, an otherwise neglected area in the resilience literature. The articles included in Table 17-1 provide an overview of much of the nursing literature on resilience. These articles are a representative sample of both theoretical and empirical efforts by nurses, including varied populations and approaches to knowledge development.

TERMINOLOGY AND ATTRIBUTES OF RESILIENCE

Most definitions in the table include the characteristic of adversity. Some definitions specifically describe the adversity as stress, loss, or illness, while others use more global terms, such as "challenging life condition" (Drummond, Kysela, McDonald, & Query, 2002) or a "disaster" (Polk, 1997). The "good" varies considerably in the definitions, as well. Several of the definitions use vague terminology, such as "go on with life" or "spring back." Few definitions of resilience provide clear descriptions of outcome variables associated with resilience.

Regarding the essential characteristics of adversity and "good" outcomes, there is the same inconsistency in the nursing literature as was found in the general resilience literature. Risk or adversity factors primarily focus on how protective factors of resilience can deter the impact that risk has on resilience outcomes. In some cases, both protective and vulnerability, or risk, factors were listed together, and it can only be assumed that in these cases, the risk factor was the absence of the protective factor identified, or on a continuum of risk to resilience. Examples of the risk factors identified in the nursing literature include survival tactics of violence (Hunter & Chandler, 1999); defensive coping and illness-related risk (Haase et al., 1999); and gender, antisocial behavior, and chronic illness (Stewart, Reid, & Mangham, 1997). No studies were found that addressed the ways that the adversity may be a "strengthener." This is puzzling because individuals often clearly credit the adversity as the important factor that influences the outcome. To illustrate, consider Lance Armstrong's quote, "The truth is that cancer was the best thing that ever happened to me. I don't know why I got the illness, but it did wonders for me, and I wouldn't want to walk away from it. Why would I want to change, even for a day, the most important, and shaping event of my life?" (Armstrong, 2000).

The positive factors of resilience reflected in Table 17-1 are numerous. In many cases, where models were specified based on literature synthesis and/or qualitative research to develop a resilience model, the relationship to and among positive factors is clearly described. Taken as a whole, the literature set provides an emerging pattern that may help distinguish positive resilience outcomes from positive outcomes of resilience. Positive resilience outcomes may include:

- Confidence, self-esteem, and self-transcendence (Haase et al., 1999)
- Self-esteem, self-efficacy, trust, connectedness, competence, and ego resilience (Hunter & Chandler, 1999)
- Maintenance of physiological and psychological health (Stewart et al., 1997)
- Self-esteem, confidence, intelligence, a toughened effect, hope, mastery, and enhanced coping (Dyer & McGuinness, 1996)
- Social competence, global self-worth, and perceived health (Heinzer, 1995).

Positive outcomes of resilience include:

- Enhanced quality of life conceptualized as well-being (Haase et al., 1999; Hockenberry-Eaton, Kemp, & DeLorio, 1994; Vinson, 2002)
- A sense of having overcome that fosters mastery (Dyer & McGuinness, 1996)
- Psychological equilibrium (Kadner, 1989)
- Global psychosocial adjustment (Stewart et al., 1997).

(text continues on page 354)

TABLE 17-1. NURSING LITERATURE ON RESILIENCE

SOURCE	METHODS OF KNOWLEDGE DEVELOPMENT	POPULATIONS STUDIED	DEFINITION OF RESILIENCE	PRIMARY BOUNDARIES
(Drummond et al., 2002)	Family Adaptation Model Development, using resilience theory (family protective factors) as underpinnings. Survey and post-test only experimental design.	Families of children with special needs and families with children in Head Start	(Borrowed) Maintenance of positive adjustment under challenging life conditions (Luthar, Cicchetti, & Becker, 2000a)	Family processes
(Dyer & McGuinness, 1996)	Concept analysis	Adults	A process whereby people bounce back from adversity and go on with their lives	Individual psychosocial process, with outcome on a continuum
(Felten, 2000; Felten & Hall, 2001)	Concept analysis	Women older than 85 who experienced illness or loss	The ability to achieve, retain or regain a level of physical or emotional health after devastating illness or loss	Individual psychosocial state influenced by external factors
(Haase, Heiney, Ruccione & Stutzer, 1999)	Triangulation using qualitative model and instrument generating and quantitative model evaluating studies	Adolescents with chronic illness, primarily cancer	The process of identifying or developing resources and stengths to manage stressors flexibly and to gain a positive outcome, i.e., a sense of confidence or mastery, self-transcendence, and self-esteem	Individual psychosocial process resulting in specific outcomes
(Heinzer, 1995)	Descriptive, model evaluation	Adults who lost a parent when an adolescent	(Borrowed) The dynamic ability or strength (both physiological and psychological in nature) that enables an individual to recover from or adjust easily to loss or misfortune and to mobilize coping resources (Garmezy et al., 1984)	Individual process Psychological variables studied, but physiological recognized in definition

COMPONENTS: ANTECEDENTS/ EXOGENOUS VARIABLES	COMPONENTS: ATTRIBUTES/ PROCESSES	COMPONENTS: OUTCOMES	KEY RELATIONAL STATEMENTS/ FINDINGS
Presence of vulnerability processes in family life that may create demands in maintenance of family protective processes	Ongoing development and successful use of protective family processes (appraisal, support, and coping)	Family adaptation	Normative adaptation is managed mostly through use of supports and through positive appraisals in the families.
Adversity and at least one caring, emotionally available person	Prosocial attitude Rebounding and carrying on Sense of self determination	Outcome a continuum of vulnerability to resilience Toughening effect Sense of having overcome that fosters mastery Enhanced coping	Accessed skills and abilities may occur within the individual or interpersonally through a supportive, caring and responsive environment
Illness or loss	Environmental factors: frailty, determination, previous experience learning to cope, access to care, cultural-based health beliefs, family support, self-care activities, caring for others and functioning efficiently External factors: Structure of the environmental factors and stress		Resilience is conceptualized as a coiled wire enclosed in a box. External factors of resilience are a configuration of environmental factors within the box and stress
Social Protective: health care resources; social integration Family Protective: family atmosphere; family support/ resources Illness-Related Risk: Illness perspective; illness-related distress	Individual Risk: defensive coping (sustained over time) Individual Protective: derived meaning; courageous coping	Resilience Self-esteem, self-trans-cendence, confidence/ mastery Quality of Life Well-being	Illness-related risk and social and family protective factors directly affect individual risk and protective factors. All these factors directly or indirectly affect resilience and quality of life outcomes.
Time since death of parent Age of adolescent at death Gender Circumstances of death (sudden or expected)	Parental attachment as basis for developing social relationships Adaptive coping	Social competence, global self-worth, perceived health	Adaptive coping consistently predicted outcome variables of resilience. Attachment was not significant

(continued)

TABLE 17-1.   NURSING LITERATURE ON RESILIENCE (*Continued*)

SOURCE	METHODS OF KNOWLEDGE DEVELOPMENT	POPULATIONS STUDIED	DEFINITION OF RESILIENCE	PRIMARY BOUNDARIES
(Hockenberry-Eaton, Kemp & Dilorio, 1994)	Quasi-experimental study of physiological and psychosocial variables	Children with cancer	(Inferred) A process of responding to life stressors that involves protective factors	Individual biological and psychological process
(Hunter, 2001; Hunter & Chandler, 1999)	Triangulation: Concept clarification through groups, phenomeno-logical analysis and journal writing. Cross-cultural comparisons Quantitative analysis using Resilience Scale	Homeless adolescents Adolescents in variety of situational settings across 2 cultures	State of being that allows a person to overcome adversity without suffering long-term negative consequences	Individual psychological state taking two forms Objective and subjective perspectives on a continuum
(Jacelon, 1997)	Synthesis of literature on resilience	Children, Adolescents, Adults in various circumstances	(Borrowed dictionary definition) Ability of people to 'spring back' in the face of adversity	Individual psychological trait and process
(Kadner, 1989)	Synthesis of literature on resilience in context of mental health services	Vulnerable populations, especially psychiatric	Ability to regain psychosocial equilibrium after a brief fragmentation in response to severe stress	Individual psychological trait, partially physically (genetically) predisposed
(Mandleco & Peery, 2000)	Review of relevant literature on resilience from developmental psychology, child psychiatry, and nursing	Children	Tendency to spring back, rebound, or recoil that involves the capacity to respond and to endure to develop and master in spite of life stressors or adversity	Individual psychological state influenced by biological trait

COMPONENTS: ANTECEDENTS/ EXOGENOUS VARIABLES	COMPONENTS: ATTRIBUTES/ PROCESSES	COMPONENTS: OUTCOMES	KEY RELATIONAL STATEMENTS/ FINDINGS
Presence of stressor	Psychological Protective: coping, self-perception, family environment, social support Physiological stress response (endocrine) Psychological stress response (state anxiety)	Well-being	Family environment and global self-worth predict epinephrine levels; social support from friends predicts norepinephrine levels; family environment and social support predict state anxiety.
Developmental independence Developed competencies Invincibility Mastery Resourcefulness Perseverance Stress	Connected Resilience: self-esteem, self-efficacy, connectedness, trust, competence, ego resilience, sociability OR Survival resilience: Psychopathology, maladaption, social and emotional withdrawal, high-risk behaviors, survival tactics of violence		Adolescents without support showed survival and self-protected resilience; those with support showed a connected form resilience
Triad of personal, family, and community factors including resources, above-average intelligence, self-reliance, independence, and positive outlook			Process is labeled "resilition." Trait is labeled resilience
Stressor as antecedent is implied	Attributes are psychological resources: ego strength, social intimacy, and resourcefulness	Outcome implied is psychological equilibrium manifested as coping	The aggregate of psychological resources promotes coping efficacy
	Internal biological factors: General health, genetic predisposition, temperament, and gender. Internal psychological factors: Cognitive capacity, coping ability, and personality characteristics. External within family factors: Home environment, parenting practices, and particular family members External outside family factors: Supportive individuals, community resources		Interactional or transactional relationship exists, with the internal and external factors affecting resilience. These relationships also exist between the internal and external factors

(Continued)

TABLE 17-1. NURSING LITERATURE ON RESILIENCE (*Continued*)

SOURCE	METHODS OF KNOWLEDGE DEVELOPMENT	POPULATIONS STUDIED	DEFINITION OF RESILIENCE	PRIMARY BOUNDARIES
(McCubbin & McCubbin, 1996; McCubbin & McCubbin, 1993)	Triangulation of qualitative and quantitative approaches for model and instrument development.	Families experiencing illness of a family member, usually a child	Positive behavioral patterns and functional competencies individuals and the family unit demonstrate under stressful or adverse circumstances, which determine the family's ability to recover by maintaining its integrity as a unit while ensuring, and where necessary, restoring the well-being of family members and the family unit as a whole	Dynamic family behavioral and functional process
(Polk, 1997)	Concept synthesis for model development using nursing model as philosophical underpinnings	No specific population	The ability to transform disaster into a growth experience and move forward.	Individual pattern that is transformative
(Rew et al., 2001)	Descriptive/exploratory correlational design	Homeless adolescents	No specific theoretical definition. Resilience operationalized by Resilience Scale (Wagnild & Young, 1993)	Individual psychological It is unclear if viewed as state or trait
(Stewart et al., 1997)	Synthesis review of literature on resilience and health	Children	Capability of individuals to cope successfully in the face of significant change, adversity, or risk	Individual physiological and psychological state that changes over time and is influenced by protective factors in the individual and environment

COMPONENTS: ANTECEDENTS/ EXOGENOUS VARIABLES	COMPONENTS: ATTRIBUTES/ PROCESSES	COMPONENTS: OUTCOMES	KEY RELATIONAL STATEMENTS/ FINDINGS
Family experienced stress and hardship	Family-developed strengths and competencies in adjustment phase, including patterns of family functioning, resources, appraisal, coping strategies, and problem-solving	Restoration and adaptation: well-functioning individual members, family sense of balance and harmony in carrying out tasks and responsibilities, and in relationship to the community.	Resiliency factors that helped families dealing with cancer recover included internal family rapid mobilization and reorganization; social support from the health care team; extended family, the community and the workplace; and changes in appraisal to make the situation more comprehensive, manageable, and meaningful.
Human and environmental energy field	Dispositional attributes, e.g., physical and ego-related attributes such as competence and sense of self Patterns of relationships and roles Situational patterns— characteristic approaches to situations or stressors Philosophical pattern of personal beliefs		Transformation manifested as specific dispositional, relational, situational, and philosophical patterns
Homelessness as condition Loneliness, hopelessness, life-threatening behaviors, and connectedness	Resilience may be an adaptive or defense strategy, rather than a protective factor		Loneliness, hopelessness, life-threatening behaviors, and connectedness were negative predictors of resilience as measured by Resilience Scale.
Transition, increased stressors	*Protective Factors* Individual Level: Coping, self-help, self-esteem, intelligence, self-efficacy Family Level: Positive parent-child attachment, future orientation, rules in the household Social support Community Level: Positive school experiences	Maintenance of physiological and psychological health such as: Global psychosocial adjustment Lack of psychopathology Self-esteem Confidence Intelligence Positive immune response	Relationship of resilience and health is clarified in discussions of risk and protective factors and resilient outcomes, in particular, psychological and physical health and health behavior.

(Continued)

TABLE 17-1.   NURSING LITERATURE ON RESILIENCE (*Continued*)

SOURCE	METHODS OF KNOWLEDGE DEVELOPMENT	POPULATIONS STUDIED	DEFINITION OF RESILIENCE	PRIMARY BOUNDARIES
(Vinson, 2002)	Inner Core Child Resilience Model Development and Testing based on resilience literature synthesis and data-based findings of descriptive correlational study	School-aged children with asthma	A combination of personality characteristics, family influences, and available social and cultural supportive environments that permits the epigenetic unfolding of adaptive processes	Individual psychosocial process
(Wagnild & Young, 1990, 1993)	Grounded theory and factor analysis of instrument.	Older adults	A personality characteristic that moderates the negative effects of stress and promotes adaptation	Individual trait
(Woodgate, 1999; Woodgate & McClement, 1997)	Synthesis of resilience literature in context of cancer to develop a model	Adolescents with cancer	Dynamic process involving the development of resources within the individual that allows the individual to gain a positive outcome in the face of significant adversity	Individual, dynamic psychological process

BOUNDARIES OF RESILIENCE

With the exception of the psychological dimension that is identified by all authors, all the other boundaries of resilience, either explicit or implied, are inconsistent. There is no consensus on whether resilience is a trait, state, process, or some combination of these dimensions. Most definitions imply that a change occurs, but there is inconsistency as to whether the resilience change is a return to a steady state or is part of growth producing process. Jacelon (1997) explicitly distinguishes and labels resilience as the trait and "resilition" as the process. Only one definition explicitly addresses a time-frame (Hunter, 2001; Hunter & Chandler, 1999).

The existence of a biological dimension was strikingly missing from most of the nursing literature, with the exception of Hockenberry's and Mandleco's works (Hockenberry-Eaton et al., 1994; Mandleco & Peery, 2000). In the context of childhood cancer, Hockenberry argued that activation of the endocrine system as a less adaptive response to stress—as indicated by an elevation of both catecholamine and cortisol—could indicate less resilience to the stressors associated with cancer (Hockenberry-Eaton, Dilorio, & Kemp, 1995). Mandleco and Peery (2000) identified four biological factors as possibly affecting resilience: general health, genetic predisposition, temperament, and gender. Re-

COMPONENTS: ANTECEDENTS/ EXOGENOUS VARIABLES	COMPONENTS: ATTRIBUTES/ PROCESSES	COMPONENTS: OUTCOMES	KEY RELATIONAL STATEMENTS/ FINDINGS
Exogenous Variables: Child Characteristics, Family Environment	Coping Patterns, Threat Appraisal	Quality of Life, Illness Indices	Paths are from family-to-child characteristics, child characteristics to appraisal, appraisal to quality of life, family to child coping, child coping to illness indices and child-perceived quality of life to illness indices.
Personal Competence, including self-reliance, independence, determination, invincibility, mastery, resourcefulness, and perseverance Acceptance of Self and Life, including adaptability, balance, flexibility, and balanced perspective of life			The Resilience Scale is of potential use as a measure of internal resources and of the positive contribution an individual brings to a difficult life event.
Stressors	*Protective Factors:* Self-concept Meaning Coping Social support from family External support from peers	Adaptation (social competence) or maladaptation (depression, low self-esteem)	Resilience is a mediating process, initiated by stressors, that results in outcomes on a continuum of adaptation and maladaptation

search supports that children with resilience are usually quite healthy and have little hereditary or chronic illness. However, hypotheses about gender and temperament need further exploration. Evidence that temperament is a factor of resilience is derived from studies examining infant temperament; however, it is not clear that temperament is biologically based. Regarding gender, although males are more vulnerable to all risk factors, one cannot assume that more vulnerability equates to less resilience.

Resilience was most frequently studied as an individual dimension rather than as a family or community aggregate. In studies focused on individuals, the family or community variables were often included as protective factors that influence outcomes for the individual. In some ways, the state-of-knowledge on family resilience is further along than individually focused research, in that the limited number of proposed models is more consistently being used and evaluated, and there is more consistency in the ways that family level measures are used.

Nurses studying resilience seem to assume the importance of obtaining subjective indicators. These subjective indicators were obtained as narratives and as self-reported quantitative measures of resilience-related concepts. As indicated in the methods section, nurse researchers have also developed creative methods for obtaining the personal meanings associated with resilience. Ways of making sense of combined, simultaneous objective, physiological measures as they relate to subjective ratings is not addressed well in either the nursing or the general literature. Because nurses focus on both physiological and psychosocial aspects of health, it would seem logical that nurse researchers would be well positioned to provide leadership in this area.

DESCRIPTION OF RESILIENCE: THE THEORY

There is agreement that models of resilience should include factors generally characterized as "protective." In addition, "risk" factors are also generally identified as influencing resilience processes and outcomes. A major problem in developing theory about resilience is that these protective and risk factors frequently resemble "laundry lists." That is, they lack an explicit description of underlying assumptions or an explicit theoretical framework that describe the mechanisms by which the protective and risk factors are linked to outcomes. Additionally, much confusion relates to whether these protective and risk factors are direct ameliorative effects or, rather, they are interactive effects reserved for individuals who have a particular attribute and who were relatively unaffected by high or low levels of adversity (Luthar & Cicchetti, 2000).

Important components that should be considered in all modeling efforts to understand and enhance resilience are context, psychological and physiological mediating units, and the patterns of mediators in relation to the context (Coyne & Downey, 1991; Freitas & Downey, 1998). Further, there is value in interventions that manipulate mediating variables, such as coping and hope, that have been found to influence resilience outcomes (Singer, 2001).

Masten (2001) provides a useful distinction between variable-focused approaches and person-focused approaches to model development. In variable-focused approaches, multivariate statistics are used to test for linkages among measures of adversity, outcomes, and environmental or individual qualities that may protect or compensate for negative consequences. Models may examine direct, indirect, and interaction effects (Luthar et al., 2000b; Masten, 2001). Direct-effects models hypothesize direct effects in multivariate correlational analyses. A direct-effects example is when the relationship of high and low scores on outcomes is directly related to high and low scores on measures of adversity, or when a path diagram directly links specific variables with an outcome. Figure 17-1 A and B illustrate the direct effects model. Indirect-effect models are those that hypothesize that the effect of variables, such as adversity or personal characteristics, is mediated by another variable, such as parental styles, as seen in Figure 17-1C. Interaction models hypothesize that the effects of adversity can be modified by individual characteristics or the environment. In general, variable-focused research indicates that adversity does not result in lasting or major effects, unless moderating and mediating systems, such as parent or social protective factors, are compromised (Masten, 2001).

Person-focused research attempts to identify and describe the patterns of variables that naturally occur, often identifying persons with either positive or poor functioning, and then examining what might contribute to these outcomes; or, using cut-off scores on selected variables to categorize adversity subgroups, and then examining outcomes in these groups. These types of person-focused designs often lack comparison low-risk groups, which are important to answer questions of whether resilient children differ from children who are doing well, but do not have high-risk char-

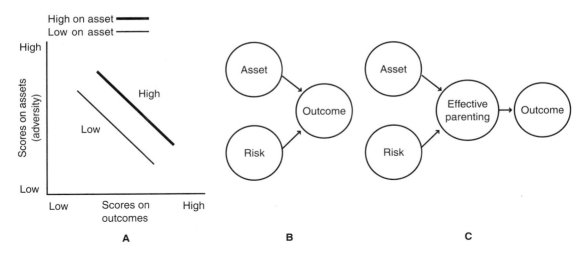

■ **Figure 17-1.** Variable-focused research models: (A) main, (B) direct, and (C) indirect effects.

acteristics. Masten (2001) also argues for more complex person-oriented models that include both health versus maladaptive pathways of development in lives studied over time, giving special attention to turning points. These pathway models have a greater potential for providing intervention frameworks.

APPROACHES TO KNOWLEDGE DEVELOPMENT ABOUT RESILIENCE IN NURSING LITERATURE

Although there is a relatively small amount of research on resilience in the nursing literature, the work accomplished to date has creatively used a variety of approaches to gain a fuller understanding of resilience. In no other discipline is such a rich combination of approaches to studying resilience found. Several of the articles in Table 17-1 are extensive analyses and syntheses of existing literature on resilience (Dyer & McGuinness, 1996; Jacelon, 1997; Kadner, 1989; Polk, 1997; Stewart et al., 1997; Woodgate & McClement, 1997; Woodgate, 1999), and many of these were used to propose models of resilience in specific health contexts. For example, Woodgate (1999) derived the Resilience Model as Applied to Adolescents with Cancer based on her synthesis of the literature on resilience within the context of cancer, and Vinson (2002) proposed a model of resilience in children with asthma. Another synthesis article used a nursing metatheory, the Science of Unitary Human Beings as the underlying framework for developing a resilience model (Polk, 1997).

In addition to literature synthesis approaches, several articles were data based. Qualitative-research approaches used to gain understanding of resilience included grounded theory and phenomenology. Qualitative methods of data collection included open-ended or phenomenological interviews, focus groups, and free-writing exercises. Some authors used triangulation of qualitative and/or quantitative empirical studies to derive models of resilience in the context of health or a specific illness. As examples, Haase, Heiney, Ruccione, and Stutzer (1999) used a decision-making process to triangulate qualitative and quantitative approaches for instrument identification or development and model testing and Hunter and Chandler (Hunter, 2001) conducted concept clarification by triangulating qualitative data collection methods, such as free-writing exercises with quantitative measures of resilience, to conduct a cross-cultural comparison of resilience.

The data-based nursing studies in Table 17-1 fall into three categories of design. First are studies describing characteristics of a sample of participants who were designated, a priori, as having resilience. Examples of such studies are: resilience in women older than 85 experiencing illness or loss (Felten, 2000; Felten & Hall, 2001); resilience in homeless adolescents (Hunter & Chandler, 1999); resilience in adult daughters of battered women (Humphreys, 2001); and modes of comfort used by a resilient survivor suffering multiple losses and severe, excruciating burn pain (Morse & Carter, 1995).

Next are studies of resilience conducted with a specific population, but without a priori designation of participants as being resilient. Examples include resilience studies of adolescents with cancer (Haase et al., 1999); resilience in a sample of adults who lost a parent when they were adolescents (Heinzer, 1995); and resilience in children with asthma (Vinson, 2002). The third design type includes studies that did not have resilience as a primary focus, but found resilience as an outcome variable. Examples of these studies include a study of women with a cardiac pacemaker (Beery, Sommers, & Hall, 2002) and a study of risk behavior in adolescents with cancer (Hollen, Hobbie, Finley, & Hiebert, 2001). While these studies fit into Masten's description of variable-focused and person-focused research, they do not reflect the complexity of design Masten recommended, to include both healthy versus maladaptive pathways of development in lives studied over time, giving special attention to turning points (Masten, 2001). By their creative approaches to clarify the patterns/processes/components of resilience, it is clear that studies conducted by nurses are headed in the "right" direction. More complex designs would seem to be a logical next phase.

SPECIFIC NURSING MODELS OF RESILIENCE

The articles in Table 17-1 that describe literature synthesis and concept analysis of resilience indicate the value that nurse scientists place on carefully developing theory. Individual-level resilience models include mastery of chronic illness with resilience as an emergent outcome (White, 1995); a "CARE" framework (containment, awareness, resilience, and engagement) to guide mental health practice (McAllister & Walsh, 2003); the Adolescent Resilience Model for adolescents with cancer and other chronic conditions (Haase et al., 1999); the Inner Core Child Resilience Model for children with asthma (Vinson, 2002); the Resiliency Model applied to adolescents with cancer (Woodgate, 1999); a model of resilience in the context of loss of a parent (Heinzer, 1995); and a model of resilience in community-dwelling women older than 85, overcoming adversity from illness or loss (Felten, 2000; Felten & Hall, 2001). Many of these models were thoughtfully developed, with underlying assumptions or philosophical perspectives explicated, and the perspectives of those experiencing the adversity taken into consideration.

Although there is less nursing literature on family or community resilience models, the work that has been done has made significant contributions to knowledge. The Family Resilience Model developed by McCubbin and McCubbin (1996) is increasingly supported in the literature on family resilience (Board & Ryan-Wenger, 2000; Smith, 1997; Svavarsdottir, McCubbin, & Kane, 2000; White, Bichter, Koeckeritz, Lee, & Munch, 2002). Other family models are also being proposed. Drummond, Kysela, McDonald, and Query (2002) proposed and tested a model of family adaptation that identified family protective factors of appraisal, support, and coping as mediators of adaptation. Appraisal was a key variable predicting adaptation. These authors identify the need for further concept clarification of the mediating variables and suggest narrative analysis as a possible method.

Across the models of resilience, the myriad of both adversity and positive concepts were inconsistently identified as antecedents, critical components, and outcomes of resilience. Antecedents usually included adversity (e.g., death, loss, illness, stressor(s), and homelessness). Protective factors were modeled as antecedents in only a few studies (Haase et al., 1999; Hunter & Chandler, 1999; Polk, 1997). Across several studies, especially those that viewed resilience as a trait, it was difficult to discern the role or order of resilience-related concepts, such as coping, hope, or mastery. These concepts were alternatively viewed as antecedent and critical component protective factors or as outcomes of resilience. For example, in some articles, coping is viewed as a mediating protective factor, while in other studies, it is an outcome of resilience. Reflective of the general literature, many protective factors do fall into broad classes of factors classified as individual, social or family.

It is clear that more work needs to be done to clarify the relationship among concepts that are correlated with resilience and those that influence resilience. To increase explanatory power, this work will most productively be done in longitudinal studies, with models that attempt to capture the full, integrative perspective of resilience.

APPLICATIONS OF THE THEORY

Research to Develop a Model and Guide the Development of Intervention

The Adolescent Resilience Model (ARM) provides one example of how a theoretical model that is grounded in contextual experiences can guide interventions. The context for the ARM was chronic illness in adolescents. Most of the work was done from the perspective of adolescents with cancer; some studies included parent and health care provider perspectives.

To develop the ARM, two series of studies were conducted: (1) *model generation* studies, using inductive approaches, and (2) *model evaluation* studies, involving instrumentation and exploratory model testing (Haase et al., 1999). The qualitative, model-generating studies provided a basis for development of the ARM through identification and clarification of salient concepts to be included in the model, and as a qualitative means of evaluating subsequent model testing results. These studies were also guided by the Haase Decision-Making Process for Model and Instrument Development (Haase et al., 1999).

Research to Evaluate Instruments

The quantitative model and instrument evaluation studies for the ARM were primarily done using latent variable structural-equation modeling approaches. The studies were done to evaluate the psychometric properties of the instruments used to measure each latent variable, and to develop an appropriate measurement model. Based on the exploratory studies of the theoretical model, factors were identified that affect the development of resilience. The resulting ARM, as it is being studied longitudinally and guiding interventions, is found in Figure 17-2.

Both protective and risk factors are included in the ARM. These factors with their related variables are highlighted in Table 17-2. Three classes of ARM protective factors are hypothesized to *positively affect* resilience outcomes. Class I Individual Protective Factors include courageous or positive coping and derived meaning. Class II Family Protective Factors include family atmosphere and support/resources available to the family. Class III Social Protective Factors include health care resources and social integration. Two classes of ARM risk factors are hypothesized to *negatively affect* resilience. The

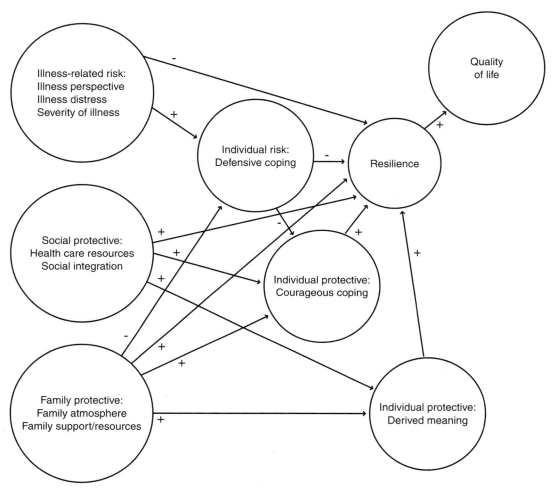

■ **Figure 17-2.** The adolescent resilience model.

Class IV Individual Risk Factor is sustained defensive coping. The Class V Illness-Related Factors include illness perspective and illness distress. The outcome factors of resilience include self-esteem, mastery/confidence, and self-transcendence, as well as quality of life, defined as a sense of well-being.

Hunter and Chandler (1999) studied the appropriateness of using the Resiliency Scale, developed by Wagnild and Young (1993) to measure resilience in adolescence. This study is described in Using Middle Range Theories 17-1.

INSTRUMENTS USED IN EMPIRICAL TESTING

Measurement is an approach to knowledge development for resilience that requires more attention. The lack of instruments to directly measure resilience may be connected with the lack of a consistent

TABLE 17-2 ADOLESCENT RESILIENCE MODEL LATENT AND MANIFEST VARIABLES

LATENT FACTOR	MANIFEST VARIABLES
I Individual Protective Courageous coping Derived meaning	Confrontive coping Optimistic coping Supportant coping Hope Spiritual perspective
II Family Protective Family atmosphere Family support/Resources	Adaptability and cohesion Parent-adolescent communication Perceived social support—family Family strengths Socioeconomic status variables
III Social Protective Health care resources Social integration	Perceived social support—health care provider Adolescent support program participation and satisfaction Adolescent support program site evaluation Perceived social support—friends
IV Individual Risk Defensive Coping	Evasive coping Emotive coping
V Illness-related Risk Illness perspective Illness distress	Uncertainty in illness Symptom distress Severity of illness
VI Resilience Quality of Life	Confidence/mastery Self-transcendence Self-esteem Sense of well-being

view as to whether resilience is a state, trait, or process. Only one direct measure of resilience was found. Wagnild and Young's measure of resilience was developed to address concerns of lack of empirical support for the relationships between resilience and psychosocial adaptation (Wagnild & Young, 1993). Resilience was conceptualized as a personality characteristic rather than a process. The instrument was developed from a grounded theory study of 24 older women who had adapted successfully to a major life event (Wagnild & Young, 1990). Five components of resilience were identified from that study. These components were validated via a review of literature and developed into a theoretical definition of resilience. In psychometric analysis of the factors in the Resilience Scale, a two-factor structure—personal competence and acceptance of self and life—was found (Wagnild & Young, 1993). This scale has been used in other studies that represent different cultural and age samples

17-1 USING MIDDLE RANGE THEORIES

This study, using a triangulated research design, examined the meaning of resilience to adolescents, and whether the Resiliency Scale can be appropriately used to measure this phenomenon in adolescents. For the study, researchers enrolled 51 students from English classes of four high schools, randomly selected from a New England city. The students selected engaged in high-risk behaviors, such as dropping out of school, becoming pregnant, or engaging in violence, and were from ethnic/racial minority groups (11.7%).

The students completed the Resiliency Scale and a demographic profile, engaged in free-writing exercises, and participated in focus discussion groups. The Resiliency Scale is a 25-item instrument, using a 7-point Likert response scale. Validity of this instrument had been established in adult populations over a 3-year period of use. The reliability coefficient of .75 and the alpha coefficient of .72 were reported. The approach to the free-writing component of the study was based on WRITE, a method in which individuals respond to a stimulus to help them express thoughts and feelings. Students wrote for 10 minutes each, during nine English class periods. Following the writing activity, the students read what they had written to a group of the other participants, who provided positive feedback. The Resiliency Scale and demographic data were analyzed using multivariate analysis, and the students' writings and field notes from the discussion groups were analyzed using a process of extracting and reformulating statements into themes.

In general, the students identified themselves as resilient, boys more so than girls, and Latinos and African Americans more so than Caucasians. For the subscores of self-esteem and self-efficacy, there were similar response patterns, boys scoring higher than girls, and Latinos and African Americans scoring higher than Caucasians. The qualitative analysis of the data revealed that adolescents had a unique perception of resilience. To them, resilience meant survival rather than possessing a healthy sense of self, a strong sense of worth, or being able to connect with and trust others.

Hunter, A. J., & Chandler, G. E. (1999). Adolescent resilience. *Image: Journal of Nursing Scholarship, 31*(3), 242–247.

(Aroian, Schappler-Morris, Neary, Spitzer, & Tran, 1997; Humphreys, 2003; Hunter & Chandler, 1999; Rew, Taylor-Seehafer, Thomas, & Yockey, 2001).

Most studies using quantitative methods in the Table 17-1 literature used existing instruments or developed instruments to measure numerous variables in proposed models. However, in many cases, it is not clear whether the instruments were derived from theories that are congruent with the conceptual frameworks or philosophical approaches being used in the studies. Haase et al. (1999) describe one approach to identifying and/or developing instruments that is clearly linked to the emerging ARM theory. Methods triangulation was done in a series of studies to develop and test the ARM and to identify or develop the instruments used to evaluate the model (Haase, 1987; Haase, Britt, Coward, Leidy, & Penn, 1992; Haase et al., 1999; Haase & Rostad, 1994). Decision trees were used to decide on labels and definitions for each model factor, and to decide whether to use existing instruments or ones developed to measure the model factors. This iterative process of decision-making sought to retain the inductively derived meanings from the qualitative studies, while taking advantage of existing theory and instruments. The result was a set of 15 instruments to measure manifest variables—8 existing instruments meeting established criteria for reliability and validity and 7 new instruments. To test the ARM and instruments, latent variable instrument and model testing studies were done (Haase et al., 1999).

It is clear that additional measurement work is essential to further the science of resilience from a nursing perspective. Cultural considerations in measurement are not well addressed. Measurement in nursing research on resilience needs to consider the issues of boundaries, including trait/process and physiological/psychological. Measurement also needs to focus on differences in resilience based on developmental factors, including age (Research Application 17-1).

17-1 RESEARCH APPLICATION

Using the Adolescent Resilience Model, interventions can be designed to target specific protective or risk factors to enhance resilience outcomes. Several studies are currently being developed and tested using the Adolescent Resilience Model. In one study, the Adolescent Resilience Model is being used to guide a music video production.

The study aims are to (1) test the efficacy of a therapeutic music video (TMV) intervention for adolescents and young adults (AYA) during the acute phase of stem-cell transplant (SCT), and (2) qualitatively examine the self-reported benefits of the TMV intervention for AYA.

For AYA undergoing SCT, participation in the TMV intervention is hypothesized to *directly*:

- Decrease illness-related distress
- Improve family environment
- Increase perceived social support
- Decrease defensive coping
- Increase positive coping
- Increase derived meaning.

Through improved family environment and perceived social support, the TMV is also hypothesized to *indirectly* affect:

- Positive coping
- Derived meaning.

As a consequence of enhancing these variables, the intervention is expected to:

- Increase resilience
- Increase quality of life.

In addition to the efficacy of the intervention for AYA, it is hypothesized that the TMV intervention is helpful and meaningful to family caregivers. This aim will be qualitatively evaluated.

The multisite study design is a two-group, randomized clinical trial. Study participants in the treatment group will receive the TMV intervention over 6 sessions, conducted by a board-certified music therapist. In the sessions, participants will select music, engage in song writing, music recording, and developing the visual content for a music video. Study participants randomized to the low-dose control group will receive six sessions conducted by a low-dose Intervener, focused on discussing content of self-selected books on tape. Sites in five states will participate in the study to increase sample ethnic, cultural, and economic diversity.

SUMMARY

The work of nurse scientists to understand resilience is in beginning stages, yet contributions to the general knowledge of resilience are considerable. Areas of strengths include the careful attention to theory, both by clarifying concepts through literature analysis and synthesis and by using qualitative methods that explore experiences of resilience from the perspectives of those who have experienced adversity. To advance the science, nurses will need to focus efforts on measurement issues, so that instruments are context and culturally sensitive, meaning based, and time sensitive. Most pressing is the need for longitudinal, prospective studies of resilience to test integrative models. Additionally, some models may be at a stage where they can be tested through manipulation of variables by developing targeted interventions to enhance resilience.

ANALYSIS EXERCISE

Using the criteria presented in Chapter 2, critique the theory, Resilience. Compare your conclusions about the theory with those found in Appendix A. A nurse scholar who has worked with the theory completed the analysis found in the appendix.

Internal Criticism
1. Clarity
2. Consistency
3. Adequacy

4. Logical development
5. Level of theory development

External Criticism
1. Reality convergence
2. Utility
3. Significance
4. Discrimination
5. Scope of theory
6. Complexity

WEB RESOURCES

1. This site provides information, education and training materials on strengths-based approaches to resilience. It features the work of Wolin and Wolin, two prominent researchers who focus on resilience:
   http://www.projectresilience.com
2. This site offers a potpourri of useful publications, forums, training information, and practical applications regarding resilience:
   http://www.resiliency.com
3. ResilienceNet provides worldwide sources of current, reviewed information about human resilience. Describes the International Resilience Project. It can be accessed at:
   http://ericps.crc.uiuc.edu/resnet/

4. American Psychological Association Help Center site on resilience:
   http://helping.apa.org/resilience
5. A chapter in Basic Behavioral Science Research for Mental Health by the National Institute of Mental Health (NIMH) on Vulnerability and Resilience can be found at:
   www.nimh.nih.gov/publicat/baschap2.cfm
6. Resilience archives on ERIC: *http://www.askeric. org/Virtual/Listserv_Archives/resilience-l.shtml*
7. A full-text guide to resilience research and application: *http://ericeece.org/pubs/books/ resguide.html*
8. The National Resilience Resource Center Web site at the University of Minnesota:
   http://www.cce.umn.edu/nrrc/index.shtml
9. Center for Effective Collaboration and Prac-

tice Web site. Describes community approach to resilience: *http://cecp.air.org/resources/ journals/ Journal.html*

10. An easily read site summarizing resilience perspectives. Focuses on resilience in early childhood: *http://homepages.picknowl.com.au/ Julietta/1-0Cont.htm*

11. Resilience/Practice, Vol 5, #1. Publication of the Center for Applied Research and Educational Improvement at the University of Minnesota. Entire volume focused on resilience and includes cultural perspectives on resilience. *http://education.umn.edu/CAREI/ Reports/Rpractice/Spring97/default.html*

12. This site provides information on community resilience programs: *http://www.cedworks.com/ bookstore/crpmain.html*

13. Discovery Health Channel resource on resilience. Includes personal stories of resilience: *http://health.discovery.com/ convergence/recovery/recovery.html*

14. General resources on family resilience: *http://www.nnfr.org/general/*

15. Gateway to links on the concepts of learned resourcefulness, resiliency, psychological hardiness, and related concepts as they apply to families and children, workplace stress, and personal development: *http://www.css.edu/ users/dswenson/web/ resilience.html*

16. Discusses resilience programs focusing on prevention: *http://www.hc-sc.gc.ca/ hecs-sesc/cds/publications/resiliency/toc3.htm*

REFERENCES

Antonovsky, A. (1979). *Health, stress, and coping.* San Francisco: Jossey-Bass.

Armstrong, L. (2000). *It's not about the bike: My journey back to life.* New York: Putnam.

Aroian, K. J., Schappler-Morris, N., Neary, S., Spitzer, A., & Tran, T. V. (1997). Psychometric evaluation of the Russian Language version of the Resilience Scale. *Journal of Nursing Measurement, 5*(2), 151–164.

Bandura, A. (1977). Self-efficacy: Toward a unifying theory of behavioral change. *Psychological Review, 84,* 191–215.

Beery, T. A., Sommers, M. S., & Hall, J. (2002). Focused life stories of women with cardiac pacemakers. *Western Journal of Nursing Research, 24*(1), 7–23; discussion 23–27.

Block, J. (1980). The role of ego control and ego resiliency in the origins of behavior. *Development of Cognition/Minnesota Symposia on Child Psychology, 13.*

Board, R., & Ryan-Wenger, N. (2000). State of the science on parental stress and family functioning in pediatric intensive care units. *American Journal of Critical Care, 9*(2), 106–122; quiz 123–124.

Bosworth, K., & Earthman, E. (2002). From theory to practice: School leaders' perspectives on resiliency. *Journal of Clinical Psychology, 58*(3), 299–306.

Coyne, J. C., & Downey, G. (1991). Social factors and psychopathology: Stress, social support, and coping processes. *Annual Review of Psychology, 42,* 401–425.

Drummond, J., Kysela, G. M., McDonald, L., & Query, B. (2002). The family adaptation model: Examination of dimensions and relations. *Canadian Journal of Nursing Research, 34*(1), 29–46.

Dyer, J. G., & McGuinness, T. M. (1996). Resilience: analysis of the concept. *Archives of Psychiatric Nursing, 10*(5), 276–282.

Felten, B. S. (2000). Resilience in a multicultural sample of community-dwelling women older than age 85. *Clinical Nursing Research, 9*(2), 102–123.

Felten, B. S., & Hall, J. M. (2001). Conceptualizing resilience in women older than 85: Overcoming adversity from illness or loss. *Journal of Gerontological Nursing, 27*(11), 46–53.

Fine, S. B. (1991). Resilience and human adaptability: Who rises above adversity? 1990 Eleanor Clarke Slagle Lecture. *American Journal of Occupational Therapy, 45*(6), 493–503.

Forsyth, G. L., Delaney, K. D., & Gresham, M. L. (1984). Vying for a winning position: Management style of the chronically ill. *Research in Nursing & Health, 7*(3), 181–188.

Freitas, A. L., & Downey, G. (1998). Resilience: a dynamic perspective. *International Journal of Behavioral Development, 22*(2), 263–285.

Garmezy, N. (1974). The study of competence in children at risk for severe psychopathology. In C. Koupernik (Ed.), *The child in his family: Children at psychiatric risk* (Vol. 3, pp. 77–97). New York: Wiley.

Garmezy, N. (1981). *Children under stress: Perspectives on antecedents and correlates of vulnerability and resistance to psychopathology:* NY: John Wiley & Sons.

Garmezy, N. (1991). Resilience in children's adaptation to negative life events and stressed environments. *Pediatric Annals, 20,* 459–466.

Garmezy, N., Masten, A. S., & Tellegen, A. (1984). The study of stress and competence in children: A building block for developmental psychopathology. *Child Development, 55*(1), 97–111.

Haase, J. (1987). The components of courage in chronically ill adolescents. *Advances in Nursing Science, 9*(2), 64–80.

Haase, J. E., Britt, T., Coward, D. D., Leidy, N. K., & Penn, P. E. (1992). Simultaneous concept analysis of spiritual perspective, hope, acceptance and self-transcendence. *Image: the Journal of Nursing Scholarship, 24*(2), 141–147.

Haase, J. E., & Heiney, S. P., Ruccione, K. S., & Stutzer, C. (1999). Research triangulation to derive meaning-based quality-of-life theory: Adolescent resilience model and instrument development. *International Journal of Cancer Supplement, 12*, 125–131.

Haase, J. E., & Rostad, M. (1994). Experiences of completing cancer therapy: Children's perspectives. *Oncology Nursing Forum, 21*(9), 1483–1492; discussion 1493–1494.

Hauser, S. T., Vieyra, M. A., Jacobson, A. M., & Wertlieb, D. (1985). Vulnerability and resilience in adolescence: Views from the family. *Journal of Early Adolescence, 5*, 81–100.

Hauser, S. T., Vieyra, M. A., Jacobson, A. M., & Wertlieb, D. (1989). Family aspects of vulnerability and resilience in adolescence: A theoretical perspective. In T. Dugan & R. Coles (Eds.), *The child in our times: Studies in the development of resiliencey.* New York: Brunner-Routledge.

Hawley, D. R., & DeHaan, L. (1996). Toward a definition of family resilience: Integrating life-span and family perspectives. *Family Process, 35*(3), 283–298.

Heinzer, M. M. (1995). Loss of a parent in childhood: Attachment and coping in a model of adolescent resilience. *Holistic Nursing Practice, 9*(3), 27–37.

Henry, D. L. (2001). Resilient children: What they tell us about coping with maltreatment. *Social Work Health Care, 34*(3–4), 283–298.

Hockenberry-Eaton, M., Dilorio, C., & Kemp, V. (1995). The relationship of illness longevity and relapse with self-perception, cancer stressors, anxiety, and coping strategies in children with cancer. *Journal of Pediatric Oncology Nursing, 12*(2), 71–79.

Hockenberry-Eaton, M., Kemp, V., & Dilorio, C. (1994). Cancer stressors and protective factors: Predictors of stress experienced during treatment for childhood cancer. *Research in Nursing & Health, 17*(5), 351–361.

Hollen, P. J., Hobbie, W. L., Finley, S. M., & Hiebert, S. M. (2001). The relationship of resiliency to decision making and risk behaviors of cancer-surviving adolescents. *Journal of Pediatric Oncology Nursing, 18*(5), 188–204.

Humphreys, J. C. (2001). Turnings and adaptations in resilient daughters of battered women. *Image: Journal of Nursing Scholarship, 33*(3), 245–251.

Humphreys, J. (2003). Resilience in sheltered battered women. *Issues in Mental Health Nursing, 24*(2), 137–152.

Hunter, A. J. (2001). A cross-cultural comparison of resilience in adolescents. *Journal of Pediatric Nursing, 16*(3), 172–179.

Hunter, A. J., & Chandler, G. E. (1999). Adolescent resilience. *Image: the Journal of Nursing Scholarship, 31*(3), 243–247.

Hymovich, D. P., & Roehnert, J. E. (1989). Psychosocial consequences of childhood cancer. *Seminars in Oncology Nursing, 5*(1), 56–62.

Jacelon, C. S. (1997). The trait and process of resilience. *Journal of Advanced Nursing, 25*(1), 123–129.

Kadner, K. D. (1989). Resilience. Responding to adversity. *Journal of Psychosocial Nursing & Mental Health Services, 27*(7), 20–25.

Kobasa, S. C. (1982). The hardy personality: Toward a social psychology of stress and health. *Social Psychology, 37*, 1–11.

Luthar, S. S., & Cicchetti, D. (2000). The construct of resilience: implications for interventions and social policies. *Development & Psychopathology, 12*(4), 857–885.

Luthar, S. S., Cicchetti, D., & Becker, B. (2000a). The construct of resilience: A critical evaluation and guidelines for future work. *Child Development, 71*(3), 543–562.

Luthar, S. S., Cicchetti, D., & Becker, B. (2000b). The construct of resilience: A critical evaluation and guidelines for future work. [see comments.]. *Child Development, 71*(3), 543–562.

Mandleco, B. L., & Peery, J. C. (2000). An organizational framework for conceptualizing resilience in children. *Journal of Child and Adolescent Psychiatric Nursing, 13*(3), 99–111.

Masten, A. S. (1994). Resilience in individual development: Successful adaptation despite risk and adversity. In E. W. Gordon (Ed.), *Educational resilience in inner-city America: Challenges and prospects* (pp. 3–35). Hillsdale, NJ: Erlbaum.

Masten, A. S. (2001). Ordinary magic. Resilience processes in development. *American Psychologist, 56*(3), 227–238.

Masten, A. S., Best, K. M., & Garmezy, N. (1990). Resilience and development: Contributions from the study of children who overcome adversity. *Development and Psychopathology, 2*, 425–444.

Masten, A. S., & Coatsworth, J. D. (1998). The development of competence in favorable and unfavorable environments. Lessons from research on successful children. *American Psychologist, 53*(2), 205–220.

McAllister, M., & Walsh, K. (2003). CARE: A framework for mental health practice. *Journal of Psychiatric Mental Health Nursing, 10*(1), 39–48.

McCubbin, H., & McCubbin, M. (1996). Resiliency in families: A conceptual model of family adjustment and adaptation in response to stress and crisis. In H. I. McCubbin, A I. Thompson, & M. A. McCubbin (Eds.), *Family assessment: Resiliency, coping and adaptation—inventories for research and practice* (pp. 1–64). Madison, WI: University of Wisconsin System.

McCubbin, M., Balling, K., Possin, P., Frierdich, S., & Bryne, B. (2002). Family resiliency in childhood cancer. *Family Relations, 51*(2), 103–111.

McCubbin, M., & McCubbin, H. (1993). Family coping with health crisis: The Resiliency Model of Family Stress, Adjustment and Adaptation. In P. Winstead-Fry (Ed.), *Families, health, and illness* (pp. 3–63). St. Louis, MO: Mosby.

Morse, J. M., & Carter, B. J. (1995). Strategies of enduring and the suffering of loss: Modes of comfort used by a resilient survivor. *Holistic Nursing Practice, 9*(3), 38–52.

Murphy, L., & Moriarty, A. (1976). *Vulnerability, coping and growth from infancy to adolescence.* New Haven, CT: Yale University Press.

Patterson, J. M. (1995). Promoting resilience in families experiencing stress. *Pediatric Clinics of North America, 42*(1), 47–63.

Patterson, J. M. (2002). Understanding family resilience. *Journal of Clinical Psychology, 58*(3), 233–246.

Pettit, G. S. (2000). Mechanisms in the cycle of maladaptation: The life-course perspective. *Prevention and Treatment, 3*(35).

Polk, L. V. (1997). Toward a middle-range theory of resilience. *Advances in Nursing Science, 19*(3), 1–13.

Rew, L., Taylor-Seehafer, M., Thomas, N. Y., & Yockey, R. D. (2001). Correlates of resilience in homeless adolescents. *Image—Journal of Nursing Scholarship, 33*(1), 33–40.

Richardson, G. E. (2002). The metatheory of resilience and resiliency. *Journal of Clinical Psychology, 58*(3), 307–321.

Rosenbaum, M. (1983). Learned resourcefulness as a behavioral repertoire for the self-regulation of internal events. In M. Rosenbaum, C.M. Franks, & Y. Jaffe (Eds.), *Perspectives on behavior therapy in the eighties* (pp. 54–73). New York: Springer Publishing Co.

Rutter, M. (1979). Protective factors in children's responses to stress and disadvantage. *Annals of the Academy of Medicine, Singapore, 8*(3), 324–338.

Rutter, M. (1987). Psychosocial resilience and protective mechanisms. *American Journal of Orthopsychiatry, 57*(3), 316–331.

Singer, B. H. & Ryff C., (2001). *New horizons in health: An integrative approach.* Washington, DC: National Academy Press.

Sinnema, G. (1991). Resilience among children with special health-care needs and among their families. *Pediatric Annals, 20*(9), 483–486.

Smith, S. D. (1997). The retirement transition and the later life family unit. *Public Health Nursing, 14*(4), 207–216.

Stewart, M., Reid, G., & Mangham, C. (1997). Fostering children's resilience. *Journal of Pediatric Nursing, 12*(1), 21–31.

Svavarsdottir, E. K., McCubbin, M. A., & Kane, J. H. (2000). Well-being of parents of young children with asthma. *Research in Nursing & Health, 23*(5), 346–358.

Vinson, J. A. (2002). Children with asthma: Initial development of the child resilience model. *Pediatric Nurse, 28*(2), 149–158.

Wagnild, G., & Young, H. M. (1990). Resilience among older women. *Image—Journal of Nursing Scholarship, 22*(4), 252–255.

Wagnild, G. M., & Young, H. M. (1993). Development and psychometric evaluation of the Resilience Scale. *Journal of Nursing Measurement, 1*(2), 165–178.

Waller, M. A. (2001). Resilience in ecosystemic context: Evolution of the concept. *American Journal of Orthopsychiatry, 71*(3), 290–297.

Wells, R., & Schwebel, A. (1987). Chronically ill children and their mothers: Predictors of resilience and vulnerability to hospitalization and surgical stress. *Developmental & Behavioral Pediatrics, 2*(2), 83–89.

Werner, E., & Smith, R. (1982). *Vulnerable but invincible: A longitudinal study of resilient children and youth.* New York: McGraw-Hill.

White, K. R. (1995). The transition from victim to victor: Application of the theory of mastery. *Journal of Psychosocial Nursing and Mental Health Services, 33*(8), 41–44.

White, N., Bichter, J., Koeckeritz, J., Lee, Y. A., & Munch, K. L. (2002). A cross-cultural comparison of family resiliency in hemodialysis patients. *Journal of Transcultural Nursing, 13*(3), 218–227.

Woodgate, R., & McClement, S. (1997). Sense of self in children with cancer and in childhood cancer survivors: A critical review. *Journal of Pediatric Oncology Nursing, 14*(3), 137–155.

Woodgate, R. L. (1999). Conceptual understanding of resilience in the adolescent with cancer: Part I. *Journal of Pediatric Oncology Nursing, 16*(1), 35–43.

Critical Analysis Exercises

Chapter 3 Analysis Exercise: Pain: A Balance Between Analgesia and Side Effects

SHIRLEY M. MOORE

INTERNAL CRITICISM

1. *Clarity.* The terms used and ideas conveyed in this theory are easy to understand. All terms are defined using words common to practicing nurses. The most unique idea expressed in the theory is the major concept of "a balance between analgesia and side effects" as a way to think about pain management. A clear definition is given of this new conceptualization of pain management. Additionally, all the propositions are expressed clearly and provide a coherent and comprehensive conceptualization.

2. *Consistency.* The description of this prescriptive theory is consistent in the use of concepts and definitions. The use of the terms and propositions are consistent with those used in other prescriptive theories. For example, the proposition specifying that nurses use appropriate multimodal interventions for pain management is prescriptive because it suggests that specific decisions and actions on the part of the nurse are likely to produce a particular outcome. In addition, consistent with prescriptive level theory, the propositions can be easily tested, using randomized controlled trials.

3. *Adequacy.* This theory presents a comprehensive approach to acute pain management. The theory addresses the affective and sensory dimensions to be considered in the management of acute pain and, as such, represents a more comprehensive approach than other current theories of acute pain management. The theory can be considered in its entirety, or regarded as discrete steps in the pain management process. Despite the comprehensive and prescriptive nature of the theory, the number of propositions is manageable for the reader.

4. *Logical development.* The description of the theory clearly chronicles the historical evolution of knowledge about pain management and explains this theory's unique contributions to the field. The theory deductively incorporates previous knowledge and theoretical perspectives of pain management and is consistent with them. For example, the gate control theory of pain can be used to explain the mechanics of effect. This theory is also an exemplar of the utility of developing middle range theory inductively from clinical practice guidelines. The arguments of the theory are well supported and the conclusions are logical.

5. *Level of theory development.* In this prescriptive theory, specific choices and actions of the nurse to promote a balance between analgesia and side effects are posed. The theory is supported by some research; it has been tested in randomized controlled trials. Dr. Good has conducted research on the

effects of nonpharmacologic adjuvants as part of pain management. Knowledge about the behavioral and social-cognitive mechanisms in some of the propositions of the theory is less developed. For example, little is known about the best ways to engage in goal setting for pain management, or timing the amount of information to provide for a patient when soliciting patient participation in acute pain management. Additionally, more research is needed about how the propositions may be influenced by cultural orientation.

EXTERNAL CRITICISM

1. *Reality convergence.*   This theory is clearly reality based. It addresses the two dimensions of pain management, affective and sensory, that nurses observe in their clients. The assumptions of the theory represent the real world, a clinical reality to which every nurse can relate.
2. *Utility.*   Acute pain management is a common problem in nursing. This is a pragmatic theory that nurses in practice and clinical researchers can easily use. Nurses can use this theory to generate testable hypotheses, both at the bedside and in full-scale research studies. Some hypotheses have been generated from this study, and the author describes empirical findings generated from them. The author suggests examples of additional hypotheses that can be tested. The theory can be used by practicing nurses to guide assessment and interventions with individual patients, as well as to guide quality assurance for groups of patients.
3. *Significance.*   This theory has high significance. Symptom management is a central function of nurses, and managing pain is particularly important. Findings from studies testing the relationships posed in the propositions of this theory will have an immediate impact on nursing care and patients.
4. *Discrimination.*   This theory is unique in that it is the only theory of pain management that focuses on the balance between analgesia and side effects. The theory has precise and clear boundaries, and the author has defined boundaries, clearly describing the phenomena that are and are not addressed by the theory. For example, the theory does not address acute pain management in children or management of chronic pain.
5. *Scope of theory.*   The scope of this theory clearly meets the criteria for a middle range theory. It is broad enough to be applicable across a number of situations requiring acute pain management, yet narrow enough to be prescriptive for use with individual patients. It is middle range in that the propositions are abstract enough to be testable using research, but concrete enough to be directly applied in practice.
6. *Complexity.*   Pain management is a complex idea. Thus, any theory that comprehensively addresses the phenomenon of pain management has the potential to be very complex and not easily understood. Dr. Good, however, has done an outstanding job of developing a parsimonious, easily understood theory. The clear descriptions of the terms, the commonly used language employed in labeling and describing the concepts, and the logical presentation of the propositions make this an easily understood theory despite the complexity of the underlying phenomenon. The use of diagrams of the propositions further reduces the complexity of the theory description.

About the Author
Shirley M. Moore, RN, PhD, FAAN is Associate Professor and Associate Dean for Research at Frances Payne Bolton School of Nursing, Case Western University, Cleveland, Ohio. She has taught nursing theory and knowledge-development courses at all levels of the nursing curriculum. Dr. Moore is a nurse researcher who, as principal investigator, has had multiple projects funded by the National Institute of Nursing Research. She has authored several articles on middle range theory development, including: Good, M., & Moore, S. (1996). Clinical practice guidelines as a source of middle range theory: Focus on acute pain. Nursing Outlook, 44(2). 74–79.

Chapter 4 Analysis Exercise: Unpleasant Symptoms

KATHERINE J. BREDOW

INTERNAL CRITICISM

1. *Clarity.* The descriptions of the five main components of the Theory of Unpleasant Symptoms (TOUS) are clearly stated. They are described in the text and defined in the definition of key terms. Focusing on unpleasant symptoms (UPS) as part of the lived experience, the theorists set out to design a model to explain the experience of UPS as they occur in a dynamic clinical situation. Management techniques also emerged as a common factor in the authors' early discussions on the development of the TOUS. Consideration should be given to including management techniques as a component of the model.

2. *Consistency.* The components are consistently used throughout the explanation of the theory. Development of the components are detailed in the references to the theorists' own symptom models (dispense and fatigue) and others symptom models (SIM and the Model of Symptom Management), and have been refined, as hypothesis testing in clinical practice and research has yielded new information. In the description of the theory there are three influencing components: physiological factors, psychological factors, and environmental factors. In the Definition of Key Terms, situational factors is the third influencing factor, of which environmental factors are a subset. Throughout the rest of the chapter, the terms are used in a congruent manner.

3. *Adequacy.* The theory explanation is succinct. The historical development of the theory was insightful and led to an understanding of the authors' intent to make the symptom experience dynamic and more reflective of the real world. The theorists' goal was to construct a model to help the nurse understand all symptoms and their management. The focus of this theory is to understand the experience of UPS. This is done by identifying antecedent factors, UPS, and their influence on performance. It is suggested that an understanding of these components and their interrelationships will help the nurse to identify possible UPS-management interventions. Though inferred, it is not

clearly stated where the management factor fits into the model. The diagram of the model is helpful in understanding the interrelationship of the factors.

4. *Logical development.* The theorists systematically set out to construct a theory to help the nurse to understand all symptoms and how to manage them. TOUS origins are founded in clinical observations, review of symptom literature, and collaboration with experts in theory development. It logically follows a line of thought of previous symptom work, expanding on it to build a theory that accounts for the antecedent factors, the dynamic experience of one or multiple symptoms, the performance and their interrelationships. The use of established reliable and valid tools to measure some UPS supports the logical foundation of TOUS. The examples of TOUS theory-based research helps to establish the usefulness and applicability to the nursing practice and research.

5. *Level of theory development.* TOUS fits the criteria of a middle range theory because it limits its scope and does not attempt to address all of the factors of the nursing metaparadigm. It provides a framework from which nurse researchers can generate hypothesis and research questions to better understand the dynamic experience of unpleasant symptoms.

EXTERNAL CRITICISM

1. *Reality convergence.* TOUS presents a comprehensive, holistic, and dynamic view of the unpleasant symptom experience. The underlying assumptions of TOUS ring true. Managing the care of people experiencing UPS is a part of the real world of nursing. Increasing insight into the reality of the unpleasant symptom experience provides direction for management of the unpleasant symptoms patients experience.

2. *Utility.* The theory supports the development of research questions and study of the five components of TOUS. It has been applied to various populations experiencing UPS and to caregivers distressed by their experience of UPS in those they care for. Examples are given for both acute and chronic experiences of UPS. Consideration of the research results led to a refinement of the TOUS. The interaction among components and their interrelationships with the other components were incorporated into the TOUS to make its utility even stronger.

3. *Significance.* Research conducted from hypothesis generated from the TOUS had a significant impact on the care that the nurses provided to patients. Since most clinical nurses deal in their practice with populations that experience UPS, this theory offers a means of investigating the whole experience of health-threatening changes to patients perceived as normal functioning. It can be useful in gaining an understanding of the UPS and management strategies.

4. *Discrimination.* The author tells the story of the development of the theory. The theorists constructed a unique theory that combined the essential components identified in earlier single-symptom models, to build a more inclusive, interactive dynamic theory for understanding the whole of UPS. No other middle range theory addresses the multiple concepts of UPS at the same time in one encompassing model. Because of the inclusion of situational factors, which are broad and have no clear boundaries, the TOUS is not as discriminating as it could be if it had not included this influencing factor. Moreover, the inclusion of culture and language, which have few definitive parameters, into the quality of symptoms, make the TOUS a less discriminating theory.

5. *Scope of theory.* The theory is useful for investigating one UPS or many UPSs. The scope of the TOUS can range from simple to complex, depending on the number of UPS and variables the investigator

chooses to study. Antecedents or influencing factors have the capability of being broad and all-encompassing, and a thorough assessment of all of these factors may be difficult.

6. *Complexity.*   Initially, the TOUS seems succinct, logical, and practical. However, if it is applied to a complex, chronically ill patient with multiple problems, the task of considering all of the possible influencing factors, their interrelationships, and their congruent relationship to the various UPS quickly becomes very complex. This is not to downplay the importance of a thorough assessment, but the more unpleasant symptoms that are entered into the model, the more complex it becomes.

About the Author

Kate Bredow, MA, RN, is a practicing school nurse, where she sees a variety of unpleasant symptoms in her patients every day. Her research experience dealt with the unpleasant symptom of sleep deprivation in the postpartum period.

Chapter 5 Analysis Exercise: Self-Efficacy

MARJORIE SIMPSON

INTERNAL CRITICISM

1. *Clarity.*   Self-efficacy is a clearly defined theoretical framework, with main concepts that include efficacy expectations and outcome expectations as the sources of self-efficacy. Theoretical clarity is supported by the well-defined constructs within the framework and their relationship to each other, with self-efficacy preceding and impacting human behavior. The constructs and concepts incorporated into the self-efficacy theoretical framework are unique to the theory, and, therefore, their meanings are less likely to be misinterpreted.

2. *Consistency.*   The relationships between the constructs included in self-efficacy remain consistently defined throughout the theoretical framework. In addition, the theme of causative capabilities as a belief that generates courses of action consistently serves as the foundation for the theory. Based on this premise, the theory of self-efficacy builds on the understanding that each individual's beliefs and past experiences influence his or her behavior.

3. *Adequacy.*   The self-efficacy framework adequately explains and predicts behavior. Individuals with higher levels of self-efficacy for a specific behavior are more likely to attempt that behavior. The concept of outcome expectations offers an explanation for failure of an individual to attempt or adopt a behavior. According to the theory, the belief that a behavior will produce a worthwhile outcome is necessary for an individual to execute the behavior, regardless of the level of self-efficacy. The completeness of the theory to predict behavior and explain situations when behaviors are not adopted supports the adequacy of the framework.

4. *Logical development.* The theory of self-efficacy was derived deductively from social cognitive theory, a model proposing that personal and environmental factors influence behavior. A basic assumption of this model is that individuals are human agents and have the ability to exercise control over their lives. This is congruent with other behavior change theories, and supports the logical development of the self-efficacy framework. In addition, the self-efficacy framework proceeds in a logical fashion. Efficacy expectations and outcome expectations are always antecedents to behavior and are reinforced when a behavior is successfully executed. In addition, the theory supports that enactive attainment is a strong influence over behavior and explains why self-efficacy for one behavior can be carried over to a different but similar behavior. These conclusions are logical and have been supported by previous nursing research.

5. *Level of theory development.* The self-efficacy theoretical model has been adapted and used in nursing research for many nursing interventions. Because the theory of self-efficacy accounts for new behaviors as well as lack of behavior change, it is predictive and can be used to explain an individual's responses to an intervention in both research and clinical settings. Therefore, self-efficacy as a middle range theory has been developed to a level that allows for purposeful nursing actions.

EXTERNAL CRITICISM

1. *Reality convergence.* An underlying assumption of the theory of self-efficacy is that most human behavior is determined by both intrinsic and extrinsic factors. Intrinsic factors include an individual's beliefs, and extrinsic factors include environmental influences that can be affected by an individual's actions. The influence of intrinsic and extrinsic factors on how people behave is reflected throughout nursing practice, and nurses frequently implement formal and informal interventions to alter these factors. For example, a rehabilitation nurse may demonstrate and instruct a patient in the use of adaptive equipment, and offer counseling or verbal persuasion to impact the patient's behavior. The actions of the nurse are altering the patient's self-efficacy for the use of adaptive equipment. In addition, addressing other physiological responses to illness, such as the unpleasant symptoms of pain and fatigue, are central to nursing and alter self-efficacy. Therefore, the theory of self-efficacy is grounded in reality and reflects the real world of nursing practice.

2. *Utility.* Core concepts that are central to the nursing profession include the interaction between nurse, patient, health, and the environment. This interaction often involves the nurse intervening to alter the intrinsic factors of the patient and the extrinsic environmental factors to facilitate behavior change and improve the patient's health. The self-efficacy theoretical framework is one that can generate researchable hypothesis on the interaction between these core nursing concepts, and can predict the outcomes of interventions, particularly those addressing the management of chronic illnesses and health promotion. Thus, it is useful both in research and practice.

3. *Significance.* Behavior change is an element that is essential to nurses in all specialties. The theory of self-efficacy is significant to the nursing profession because it offers a framework to generate hypothesis and conduct research to test behavioral change interventions. The research results derived from the self-efficacy framework can directly impact the way nurses practice. Self-efficacy measures can be used in clinical settings to identify individuals with low self-efficacy, and nurses can then develop approaches to increase self-efficacy to promote certain behaviors.

4. *Discrimination.* The self-efficacy theory can be used to generate and to test hypotheses that are unique to the diverse nursing profession. Because the framework is flexible, it can be adapted by all

nursing specialties to the specific behaviors and conditions that are central in research and practice. Self-efficacy is operationalized using scales that measure strength and magnitude of self-efficacy for a specific behavior, as defined by the nurse researcher. The self-efficacy theory, therefore, is not only able to differentiate nursing from other disciplines, but it is able to distinguish and define the parameters of nursing specialties.

5. *Scope of theory.*   The scope of the theory of self-efficacy is narrowly focused on the elements that influence behavior. Although the concept of behavior is comprehensive, the four sources of efficacy expectations and outcome expectations account for all of the factors that influence behavior. Therefore, self-efficacy is a middle range theory with a framework that is practical and applicable to all behavior-focused nursing research and practice.

6. *Complexity.*   The theory of self-efficacy is complex enough to account for all intrinsic and extrinsic factors that influence human behavior. However it is parsimonious enough that the relationships between the constructs within the theory are easily understood. The theoretical framework clearly defines and explains the concepts self-efficacy and behavior, as well as the constructs that include outcome expectations and the four sources of efficacy expectations. These variables that are incorporated into the theory are precise enough that they are easily understood and extensive enough to account for all human behavior.

About the Author
Marjorie Simpson, MS, CRNP, is a doctoral student and Clinical Instructor, School of Nursing, at the University of Maryland, Baltimore. Her research for her dissertation is on self-efficacy expectations in performance of restorative-care activities for nursing assistants. She has recently coauthored an article on measurement related to her research topic: Resnick, B., & Simpson, M. (2003). Reliability and validity testing self-efficacy outcome expectations scales for performing restorative care activities. Geriatric Nursing, 24(2), 2–7.

Chapter 6 Analysis Exercise: Reasoned Action and Planned Behavior

WILLIAM BREEN

INTERNAL CRITICISM

1. *Clarity.* Definitions of major concepts are clearly described. Descriptions are logical and consistent with definitions included in health-behaviors literature. The major constructs represent distinctly different aspects of the theory and do not overlap conceptually. For example, the major constructs

of attitude, subjective norms, and perceived behavioral control represent unique and separate aspects of behavioral intention. Similarly, three types of beliefs, behavioral, normative, and control, are defined and described as determinants of attitude, subjective norm, and perceived behavioral control, respectively (see model).

Behaviors of interest are described in terms of target, action, context, and time. The theorist describes the importance of considering these factors in behavior measurement. It is not clear how target, action, context, and time fit within the theory or influence the major theory constructs of attitude, subjective norm, and perceived behavioral control.

2. *Consistency.* Definitions of terms are consistent throughout the description of the theory. Information obtained from the theorist's Web site supports consistency between the theoretical definitions and measurement in clinical practice and research. The Web site includes specific illustrations that clarify each major construct and appropriate measurement considerations. All measurement examples are consistent with the construct definitions.

3. *Adequacy.* The theorist describes basic factors influencing one's decision to change behavior and comply with or adapt to others' expectations. The constructs of attitude, subjective norms, and perceived behavioral control influence the decision to change behavior or "behavioral intention." Antecedents to these constructs are one's behavioral beliefs, normative beliefs, and control beliefs.

The definitions and descriptions of the three belief constructs do not include a number of affective and cognitive factors identified in the literature that may influence attitude, subjective norms, and perceived behavioral control; behavioral intention; and ultimately, behavior.

These areas include the constructs and variables of:

Anticipated grief: the perceived degree and nature of loss if the new behaviors are implemented
Perceived moral obligation: the obligation felt by the person to comply with prescribed behaviors because compliance has moral or ethical implications
Self-image: one's perception of self; for example, how does the "fit" between the specific behavior and one's self perception influence attitude?
Perceived seriousness: the perceived seriousness of the actual or potential consequences of not changing behavior
Definition of health: one's conceptualization of what is healthy; for example, is a person with a lower standard or perception of what is healthy less likely to engage in prescribed behaviors?
Knowledge: one's understanding of the behavior to be performed. While the research literature identifies that knowledge of the behavior to be accepted is not an antecedent to behavioral intention, the question of whether or not knowledge is needed to implement prescribed behaviors regardless of intent is not addressed in the theory. Knowledge may be an antecedent to perceived behavioral control.

4. *Logical development.* The relationship of the constructs attitude, subjective norm, and perceived behavioral control to behavioral intention and, ultimately, behavior are logically developed. The three antecedents to behavioral intention are independent of each other yet represent factors influencing behavior decisions.

The aforementioned aspects of behavioral change that are not clearly addressed in the theory description would add to the logical development of the theory. For example, the perceived seriousness of not adapting a behavior is not clearly identified in the description of the theory and in the definitions of the major constructs, yet an example of a measurement question provided at the theorist's Web site asks the participant to identify the seriousness of potential consequences of not exercising (i.e., blood pressure).

5. *Level of theory development.*   The Theory of Planned Behavior provides a conceptual description of factors that contribute to the decision of whether or not to perform or adopt a healthy behavior. The antecedents to the primary theoretical construct, behavioral intention, are logical and fit with the findings of health behaviors research. Because the theory is logically developed and consistent, it can serve as an excellent framework for selected health behaviors and/or beliefs research.

The level of theory development is hampered by the complexity of the topic area (behavior). Without clear descriptions of the contribution of the concepts described as missing in the "adequacy" section of this evaluation, the theory is somewhat limited in its utility for research and development of knowledge in the area of health behaviors.

EXTERNAL CRITICISM

1. *Reality convergence.*   The Theory of Planned Behavior has reality convergence in the sense that the major assumptions of the theory and its constructs fit with the practice experiences of health professionals. Similarly, the theoretical constructs and their respective definitions are consistent with current research findings and general health behaviors literature.

The reality convergence of this theory is hampered by the complexity of the determinants of behavior. The experience of health providers and the research indicate that the decision to adopt a recommended health behavior involves more than what is described in the constructs of the theory, particularly regarding beliefs.

2. *Utility.*   The theory serves as a basis for hypothesis generation in health behaviors research, and supports development and investigation of researchable questions that lie within the scope of the theory. Examples of research topics that would be supported by the Theory of Planned Behavior include but are not limited to perceived control (self efficacy) and acceptance of health behaviors; or influence of family and social support upon health behavior. Evidence of the utility of the theory is provided by the number and scope of research studies using the theory as a conceptual basis.

3. *Significance.*   Research conducted using hypotheses and research questions supported by the theory have considerable significance providing important insights into factors contributing to health-behavior decision-making. Research results provide specific recommendations for considerations and nursing actions that will promote healthy behaviors.

4. *Discrimination.*   There are a variety of middle range theories that address health behaviors and related constructs. These theories describe constructs that parallel those included in the Theory of Planned Behavior (e.g., health beliefs, health promotion activities, perceived control, self-efficacy, and formal and informal support).

The major constructs of the Theory of Planned Behavior are unique in their definitions, antecedents (beliefs), and consequences (behavioral intention). The particularly unique or discriminating aspect of the theory is construct-behavioral intention. Other health behavior theories do not identify intention as a preliminary step to behavior.

Describing behaviors within terms of target, action, context, and time is a unique aspect of the theory. The theorists identify that measurement using the theory should include definitions of behaviors in terms of these factors.

5. *Scope of theory.* The scope of the Theory of Planned Behavior is relatively narrow. It provides a basis for research and measurement that is specific to determinants of behavior. The theory also provides specific considerations for nursing care. The theory and the related research provide a basis for development of health protocols and procedures that can improve patient acceptance of recommended health behaviors.

6. *Complexity.* On the continuum from parsimony (limited number of variables) to complex (extensive number of variables), the Theory of Planned Behavior is relatively simple. The theoretical model involves three categories of behaviors that are antecedent to the major constructs of attitude, subjective norms, and perceived behavioral control. The three major constructs are antecedent to behavioral intention and behavior. The relative simplicity of the theory raises questions of its adequacy as a theory addressing the complex topic of behavior.

About the Author
William McBreen, PhD, RN, is Director of the Master's Program in Nursing at Winona State University, Winona, Minnesota.

Chapter 7 Analysis Exercise: Empathy

SUSAN RAY

INTERNAL CRITICISM

1. *Clarity.* Olson's Theory of Empathy clearly defines at the beginning of the manuscript the main concepts of the theory: nurse-expressed empathy, patient-perceived empathy, and patient distress.

2. *Consistency.* The definitions of the key concepts are consistent throughout the explanation of the theory. Olson is consistent in the definitions of empathy and the actual measurements of empathy. There is congruence between concepts, principles, interpretations, and methods throughout the theory. Olson's theory is based on reciprocal principles that are consistent with Orlando's model. The nurse observes the patient's behavior, interprets it, and then checks her or his reaction with the patient. Only after the patient confirms or clarifies the meaning of the behavior, does she or he act on the behavior to solve the patient's problem.

   Olson is consistent throughout the description of her theory in her interpretation of the reality of the phenomenon under consideration. Her thought follows logistic, deductive discriminations. Olson's argument moves by telling what the nurse sees, what is interpreted, and what is verified or meant by the patient. A downward, deductive pattern of argument is discernible throughout the discussion of her theory.

3. *Adequacy.* Olson's theory is about the intimate, professional relationship that forms between a nurse and a patient. She includes a thorough account of the historical background from various disciplines on the topic of empathy. In addition, the definitions of empathy in the nursing literature are explored over the past 10 years. Olson conceptualizes empathy as a three-step therapeutic communication process in the nurse–patient relationship. She differentiates nursing from other helping professions by its functioning in the immediate present to ascertain and meet the patients' needs. Any theory that locates its principles in the nature of the exchange between the patient and the nurse is an interaction theory. Olson focuses nursing in communication, both verbal and behavioral. The theory is adequate because its scope includes any professional communication relevant to meeting patients' needs at any level within and throughout the health care system.

4. *Logical development.* Olson presents a deductive mode of reasoning in which conclusions proceed in a logical fashion. Her arguments are well supported by previous work on empathy in nursing and other disciplines. Olson's theory logically follows a line of thought and draws conclusions from the previous work of Orlando's more abstract model. Orlando describes a process of verification in a therapeutic encounter whereby nurses have their perceptions validated or corrected by patients. Olson logically concludes that the process of verification as defined by Orlando can be equated to expressed empathy, the communicative component of empathy.

   Olson links nurses' therapeutic levels of empathy to Orlando's disciplined professional response. Orlando did not specifically discuss the development of empathy skills in relation to a disciplined professional response. However, Olson logically argues that the professional response as described by Orlando would be difficult to achieve without high levels of empathy.

   Olson uses a deductive process to derive a set of propositions from Orlando's model. She outlines the relational statements in Orlando's model and deduces propositions for her middle range theory. Olson selected three relevant relational statements in Orlando's model for the development of three middle range theory propositions. The three propositions were developed logically from premises and assumptions.

   The flow of the connections of Orlando's relational statements to the propositions of the middle range theory is logically presented. In addition, Olson includes a diagram that links the concepts from Orlando's model to the concepts and propositions of her middle range theory. Olson argues that exploring the patient's thoughts and feelings, which is part of being empathic, links theoretically to Orlando's description of the assessment of a patient's immediate needs and immediate experiences (Orlando's proposition number two). In addition, Olson links Orlando's proposition number three and the patient's feeling of being understood. Olson's middle range theory links these feelings of being understood theoretically to decreased distress, decreased helplessness, and increased comfort in Orlando's proposition number two. Olson's theory demonstrates a logical development from its premises to its outcome because the flow of logic explicitly used in the empathic process reasonably leads one to the conclusion or outcome, decreased patient distress.

5. *Level of theory development.* Olson's Theory of Empathy is a middle range theory. Olson's theory meets the following middle range characteristics: not comprehensive, but not narrowly focused; some generalizability across settings and specialties; limited number of concepts; propositions that are clearly stated and that generate testable hypotheses (McEwen & Wills, 2002). In addition, Olson followed the specific recommendations by Liehr and Smith (1999) in the development of a middle range theory as follows: clearly articulate the theory name; succinctly describe approaches used for generating the theory; clarify the conceptual linkages of the theory in a diagrammed model; eluci-

date the research-practice links of the theory; and explain the association between the theory and the discipline of nursing.

The function of middle range theories is to describe, explain, or predict phenomenon (Blegen & Tripp-Reimer, 1997). The Theory of Empathy is predictive in that its concepts or variables are associated with a change in the value of another variable or concept.

EXTERNAL CRITICISM

1. *Reality convergence.* Reality convergence will be considered as it relates to principle, interpretation, and method. Principles are the crucial premises of a theory. Olson locates her theory's principles in the nature of the exchange between the nurse and the patient. Olson begins with the premise that empathy is one of the most essential variables in the nurse–patient relationship. Nurse-expressed empathy is likened to the process of verification that is part of Orlando's disciplined professional response. Empathic communication skills are essential for nurses to understand the immediate needs and experiences of patients. Therefore, it is the responsibility of nurses to develop empathic communication skills to explore with clients their immediate needs and experiences (i.e., thoughts and feelings). The accurate perceptions of nurses verbally shared with patients can lead to patient-perceived empathy that, in turn, can result in lower patient distress. These underlying assumptions represent the real world of nursing. The Theory of the Empathic Process can be used in any communication relevant to patient needs anywhere in the health care system. Olson's interpretation locates nursing in empathic communication with the patient as a crucial participant in the process. This interpretation reflects the real world of nursing from the writer's viewpoint. Olson's deductive method lends itself readily to the traditional scientific (quantifiable) method. The theory provides a structure from which the relationships among nurse-expressed empathy, patient-perceived empathy, and patient outcomes can be studied further in future research. The theory is pragmatic because it can be operationalized with instruments used for empirical testing in a variety of real life settings.

2. *Utility.* The theory has utility in nursing research, practice, education, and administration. Further understanding of the antecedents and the outcomes related to empathy could be discovered by the use of this theory in research and practice.

Olson and Hanchett (1997) demonstrated how the middle range theory was developed and tested through research. The results supported the relationships that Orlando proposed to exist between accurate perceptions of patients' needs and patient distress. In addition, the findings supported the hypotheses generated by Olson's theory of the Empathic Process. The findings also supported the need to develop empathic communication skills in nursing students and practicing nurses.

Olson suggests other ways that nurse researchers could examine the three concepts in the empathic process in future research, both in education and practice. She clarifies that although one patient outcome (patient distress) was selected for her theory, other measures of patient outcome could be substituted for patient distress, without modifying the model significantly. For instance, patient satisfaction could be substituted, allowing the theory to be used in multiple client situations and health care settings.

The theory builds on Orlando's process of verification in a therapeutic encounter whereby nurses have their perceptions validated or corrected by patients to ascertain and meet patient needs. The theory conceptualizes empathy as a three-step communication process. However, the theory does not offer an explicit way to communicate empathically with patients to meet their needs. Further research is needed to develop a prescriptive theory that would offer explicit empathic communication skills useful to educators, student nurses, practicing nurses, and administrators.

3. *Significance.* The theory focuses on the understanding of empathy in the nurse–patient relationship that provides the basis for all other nurse–patient activity. The theory contributes to nursing knowledge by offering a structure to facilitate understanding the relationships among nurse-expressed empathy, patient-perceived empathy, and patient outcome. The three hypotheses generated by the theory have an impact on the way nurses carry out nursing interventions in the real world. The three concepts of the theory can be taught and operationalized for further research. Nurses may use the theory to further develop explicit empathic communication skills and interventions. Empathy is indispensable to effective nurse–patient relationships; therefore, understanding the empathic process is key to understanding as the essential core of nursing (Bennet, 1995). Thus, the theory has immense significance for the nursing profession.

4. *Discrimination.* A number of grand theories describe nursing as a relationship between a nurse and a patient. However, Orlando's model emerged as the most suitable for the development of the Theory of Empathy (Olson & Hanchett, 1997). In particular, Orlando's process of verification was likened to expressed empathy, the communicative component of empathy. Therefore, the hypotheses generated by the theory are unique and could not be arrived at by another nursing theory. In particular, the theory addresses the discipline's professional response (i.e., nurse expressed-empathy), patient-perceived empathy, and patient distress as an outcome measure of nursing care.

The theory offers precise, clear boundaries and definitive parameters regarding the empathic process.within the nurse–patient relationship. The theory constructs a unique professional nursing function, that is, the empathic process to ascertain and meet patients' immediate needs for help. The product or outcome is to relieve patients' distress, which differentiates nursing from other health professions.

5. *Scope of the theory.* The scope of the theory is broadly applicable because it includes the nursing empathic communication process relevant to meeting patients' needs in all specialties, whether in nursing administration, education, or practice.

6. *Complexity.* The theory strikes a balance between complexity and parsimony. It is parsimonious in that it describes three empathy-related definitions as the key components in the theory. The theory is understandable without lengthy descriptions and explanations of the three key concepts. However, the theory is complex, given that the empathic communication process within the dynamics of the nurse–patient relationship can be complex. Overall, Olson's Theory of Empathy is a middle range theory that contributes significantly to nursing knowledge and the discipline of nursing.

REFERENCES

Bennett, J. (1995). "Methodological notes on empathy": Further considerations. *Advances in Nursing Science, 18*(1), 36–50.

Blegen, M. A., & Tripp-Reimer, T. (1997). Implications of nursing taxonomies for middle range theory development. *Advances in Nursing Science, 19*(3), 37–50.

Liehr, P., & Smith, M. J. (1999). Middle range theory: Spinning research and practice to create knowledge for the new millennium. *Advances in Nursing Science, 21*(4), 81–91.

McEwen, M., & Wills, E. M. (2002). *Theoretical basis for nursing.* Philadelphia, PA: Lippincott Williams & Wilkins.

Olson, J. K., & Hanchett, E. (1997). Nurse-expressed empathy, patient-perceived empathy and patient distress. *Image: Journal of Nursing Scholarship, 29*, 73–76.

About the Author

Susan Ray, RN, MScN, is a Clinical Nurse Specialist/Nurse Practitioner in Psychiatric-Mental Health Nursing. She has taught the theory of empathy to both RN and RPN students, and uses the theory in her practice with veterans diagnosed with posttraumatic stress disorder. She is also a doctoral student, Faculty of Nursing, University of Alberta, Edmonton, Alberta, Canada.

Chapter 8 Analysis Exercise: Chronic Sorrow

ANN M. SCHREIER

INTERNAL CRITICISM

1. *Clarity.*   The description of the key concepts of theory are clearly described and easily understood by the reviewer. The definition of chronic sorrow identifies it as a pervasive, permanent, periodic, and potentially progressive experience. The key concepts of loss, disparity, trigger events, and management methods are clearly defined, as well as the proposed relationship between these concepts. The theory is useful in understanding and anticipating various individuals' reactions to trigger events, such as the anniversary of a cancer diagnosis.
2. *Consistency.*   The author consistently maintains the definitions of the key terms of loss experience, disparity, trigger events, and management methods. These key terms are congruent with the described research studies.
3. *Adequacy.*   This theory explains what chronic sorrow is, as well as some of the common loss experiences that lead to chronic sorrow. However, it does not address why some individuals who have a loss experience do not experience chronic sorrow. In the example of bereaved individuals, 97% of the bereaved had symptoms of chronic sorrow (Eakes, Burke, & Hainsworth, 1999). Given that few of the subjects did not experience the symptoms labeled as chronic sorrow, the theory does address the experience of loss adequately. Future studies could examine whether there are predictors of those who will not experience chronic sorrow. Do individuals who do not experience chronic sorrow have different personality characteristics, or receive different health care interventions at the time of the loss? Another area that is open to future research is the identification of other conditions that commonly lead to chronic sorrow.
4. *Logical development.*   The theoretical model of chronic sorrow is logically developed from the 10 qualitative studies conducted by the Consortium for Research on Chronic Sorrow. Because of the excellent base of qualitative studies, the theory aids in the understanding of the loss experience. With this research, the authors are able to draw conclusions and make arguments that are well supported by clinical and research data.

5. *Level of theory development.*   The theory is appropriate to a middle range theory because it has a scope that is limited to the explanation of a single phenomena, that of response to loss.

EXTERNAL CRITICISM

1. *Reality convergence.*   In clinical work with oncology patients, the theory makes sense of the reactions that nurses see, for example, in patients with a recurrence of the diagnosis of cancer, or to the stress patients experience when awaiting results from routine diagnostic tests during the remission period.
2. *Utility and discrimination.*   Researchers could generate hypotheses based on the theoretical model. For instance, an appropriate hypothesis might be that parents of diabetic children, who participate in a 6-week support group, will demonstrate less discomfort from chronic sorrow than parents who do not participate in a support group. In addition, the authors' work on an assessment instrument and its inclusion in this book clearly enhances the utility of the theory both for research and clinical practice. The theory of chronic sorrow is unique and specifically addresses grieving needs and the experience of loss.
3. *Significance.*   This theoretical model lends itself to research on effectiveness of interventions for both caregivers and patients. In addition, the model can be used to determine what conditions are more likely to trigger an exacerbation of chronic sorrow and begin a chronic sorrow experience. With this knowledge, nurses will be able to anticipate needs and respond to these needs in an effective manner.
4. *Scope of theory.*   The concepts and hypothesized relationships can easily be applied in clinical settings, and the score is narrow enough to fit the expectations of a middle range theory.
5. *Complexity.*   The major concepts include loss experience, disparity, trigger events, chronic sorrow, and management methods. The conceptualization of the model is easily displayed in Figure 8-1 (Theoretical Model of Chronic Sorrow). Because the model is logical and cyclical, this figure enhances the reader's understanding of the relationship between the variables. The model clearly delineates the subconcepts of internal versus external management, ineffective versus effective management, and discomfort versus increased comfort, as well as where appropriate intervention by nurses and other health care providers can occur. There are a limited number of variables, and the number appears to be sufficient to explain the phenomena. The description accompanying the theory is succinct and readily understood.

About the Author
Ann M. Schreier, RN, PhD, is Assistant Professor of Nursing, Department of Adult Health, East Carolina University, Greenville, North Carolina. She has served as a consultant and clinical director at the Hospice Society in Bethesda, MD. She has received external funding to conduct nursing research in the area of self-care and chronicity. She also has several research-related publications in the area of self-care, pain control, and patient education.

Chapter 9 Analysis Exercise: Social Support

JOANN P. WESSMAN

Dr. Schaffer presents several social support theories in her chapter. The present critique is focused on the *body* of middle range social support theories that she presents. Therefore, some criteria for the critique have been modified.

INTERNAL CRITICISM

The present critique will focus on clarity, consistency, adequacy, and level of theory development. The issue of logical development will not be considered inasmuch as this criterion is specific to one particular theory.

1. *Clarity.* The lack of a clear definition of social support is cited and evident throughout the chapter. Specifically, definitions lack the clarity to differentiate if social support encompasses interactions where (1) negative consequences occur for provider or recipient, or (2) support providers are in "formal" categories such as professionals. It is unclear from the chapter discussion if social support can be considered to have occurred when it is not the intention of the provider to be helpful, but, indeed, support inadvertently is given. The author gives clear examples that differentiate meaning among emotional, information, instrumental, and appraisal kinds of support. Not as clear are the uses of the subconcepts structure and function.

2. *Consistency.* The lack of consistent use of the construct social support is identified in the chapter. When definitions vary widely, as they do, interpretations, principles, and methods will likewise lack consistency. The chapter section on clinical applications, particularly the use of social support as nursing intervention, highlights the diversity in conceptualizations of social support.

3. *Adequacy.* How adequate is the body of theories reviewed? Certainly the lack of definitional clarity and inconsistent use of definitional qualities diminishes adequacy. Yet, given these limitations, the robust nature of the concept, social support, is evident throughout the discussion. Yes, some definitional areas are ambiguous and inconsistent. However, the collection of theories reviewed does permit the nursing community to enter into meaningful dialog about the nature of social support. In this sense, the body of current theories possesses at least a degree of adequacy—meaningful conversations are evoked.

4. *Level of theory development.* It is interesting to note that among the theories of social support are elements of factor-isolating, explanatory, predictive, and prescriptive levels. Each theory cited attempts definition of the concept. Identification of variables related to social support, such as perceptions, timing, motivation, duration, direction, life stage, and source, offer a sense of factor-relating level of theory (explanation). The variability among instances of social support can be explained, at least to some degree, by these variables. We get a sense of explanation as to why not all

instances of social support look identical, and relationships within the construct social support begin to emerge. Some social support theorists such as Norbeck clearly are mapping out relationships that can predict outcomes of nursing interventions aimed at enhancing social support. Clinical situations where social support interventions should be prescribed in a defined manner (predictive and prescriptive theory) are being identified.

EXTERNAL CRITICISM

Each of the six specific criteria of external criticism will be approached from the view of the *body* of several social support theories available to the nurse in practice and research applications. At times, specific social support theories will be isolated.

1. *Reality convergence.*   Several of the social support theories converge well with "real world" nursing experiences. Chronically ill clients thrive when surrounded by supportive families and communities. Nursing's systems succeed when embedded in nurturing broader societal structures.

   The idea inherent in the buffer theory that social support modulates life stressors is one threaded throughout nursing literature. Design of care structures and referrals to type of care-giving facilities are shaped, in part, by the social supports available to the client to modulate stressors.

   Norbeck's model for using social support as intervention to improve health outcomes "rings true" with common nursing practices. Nurses routinely include family in client-education programs because they expect family members to reinforce learning. Nurses often suggest support groups for clients experiencing complex, intense, and/or prolonged health challenges, believing that the group will be a source of healing and growth.

   Many more examples could be given. Social support theories have a high degree of reality convergence with lived nursing experiences.

2. *Utility.*   How useful are present social support theories when applied in practice and research? Dr. Schaffer offers several specific examples to support the utility of social support theories for nursing. Her Table 10-2 offers specific clinical applications of social support theories that, in shaping meaningful interventions, reduce client stress and promote effective client coping. Examples are offered on individual, dyadic, group, community, and systems levels. Clearly, social support theories are useful in a variety of clinical situations.

   The examples of social support instruments described in Table 10-3 demonstrate the ability to operationalize social support theories in a way useful for research. The availability of specific instruments to measure social support in a valid and reliable manner is both useful and crucial to the researcher conducting quantitative studies. Schaffer and Lia-Hoagberg's study of the effects of social support on prenatal care and health behaviors of low-income women demonstrates the usefulness of present social support theories in guiding research. Present social support theories clearly are "birthing" useful instruments and studies.

3. *Significance.*   Dr. Schaffer supports well her strong assertion that middle range social support theories are of significance to nursing. Social support influences health status, health behavior, use of health services, and health outcomes. Current social support theories help to explain this influence in a manner that permits meaningful intervention. The theories offer a way to apply the nursing process in the arena of interpersonal relationships of the client with supportive "others." Theories

place the client within a relevant social context. Social support theories reflect the tradition within nursing to view the individual or family as an integral part of a rich fabric of relationships that define and reflect health.

4. *Discrimination.* The lack of definitional clarity and inconsistent use of the term "social support" among various theories adversely reflects on these theories' ability to discriminate social support from other related concepts. Perhaps this is the greatest limitation of the body of theories taken as a whole. (Individually, each social support theory may discriminate at a commendable level.)

   Norbeck's work reflects a strong attempt to develop social support theory in a manner that is unique to nursing. But many of the theorists are not nurses, and do not aim to develop the construct in a manner that discriminates nursing applications from those of other disciplines. This lack of discrimination is also a limitation of many social support theories.

5. *Scope of theory.* The social support theories discussed by Dr. Schaffer clearly are of appropriately circumscribed scope to be considered middle range theories. Their application to practice situations is direct because of this limited scope. Yet the theories are broad enough to encompass a specific type of interpersonal relationships at several levels from the individual to a given society.

6. *Complexity.* The complexity varies among the present social support theories. Some develop a limited number of variables; some, an extensive array. Dr. Schaffer notes that Brown's theory of social support develops one broad factor; in contrast, the model of Barerra is multidimensional. The lack of definitional consensus among social support theories creates an artificial complexity that functions in a negative manner.

SUMMARY

The present body of social support theories lacks a clear definition of the phenomenon. Like clarity, the criterion of consistency is not met. Even with these limitations, there is a sense in which the theories are adequately serving nursing to influence practice and research. Among the theories are elements of factor-isolating, explanatory, predictive, and prescriptive levels of theory development.

Looking at the criteria for external criticism, a positive picture is seen. There is strong reality convergence with the "real world" of nursing. The theories are proving to be useful both to practice and to research. Significance seems evident when looking at social support theories from the perspective of health status, health behaviors, use of health services, and health outcomes. Scope of theories seems clearly to be midrange. Only discrimination is a criterion unmet, and complexity, a criterion difficult to assess.

About the Author
Joann P. Wessman, RN, PhD, is a Professor at Bethel College, St. Paul, Minnesota. She teaches nursing theory development and analysis at the graduate level. She has served as dissertation or thesis advisor to doctoral and master's students using middle range theory. Her recent research is in faith/health integration in church-affiliated frail elderly.

Chapter 10 Analysis Exercise: Interpersonal Relations

SONJA J. MEIERS

KATHLEEN SHERAN

INTERNAL CRITICISM

1. *Clarity.* This theory is rather complex when all aspects are considered. The major concepts are clearly defined, readily understandable, but numerous. The major concepts are nurse–patient relationship, phases of the nurse–patient relationship, roles of the nurse, psychobiological experiences, and psychological tasks. All concepts are generally at a high level of abstraction. The role of and importance of the nurse's self-understanding in the therapeutic relationship is clearly outlined.

2. *Consistency.* The theory is consistent and congruent in defining concepts throughout the original work. The focus on the nurse–patient relationship as central to practice and the concept of how the nurse intervenes are consistent with a theory based on interpersonal relations focus. Phases of the nurse–patient relationship, as originally defined, have been subsequently altered. This alteration has been from the defined phases of orientation, identification, exploitation, and termination, to orientation, working, and resolution phases, with identification and exploitation now considered as subphases of the working phase. Concepts of anxiety, tension, unmet needs, frustration, and conflict are consistently presented as targets for the counseling role of the nurse. The worldview is phenomenological in nature and reinforced throughout the theory.

3. *Adequacy.* The theory is adequate in its ability to transfer to settings that allow the nurse time and opportunity to interact with the patient. Since the major foundations of the theory are deducted from disciplines other than nursing, the uniqueness is not found in the body of knowledge but, rather, in the therapeutic role of the nurse in interaction with the patient. Current weaknesses are its emphasis upon the individual patient to the exclusion of family and community, the absence of pathophysiology, and a narrow set of cultural assumptions surrounding interpersonal interaction.

4. *Logical development.* Both inductive and deductive methods are used in development of the theory. The works of Freud, Havighurst, Sullivan, Maslow, and Rogers formed the deductive integration base for the hypothesis statements. Additionally, and most beneficial to nursing, Peplau's inductive approach is a well-formulated theory-development process where observation of nursing practice with patients has resulted in identification of concepts of interest. Theoretical relationships between concepts are clearly presented in the statements of assumptions throughout the historical development of the theory. Within the theory, the role of the nurse is to facilitate the individual in their movement through the steps of the nursing process.

5. *Level of theory development.* This middle range theory is at the descriptive level. Classification of the phases of interpersonal relations between the nurse and patient is its focus. Specifically, interactional phenomena and intrapersonal and interpersonal phenomena of nursing situations and psychosocial phenomena are described.

EXTERNAL CRITICISM

1. *Reality convergence.* The basic underlying assumptions ring true and represent the real world of nursing, particularly in the specialty of psychiatric nursing. Definitions of major tradition domains of nurse, patient, health, and environment are similar to those used in practice. Elements of developmental psychology, humanistic psychology, and learning theory used in the theory are widely accepted premises within the discipline of nursing. The influence of Freud regarding the unconscious motivation of the patient as important to the nurse's role of assisting patients with management of anxiety is evident. These deductions from Freud, Sullivan, and others as they pertain to the nurse–patient interpersonal process are generally accepted, but may not be commonly understood or applied by the nurse generalist. The behaviorist perspective does provide an alternative and popular view of therapist–patient relationships.

2. *Pragmatic.* The theory can be operationalized in nursing-practice settings that value the primacy of the interpersonal process intended to be therapeutic. It is most helpful for viewing and understanding the patient's psychobiological needs, and provides a method for assessing and intervening with these issues. The theory is applicable as a framework to teach the essential elements of therapeutic communication in nursing education.

3. *Utility.* This theory has not yet generated large numbers of research studies, though it meets the criteria of empirical adequacy for a middle range theory. Research that has been completed focuses on factors that influence the development of the nurse–patient relationship. Because many of the practice aspects of the theory have been inductively derived, instrument development has been limited. Therefore, measurement of variables within the theory has not been broadly achieved. Further demonstration of the link between the nurse–patient relationship, symptom relief, and the ultimate well-being of patients is needed.

4. *Significance.* The theory meets the criterion of significance for the discipline. The theory has been published, unchanged since 1952 and continues to be useful, specifically in contemporary mental health nursing. Other nurse scientists have expanded use in areas such as therapeutic milieu, crisis, and family theory. The frequency of reference to the importance of and phases of the nurse–patient relationship in nursing textbooks and empirical studies attests to its continued utility.

5. *Discrimination.* Though the theorist is clear in distinctions between professional nursing practice and medicine in original works, there is not clear distinction between the important content of the nurse–patient relationship and the physician–patient relationship. The basic theory is easily applicable to a variety of helping professions and, though contributing its focus on the interaction to disciplinary development in nursing, is not limited uniquely to nursing.

6. *Scope of theory.* The theory is broad and can be applied in many practice domains, especially those nursing roles that assist the patient with interpersonal or intrapersonal difficulty. It does not provide concepts about pathophysiological or biological phenomena.

7. *Complexity.* The theory has breadth, life, and fluidity. The core of the theory is parsimonious (the relationship between the nurse and the patient). However, the theory describes several important related concepts that explain how to understand the nurse–patient interaction, creating complexity. If these concepts are considered part of the Theory of Interpersonal Relations, it meets the criterion for complexity. Application of the theory requires the nurse be able to be both inductive and deductive when reasoning.

About the Authors

Sonja J. Meiers, PhD, MS, RN, is Associate Professor and Director of the Graduate Program at Minnesota State University, Mankato. Theory development is one of her areas of research interest. Kathleen Sheran, MS, RN, CNS, is Assistant Professor at Minnesota State University, Mankato. Her education, practice, and teaching background is in psychiatric–mental health nursing, all of which have made use of Peplau's Theory of Interpersonal Relations.

Chapter 11 Analysis Exercise: Modeling and Role-Modeling

MARTHA SOFIO

INTERNAL CRITICISM

1. *Clarity.* The theory is easy to understand. The language is simple and the concepts are clearly defined and used with consistency throughout the theory. The coined concept of affiliated individuation is one that does not immediately generate semantic clarity for the reader; however, it is clearly defined in this framework. It calls for further validation and concept analysis. The concept of self-care has a meaning in this framework that varies greatly from its general use, or use in other nursing theories. The concept of self-care knowledge as a subconscious component of person requires validation.

2. *Consistency.* Concepts remain consistently defined throughout the theoretical content. The concept of adaptation as an equilibrium level on a continuum of health and illness is consistent with the interpretation of person as a system adjusting in response to environmental stimuli. Stress is consistently presented as response to a stressor, and adaptation as a holistic response to experienced stressors. Other conceptual definitions of nurturance, object attachment, unconditional acceptance, self-care, holism, and health remain constant throughout the theory. The worldview is that of holistic human experience as related to mind–body interaction; however, it is not proposed to the extent of person/environment unity. The conceptualization of holism is addressed with consistency in reference to both client and nurse.

3. *Adequacy.* This theory is adequate in that its concepts and principles transfer readily into a variety of practice settings. The authors do not specify clinical situations for the use of this theory, and it is readily applicable to the care of individuals in almost all clinical settings. It is challenging, however, to extrapolate it to situations of family assessment and intervention. Because of the major use of theories from other disciplines, its exclusive differentiation for nursing is questionable.

4. *Logical development.* The theory evidences logical development. Deductively using differing external theoretical bases in the description of person, the authors systematically present theoretical relationships. Initially, theories are presented supporting how people are alike, followed by theoretical support for how people are different. These theoretical bases are then described in relationships called "linkages," which offer rich ground for hypothetical deductive research and development of nursing interventions. The theoretical bases and linkages are synthesized to aid in developing a conceptualization of the client's world, the process of which is called modeling. The nursing process is explicated through the use of role-modeling the developed model of the client's world. Specific interventions are subsumed under five generalized aims, all oriented to fulfilling the purpose of the model. All logical steps of the nursing process are intact.

5. *Level of theory development.* This theory is at the explanatory level. It provides clarity as to how to develop a model of the client's world, and proposes that use of that unique model in the role-modeling process will facilitate the client's adaptation. It is in this sense that role-modeling or nurturance provides the basis for predictive and prescriptive nursing theory development.

EXTERNAL CRITICISM

1. *Reality convergence.* The basic premises of the theory easily converge with reality. The principles of growth and development, basic human needs, and adaptation to change and loss are commonly understood and generally accepted. The theory purports to be holistic, and the understanding of mind–body–spirit interaction is widely accepted within the discipline. The conceptualization of mutual goal planning is congruent with the values system of today's practitioners. The conceptualization of self-care knowledge, however, where the client knows what made him ill, and what will make him better might offer some difficulty in this regard.

2. *Utility.* The theory fulfills the criterion of utility. It readily gives the practicing nurse a framework with which to view the client, and from which to facilitate the client's plans for care. Detailed processes for collecting, aggregating, analyzing, and synthesizing data are provided. The theory easily lends itself to curricular development and student education. Adaptive potential, self-care, affiliated individuation, role-modeling, and multiple other conceptualizations offer important subject matter for the execution of nursing research.

3. *Significance.* The theory addresses essential issues in nursing, namely those of client assessment and intervention. Its most significant foci are those of mind–body interaction and mutual goal planning, which compel the nurse to respectively envision the client holistically and to empower him or her. The theory proposes multiple content areas supportive of research in the development of the discipline's body of knowledge.

4. *Discrimination.* A major limitation of the theory is its lack of capacity to discriminate nursing from other health professions and its interventions from other care-tending acts. It would be possible for a physician, psychologist, or social worker to implement this theory. The boundaries are open, and the extant acts and practices can flow inside or outside the discipline.

5. *Scope.* The theory is broad in scope and can be used in diverse practice domains.

6. *Complexity.* The theory is not parsimonious. It is complex and composed of multiple descriptive and explanatory components. The subject matter is rich and presented in great depth. The concept of person is dominant and the inter-relationship of theoretical variables is numerous.

About the Author

Martha Sofio, MS, RN, Assistant Professor at Metropolitan State University, St. Paul, Minnesota is a certified nurse practitioner and certified hypnotherapist who studied with Helen Erickson. She teaches in both the graduate and undergraduate nursing programs at Metropolitan State University. Modeling and Role-Modeling is the theoretical foundation of its undergraduate curriculum.

Chapter 12 Analysis Exercise: Comfort

LINDA WILSON

INTERNAL CRITICISM

1. *Clarity.*   The criterion of clarity is evaluated by how clearly the theory is presented and how easily it is understood by the reader (Barnum, 1990). Comfort Theory is clearly presented in the literature and can be easily read and understood by any reader. Through her program of research and numerous publications, Dr. Kolcaba clearly presents the development and evolution of the Comfort Theory.

2. *Consistency.*   The criterion of consistency is evaluated by examining the definitions and repeated use of the terms of a theory (Barnum, 1990). Comfort Theory has several key concepts that are defined throughout the literature. In every publication, these key concepts are clearly and uniformly defined.

3. *Adequacy.*   The criterion of adequacy is evaluated by how the theory accounts for the specialty to which it applies (Barnum, 1990). Comfort Theory can be applied to all populations. The three senses of comfort (ease, relief, and transcendence) and the contexts in which they occur (physical, social, psychospiritual, environmental) account for comfort care with any patient.

4. *Logical development.*   The criterion of logical development prescribes that the reasoning and conclusions of a theory be clearly presented (Barnum, 1990). Throughout the literature, the ongoing development of Comfort Theory is clearly presented in a reasonable and valid manner. In each of her publications, Dr. Kolcaba presents the theory and the logical reasoning that supports its evolution.

5. *Level of theory development.*   To assess the level of theory development, the researcher needs to evaluate the research that has been completed using the theory (Barnum, 1990). At the time of this author's dissertation research (1998–2000), comfort and Comfort Theory had been clearly defined in the literature; therefore, studies testing explanatory theory using a correlational design were in order. Since that time, Dr. Kolcaba has published the development of the middle range Theory of Comfort. Comfort Theory meets the description of a middle range theory because it consists of several well-defined concepts and can be viewed as both general and complex (Fawcett & Downs, 1992).

EXTERNAL CRITICISM

1. *Reality convergence.* The criterion of reality convergence can be evaluated by examining the principles, interpretations, and method of a theory (Barnum, 1990). Both the concept of comfort and Comfort Theory have practical application to many populations. The essential principles and assumptions of Comfort Theory are clearly defined in the literature by Dr. Kolcaba and can easily be applied to any patient population. The logical development and presentation of the theory allows for easy interpretation and application of the theory in nursing research. Dr. Kolcaba's perception of the nursing world presents the patient and family who are cared for holistically.

2. *Utility.* The criterion of utility refers to the usefulness of the theory by nursing in any practice setting (Barnum, 1990). Comfort Theory can be applied to patients of all ages and in any practice setting. During dissertation research, this author was able to easily apply Comfort Theory to the population of hospitalized medical patients.

3. *Significance.* The criterion of significance is met if the theory contributes to the further development of nursing knowledge, and if it addresses essential nursing issues (Barnum, 1990). Comforting patients is a fundamental part of nursing care because comfort is a desired and expected patient outcome. Comfort Theory provides the basis for comfort care by presenting the three senses (ease, relief, transcendence) and contexts (physical, social, psychospiritual, environmental) in which the outcome of comfort occurs.

4. *Discrimination.* The criterion of discrimination is evaluated by the ability of the theory to differentiate nursing from other health professions and other caring acts (Barnum, 1990). Nurses care for patients holistically and in four contexts of human experience (physical, social, psychospiritual, environmental) from which the outcome of comfort occurs.

5. *Scope of theory.* The criterion of scope of theory evaluates if the theory is broad or limited in scope (Barnum, 1990). The Theory of Comfort is broad in scope because it can be applied to patients of all ages and in various practice settings.

6. *Complexity.* The criterion of complexity allows the researcher the opportunity for explanation and interrelationship of multiple variables (Barnum, 1990). Comfort Theory allows the researcher the opportunity to examine comfort through the three senses of comfort (ease, relief, transcendence) and the four contexts (physical, social, psychospiritual, environmental) in which the outcome of comfort occurs. Any or all of these variables can be measured at one time. In addition, Comfort Theory posits relationships between nursing interventions, patient comfort, health-seeking behaviors, and institutional integrity. Any or all of these relationships can be tested through nursing research.

REFERENCES

Barnum, B. J. (1990). *Nursing theory: Analysis, application, evaluation.* Glenview, IL: Scott, Foresman, Little, Brown.

Fawcett, J., & Downs, F. S. (1992). *The relationship of theory and research* (2nd ed.). Philadelphia: F. A. Davis.

About the Author
Linda Wilson, RN, PhD, CPAN, CAPA, BC, is an Education Specialist for Nursing Continuing Education and Perianesthesia at Thomas Jefferson University Hospital in Philadelphia. Dr. Wilson used the Comfort Theory during her dissertation research, while studying adult hospitalized medical patients.

Chapter 13 Analysis Exercise: Health-Related Quality of Life

LYNNE PLOETZ

INTERNAL CRITICISM

1. *Clarity.*   The detailed description of Wilson and Cleary's model of Health-Related Quality of Life (HRQOL) allows the reader to develop a clear understanding of the components and concepts involved in the theory. With a focus on patient outcomes, the authors (both physicians) indicate that health measures exist on a continuum of increasing complexity. They spell out five domains, including biophysiological factors, symptoms, functioning, general health perceptions, and overall quality of life. They explain the health concepts involved in each level and relate these to general health perceptions and overall quality of life. In addition, they discuss the role of patient preferences and the emotional or psychological factors involved in HRQOL (Wilson & Cleary, 1995).
2. *Consistency.*   The terminology used by Wilson and Cleary (1995) in explaining and discussing HRQOL is consistent throughout their paper. Because they are medical doctors, their terminology is congruent with nursing terminology and can readily be understood by nurses.
3. *Adequacy.*   The questions asked by HRQOL are highly relevant to nursing research and practice, and exist on both individual and global scales. Using Wilson and Cleary's model, HRQOL thoroughly addresses the issues relevant to one's health perceptions and quality of life.
4. *Logical development.*   Wilson and Cleary (1995) provide a well-researched argument that proceeds logically from their initial discussion on the role of HRQOL in research outcomes and how this can be used to improve patient outcomes. They identify the lack of a conceptual model of how different types or levels of patient outcomes relate to each other and to overall HRQOL, and propose a model that considers five main factors and their relationship to each other in determining overall HRQOL. The systems-type model flows logically from the description of these factors to define causal relationships between the factors.
5. *Level of theory development.*   HRQOL is sufficiently defined and narrow to be considered an explanatory middle range theory. The practical nature of the theory allows the researcher to develop testable hypotheses regarding HRQOL in different patient populations.

EXTERNAL CRITICISM

1. *Reality convergence.* The HRQOL theory immediately "makes sense" to the nurse. This theory provides a framework for better understanding the relationship of illness and nursing interventions to patients' quality of life.
2. *Utility.* The HRQOL model is useful for nurses in both research and practice. Nurses in any discipline can identify hypotheses that can be tested by using the HRQOL model.
3. *Significance.* HRQOL is highly significant to nursing research and practice. As patients live longer with chronic illness because of improved diagnostics and therapeutics, research into nursing interventions that improve HRQOL becomes even more significant.
4. *Discrimination.* Because HRQOL is a multidisciplinary concept, boundaries could extend beyond nursing practice. When HRQOL is used as a framework for nursing research, care must be taken to provide clear boundaries regarding nursing interventions.
5. *Scope.* This model is sufficiently narrow in scope that research can focus on individuals as well as groups. However, studies could be designed that allow a broader scope, if desired.
6. *Complexity.* The HRQOL model by Wilson and Cleary is quite complex, with five determinants, each having multiple variables. However, the model allows the researcher to identify specific variables for study. Control of extraneous variables is necessary in any research study, and the thorough explanation of variables in the model would facilitate identification and control of those considered extraneous.

REFERENCE

Wilson, I. B., & Cleary, P. D. (1995). Linking clinical variables with health-related quality of life: A conceptual model of patient outcomes. *Journal of the American Medical Association, 273*(1), 59–65.

About the Author
Lynne Ploetz, RN, BS, is President and CEO of Matrix Advocare Network, Minneapolis, MN. She is a nurse entrepreneur who works to improve her patients, health-related quality of life through innovative nursing practice. Ms. Ploetz is certified in gerontological nursing by American Nurses Credentialing Center and is a certified case manager through the Commission for Case Management Certification. Several years ago, she started a geriatric case-management company, Matrix Advo-Care Network. Today she employs 20 registered nurse, care consultants throughout Minnesota, who provide health advocacy and care-consulting services to frail elderly and people with mental and physical disabilities.

Chapter 14 Analysis Exercise: Health Promotion

MADELEINE J. KERR

INTERNAL CRITICISM

1. *Adequacy.*   The model broadly describes several factors that have relationships to health-promoting behavior. In comparison to some other models, the Pender Health Promotion Model is broader, in that the model includes a number of intrapersonal factors (such as perceived barriers to the behavior), interpersonal factors (such as social norms), and situational influences (such as availability of healthful options). A possible gap is the model's focus on individual health promotion. The model has implications for the health promotion of families and communities, however, use of multiple models would be ideal to address these populations. Tests of the initial Health Promotion Model in 38 studies have accounted for considerable variance in health-promoting lifestyle and several specific behaviors, such as exercise. The revised Health Promotion Model needs to be tested empirically.

2. *Clarity.*   The phenomenon that the model seeks to explain is health-promoting behavior. This phenomenon has multiple definitions, but Pender's definition carefully circumscribes the limits of this phenomenon. Some readers may struggle with the concept, particularly in light of the traditional medical model with which so many nurses are familiar. While Pender offers that one major distinguishing feature between health promotion and health protection is motivation for the behavior, these may not be easily distinguished in practice. For instance a client may engage in exercise for the dual benefits of increasing energy and avoiding cardiovascular disease and obesity. It is not clear how these dual motivations may affect the model.

   Pender's model is presented in a language and style that is easily understood by nurses and other health professionals. A schematic illustrates relationships between concepts. She provides clear definitions of terms. Relationship statements are established in Pender, Murdaugh, & Parson's (2002) *Health Promotion in Nursing Practice* (4th ed.).

3. *Consistency.*   Model terminology in definitions corresponds with use in relationship statements and throughout the description of the theory.

4. *Logical development.*   The revised model includes clearly established assumptions, concepts, and relationships. Each of these is clearly labeled and presented to the reader.

   The theoretical foundations of the model are attributed to several well-established theories of behavior. These theories include Feather's Expectancy-Value Theory and Bandura's Social Cognitive Theory. Concepts that did not receive empirical support in the initial Health Promotion Model were dropped in the revised model. The rationale for each of the model revisions is explained, and detailed results of previous model-testing empirical studies are clearly presented in *Health Promotion in Nursing Practice* (4th ed.).

5. *Level of theory development.* The model represents a middle range theory in that it addresses a specific phenomenon. It is intended for use in providing health-promotion services to clients.

EXTERNAL CRITICISM

1. *Reality convergence.* Pender's model describes phenomena of interest to nurses, and includes a variety of factors that are well known to experienced health professionals, such as client perceptions of barriers and benefits. The theory has been supported in a number of model-testing studies.
2. *Utility.* The theory can be operationalized to provide interventions in real life settings. For example, Lusk (1999) used the Pender health-promotion model to identify factors influencing workers' use of hearing protection. This information was subsequently used to develop an educational intervention that increased this health behavior 20% from baseline. The model also is potentially useful for individually tailoring behavior change interventions to individuals with interactive computer communications.

   Research shows the model to be useful for explaining and predicting client behavior in several important areas, including exercise, and nutrition. The model has only recently begun to be used in the design of interventions, but may prove useful in guiding nurses to design cost-effective strategies to improve client health. The model provides a "framework for understanding the dimensions on which health promotion interventions can be based" (Pender, Murdaugh, & Parsons, 2002, p. 75). However, the model does not guide the nurse using the framework in methods to develop interventions.
3. *Significance.* Health promotion as a phenomenon has enormous potential for the discipline of nursing. A change in focus from disease prevention to health promotion expands the role of nursing in society, and has potential for greatly enhancing the well-being of society. Investment in diagnosis and treatment of disease has been the dominant model of health care until recently. However, the limitations of this model are now recognized more than ever, while the role of health behavior as a determinant of health is growing in recognition. The economic and nontangible advantages of investing in health promotion are gaining popularity in business and government. Because health behavior is a large and growing concern, having far-reaching consequences for the health and prosperity of society, the Health Promotion Model has great potential significance.
4. *Discrimination.* The Pender Health Promotion Model is unique within nursing, although it does bear some resemblance to theories of health behavior in the social and psychological sciences. However, its unique approach-oriented nature distinguishes it from other theories of health behavior that have an avoidance orientation. The model provides a framework for discriminating which concepts are relevant to specific health behaviors. Much work remains to be done to determine how the model can be applied to different behaviors, and in various cultural, developmental, and gender-based populations. The model focuses more on health promotion for individuals than on families, communities, and society.
5. *Scope.* The espoused scope of the theory is health-promoting behavior. Health-promoting behavior is directed toward increasing the level of well-being and self-actualization of a given individual or group (Pender, Murdaugh, & Parsons, 2002, p. 34). Examples of health-promoting behavior provided by the authors include physical activity, nutrition, stress management, and social support. This range of behaviors is appropriate to middle range theory. However, the authors also describe

the application of the model to health behavior beyond the scope of health promotion (e.g., use of hearing protection and environmental tobacco-smoke exposure). The success of the model in describing and explaining these client behaviors suggests that the model may have a scope of application beyond its original intent.

6. *Complexity.* The Pender Health Promotion Model uses relatively few (11, to be exact) concepts to address the complex phenomenon of health-promoting behavior. Relationships between even this small number of concepts is potentially large, however, because a single factor may have multiple relationships to other factors within the model. The authors seem to have achieved a balance between thoroughness and parsimony.

REFERENCES

Lusk, S., Kerr, M., Ronis, D., & Eakin, B. (1999). Applying the health promotion model to development of a worksite intervention. *American Journal of Health Promotion, 13*(4), 219–226.

Pender, N., Murdaugh, C., & Parsons, M. (2002). *Health promotion in nursing practice* (4th ed.). Upper Saddle River, NJ: Prentice Hall.

About the Author

Madeleine J. Kerr, PhD, RN, is Associate Professor in Public Health Nursing at the University of Minnesota School of Nursing, Minneapolis. She applies Pender's Health Promotion Model to the study of construction worker's hearing health behavior, and to the design of computer-based tailored educational interventions to promote use of hearing protection devices. She has also conducted one of the first cross-cultural tests of the Health Promotion Model with Mexican-American workers.

Chapter 15 Analysis Exercise: Deliberative Nursing Process

MIMI DYE

INTERNAL CRITICISM

1. *Clarity.* The theory demonstrates clarity in its specific definition of easily understood terms, and in its specific use of those terms as they are involved in the flow of communication and activities inherent in the Deliberative Nursing Process.

2. *Consistency.* The theory demonstrates consistency because the definition, use of terms, and formulation remain the same throughout.

3. *Adequacy.* The theory demonstrates adequacy because its scope includes any professional communication relevant to meeting patient needs at any level within and throughout the health care

system. Implicit in the theory is that the nurse will validate the needs of a patient who is mute, cognitively impaired, or cognitively compromised, by means other than direct verbal communication, such as observations by the nurse or information provided by significant others.

4. *Logical development.*   The theory demonstrates logical development from its premises to its product or outcome because the flow of ingredients explicitly used in the Deliberative Nursing Process reasonably leads one to the product, or outcome, that is, improvement in the patient's immediate behavior.

5. *Level of theory development.*   Because this theory is situation-producing or prescriptive theory, it is Level IV theory. For instance, the nurse's greater understanding of the patient's need for help results in alleviating the patient's distress more effectively.

EXTERNAL CRITICISM

1. *Reality convergence.*   The theory begins with the premise that the patients may have needs that they may not be able to express or meet without professional nursing assistance. Therefore, it is the responsibility of nurses to explore with patients whether or not they have such needs, and whether or not their nursing activities meet those needs. This theory includes using the Deliberative Nursing Process in any communication relevant to patient needs anywhere in the health care system. Essentially, it involves the patient as a crucial member of this communication system. Meeting patient needs with patients is widely accepted in nursing.

2. *Utility.*   Since the theory offers the Deliberative Nursing Process as an explicit way to keep communication clear and has as its purpose ascertaining and meeting patient needs, it is useful to the administrator as well as to the practitioner. It is useful to the educator because it can be taught and practiced within the educational system. It is useful to the researcher because its variables lend themselves to research. The theory, therefore, has a high degree of utility for the nursing profession.

3. *Significance.*   Since the theory focuses on nurse–patient communications and communications within the health care system relevant to meeting patients' health care needs, specifically, responding to and relieving patients' immediate distress, the theory addresses the essential core issue in nursing—responding to and meeting patients' needs that cannot be met without professional nursing assistance. The theory contributes to nursing knowledge by offering the Deliberative Nursing Process, designed to ascertain and meet patients' needs and relieve patients' immediate distress. The theory can be taught. Its variables lend themselves to research. Therefore, the theory has immense significance for the nursing profession.

4. *Discrimination.*   The theory constructs a system of nursing practice for nurses to fulfill a distinct professional function wherever they practice. The theory is inclusive for nurses in administration, education, and clinical practice in all specialties. The unique professional nursing function is to ascertain and meet patients' immediate needs for help when patients are unable to do so without professional nursing assistance. The product or outcome of this function is to relieve patients' distress. Therefore, this theory differentiates nursing from health professions.

5. *Scope of theory.*   The scope of the theory is broadly applicable because it includes nursing communications relevant to meeting patients' health care needs in all specialties, wherever and however nurses are practicing, whether in administration, education, practice, or research.

6. *Complexity.*   The theory offers a balance between parsimony and complexity. It is parsimonious in that its elements are few and includes only those needed to describe and explain the theory. It is complex because communication between and among people can be complex and the dynamics of relationships including nurse–patient relationships can be complex.

About the Author
Mimi Dye, MSN, ARNP, is a former student and longtime friend of Ms. Orlando. She has recently served as a consultant to the New Hampshire Hospital Orlando Project.

Chapter 16 Analysis Exercise: Planned Change

SAGRID E. EDMAN

INTERNAL CRITICISM

1. *Clarity.*   The theories covered are primarily stage theories. Terminology that is not common to nursing is defined and can be applied to nursing situations. The theories vary in level of abstraction from relatively concrete terms to fairly abstract terms, such as the stages described by DiClemente and Prochaska (1998). Several of the theories rely on a basic problem-solving process, with some variation in terminology

2. *Consistency.*   The approaches of the theorists are consistent in that they all use a stage theory approach derived from observations and descriptions of actual situations involving change. Most of the theories take a qualitative approach and rely on anecdotal evidence as the source of the data. There is not a great deal of consistency in the terms or interpretations described. Each theorist has his or her own terminology for the stages or has expanded on another theorist's work. However, all of the stage theories have some common characteristics and, with some careful analysis, could be condensed into one mega stage set. Differences occur because some of the stage theories divide up the change process into many stages, and other theories include only three or four stages.

    In addition to stage theories, some studies reported describe reactions to change and are not at the level of a true theory, but are anecdotal or conceptual in nature.

3. *Adequacy.*   The theories are adequate only up to a point. They do provide for a framework for planning a change event or analyzing a change that has occurred. However, they do not adequately take into account the unintended occurrences that usually occur in any complex change project. The theories imply that individuals and organizations move through the stages one by one. Problems such as resistance and other negative consequences are mentioned, but the theories do not provide any real direction for managing situations that involve difficult circumstances.

4. *Level of theory development.* These middle range theories are descriptive and rely on a set of stages that a planned change event goes through. Research projects that are based on the existing change theories are often qualitative studies relying on interviews and observation. The theories are applied to a situation so that they become a deductive framework that often just affirms the stages of the theory, rather than providing a rigorous evaluation of it.

EXTERNAL CRITICISM

1. *Reality convergence.* Change is a daily occurrence in health care and nursing. But most change theories are not specific to nursing. They are neutral in relation to a specific profession. They do, however, represent stages that are present in almost every large-scale change project. Most authors use terminology that would be familiar to nurses and could form the conceptual framework for nursing research.

   The problem, however, is that in many cases nurses engage in planned-change projects without using any of the change theory knowledge base that is available. Further, they may not be aware of the wide variety of change models that are present in the literature, thus limiting the resources available to them.

2. *Utility.* The theories can be useful in both practice and research if applied with proper analysis and discrimination. They are, however, limited in their application. Stage theories do not take into account the many variables that can occur in a complex or large-scale change project. They are limited to some types of planned change but do not reflect some of the real-world situations such as:

   - Other changes taking place in the organization that may affect the conduct of the project
   - Unintended consequences that arise out of the woodwork and force revisions that may delay or undermine the goals of the original project
   - Unexpected resistance or political compromises that may have to be made to move the project forward
   - The fact that many change situations are not planned but are crisis events or changes that are imposed by legislation, financial exigency, demographic change, technological innovation, etc.

   In addition, most of the theories do not adequately account for the need or requirement for:

   - A change agent who is respected and has both the authority and the political know-how to work through problems (Lippitt's work does identify the importance of the role and definition of the change agent)
   - A constant feedback loop and internal or external problem-solving process to allow revisions as the project moves ahead—as described by Havelock (1976) in his work on diffusion of innovation. His terminology for this feedback loop is "linkage."

Many nursing research projects have used change theories as conceptual frameworks, but little work has been done to begin to develop a unique theory of change for nursing. Indeed, it is questionable whether the profession needs its own theory of change. The existing theories are process constructs that can be applied to many situations and planned change projects.

3. *Significance.*   The theories do reflect issues related to change, but they are not nursing theories. They are neutral in relation to a specific content area or knowledge base. The theories are more accurately described as conceptual frameworks that provide a basis for understanding, planning, and evaluating the dynamics of change.

The theories presented do not represent some of the most recent work on change, such as chaos theory, that has been done in the field of organizational studies. There is a vast field of change literature that has not shown up in the work of the profession.

4. *Discrimination.*   These theories, for the most part do not overlap interpersonal processes. Because they are stage theories they describe the steps that need to occur in the development or implementation of a change process. Studies that do describe interpersonal processes are descriptive in nature and report on human responses to change, such as the work by Yoder-Wise (2003) or Perlman and Takas (1990). These are not empirically tested studies. The theories do not attempt to discriminate as to the discipline of nursing.

5. *Scope of theory*   The existing change theories can be applied to many aspects of the nursing practice arena. Though they are not nursing theories, they do have utility in the planning of change projects in nursing.

6. *Complexity.*   As a group, the theories are fairly complex. They take into account many aspects of the change process. However, the change agent or agents need to be cognizant of the assumptions that form the basis for each theory or stage set. Not every theory would be appropriate to plan for or evaluate a change event.

Newer theories and more recent literature, however, reflect the complexity or organizational change to a much higher degree.

REFERENCES

DiClemente, C., & Prochaska, J. (1998). Toward a comprehensive transtheoretical model of change. In W. R. Miller & N. Healther (Eds.), *Treating addictive behaviors* (pp. 3-24). New York: Plenum Press.

Havelock, R. G. (1976). *Planning for innovation through dissemination and utilization of knowledge.* Ann Arbor, MI: University of Michigan, Center for Research on Utilization of Scientific Knowledge, Institute for Social Research.

Perlman, D., & Takacs, G. (1990). The ten stages of change. *Nursing Management, 21* (4), 33-38.

Yoder-Wise, P. S. (Ed.). (2003). *Leading and managing change in nursing* (3rd ed.). St. Louis, MO: Mosby.

About the Author

Sagrid E. Edman, PhD, MA, RN, is Professor Emeritus, Bethel College, St. Paul, Minnesota. She has been involved in research on the "Impact of the Changing Health Care System on Nurses: Response of Clinical Managers to Merger and Massive Organizational Change" for more than a decade. She has presented "Managing the Whirlwind of Change," nationally to many different nursing audiences.

Chapter 17 Analysis Exercise: Resilience

MARSHA L. ELLETT

INTERNAL CRITICISM

1. *Clarity.*   According to the Adolescent Resilience Model (ARM), resilience may occur as a result of a process that includes deriving meaning from an adverse experience through interaction with others. The ARM is parsimonious, given the widespread agreement among researchers that resilience is a complex, multidimensional construct. The concepts of the model are named but are not explicitly defined. They are operationalized clearly by instruments derived from decision trees for the qualitative work. Three classes of protective factors—individual, family, and social are hypothesized to positively affect resilience outcomes. The individual protective factors include courageous or positive coping and derived meaning. The familial protective factors include family atmosphere and support/resources available to the family. The social protective resources include health care resources and social integration. Two classes of factors are hypothesized to negatively affect resilience—individual risk factor and illness-related stress factors. The individual risk factor is sustained defensive coping, and the illness-related stress factors include illness perspective and illness distress. The outcome factors of resilience include self-esteem, mastery/confidence, and self-transcendence, as well as quality of life, defined as a sense of well-being.
2. *Consistency.*   There is consistency between the text and the model (Figure 17-2) in the social and family protective factors. However, the illness-related stress factors, including illness perspective and illness distress, in the text are referred to as symptom-related risk in the model and include illness perception, symptom distress, and severity of illness. This inconsistency in wording between the text and the model is somewhat confusing. Also, the only outcome variable depicted in the model is quality of life, so the relationships of self-esteem, mastery/confidence, and self-transcendence to quality of life are unclear.
3. *Adequacy.*   A strength of the ARM is that it is an emerging model grounded in contextual experiences. It appears that defensive coping is an individual risk factor only if it is sustained. Progression to courageous coping can occur, which is positively related to resilience. Further refinement of the concepts will occur with continued use of the model.
4. *Logical development.*   The Adolescent Resilience Model was developed first through qualitative studies that allowed the identification and clarification of concepts to be included in the model. Next, quantitative structural equation modeling was used to identify relationships among concepts. Then, qualitative methods were again used to evaluate these identified relationships.
5. *Level of theory development.*   The ARM is only beginning to be used to guide nursing interventions; therefore, it is an emerging middle range theory.

EXTERNAL CRITICISM

1. *Reality convergence.* The assumptions underlying the ARM were not specifically stated as such; however, one assumption may be that persons with resilience require time to reflect on the meaning of their actions. Thus, Haase and colleagues state that resilience may occur through a process that includes deriving meaning from the experience through interaction with others. The ARM appears to reflect the real world of nursing and makes inherent sense to this reader. This model's ability to guide interventions is just beginning to be tested. The one described study testing the ARM aims to test the efficacy of a therapeutic music video intervention for adolescents and young adults during the acute phase of stem-cell transplant. This indicates that the model has the potential to be useful in real-life settings.

2. *Utility.* The researchers state that several studies are currently being developed using the ARM, but only the study mentioned was described. In this study, the ARM was being used to generate hypotheses.

3. *Significance.* Any model that can guide nursing interventions to enhance resilience outcomes in adolescents and young adults faced with cancer would be highly significant.

4. *Discrimination.* Whether the ARM will guide hypothesis generation that could not be generated by other models of resilience is not known presently. At this time, the boundaries of resilience are inconsistent.

5. *Scope.* The scope of the ARM currently is narrow in that it is being studied in chronically ill adolescents, mostly those with cancer, and is being tested in practice. If the initial intervention research is successful, this reader can see expanding the scope of this model slightly to include adolescents with other serious chronic illnesses and then, later, to chronically ill participants in different age groups facing different developmental tasks. The ARM has the potential to become more global in time with continued refinement.

6. *Complexity.* Given that resilience is a complex, multidimensional construct, the ARM is parsimonious, with few concepts that can be fairly easily understood without lengthy descriptions or explanations.

About the Author

Marsha Ellett, DNS, RN, is an Associate Professor at Indiana University School of Nursing, Indianapolis and a pediatric clinical nurse specialist. She teaches pediatrics in both the baccalaureate and master's programs (Pediatric Clinical Nurse Specialist Program). Her research has focused on enteral tube placement in children and colic in infants. It is through her association with her colleague, Joan Haase, that she became familiar with the Adolescence Resilience Model. She identifies the model's utility to the practice of her specialty, in work with young people with chronic illnesses, such as Crohn's disease, ulcerative colitis, and chronic aggressive hepatitis.

Instruments

BURKE/EAKES CHRONIC SORROW ASSESSMENT TOOL©

The questions below are asked about the effects that certain life events or situations may have on people over a period of time so that helping professionals can better meet their needs. In answering these questions, please focus on the impact that these life events or situations continue to have on your life. There are no right or wrong answers. You do not have to answer any or all of the questions and can stop without penalty of any kind. Thank you for taking the time to answer these questions.

DEMOGRAPHICS/BACKGROUND

1. Which of the following best describes your situation? (Please check only one)

a) _____ Parent of disabled child (please specify the disability) _____

b) _____ Person with a chronic condition (please specify the condition) _____

c) _____ Caregiver of someone with a chronic or life-threatening illness (please specify the condition) _____

d) _____ Bereaved person (please specify the relationship of deceased to you) _____

2. I have been dealing with this situation/loss for_____ years. (Please write in number of years)

3. Please provide the following information about yourself:

a) Sex: _____ male _____ female

b) Age: _____ years

c) Marital status: _____ single _____ married _____ widowed _____ divorced _____ separated

3. (continued)

    d) Religion: _____ Protestant _____ Catholic _____ Jewish

       Other (Please write in): _____

    e) Ethnic origin: _____ Caucasian _____ Hispanic _____ African American

       _____ American Indian _____ Asian

       Other (Please write in): _____

    f) Please indicate your highest completed level of education:

       a. Less than high school

       b. High school graduate

       c. Associate/technical degree

       d. Bachelor's degree

       e. Master's degree

       f. PhD/MD or equivalent

    g) Total family income per year from all sources before taxes:

       a. Below $5,000

       b. $5,001–10,000

       c. $10,001–15,000

       d. $15,001–20,000

       e. $20,001–25,000

       f. $25,001–30,000

       g. $30,001–40,000

       h. Over $40,000

DISPARITY

4. Even though some time may have passed since you began dealing with your situation/loss, you may still be coping with some ongoing issues and reactions. Please read the following statements and indicate if this is true for you. Remember, there are no right or wrong answers.

   a) I recognize the hole this situation/loss has created in my life.   ☐ True   ☐ False

   b) I think about the difference this situation/loss has made in my life.   ☐ True   ☐ False

   c) I experience changes in my life as a result of the situation/loss.   ☐ True   ☐ False

   d) I feel its effects in bits and pieces.   ☐ True   ☐ False

GRIEF-RELATED FEELINGS

The following are feelings you may have experienced as a result of your situation/loss.

5. At those times when you experience these feelings associated with your situation/loss, please indicate how upsetting they are for you. Remember, there are no right or wrong answers.

	Have Not Experienced	Have Experienced But Not Upsetting	Have Experienced, Somewhat Upsetting	Have Experienced, Very Upsetting
a) sad				
b) anxious				
c) angry				
d) overwhelmed				
e) heartbroken				
f) other (please specify):				

CHARACTERISTICS OF CHRONIC SORROW
(Pervasive, Permanent, Periodic, Potentially Progressive)

The questions below ask more about the feelings you may experience related to your situation/loss. Please mark the extent to which each statement below is true for you.

6. In describing my feelings about my situation/loss, I:

    a) have ups and downs. ☐ True ☐ False

    b) feel their effects on other parts of my life. ☐ True ☐ False

    c) feel them more strongly now than at first. ☐ True ☐ False

    d) believe they will impact on me the rest of my life. ☐ True ☐ False

TRIGGERS

There may be certain times when you tend to experience the feelings associated with your situation/loss. Please read the following statements and indicate which are true for you.

7. These feelings about my situation/loss come up when I:

    a) have to seek medical care. ☐ True ☐ False

    b) realize all the responsibilities I have. ☐ True ☐ False

    c) compare where I am now with where others are in their lives. ☐ True ☐ False

    d) think of all I now have to do. ☐ True ☐ False

    e) meet someone else in the same situation. ☐ True ☐ False

    f) experience the anniversary of when this began. ☐ True ☐ False

    g) have a "special day" such as a birthday or holiday. ☐ True ☐ False

    h) other (please specify):_____

INTERNAL COPING MECHANISMS

The statements below are things you may have found helpful to you in managing the feelings associated with your situation/loss. Please indicate which is true for you.

8. It helps me deal with my feelings when I:

	Never Tried	Have Tried, But Not Helpful	Have Tried, Somewhat Helpful	Have Tried, Very Helpful
a) keep busy				
b) take one day at a time				
c) talk to someone close to me				
d) pray				
e) exercise				
f) count my blessings				
g) work on my hobbies				
h) express my feelings				
i) go to church, synagogue, or other place of worship				
j) talk with others in similar situations				
k) take a "can do" attitude				
l) talk with a minister, rabbi, or priest				
m) talk with a health professional				
n) focus on the positive				

o) other (please specify): _____

EXTERNAL COPING MECHANISMS

The following questions are to find out how helping professionals can assist people who are dealing with situations/losses such as yours. Please indicate which is true for you. Remember, there are no right or wrong answers.

9. It helps me deal with my feelings when helping professionals:

	Never Tried	Have Tried, But Not Helpful	Have Tried, Somewhat Helpful	Have Tried, Very Helpful
a) listen to me				
b) recognize my feelings				
c) answer my honestly				
d) allow me to ask questions				
e) take their time with me				
f) provide good care				

g) other (please specify): _____

Friends and family may also be helpful to you as you deal with the feelings associated with your situation/loss. Please read the following and indicate which is true for you.

10. It helps me deal with my feelings when family and friends:

	Never Tried	Have Tried, But Not Helpful	Have Tried, Somewhat Helpful	Have Tried, Very Helpful
a) listen to me				
b) have a positive outlook				
c) accept my feelings				
d) provide emotional support				
e) offer a helping hand				
f) acknowledge my situation/loss				

g) other (please specify): _____

Thank you for answering these questions. Please return the questionnaire at this time.

GENERAL COMFORT QUESTIONNAIRE

Thank you VERY MUCH for helping me in my study of the concept COMFORT. Below are statements that may describe your comfort right now. Four numbers are provided for each question; please circle the number you think most closely matches what you are feeling. Relate these questions to your comfort *at the moment you are answering the questions.*

	Strongly Agree			Strongly Disagree
1. My body is relaxed right now	4	3	2	1
2. I feel useful because I'm working hard	4	3	2	1
3. I have enough privacy	4	3	2	1
4. There are those I can depend on when I need help	4	3	2	1
5. I don't want to exercise	4	3	2	1
6. My condition gets me down	4	3	2	1
7. I feel confident	4	3	2	1
8. I feel dependent on others	4	3	2	1
9. I feel my life is worthwhile right now	4	3	2	1
10. I am inspired by knowing that I am loved	4	3	2	1
11. These surroundings are pleasant	4	3	2	1
12. The sounds keep me from resting	4	3	2	1
13. No one understands me	4	3	2	1
14. My pain is difficult to endure	4	3	2	1
15. I am inspired to do my best	4	3	2	1
16. I am unhappy when I am alone	4	3	2	1
17. My faith helps me to not be afraid	4	3	2	1
18. I do not like it here	4	3	2	1
19. I am constipated right now	4	3	2	1
20. I do not feel healthy right now	4	3	2	1
21. This room makes me feel scared	4	3	2	1
22. I am afraid of what is next	4	3	2	1

	Strongly Agree			Strongly Disagree
23. I have a favorite person(s) who makes me feel cared for	4	3	2	1
24. I have experienced changes that make me feel uneasy	4	3	2	1
25. I am hungry	4	3	2	1
26. I would like to see my doctor more often	4	3	2	1
27. The temperature in this room is fine	4	3	2	1
28. I am very tired	4	3	2	1
29. I can rise above my pain	4	3	2	1
30. The mood around here uplifts me	4	3	2	1
31. I am content	4	3	2	1
32. This chair (bed) makes me hurt	4	3	2	1
33. This view inspires me	4	3	2	1
34. My personal belongings are not here	4	3	2	1
35. I feel out of place here	4	3	2	1
36. I feel good enough to walk	4	3	2	1
37. My friends remember me with their cards and phone calls	4	3	2	1
38. My beliefs give me peace of mind	4	3	2	1
39. I need to be better informed about my health	4	3	2	1
40. I feel out of control	4	3	2	1
41. I feel crummy because I am not dressed	4	3	2	1
42. This room smells terrible	4	3	2	1
43. I am alone but not lonely	4	3	2	1
44. I feel peaceful	4	3	2	1
45. I am depressed	4	3	2	1
46. I have found meaning in my life	4	3	2	1
47. It is easy to get around here	4	3	2	1
48. I need to feel good again	4	3	2	1

Available at www.uakron.edu/comfort. No permission needed.

Code # _____   **Date** _____   **Time** _____

Comfort Behaviors Checklist: *How is patient acting right now?*
Please circle best response. *NA* = not applicable

. . . .

	NA	No	Somewhat	Moderate	Strong
Vocalizations					
1. complaining	0	1	2	3	4
2. awake	0	1	2	3	4
3. moaning	0	1	2	3	4
4. content sounds/talk	0	1	2	3	4
5. crying/shouting	0	1	2	3	4
Motor Signs					
6. peaceful	0	1	2	3	4
7. agitated	0	1	2	3	4
8. rapid pacing	0	1	2	3	4
9. fidgety	0	1	2	3	4
10. muscles relaxed	0	1	2	3	4
11. rubbing an area	0	1	2	3	4
12. guarding	0	1	2	3	4
Behaviors					
13. anxious	0	1	2	3	4
14. accepts kindness	0	1	2	3	4
15. likes touch/ hand holding	0	1	2	3	4
16. appears depressed	0	1	2	3	4
17. able to rest	0	1	2	3	4
18. able to eat	0	1	2	3	4
19. calm, at ease	0	1	2	3	4

20. purposeless movements	0	1	2	3	4

Facial . . . .

21. grimaces/winces	0	1	2	3	4
22. relaxed expression	0	1	2	3	4
23. wrinkled brow	0	1	2	3	4
24. appears frightened or worried	0	1	2	3	4
25. smiles	0	1	2	3	4

Miscellaneous . . . .

26. unusual breathing	0	1	2	3	4
27. focuses mentally	0	1	2	3	4
28. converses	0	1	2	3	4
29. awakens smoothly	0	1	2	3	4

If this is the *only* comfort/pain instrument being used, ask the patient:

30. Do you have any pain? No_____Yes _____ [Please rate your pain from 1 to 10, with 10 being the highest possible pain]. _____ (rating)

31. Taking everything into consideration, how comfortable are you right now? [Please rate your total comfort from 1 to 10, with 10 being the highest possible comfort.] _____ (rating)

Other open-ended comments . . . .

(change in medication use, recent injury, recent decline in functional status, staff reports of comfort/discomfort, changes in appetite, ambulation, etc.)

Adapted by K. Kolcaba from: Volicer, L. (1988). Management of advanced Alzheimer's dementia/The comfort checklist. In L. Volicer (Ed.). *Clinical management of Alzheimer's disease.* Rockville, MD: Aspen Publications.

Scoring of the Behaviors Checklist

1. *Subtract* number of "not applicable" (NA) from 29, to obtain **total answered.**

2. *Multiply* total answered (step 1) by *4*, to obtain **total possible score.**

3. *Reverse code:* numbers 1, 3, 5, 7, 8, 9, 11, 12, 13, 16, 20, 22, 23, 25 to obtain **raw comfort responses.**

4. *Add* **raw comfort responses** (step 3) for all questions not marked NA, to obtain actual comfort score.

5. *Divide actual comfort score* (step 4) *by total possible score* (step 2) and round to two decimal places. (If the third decimal place is a 5 or greater, round the second decimal place up to the next number.)

6. *Report score* as a **2-digit number** (rounded percent without the % sign or decimal) *Higher scores* indicate *higher Comfort.*

Comfort Behaviors Checklist © K. Kolcaba (2002)
Available at www.uakron.edu/comfort. No permission needed.

PAEDIATRIC ASTHMA QUALITY OF LIFE QUESTIONNAIRE WITH STANDARDISED ACTIVITIES (PAQLQ(S))

SELF-ADMINISTERED

© 1999

QOL TECHNOLOGIES LTD.

TM

For further information:

Elizabeth Juniper, MCSP, MSc
Professor
20 Marcuse Fields,
Bosham,
West Sussex,
PO18 8NA. UK
Tel: + 44 (0) 1243 572124
Fax: + 44 (0) 1243 573680
E-mail: juniper@qoltech.co.uk
Web: www.qoltech.co.uk

**PAEDIATRIC ASTHMA
QUALITY OF LIFE QUESTIONNAIRE (S)
SELF-ADMINISTERED**

PATIENT ID _____

DATE _____

Please complete **all** questions by circling the number that best describes how you have been during the **past week as a result of your asthma.**

HOW **BOTHERED** HAVE YOU BEEN DURING THE LAST WEEK DOING:

	Extremely Bothered	Very Bothered	Quite Bothered	Somewhat Bothered	Bothered a Bit	Hardly Bothered at All	Not Bothered
1. PHYSICAL ACTIVITIES (such as running, swimming, sports, walking uphill/ upstairs and bicycling)?	1	2	3	4	5	6	7
2. BEING WITH ANIMALS (such as playing with pets and looking after animals)?	1	2	3	4	5	6	7
3. ACTIVITIES WITH FRIENDS AND FAMILY (such as playing at recess and doing things with your friends and family)?	1	2	3	4	5	6	7
4. COUGHING	1	2	3	4	5	6	7

IN GENERAL, **HOW OFTEN** DURING THE LAST WEEK DID YOU:

	All of the Time	Most of the Time	Quite Often	Some of the Time	Once in a While	Hardly Any of the Time	None of the Time
5. Feel FRUSTRATED because of your asthma?	1	2	3	4	5	6	7

PAEDIATRIC ASTHMA
QUALITY OF LIFE QUESTIONNAIRE (S)
SELF-ADMINISTERED

PATIENT ID _____

DATE _____

	All of the Time	Most of the Time	Quite Often	Some of the Time	Once in a While	Hardly Any of the Time	None of the Time
6. Feel TIRED because of your asthma?	1	2	3	4	5	6	7
7. Feel WORRIED, CONCERNED OR TROUBLED because of your asthma?	1	2	3	4	5	6	7

HOW **BOTHERED** HAVE YOU BEEN DURING THE LAST WEEK BY?

	Extremely Bothered	Very Bothered	Quite Bothered	Somewhat Bothered	Bothered a Bit	Hardly Bothered at All	Not Bothered
8. ASTHMA ATTACKS	1	2	3	4	5	6	7

IN GENERAL, **HOW OFTEN** DURING THE LAST WEEK DID YOU:

	All of the Time	Most of the Time	Quite Often	Some of the Time	Once in a While	Hardly Any of the Time	None of the Time
9. Feel ANGRY becauseof your asthma?	1	2	3	4	5	6	7

HOW **BOTHERED** HAVE YOU BEEN DURING THE LAST WEEK BY?

	Extremely Bothered	Very Bothered	Quite Bothered	Somewhat Bothered	Bothered a Bit	Hardly Bothered at All	Not Bothered
10. WHEEZING	1	2	3	4	5	6	7

IN GENERAL, **HOW OFTEN** DURING THE LAST WEEK DID YOU:

	All of the Time	Most of the Time	Quite Often	Some of the Time	Once in a While	Hardly Any of the Time	None of the Time
11. Feel IRRITABLE (cranky/grouchy) because of your asthma?	1	2	3	4	5	6	7

**PAEDIATRIC ASTHMA
QUALITY OF LIFE QUESTIONNAIRE (S)
SELF-ADMINISTERED**

PATIENT ID _____

DATE _____

HOW **BOTHERED** HAVE YOU BEEN DURING THE LAST WEEK BY?

	Extremely Bothered	Very Bothered	Quite Bothered	Somewhat Bothered	Bothered a Bit	Hardly Bothered at All	Not Bothered
12. TIGHTNESS IN YOUR CHEST	1	2	3	4	5	6	7

IN GENERAL, **HOW OFTEN** DURING THE LAST WEEK DID YOU:

	All of the Time	Most of the Time	Quite Often	Some of the Time	Once in a While	Hardly Any of the Time	None of the Time
13. Feel DIFFERENT OR LEFT OUT because of your asthma?	1	2	3	4	5	6	7

HOW **BOTHERED** HAVE YOU BEEN DURING THE LAST WEEK BY?

	Extremely Bothered	Very Bothered	Quite Bothered	Somewhat Bothered	Bothered a Bit	Hardly Bothered at All	Not Bothered
14. SHORTNESS OF BREATH	1	2	3	4	5	6	7

IN GENERAL, **HOW OFTEN** DURING THE LAST WEEK DID YOU:

	All of the Time	Most of the Time	Quite Often	Some of the Time	Once in a While	Hardly Any of the Time	None of the Time
15. Feel FRUSTRATED BECAUSE YOU COULDN'T KEEP UP WITH OTHERS?	1	2	3	4	5	6	7
16. WAKE UP DURING THE NIGHT because of your asthma?	1	2	3	4	5	6	7
17. Feel UNCOMFORTABLE because of your asthma?	1	2	3	4	5	6	7

PAEDIATRIC ASTHMA
QUALITY OF LIFE QUESTIONNAIRE (S)
SELF-ADMINISTERED

PATIENT ID _____

DATE _____

	All of the Time	Most of the Time	Quite Often	Some of the Time	Once in a While	Hardly Any of the Time	None of the Time
18. Feel OUT OF BREATH because of your asthma?	1	2	3	4	5	6	7
19. Feel you COULDN'T KEEP UP WITH OTHERS because of your asthma?	1	2	3	4	5	6	7

IN GENERAL, **HOW OFTEN** DURING THE LAST WEEK DID YOU:

	All of the Time	Most of the Time	Quite Often	Some of the Time	Once in a While	Hardly Any of the Time	None of the Time
20. Have trouble SLEEPING AT NIGHT because of your asthma?	1	2	3	4	5	6	7
21. Feel FRIGHTENED BY AN ASTHMA ATTACK?	1	2	3	4	5	6	7

THINK ABOUT ALL THE ACTIVITIES THAT YOU DID IN THE PAST WEEK:

	Extremely Bothered	Very Bothered	Quite Bothered	Somewhat Bothered	Bothered a Bit	Hardly Bothered at All	Not Bothered
22. How much were you bothered by your asthma during these activities?	1	2	3	4	5	6	7

**PAEDIATRIC ASTHMA
QUALITY OF LIFE QUESTIONNAIRE (S)
SELF-ADMINISTERED**

PATIENT ID _____

DATE _____

IN GENERAL, **HOW OFTEN** DURING THE LAST WEEK DID YOU:

	All of the Time	Most of the Time	Quite Often	Some of the Time	Once in a While	Hardly Any of the Time	None of the Time
23. Have difficulty taking a DEEP BREATH?	1	2	3	4	5	6	7

DOMAIN CODE:

**Symptoms: 4, 6, 8, 10, 12, 14, 16, 18, 20, 23
Activity Limitation: 1, 2, 3, 19, 22
Emotional Function: 5, 7, 9, 11, 13, 15, 17, 21**

Index

Page numbers followed by "t" denote tables; those followed by "f" denote figures; those followed by "b" denote boxes.